CLINICAL
NEUROENDOCRINOLOGY

CONTEMPORARY NEUROLOGY SERIES AVAILABLE:

Fred Plum, M.D., *Editor-in-Chief*
J. Richard Baringer, M.D., *Associate Editor*
Sid Gilman, M.D., *Associate Editor*

CLINICAL
NEUROENDOCRINOLOGY

JOSEPH B. MARTIN, M.D., Ph.D., F.R.C.P.(C)

Julieanne Dorn Professor of Neurology
Harvard Medical School
Chief, Neurology Service
Massachusetts General Hospital
Boston, Massachusetts

SEYMOUR REICHLIN, M.D., Ph.D.

Professor of Medicine
Director, Endocrine Division
Department of Medicine
Tufts New England Medical Center
Boston, Massachusetts

EDITION 2

F. A. DAVIS COMPANY • Philadelphia

NOTE: As new scientific information becomes available through basic and clinical research, recommended treatments and drug therapies undergo changes. The author(s) and publisher have done everything possible to make this book accurate, up-to-date, and in accord with accepted standards at the time of publication. However, the reader is advised always to check product information (package inserts) for changes and new information regarding dose and contraindications before administering any drug. Caution is especially urged when using new or infrequently ordered drugs.

Library of Congress Cataloging-in-Publication Data

Martin, Joseph B., 1938–
  Clinical neuroendocrinology.

  (Contemporary neurology series ; 28)
  Includes bibliographies and index.
  1. Nervous system—Diseases.   2. Endocrine glands—
Diseases.   3. Neuroendocrinology.   I. Reichlin, Seymour,
1924–   . II. Title. III. Series. [DNLM:
1. Endocrine Diseases. 2. Endocrine Glands—physiology.
3. Nervous System Diseases.   W1 CO769N v.28 /
WL 100 M381c]
RC361.M33 1987   616.8   87-563
ISBN 0-8036-5886-9

This book is dedicated to our wives.

PREFACE

The concept of neurosecretion, the portal-vessel chemotransmitter hypothesis of anterior pituitary regulation, the role of neurotransmitters in the control of hypophysiotropic neurons, and the chemical structures of three of the hypophysiotropic hormones had been established when the first edition of this book was published in 1977. Since then, all of the recognized anterior pituitary regulating factors have been identified chemically, several previously unrecognized regulatory factors have been discovered, the molecular bases of biosynthesis of all of the known hypophysiotropic hormones have been characterized, and each of the hypophysiotropic hormones has been introduced into clinical medicine.

These leaps forward have corresponded in time with the emergence of biology of the central nervous system, with the new understanding of the neuropeptides, and some comprehension of their relevance to brain function, their phylogenetic significance, their role in extrahypothalamic function, and their involvement in neurologic and psychiatric disease.

The rapid pace of discovery and the extraordinary broadening of the fundamental science base of neuroendocrinology to include neural science as well as endocrinology have made difficult the tasks of keeping abreast of developments in the field and of maintaining a continuing interaction with clinical medicine. As in the first edition, our purpose in writing this book is to summarize and integrate current knowledge of neuroendocrinology derived from laboratory and clinical investigations and to apply it to the understanding of pathogenesis, diagnosis, and management of disease of pituitary regulation and of the hypothalamus, as well as to disorders of brain function and behavior secondary to hormone disturbance.

The authors acknowledge with gratitude the dedicated efforts of Barbara Chamberlain, Patricia Clougherty, and Kathy Kreatz.

Joseph B. Martin, M.D., Ph.D.
Seymour Reichlin, M.D., Ph.D.

CONTENTS

PART 1

Fundamental Aspects of Neuroendocrinology

Chapter 1

INTRODUCTION AND DEFINITIONS

Essential elements of what is now called neuroendocrinology were recognized long before the dawn of civilization, many eons before any concept of either a nervous system or of glandular function had been formulated. Primitive herdsmen recognized the seasonal breeding of domestic animals, the differences in behavior between male and female animals, the effect of castration on the docility of cattle, horses, and pigs, and various aspects of the suckling reflex and of maternal behavior. Some species of wild animals preserved their food stores by hibernation. The deliberate castration of prepubertal boys to change their behavior was practiced in antiquity, and the periodicity of the menstrual cycle is well described in the Old Testament. All these phenomena involve the interaction of the nervous system and the endocrine system; the mechanisms of these phenomena continue to be the subject of intense neuroendocrine study. As one considers the long history of interest in these matters, it is somewhat sobering to recall that the first experimental demonstration of an endocrine secretion was reported in 1849, by Berthold,[1] and that the year 1986 was the 100th anniversary of the first report of a pituitary hyperfunctional disease, acromegaly, published by Pierre Marie.[14]

Neuroendocrinology has traditionally been defined as the study of the relationship between the nervous system and the endocrine system. Operating together, the two systems regulate almost all of the metabolic and homeostatic activities of the organism. Neuroendocrine mechanisms are involved in the regulation of growth, of differentiation of tissues, of reproduction, and of a wide variety of behaviors and drive states. The two regulatory systems interact: Every hormone can act on the central nervous system, and the secretion of virtually every hormone is regulated directly or indirectly by the brain. Dysfunction of these systems is involved primarily or secondarily in an extraordinary range of human diseases.

Although interactive, the endocrine and nervous systems were considered in the past to be separate, but a number of recent advances have blurred these older distinctions. Many of the neuroregulators identified in the nervous system of higher animals also are found in endocrine glands and in the gastrointestinal tract.[3,9,10,21] Many of the same kinds of substances — hormones, neuropeptides, and neurotransmitters — have been identified in simple invertebrate organisms, including single-celled animals. Embryologic studies have shown that several glandular structures arise developmentally from primitive ectoderm, as does the nervous system. Molecular biologic techniques have shown that the prohormones of several neuropeptides are present throughout most of the animal kingdom.[15,16] Taken in the context of contemporary biology, these findings now strongly suggest that the two principal regulatory systems of higher animals, *endocrine* and *nervous,* have evolved in parallel from primitive, single-celled organisms, that the various parts of the two systems often use interchangeable components and messengers for communication, and that the higher functions of advanced animals have adapted primitive signalling devices to carry out complex, ordered, regulatory functions. For these reasons, in part, neuroendocrinology has expanded to include the study of the secretions of neurons whether or not those secretions enter the bloodstream, which is the essential definition of a true *hormone.*

Having called attention to certain of the fundamental similarities of the two systems, it is still important to point out that the basic functional unit of the endocrine system is the secretory cell, which provides its regulatory influence through the circulating blood, and that the basic functional unit of the nervous system is the neuron, which provides an organized network of point-to-point connections. Specificity within the endocrine system is conveyed by the appearance of specialized receptors on target cells; specificity within the central nervous system is conveyed by neurotransmitter specificity, receptor specificity, and by point-to-point hard wiring. An important feature of neuropeptide and neurotransmitter cells is that the particular site in which neurotransmitters and neuropeptides are found determines their functional role though not their mechanisms of action.

This book deals with the secretory functions of nervous tissue (neurosecretion), with the neuroendocrine control of glandular function — especially with the regulation of the pituitary and of its target organs — with the pineal gland, and with the pathophysiology, diagnosis, and treatment of diseases of neuroendocrine significance.

NEURAL CONTROL OF GLANDULAR SECRETION

Secretory cells can be classified into three types: *exocrine,* which secrete into a hollow lumen that communicates with the exterior of the body; *endocrine,* which secrete into the circulation; and *neuronal,* which can secrete into the circulating blood (neurohormonal) or at synaptic contacts (neurotransmitters, neuromodulators). All secretory cells are regulated directly or indirectly by neural impulses. Exocrine glands are regulated mainly by *secretomotor* fibers; the classical endocrine system is regulated by the pituitary, which in turn is regulated by *neurosecretory* cells of the hypothalamus; and neurons are regulated by neurotransmitters (and neuromodulators). In addition to neural regulation, virtually all glands also are influenced by circulating hormones and metabolic factors (Figs. 1 and 2).

SECRETOMOTOR

Secretomotor control is mediated through nerves that end directly by defined synapses on secretory cells. Regulation of the flow of saliva, tears, sweat, sebum, gastric juice, and release of epinephrine, melatonin (secreted by the pineal gland), renin (secreted by renal juxtaglomerular cells), and

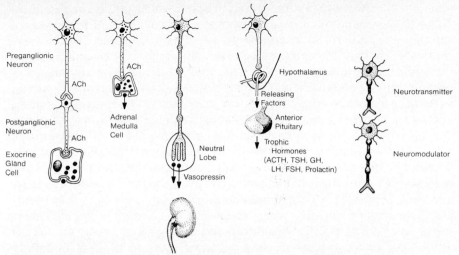

FIGURE 1. Examples of neuroendocrine systems are shown here. *(Left)* Neurosecretomotor neurons are illustrated. Postganglionic or preganglionic sympathetic fibers make direct synaptic contact with exocrine glands or hormone-secreting cells of the adrenal medulla. *(Center)* Hypothalamic neurosecretory neurons are illustrated. Neurosecretory neurons of the supraoptic system that release ADH (vasopressin) into the blood are shown. Hypothalamic tuberoinfundibular neurons release hypophysiotropic hormones (releasing factors) into the pituitary portal system to regulate secretion of hormones from the anterior pituitary. *(Right)* Neurons in the brain secrete peptides at synaptic sites. Ach, acetylcholine; ACTH, adrenocorticotropin; TSH, thyroid-stimulating hormone (thyrotropin); GH, growth hormone (somatotropin); LH, luteinizing hormone; FSH, follicle-stimulating hormone.

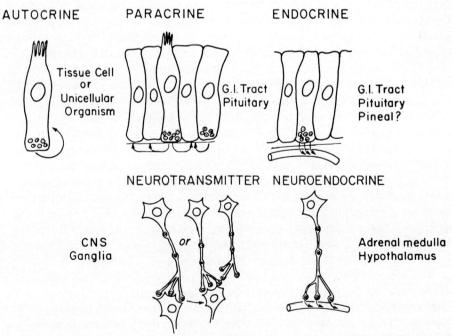

FIGURE 2. Modes of secretion and action of peptide hormones are illustrated here. Abbreviations: GI, gastrointestinal; CNS, central nervous system. (From Krieger,[9] with permission.)

pancreatic hormones (secreted from pancreatic islets) are examples of the range of secretomotor control. Secretomotor nerve fibers form part of the sympathetic and the parasympathetic nervous systems and thus can be controlled directly by central nervous system pathways. Traditionally, secretomotor control has been attributed to the release at nerve endings of norepinephrine (sympathetic nerves) and acetylcholine (parasympathetic nerves), but more recently it has been recognized that neuropeptide transmitters may coexist in the same fibers as the catecholamines and acetylcholine, and that the effects of nerve stimulation often are due to the synergistic action of the two transmitters.[5,6,11,12,13,19,20] The best example of this relationship is the parasympathetic neuronal control of the parotid gland and the sweat glands which is mediated both by acetylcholine and vasoactive intestinal peptide (VIP).[6,19] Stimulation of the nerve supply to these structures releases both factors. Administered by itself, acetylcholine stimulates secretion of enzyme-rich saliva or salt-containing sweat; by itself, VIP has little effect on salivary or sweat production but stimulates blood flow. Administered together, VIP and acetylcholine bring about an increase in secretion that is much greater than that caused by acetylcholine alone.[5,11,12]

Preganglionic sympathetic fibers (which terminate in sympathetic ganglia) were traditionally classified as cholinergic but are now known also to contain biologically active peptides. For example, preganglionic sympathetic nerve stimulation in higher vertebrates probably releases VIP as well as acetylcholine.[7] In amphibia, a peptide similar to mammalian gonadotropin-releasing hormone is a major preganglionic neurotransmitter.[8]

NEUROSECRETION

Strictly defined, the term neurosecretion refers to the release of a hormone into the blood from a nerve terminal.[17] In 1928, Ernst Scharrer proposed the idea that a neuron could possess secretory functions, based on morphologic study of certain hypothalamic cells in fish.[17,18] Later, he and his colleagues observed analogous structures in the mammalian hypothalamus, recognized that the appearance of certain groups of neurons was modified by changes in the state of hydration, and showed that extracts of the hypothalamus contained bioassayable antidiuretic hormone.[17] They proposed that the secretions of the neural lobe actually arose in the hypothalamus.

The classic example of a neurosecretory gland in the mammal is the neurohypophysis. In this structure, neurosecretions (vasopressin and oxytocin) formed in cell bodies located in the hypothalamus and transported to the neural lobe by axoplasmic flow are released into the blood and, as true hormones, they regulate the function of organs at a more remote site. Because neurons analogous to those of the neurohypophysis (and containing vasopressin or oxytocin) can terminate in synapses on other neurons *within* the neuraxis, the concept of neurosecretion now includes the release of any neuronal secretory product from a nerve ending; the secretion can serve as a neurohormone, a neurotransmitter, or a neuromodulator (Fig. 3). The distinction between a neurotransmitter and a neuromodulator is not hard and fast; many workers consider that a neuromodulator has a longer latency of onset of effect, persists longer, and may function mainly to modify the responsiveness of the target neuron to the action of a classical

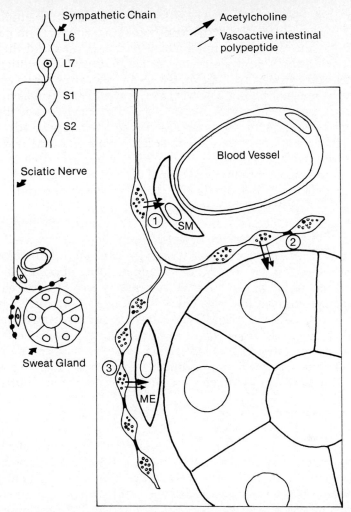

FIGURE 3. This is a schematic illustration of the effects of sympathetic innervation of sweat glands. Acetylcholine *(thick arrow)* and vasoactive intestinal polypeptide *(thin arrow)* are released from the same nerve endings. Whereas VIP mainly causes vasodilation by relaxing smooth muscle cells (SM) around blood vessels, acetylcholine mainly causes secretion by direct stimulation of secretory cells or indirectly through myoepithelial cells. (From Lundberg et al,[12] with permission.)

neurotransmitter.[2] Inasmuch as communication within the nervous system is almost exclusively through chemical messengers, neurosecretion generally is considered a fundamental property of all neurons. The ultimate route taken by the secretory product of an axon and its site of action depends upon its special topographic relationships to other structures.

Discovery of the widespread distribution of extrahypothalamic peptidergic neuron systems has led to the recognition that many important brain functions are modulated by the secretions of specific neurons. Guillemin has referred to this insight as "the new endocrinology of the neuron."[4] Detailed description of these patterns of neurosecretion is covered in chapter 18. Regardless of their location, neurosecretory cells retain the functional and structural properties of neurons (Figs. 4 and 5). They display electrophysiologic characteristics similar to other neurons, have neuron-type organelles and other cell constituents, are acted upon by other neurons through synapses, and react to neurotransmitter substances such as acetylcholine. The specialized neurons that secrete hormones into the blood serve as one of the major links by which the brain regulates metabolic and reproductive activities. Wurtman and Anton-Tay[22] applied the term "neuroendocrine transducer" to nerve cells of this type because they are capable of translating neural activity to a hormonal output. They provide a final common pathway for endocrine regulation, analogous to the anterior horn cell, which, as formulated by Sherrington, forms the final common pathway from the nervous system to the locomotor system. Neurons affecting glandular function are in turn governed by other neurons and by their

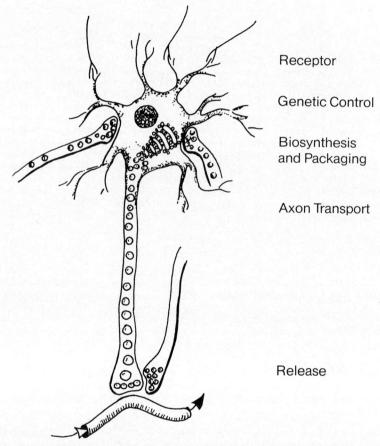

Receptor

Genetic Control

Biosynthesis
and Packaging

Axon Transport

Release

FIGURE 4. Neurobiology of the peptidergic neuron is shown here. Neurosecretory neurons can be looked on as having secretory functions in many ways analogous to glandular cells. A secretory product, formed on endoplasmic reticulum under the direction of mRNA, is packaged in granules and transported along the axon by axoplasmic flow to reach nerve terminals, where they are released. Virtually all neurons carry out similar functions: Some secrete neurotransmitters, such as acetylcholine or noradrenaline; others, such as motor nerves, secrete myotrophic factors. In all neurons there is a constant orthograde (forward) flow of cytoplasm and formed elements such as mitochondria. Retrograde flow also takes place to bring substances that enter nerve endings back to the body of the cell. (From Reichlin, S: Summarizing comments. In Gotto, AM, Jr, Peck, EJ, Jr, Boyd, AE, III, et al (eds): *Brain Peptides: A New Endocrinology.* Elsevier, Amsterdam, 1979, 379–403.)

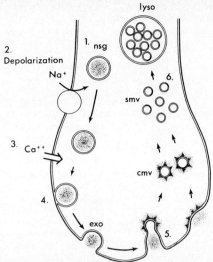

FIGURE 5. This diagram of a neurohypophysial nerve terminal illustrates mechanisms of hormone secretion. The numbers show the sequential steps in transport and release of hormone and the recapture of granule membrane to form small synaptic vesicles. 1, Neurosecretory granules, synthesized in the perikaryon of the cell are transported to the nerve terminal. 2, Depolarization of the terminal is associated with sodium uptake. 3, Depolarization triggers increased permeability to calcium. Uptake of calcium is essential to the secretory process. 4, Membrane of neurosecretory granule fuses with external membrane of terminal. 5, Entire contents of granule are extruded from the cell. 6, The membrane of the empty vesicle is reincorporated into the terminal to form synaptic vesicle. Lysosomes take up a portion of the empty vesicles, and enzymatic degradation ensues. Abbreviations: nsg, neurosecretory granule; exo, exocytosis; cms, coated microvesicles; smv, synaptic microvesicles; lyso, lysosomes. (Modified from Douglas, WW: *Mechanism of release of neurohypophysial hormone: Stimulus-secretion coupling.* In Greep, RO, and Astwood, EB (eds): *Handbook of Physiology, Section 7: Endocrinology,* vol. 4, part 1. American Physiological Society, Williams & Wilkins, Baltimore, 1974, p 211.)

metabolic and hormonal environments. Specialized neuronal receptors reactive to changes in both the internal and the external environments thus can modulate endocrine function. These receptors also serve to generate adaptive and sexual behavior. At the highest level, the central nervous system integrates the varied neural and hormonal mechanisms to maintain the integrity of the individual organism and to perpetuate the species.

REFERENCES

1. BERTHOLD, AA: *Transplantation der Hoden.* Arch Anat Physiol Wiss Med (Leipzig) 1849:42–46.
2. BLOOM, FE: *Contrasting principles of synaptic physiology: Peptidergic and non-peptidergic neurons.* In FUXE, K, HÖKFELT, T, LUFT, R (EDS): *Central Regulation of the Endocrine System.* Plenum Press, New York, 1979, pp 173–187.
3. BUCHANAN, KD: *Gut hormones and the brain.* In BESSER, GM, MARTINI, L (EDS): *Clinical Neuroendocrinology,* vol. II. Academic Press, New York, 1982, pp 332–359.
4. GUILLEMIN, R: *Peptides in the brain: The new endocrinology of the neuron.* Science 202:390–402 (Nobel Lecture), 1978.
5. HOKFELT, T, JOHANSSON, O, LJUNGDAHL, A, ET AL: *Peptidergic neurons.* Nature 284:515–521, 1980.
6. HOKFELT, T, LUNDBERG, JM, SCHULTZBERG, M, ET AL: *Coexistence of peptides and putative transmitters in neurons.* Adv Biochem Psychopharmacol 22:1–23, 1980.
7. IP, NY, PERLMAN, RL, ZIGMOND, RE: *Acute transsynaptic regulation of tyrosine 3-monoxygenase activity in the rat superior cervical ganglion: Evidence for both cholinergic and noncholinergic mechanisms.* Proc Natl Acad Sci USA 80:2081–2085, 1983.

8. JAN, YN, JAN, LY, KUFFLER, SW: *A peptide as a possible transmitter in sympathetic ganglia of the frog.* Proc Natl Acad Sci USA 76:1501–1504, 1979.
9. KRIEGER, DT: *Brain peptides: What, where, and why.* Science 975–985, 1983.
10. KRIEGER, DT, MARTIN, JB: *Brain peptides.* N Engl J Med 304:876–885, 944–951, 1981.
11. LUNDBERG, JM, ANGGARD, A, FAHRENKRUG, J. *Complementary role of vasoactive intestinal polypeptide (VIP) and acetylcholine for cat submandibular gland blood flow and secretion.* Acta Physiol Scand 3:329–337, 1982.
12. LUNDBERG, JM, ANGGARD, A, FAHRENKRUG, J, ET AL: *Vasoactive intestinal polypeptide in cholinergic neurons of exocrine glands: Functional significane of coexisting transmitters for vasodilation and secretion.* Proc Natl Acad Sci USA 77:1651–1655, 1980.
13. LUNDBERG, JM, HOKFELT, T, ANGGARD, T, ET AL: *Organizational principles in the peripheral sympathetic nervous system: Subdivision by coexisting peptides (somatostatin-, avian pancreatic polypeptide- and vasoactive intestinal polypeptide-like immunoreactive materials).* Proc Natl Acad Sci USA 79:1303–1307, 1982.
14. MARIE, P: *Sur deux cas d'acromegalie; hypertrophie singuliere non congenitale, des extremites superieures, inferieures et cephalique.* Rev de med Par 297–333, 1886.
15. ROTH, J, LeROITH, D, SHILOACH, J, ET AL. *The evolutionary origins of hormones, neurotransmitters, and other extracellular chemical messengers.* N Engl J Med 306:523–527, 1982.
16. ROTH, J, LeROITH, D, SHILOACH, J, ET AL: *Intercellular communication: An attempt at a unifying hypothesis.* Clin Res 31:354–363, 1983.
17. SCHARRER, E, SCHARRER, B: *Secretory cells within the hypothalamus.* In *The Hypothalamus. Association for Research in Nervous and Mental Disease.* Hafner Publishing, New York, 1940, pp 170–194.
18. SCHARRER, E, SCHARRER, B: *Neuroendocrinology.* Columbia University, New York, 1963.
19. SCHULTZBERG, M, HOKFELT, T, LUNDBERG, JM: *Peptide neurons in the autonomic nervous system.* Adv Biochem Psychopharmacol 25:341–348, 1980.
20. SCHULTZBERG, M, HOKFELT, T, LUNDBERG, JM: *Coexistence of classical transmitters and peptides in the central and peripheral nervous system.* Br Med Bull 38:309–313, 1982.
21. SYNDER, SH: *Drug and neurotransmitter receptors in the brain.* Science 224:22–31, 1984.
22. WURTMAN, RJ, ANTON-TAY, F: *The mammilian pineal as a neuroendocrine transducer.* Rec Prog Horm Res 25:493–522, 1969.

Chapter 2

HYPOTHALAMIC-PITUITARY UNIT

Early in the twentieth century, clinicians recognized that pituitary insufficiency resulted from disease in the region of the hypothalamus, but they were unable to resolve whether the effects were due to direct damage to the adjacent pituitary gland.[5,27] On the basis of careful pathologic study, Erdheim[26] concluded that these changes could be caused by hypothalamic damage alone; and Aschner[6] in 1909 demonstrated that gonadal deficiency (now recognized as being due to gonadotropin failure) could be produced in dogs by hypothalamic lesions which spared the pituitary. Over the following four decades, many workers studied the effects of "isolation" of the pituitary by surgical section of the pituitary stalk, but the results were ambiguous and controversial. In a series of classic experiments, Harris and Jacobsohn[40] demonstrated the crucial role of the blood vessels of the stalk in this regulation. Stalk section in the rat caused loss of sexual function, which returned when the hypophysial-portal vessels regenerated. When a paper plate was inserted into the stalk region to prevent regeneration of the vessels, sexual function failed to return. They also showed that pituitaries transplanted to the pituitary fossa function normally, whereas pituitary transplants in other sites remained devoid of activity. These observations showed that the pituitary fossa was a privileged site for the growth and function of the pituitary and indicated that the crucial factor was the special blood supply from the hypothalamus. Some criticized the results of the Harris-Jacobsohn experiments as being due to damage to the pituitary caused by transplantation, but this reservation was resolved convincingly in the double transplantation experiments of Nikitovitch-Winer and Everett,[72] who demonstrated in rats that the pituitary failure resulting from transplantation of the gland to the renal capsule was corrected by retransplantation of the same pituitary to the region beneath the basal hypothalamus, if anatomic reconnection of the blood vessels occurred. Reconstitution of pituitary function did not occur in control experiments in which the pituitary was retransplanted to the temporal lobe.

The hypophysial vessels, now known to be the conduit of the hypothalamic hypophysiotropic hormones, were first described in 1930 by a Hungarian medical student, Popa,[82] following the lead given by his teacher, Ranier. The vessels were characterized by a peculiar group of coiled capillaries at the inferior extent of the hypothalamus that left the brain and joined to form long vessels that traversed the pituitary stalk. Popa and his subsequent coworker Fielding incorrectly asserted that the blood in

11

these vessels flowed from the pituitary upward to the base of the brain. In 1936, Wislocki and King[99] described similar vessels in the monkey and suggested on the basis of anatomic features that blood probably flowed from the hypothalamus to the pituitary. In 1947, Green and Harris[31-33] confirmed this suggestion by direct observation in the rat that blood in the hypothalamic portal veins did indeed flow to the anterior pituitary, an observation that had been made previously in the toad by Houssay and coworkers.[46] Green and Harris proposed that the hypothalamus secretes specific pituitary-regulatory substances into the portal capillaries of the median eminence to be transported to the adenohypophysis by the portal vessels. This portal vessel-chemotransmitter hypothesis has continued to serve as the model for studies undertaken to clarify the details of this control.[32-34] A similar proposal was also made in 1936 by Friedgood[29] in a then unpublished lecture, and the earliest germs of this idea may be found in the writings of Hinsey and Markee, in 1933.[5]

As it is so often the case in science, contemporary ideas can often be seen as reflections of the speculations of antiquity. In *De Humani Corporis Fabrica* (1543), Vesalius described the drainage of cerebrospinal fluid through the floor of the third ventricle (which he named *infundibulum* because of its resemblance to a funnel) into the pituitary and thence into the nose to form mucus *(pituita)* from which our modern term pituitary is derived. Indeed, more recent studies utilizing sophisticated radioimmunoassays show that several hypophysiotropic hormones may find their way to the anterior pituitary by way of the cerebrospinal fluid through the floor of the third ventricle and median eminence (see below).

Athough the anterior pituitary gland lacks a direct nerve supply, the secretion of each of its hormones is under the control of the central nervous system. The pituitary and, in turn, its target glands respond to changes in the external and internal environments through specialized secretory neurons localized in the ventral hypothalamus. In addition, the neurohumoral connections of the anterior pituitary are important in the feedback regulations of a number of hormones — such as cortisol, the gonadal steroids, and thyroxine — and serve as part of the integrated mechanism by which behavior and metabolism are adapted to the external environment.

THE PITUITARY

The pituitary gland, or hypophysis, lies close to the medial basal hypothalamus, to which it is connected by a highly vascular stalk (Figs. 1 and 2). It is divided into two lobes, the anterior, or *adenohypophysis*, and the posterior, or *neurohypophysis*.[16,28,30,41,54] The adenohypophysis develops from Rathke's pouch, which arises from primitive buccal endoderm. The neurohypophysis, which forms as a diverticulum from the base of the hypothalamus, consists of the neural lobe and the neural stalk.

The adenohypophysis is made up of three parts. The *pars distalis* is the primary source of the classical anterior pituitary hormones (Table 1), thyrotropin (thyroid-stimulating hormone, TSH), adrenocorticotropin (ACTH), growth hormone (GH; somatotropin), prolactin (PRL; luteotropic hormone), luteinizing hormone (LH; interstitial cell-stimulating hormone, ICSH), and follicle-stimulating hormone (FSH); several other pituitary

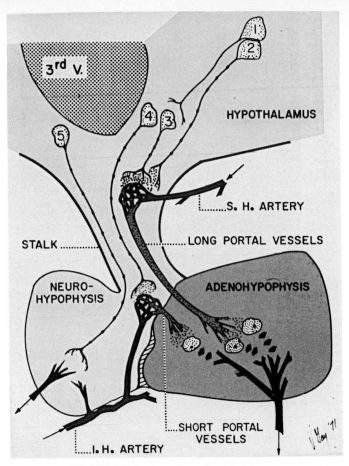

FIGURE 1. This figure summarizes the types of neural input in pituitary regulation. Neuron 5 represents the peptidergic neurons of the supraopticohypophysial and paraventriculohypophysial tracts, with hormone-producing cell bodies in the hypothalamus and nerve terminals in the neural lobe. Neurons 4 and 3 are the neurons of the tuberoinfundibular tract that secrete the hypophysiotropic hormones into the substance of the median eminence in anatomic relationship to the primary plexus. Neuron 1 represents a monoaminergic neuron ending in relation to the cell body of the peptidergic neuron. Neuron 2 represents a monoaminergic neuron ending on terminals of the peptidergic neuron to give axoaxonic transmission. Neurons 1 and 2 are the functional links between the remainder of the brain and the peptidergic neuron. Not shown are the fibers of the tuberohypophysial tract. These fibers in certain animal species, but not in humans, arise in the arcuate nucleus of the hypothalamus and terminate on the cells of the intermediate lobe. In adult humans the intermediate lobe is vestigial. (From Gay, VL: *The hypothalamus: Physiology and clinical use of releasing factors.* Fertil Steril 23:50–63, 1972.)

hormones and growth factors also have been described. The *pars intermedia,* or intermediate lobe,[97] is vestigial in the adult human, but it is quite well defined in the human fetus and in lower mammals, including rodents. It is the source of melanocyte-stimulating hormone (MSH) in lower mammals, whereas in the adult human, MSH is not secreted as such by the pituitary.[50] The *pars tuberalis,* consisting of secretory cells similar in appearance to those of the *pars distalis,* envelops the pituitary stalk and covers the surface of the median eminence.

Microscopically, the *pars distalis* consists of cuboidal secretory cells arranged around sinusoids lined with fenestrated endothelium. Immuno-

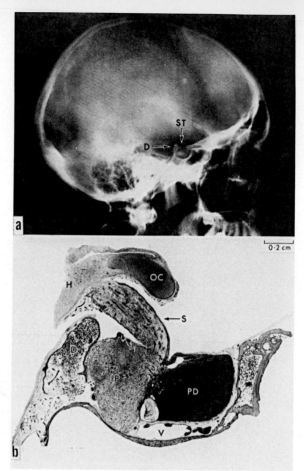

FIGURE 2. *(a)* This is a lateral roentgenogram of the skull to show the sella turcica. ST shows the position of pituitary stalk; D, the dorsum sella. *(b)* This is a sagittal section of human pituitary and stalk (S) attached to the hypothalamus (H). The pars intermedia is not shown. Abbreviations: OC, optic chiasm; IP, infundibular process or neurohypophysis; PD, par distalis or adenohypophysis; D, dorsum sella. (From Daniel, PM, and Prichard, MML: *Studies of the hypothalamus and the pituitary gland.* Acta Endocrinol (Suppl) 201, 1975, with permission.)

cytochemical studies have demonstrated that each of the anterior pituitary hormones is produced by a separate set of cells.[45,55,56] The exceptions are some cells that contain both LH and FSH, and cells that produce ACTH also produce other peptides of the opiomelanocortin family (see below). Each cell type has a distinctive appearance by electron microscopy, distinguished primarily on the basis of the size, shape, and electron density of the secretory granules. In pituitary tumors, however, the same cell may secrete more than one hormone[55,56] (see chapter 12).

HYPOPHYSIAL-PORTAL CIRCULATION

Anterior pituitary neural innervation is sparse, consisting primarily of postganglionic sympathetic fibers ending on blood vessels. The anterior pituitary is highly vascular and receives the highest blood flow of any organ in

TABLE 1. Anterior Pituitary and Hypophysiotropic Hormones

Pituitary Hormone	Hypophysiotropic Hormones	
	Name	**Structure**
Thyrotropin (TSH)	Thyrotropin-releasing hormone (TRH)	Tripeptide
Adrenocorticotropin (ACTH)	Corticotropin-releasing hormone (CRH)	41 Amino acids
Luteinizing hormone (LH)	Luteinizing hormone releasing hormone (LHRH)	Decapeptide
	or	
Follicle stimulating hormone (FSH)	Gonadotropin-releasing hormone (GnRH)	44 Amino acids
Growth hormone (GH)	Growth hormone-releasing hormone (GHRH)	14 Amino acids
	Growth hormone release-inhibiting hormone* (somatostatin GIH)	
Prolactin	Prolactin release-inhibiting factor (PIF)	Dopamine
	Prolactin-releasing factor (PRF)†	(? Vasoactive intestinal peptide)

*Somatostatin also inhibits TRH-stimulated TSH release
†TRH also stimulates prolactin release

the body, 0.8 ml/gm/min.[75,76] This blood supply is not directly arterial but courses from the portal vessels of the pituitary stalk (Figs. 3 and 4).

Portal vessels (6 to 10 in number) are formed by the confluence of capillary loops of the median eminence. These loops extend through both the external and internal zones of the median eminence.[33,99,100] Veins collect blood from these loops and join to form the portal vessels, which descend along the anterior surface of the pituitary stalk to the adenohypophysis. Portal vessels anastomose with capillaries of the neurohypophysis, which in turn receive a direct arterial supply from the inferior hypophysial

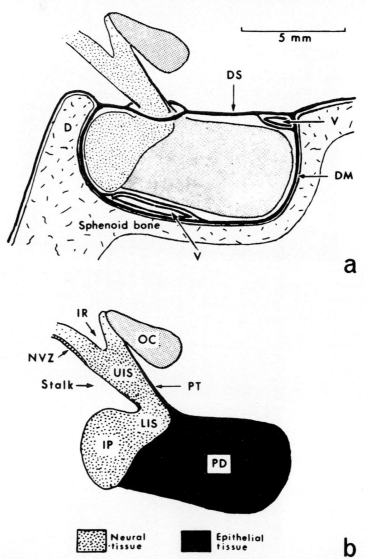

FIGURE 3. *(a)* and *(b)* Shown here is a diagram of human pituitary gland within sella turcica. The upper infundibular stalk (UIS), lower infundibular stalk (LIS) and infundibular process (IP) are all of neural origin. The pars distalis (PD) and pars tuberalis (PT) arise from epithelial tissue. Abbreviations: DS, diaphragma sella; V, veins; DM, dura mater lining sella turcica; IR, infundibular recess of third ventricle; NVZ, neurovascular zone of median eminence; OC, optic chiasm. (From Daniel, PM, and Prichard, MML: *Studies of the hypothalamus and the pituitary gland.* Acta Endocrinol (Suppl) 201, 1975, with permission.)

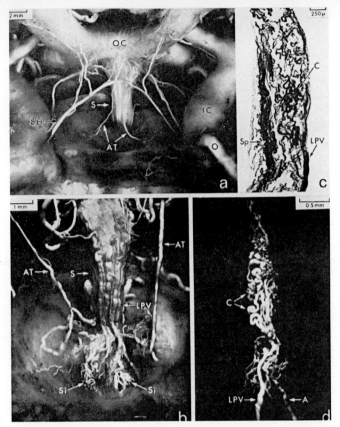

FIGURE 4. Shown here are pituitary portal vessels of human gland. (*a*) View from above of superior hypophysial artery (SH), arising from internal carotid (IC). Abbreviations: OC, optic chiasm: S, stalk of pituitary; AT, artery of the trabeculum, O, ophthalmic artery. (*b*) Higher magnification of stalk vessels and long portal veins (LPV) are shown here. Abbreviation: Si, sinusoidal capillaries in pituitary. (*c*) This is a sagittal section of stalk-median eminence junction to show primary capillaries (C) and long portal veins (LPV). Abbreviation: Sp, short portal vessels. (*d*) This shows a cluster of capillaries and long portal vein. (From Daniel, PM, and Prichard, MML: *Studies of the hypothalamus and the pituitary gland.* Acta Endocrinol (Suppl) 201, 1975, with permission.)

artery.[32,90,99] Direct observation in anesthetized animals[33] indicated that the predominant direction of blood flow in these vessels was downward from hypothalamus to anterior pituitary, but Bergland and Page[8,9] marshalled anatomic evidence for other patterns of flow, including flow from the pituitary upward to the hypothalamus. This pattern of blood flow has not been proven by direct study, and, indeed, recent observations by Page in the pig have confirmed the traditional view of the downward direction of blood flow.[75]

THE HYPOTHALAMUS

GROSS ANATOMY

Seen from below, the ventral surface of the hypothalamus forms a convex bulge termed the tuber cinereum (gray eminence)[70] (Fig. 5). Its gray color

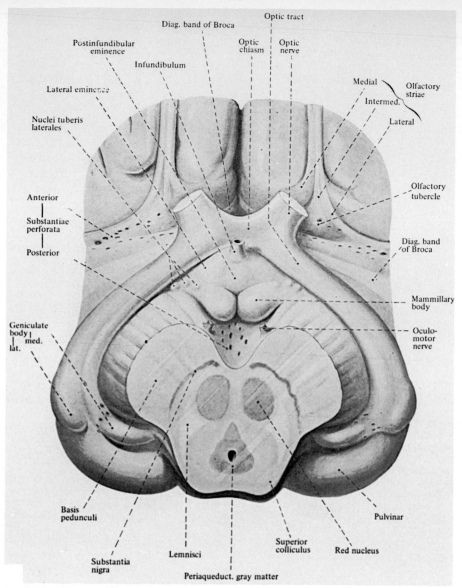

FIGURE 5. Illustrated here is the base of human brain, showing hypothalamus and neighboring structures. (From Nauta and Haymaker,[70] with permission.)

derives from the richness of cell bodies and unmyelinated fibers. Arising from it in the midline is the median eminence, readily recognized by its intense vascularity which corresponds to the distribution of the primary hypophysial-portal plexus.[23,70] The median eminence also forms the floor of the third ventricle and constitutes the infundibulum. The pituitary stalk is attached to and forms a direct extension of the infundibulum. Other prominent gross features of the hypothalamus are its anterior border with the optic chiasm, and its posterior limit, the mammillary bodies, so called because of their resemblance to miniature breasts. These structures contain the mammillary nuclei.

18   FUNDAMENTAL ASPECTS OF NEUROENDOCRINOLOGY

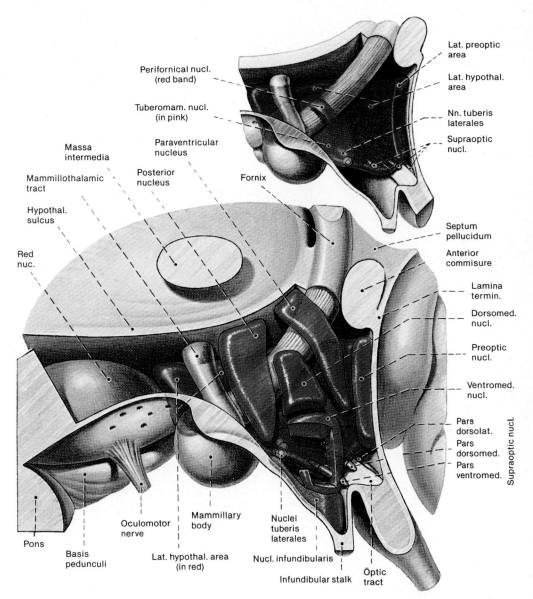

FIGURE 6. Diagram of dissected human brain, showing the major hypothalamic nuclei. Lateral to the fornix and the mammillothalamic tract is the lateral hypothalamic area *(in red)*, in which the tuberomammillary nucleus *(in pink)* is situated. Situated rostrally in this area is the lateral preoptic nucleus. Surrounding the fornix is the perifornical nucleus *(represented as a red band)*, which joins the lateral hypothalamic area with the posterior hypothalamic nucleus. The medially situated nuclei *(in yellow)* fill much of the region between the mammillothalamic tract and the lamina terminalis. The nuclei tuberis laterales *(in blue)* are situated at the base of the hypothalamus, mostly in the lateral hypothalamic area. The supraoptic nucleus *(in green)* consists of three parts. (From Haymaker, W., et al. (eds.): *The Hypothalamus.* Charles C Thomas, Springfield, Illinois, 1969, with permission.)

Hypothalamic boundaries are somewhat arbitrary, as they merge imperceptibly with surrounding areas.[70] The anterior limits of the hypothalamus are defined as the optic chiasm and lamina terminalis, where it is continuous with the preoptic area (which is developmentally and functionally similar to the hypothalamus) and with the substantia innominata and the septal region. Posteriorly, the hypothalamus is bounded by an imaginary plane defined by the posterior border of the mammillary bodies ventrally and by the posterior commissure dorsally. Caudally, the hypothalamus merges with the midbrain periaqueductal gray and tegmental reticular formation. The dorsal limit of the hypothalamus is taken to be the horizontal level of the hypothalamic sulcus on the medial wall of the third ventricle, roughly at the horizontal level of the anterior commissure. Here the hypothalamus is continuous with the subthalamus and zone incerta. Laterally, the hypothalamus is bounded by the internal capsule and the basis pedunculi, being continuous with the subthalamus caudodorsally.

The arterial blood supply of the hypothalamus varies in its detail from species to species, but it is similar in all mammals in being derived from small branches of the internal carotid artery.[8,23] In man, the median eminence is supplied by the paired superior hypophysial arteries.

NUCLEAR GROUPS

On cytoarchitectonic grounds the hypothalamus may be divided into nuclear groups (Fig. 6). Generally groupings of the hypothalamic nuclei are fairly constant in all vertebrates, but the nuclei are less clearly demarcated in humans and primates than in rodents. On cytologic and phylogenetic grounds, Nauta and Haymaker[70] divided the hypothalamus longitudinally into three zones (Table 2). The medial hypothalamus is cell dense and is separated from the lateral hypothalamus by the plane of the fornix. A longitudinal trajectory of fibers, the median forebrain bundle (MFB), among which lie the neuronal perikarya of the region, are the dominant features of the lateral hypothalamus. Medial and periventricular divisions of the hypothalamus contain pituitary-related neurosecretory cells and those involved directly in visceral functions; and the lateral hypothalamus is a relay station enmeshed in a multineuronal, multisynaptic system connecting the limbic forebrain and midbrain. Medial and lateral divisions of the hypothalamus are strongly and reciprocally interconnected. The limbic system communicates with the medial hypothalamus primarily via the lateral hypothalamus.

Forming a rather loose system of largely unmyelinated fibers running among the cell bodies of the lateral hypothalamus, the MFB conducts both caudally and rostrally. In general, cells associated with the MFB have dendritic arborizations that ramify in planes perpendicular to the MFB. Rostrally the MFB connects with the septal area, substantia innominata, nucleus accumbens, amygdala, and piriform cortex. Caudally it connects with the midbrain tegmentum, in particular the periaqueductal gray and the tegmental reticular formation. Throughout the hypothalamus, the MFB gives and receives fibers from the medial hypothalamus. Median forebrain bundle fibers make numerous axodendritic synapses onto lateral hypothalamic neurons.

TABLE 2. Major Hypothalamic Cell Groups*

Periventricular Zone	Medial Zone	Lateral Zone
preoptic	medial preoptic area	lateral preoptic area
periventricular area		
anterior	medial preoptic nuclear	lateral hypothalamic area
periventricular nucleus		
suprachiasmatic nucleus		supraoptic nucleus
paraventricular-periventricular nucleus	anterior hypothalamic area	
arcuate nucleus	paraventricular nucleus	
(infundibular nucleus)	ventromedial nucleus	
dorsomedial n.		
tuberal magnocellular n.	periformical nucleus	
	posterior hypothalamic area	
	medial mammillary nucleus	

*Adapted from Bleir, Cohn and Siggelkow: *A cytoarchitectonic atlas of the hypothalamus and hypothalamic third ventricle of the rat.* In Morgane, PJ, and Panskeep, J (eds): *Handbook of the Hypothalamus,* vol 1. Dekker, New York, 1979, pp 137–220.

The other important conduction system of the medial hypothalamus is the stria terminalis, a compact bundle of fibers which originates in the amygdala, follows the curve of the caudate around the margin of the lateral ventricle, and enters the hypothalamus at the anterior commissure. Its primary projection is to the bed nucleus of the stria terminalis.[24,42,70] It divides into two loose bundles at the anterior commissure, the supracommissural and postcommissural fibers, respectively, both of which provide strong projections to the region of the ventromedial nucleus (VMN).

> Postcommissural components of the stria terminalis contain fibers which originate in the medial and basomedial nuclei of the amygdala[24,42,57] and terminate in the core of the VMN.[47,57] The capsule of the VMN receives fibers which travel via the supracommissural branch of the stria terminalis and which do not originate from the amygdala proper, but from the subiculum and from the amygdalo-hippocampal area.[57]

Because of the rich interconnections of VMN with the arcuate nucleus (ARC) and because of the profound endocrine effects of VMN lesions, the stria terminalis is an important pathway from limbic forebrain to the tuberoinfundibular system.

The paired suprachiasmatic nuclei (SCN), located above the optic chiasm, are known to be important in determining circadian rhythmicity. They receive direct input from the retina (retinohypothalamic tract) and function to determine activity cycles, feeding and drinking behavior, and hormonal rhythms. Well defined anatomically in rodents, a nucleus corresponding to the SCN also has been identified in human brain.[68,69]

The Median Eminence

As noted above, the median eminence, or *infundibulum*, is a specialized region of the floor of the third ventricle that gives rise to the pituitary stalk. Stalk and median eminence contain the *contact zones* between the terminals of the tuberoinfundibular neurons and the capillaries of the hypophysial portal circulation. High vascularity and blood flow, virtually complete lack of neuronal perikarya, and specialized ependymal cells known as *tanycytes* characterize these structures.

Like other circumventricular organs, the median eminence contains capillaries with fenestrated endothelia, and unlike most of the brain, it has no barrier to the diffusion of substances from the circulation such as protein-bound hormones (thyroxine, cortisol, estradiol) or peptide and protein hormones.[14] For example, horseradish peroxidase (HRP), molecular weight 43,000, injected into the systemic circulation is excluded from the brain substance except for the median eminence and the circumventricular organs. Thus, intracellular spaces of the median eminence are sites potentially available to circulating substances that can modulate release of the hypothalamic releasing factors. Experiments with the direct application of HRP to the median eminence[61,63,96] suggest the presence of a diffusion barrier between the median eminence and the adjacent medial basal hypothalamus. This observation indicates that the releasing factors released into the extracellular space of the median eminence are not able to diffuse into the arcuate nuclei or into other regions of the adjacent brain.

The median eminence is composed of three zones, or layers: the *inner ependymal zone*, and two palisade zones, the *inner palisade zone* and the *outer palisade zone.*[49,52,53,80] The outer palisade zone contains unmyelinated nerve fibers, axon terminals, glial cells, and basal processes of tanycytes (Fig. 7). Few or no synapses are seen between neuronal processes. The nerve terminals are separated from the capillary lumen by the fenestrated endothelium and by two basement membranes that surround the capillary and that of the neuroepithelium (Fig. 8).

Axon terminals within the median eminence contain both dense core and small clear vesicles.[49,52,80] About 20 percent of the terminal boutons in the median eminence contain catecholamines and catecholamine-synthesizing enzymes packaged in dense core vesicles of about 60 nm diameter. These terminals are concentrated in the lateral third of the median eminence.[3] Another population of terminals contains larger dense core vesicles, up to 150 nm in diameter, shown by differential centrifugation and immunohistochemistry to contain the peptide-releasing factors.[47] Other nerve terminals of the external palisade zone also contain electron-dense, 170-260 nm diameter secretory granules typical of the vasopressin and oxytocin magnocellular systems and reactive immunocytochemically with antibodies to vasopressin, oxytocin, and neurophysin.[103] These findings imply that the neurohypophysial hormones themselves also may be released into the hypophysial portal circulation to act on the anterior pituitary as releasing factors. Indeed, vasopressin is an important component in

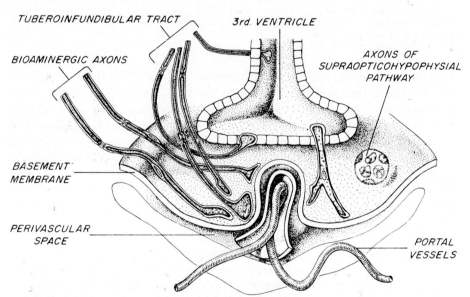

FIGURE 7. This is a diagram of the anatomic relationships of important secretory structures in the median eminence, visualized as if one were looking rostrally at a cut section. The interstitial space in which all the nerve endings terminate is a free pool without a blood-brain barrier. It is separated from the lumen of the third ventricle by ependyma whose tight junctions prevent direct diffusion from medial eminence to third ventricle lumen. Tuberoinfundibular neurons, some peptidergic, some bioaminergic, end in the interstitial space; many, but not all, end directly on capillary loops. Few if any true axoaxonic synapses are found here. Stretching between lumen and outer third of median eminence are tanycytes, specialized cells that may have transport functions. The supraopticohypophysial pathway is shown as a cut section of fibers in passage, but it should be recognized that some of the neurohypophysial neurons end in the median eminence.

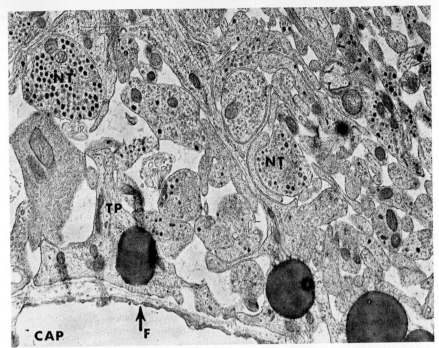

FIGURE 8. This is an electron photomicrograph of the median eminence of the rat. A capillary lumen (CAP) is evident in the lower left part of the figure. Fenestrations (F, *arrow*) of the capillary endothelium can be identified. The lipid droplets are contained in tanycyte processes (TP) which together with nerve terminals (NT) abut on the capillary. Dense core and "synaptic" vesicles are evident in the nerve terminals of neurosecretory neurons. These terminals are believed to contain the hypophysiotropic hormones and the catecholamines norepinephrine and dopamine. (× 18,000) (Courtesy of J. Brawer.)

regulating release of ACTH, β-endorphin, and GH.[91,92,101] A role for oxytocin in anterior pituitary function has not been established. All of the terminal boutons of the external palisade zone, plus those of the neurohypophysis, contain small clear vesicles whose composition and functions are unknown.

The inner *palisade* zone of the median eminence contains the unmyelinated axons of the magnocellular neurosecretory neurons en route from the hypothalamus to the neurohypophysis. This zone is also highly vascular, containing capillary loops which communicate with those of the external zone.

The inner *ependymal* zone forms the floor of the third ventricle. It contains a capillary plexus separate from that of the palisade zones[4] and is composed primarily of the cell bodies of the tanycytes, the specialized ependymal cells lining the ventral part of the third ventricle. Unlike the ependyma of the dorsal third ventricle, the ventricular surface of the tanycytes is not ciliated but, rather, is covered with microvilli. Numerous blebs are apparent in scanning electron micrographs of tanycyte membranes lining the ventricle; these blebs have been taken as evidence for secretory activity. The tanycytes are connected by tight junctions and thereby form a barrier to diffusion between the ventricular cerebrospinal fluid (CSF) and the extracellular space of the median eminence. They have long basal processes which pass through both palisade zones of the median eminence to end on capillaries, where the basal surface of the processes contains numerous infoldings. The tanycyte processes contain numerous vacuoles and vesicles, but little direct evidence of pinocytotic activity is seen in electron micrographs. Terminal boutons of axons in the outer palisade zone occasionally make synapse-like contacts with tanycyte processes, suggesting a cellular interaction between these supporting cells and neurons.

The function of the tanycytes remains a matter of speculation. Because of their striking morphology, they have been invoked as potential conduits for transfer of hormones from CSF to capillaries of the median eminence[7] and vice versa.[59] However, as Mezey and Palkovits[66] point out, the anatomy of tanycytes is more suggestive of a barrier than of a conduit.

TUBEROINFUNDIBULAR NEURONS

The location of neurons whose terminals project to the external zone of the median eminence (thus constituting the *tuberoinfundibular neurons*) has been studied using a variety of techniques.[62,63,84] Most of the cell bodies are located in the medial basal hypothalamus in the arcuate nucleus (ARC), the anterior periventricular area, and the medial preoptic area (mPOA) (Fig. 9). Using sensitive techniques, including the application of the tracer wheat germ agglutinin[63] to the median eminence, it has been possible to show that cells in the medial septum and diagonal band of Broca also are labeled, as well as some cells in the magnocellular cluster of the paraventricular nucleus, presumably those containing vasopressin and oxytocin. Retrograde flow studies have failed to reveal projections from the amygdala, ventro-

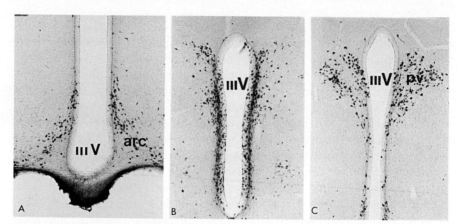

FIGURE 9. Shown here is the tuberoinfundibular neuronal system revealed by retrograde transport of wheat germ agglutinin. Location of cell bodies of neurons projecting to the median eminence of the hypothalamus can be traced (as in this study by Lechan and colleagues[63]) by injecting a minute amount of wheat germ agglutinin into the median eminence of the rat *(A)*. This tracer, which is a lectin, binds to carbohydrate receptors on nerve endings, is taken up into the cell by endocytosis, and is transported in retrograde fashion to be localized in cell bodies. Principal groups are *(A)* the arcuate nucleus (arc); *(B)* periventricular nucleus (which forms a feltwork of fibers and cells around the third ventricle) (IIIV); and *(C)* the small cell division of paraventricular nucleus (pv). Note that the distribution of cell bodies in the pv nucleus differs somewhat from that shown for the neurohypophysial peptides. Those projecting to the neural lobe are larger, are located laterally in the nucleus, and do not contain the retrograde tracer that was injected into the median eminence. (From Lechan, Nestler, Jacobson[63] with permission.)

medial nucleus, or aminergic nuclei of the brainstem, but studies using specific antisera directed against growth hormone releasing hormone (GHRH) have shown neurons in VMN with projections to the median eminence.[10,61]

Lesion studies have partially confirmed the retrograde transport results. Rethelyi and Halasz[85] found that surgical isolation of the medial basal hypothalamus, including the suprachiasmatic area, led to no degeneration of terminals in the external zone of the median eminence as judged by electron microscopy. Zaborszky and Makara[102] made focal electrolytic lesions in various hypothalamic nuclei and examined the median eminence for degenerating terminals. They observed degeneration following lesions of the ARC and anterior periventricular nuclei, confirming HRP studies, but also after lesions of VMN and the premammillary and posterior hypothalamic nuclei. Neither retrograde[63] nor anterograde labeling[21] techniques confirm the VMN to median eminence projection. It is likely that the VMN lesions interrupt axons of passage from the anterior periventricular region to the median eminence.[79] The possibility that cells in the limbic system might project directly to the median eminence[22] has not been confirmed by retrograde tracing techniques.

Tuberoinfundibular neurons have also been identified electrophysiologically.[84] Using extracellular single unit recordings, cells can be located which respond antidromically with short latency to electrical stimulation of the surface of the median eminence.

In addition to the axons of the median eminence, tuberoinfundibular neurons give rise to other axon collaterals that either terminate within the nucleus of origin or project to other hypothalamic, and possibly extrahypothalamic, nuclei. Van den Pol and Cassidy[93] performed a careful Golgi analysis of the ARC neurons of the rat. They found cells with one axon branch entering the median eminence and another collateral branch terminating within the ARC. These collaterals were found in a minority of those cells with axons entering the median eminence. However, quantitative assessments of axonal branching patterns are made difficult by the capricious nature of Golgi impregnation of axons. The same authors also found cells with axon branches terminating within the ARC and collateral branches leaving the ARC dorsally. The results of Rethalyi and Halasz[85] are consistent with these findings. These latter authors, on the basis of lesion studies, provide evidence of particularly strong projections of ARC to VMN and to the lateral hypothalamic area.

Electrophysiologic studies have demonstrated single units which could be activated antidromically by stimulation of both median eminence and other hypothalamic regions, including PVN and the anterior hypothalamic nucleus.[84] Moreover, stimulation of the median eminence induces, in addition to antidromic invasion of tuberoinfundibular neurons, a post-stimulation inhibition of activity lasting 100 to 150 msec, consistent with recurrent inhibition by axon collaterals. The presence of recurrent collaterals from tuberoinfundibular neurons also is important in providing evidence for a central nervous system neurotransmitter function for hypothalamic releasing peptides. If Dale's principle holds, the same neurohumors released into portal vessels by tuberoinfundibular neurons will be released by their axon collaterals ending on other neurons.

HYPOPHYSIOTROPIC HORMONES OF THE HYPOTHALAMUS

The task of identifying the chemical structures of the hypophysiotropic releasing factors was taken up by Andrew Schally and Roger Guillemin and their collaborators beginning in the mid-1950s. The Guillemin group used sheep hypothalami[36] as their starting material; the Schally group used hypothalami from the pig.[88] Their success depended on their organizing massive and well-focused efforts, on the development of convenient and reliable bioassays for the releasing factors, and on the application of innovative techniques of peptide chemistry. Five peptides have been isolated from hypothalamic extracts on the basis of their specific and potent actions to stimulate or to inhibit the release of anterior pituitary hormones *in vitro* (see Table 1). One of the releasing factors, growth hormone releasing hormone (GHRH), was first identified as an ectopic secretion of a pancreatic adenoma that caused acromegaly[37,86] (Fig. 10), but an identical factor was subsequently demonstrated in human hypothalamus.[35] The first to be identified was thyrotropin-releasing hormone (TRH), whose structure was reported virtually simultaneously by the two laboratories in 1969[11,36,88] (Fig. 11). In 1971, Schally and coworkers characterized luteinizing hormone-releasing hormone (LHRH), now most often termed gonadotropin-releasing hormone (GnRH)[88] (see Fig. 11). In 1973, Guillemin and his coworkers characterized somatostatin (somatotropin release inhibiting factor [SRIF]), which inhibits growth hormone release[13] (see Fig. 11). The structures of all three of these small peptides proved identical in sheep and pigs. In 1981, Vale and coworkers[91] reported the sequence of corticotropin-releasing hormone (CRH, CRF), a 41-amino-acid peptide from sheep hypothalami that stimulates corticotropin (ACTH) and beta-endorphin release *in vitro*. More recently, rat CRH has been characterized and is known to be identical[89] in structure to human CRH (Fig. 12). In the case of pituitary

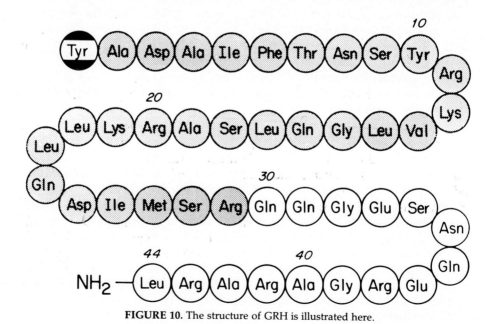

FIGURE 10. The structure of GRH is illustrated here.

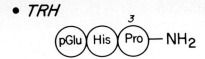

• *TRH*

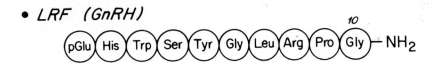

• *LRF (GnRH)*

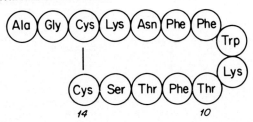

• *SOMATOSTATIN*

FIGURE 11. This is an illustration of amino acid structures of TRH, LHRH (LRF, GnRH), and somatostatin.

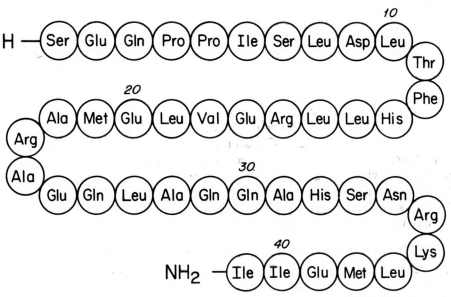

FIGURE 12. Illustrated here is the amino acid sequence of human CRH.

prolactin, which is under a tonic inhibitory influence by the hypothalamus, current evidence indicates that dopamine serves as the principal prolactin release-inhibiting factor (PIF).[65,71] Very recently, a peptide PIF has been identified in the prohormone for GnRH.[73,81] This remarkable finding suggests that a common precursor may give rise to two active peptides with different biologic effects. The one, GnRH, acts to stimulate gonadotropin release, and the other, called GAP (GnRH-associated peptide), inhibits prolactin secretion (see chapter 7 for structure and further discussion). There is also evidence for the existence of prolactin-releasing factor(s),[94] the principal candidates being vasoactive intestinal polypeptide (VIP),[1] PHI (peptide histidine isoleucine),[44,48,95] and TRH.[65]

The availability of pure hypothalamic hormones has permitted the development of immunoassays and immunohistochemical studies (Figs. 13–16), the demonstration of substantial amounts of releasing hormone in extrahypothalamic tissues, and extensive clinical trials in diagnoses and in therapy.

Although it was initially thought that the releasing factors were entirely specific, it is now clear that several of the factors may influence the secretion of more than one hormone. Thyrotropin releasing hormone is a potent stimulus for prolactin release and may also function physiologically as a prolactin-releasing factor. It does not cause release of GH, ACTH, FSH, or LH in normal individuals. Thyrotropin releasing hormone releases GH in persons with acromegaly and in others with certain clinical conditions (see chapter 8). Somatostatin, which inhibits GH release, also inhibits TSH secretion and prevents TRH-stimulated TSH release without affecting TRH-induced prolactin release. Somatostatin also has effects on other hormone-secreting tissues, such as the gut and pancreas.

These observations, which indicate more widespread effects of the hypothalamic hormones, have added to the complexity of hypothalamic-pituitary control. In the case of several anterior pituitary hormones, the effects of the hypothalamus are mediated by the interaction of several factors. Growth hormone secretion is stimulated by GHRH and inhibited by somatostatin; prolactin release is stimulated by several PRFs and inhibited by dopamine; and the secretion of ACTH is mediated by CRH, interacting in a synergistic way with vasopressin and epinephrine.[92] As far as is now known, there is only a stimulatory hypothalamic control for gonadotropin secretion. The effects of the hypothalamic factors interact at the level of the pituitary with the feedback effects of circulating target gland hormones. For example, TSH secretion is inhibited by thyroxine, ACTH secretion is inhibited by cortisol, GH secretion is sensitized by estrogens and thyroxine, and the secretion of the gonadotropins is regulated by a complex interaction with estrogens, progesterone, and androgens. In addition, the secretion of each of the hypothalamic releasing hormones is subject to feedback control by peripheral hormones, interacting with central neurotransmitters and neuroregulators.

BIOSYNTHESIS OF THE HYPOPHYSIOTROPIC HORMONES

The precursor (prohormone) for each of the hypothalamic hypophysiotropic hormones has now been characterized. The structures for each are shown in chapter 18.

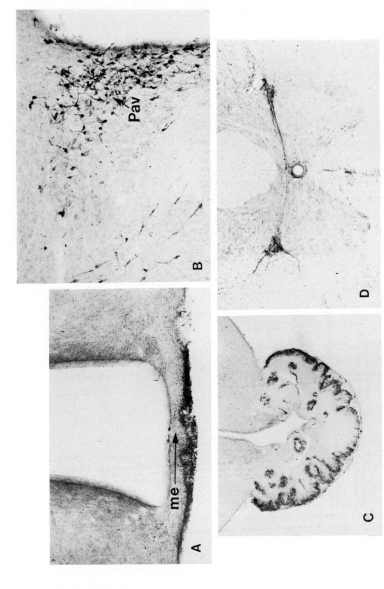

FIGURE 13. (A) Shown here is the distribution of thyrotropin-releasing hormone immunoreactivity in the stalk-median eminence (me) of the rat. (B) TRH-immunoreactive cell bodies in the medial division of the paraventricular nucleus (Pav) of the rat. (C) TRH-immunoreactive nerve endings in the medial eminence of rhesus monkey. (D) Transverse section of the upper thoracic spinal cord of the rat to show distribution of TRH-immunoreactive fibers terminating in the intermediolateral column (site of the preganglionic sympathetic nervous system). (All figures courtesy of Dr. Ronald M. Lechan. A and B are from Lechan, RM, and Jackson, IM: *Immunohistochemical localization of thyrotropin-releasing hormone in the rat hypothalamus and pituitary.* Endocrinology 111:55–65, 1982. Reproduced with permission. C is from Lechan,[61] with permission. D is from Jackson, IM: *Thyrotropin-releasing hormones.* N Engl J Med 306:145–155, 1982, reproduced with permission.)

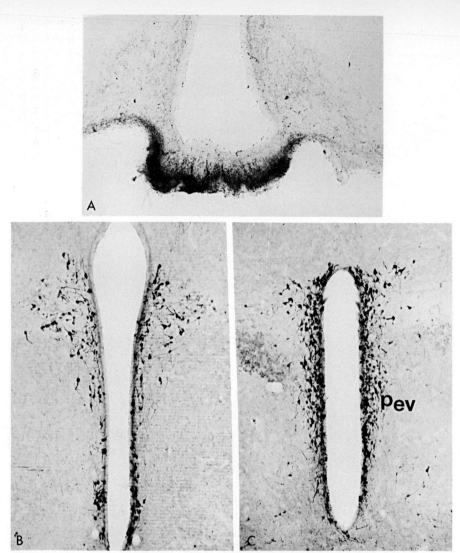

FIGURE 14. *(A)* Shown here is the external median eminence of rat, showing immunoreactive somatostatin in nerve terminals. (From Lechan, RM, Goodman, RH, Rosenblatt, M, et al: *Prosomatostatin-specific antigen in rat brain: Localization by immunocytochemical staining with an antiserum to a synthetic sequence of preprosomatostatin.* Proc Natl Acad Sci USA 80:2780–2784, 1983 with permission.) *(B)* This is the periventricular plexus (Pev) of somatostatin-containing cells in the anterior hypothalamus of the rat. Distribution corresponds well with the location of the periventricular plexus that contains retrogradely transported wheat germ agglutinin (see Figure 9). *(C)* The median division of paraventricular nucleus contains many somatostatin-positive cells. Note again the close resemblance of these cells to the location of those that project to the median eminence.

Mechanism of Hypophysiotropic Hormone Action on the Anterior Pituitary

In addition to their effects in stimulating the release of preformed hormone, the hypothalamic regulating factors are authentic tropic hormones to the anterior pituitary. They stimulate the synthesis of new hormones by inducing the transcription of mRNA, and they bring about the anatomic differ-

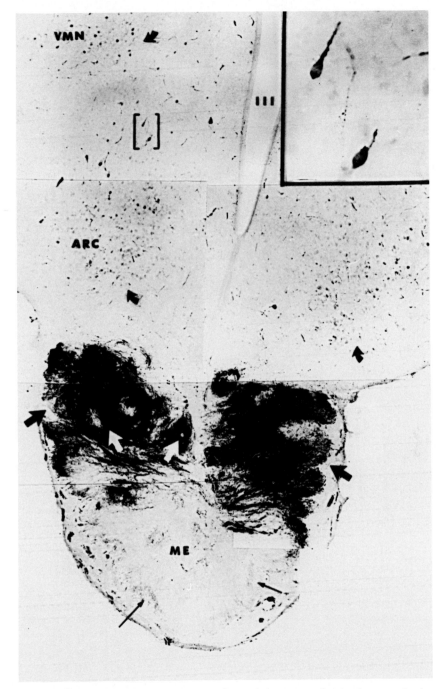

FIGURE 15. This figure shows the anatomy of growth hormone-releasing hormone in rhesus monkey delineated by immunohistochemical staining using an antibody directed against GHRH-1-44. Note the heavy distribution of fibers in the lateral margins of the median eminence (ME) and the scattering of cells in the arcuate nucleus (ARC). Inset shows cells in the arcuate nucleus. (From Lechan et al,[61] with permission.)

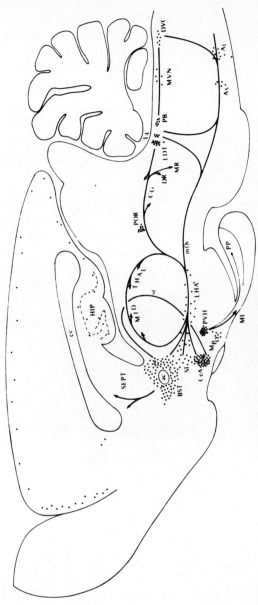

FIGURE 16. CRF-immunoreactive cells in the rat brain. The principal fibers regulating the anterior pituitary gland are shown as rising from the periventricular nucleus (PVH), but there is an extensive distribution elsewhere, especially around the hypothalamus. A_1, noradrenergic cell group 1; A_5, noradrenergic cell group 5; BST, bed nucleus of the stria terminalis; CC, corpus callosum; Cea, central nucleus of the amygdala; CG, central gray; DR, dorsal raphe; DVC, dorsal vagal complex; HIP, hippocampus; LC, locus coeruleus; LDT, laterodorsal tegmental nucleus; LHA, lateral hypothalamic area; ME, median eminence; Mid Thal, midline thalamic nuclei; MPO, medial preoptic area; MVN, medial vestibular nucleus; PB, parabrachial nucleus; POR, perioculomotor nucleus; PP, posterior pituitary; PVH, periventricular nucleus; SEPT, septal region; SI, substantia innominata. (From Swanson, LW, Sawchenko, PE, Rivier, J, et al: *Organization of ovine corticotropin-releasing factor immunoreactive cells and fibers in the rat brain: An immunohistochemical study.* Neuroendocrinology 36:165–186, 1983, with permission.)

entiation of the cells of the pituitary. Dopamine, which is the principal prolactin release-inhibiting factor, and somatostatin, the principal inhibitor of GH and TSH secretion, act to inhibit many aspects of cell function (Fig. 17). All of the hypophysiotropic factors act by binding to individual populations of well-defined receptors on the plasma membrane of the cell.[20,38] Subsequent "postreceptor" effects follow one of two general activation pathways. The first involves the stimulation of membrane-bound adenylate cyclase, an enzyme that generates cyclic 3',5'-adenosine monophosphate (cyclic AMP), which in turn stimulates a cascade of cellular events mediated by phosphorylations of specific protein kinases (Fig. 18). These phosphorylated compounds activate cellular enzymes and stimulate the release process and the formation of new protein.

The second important pathway of postreceptor activation of pituitary

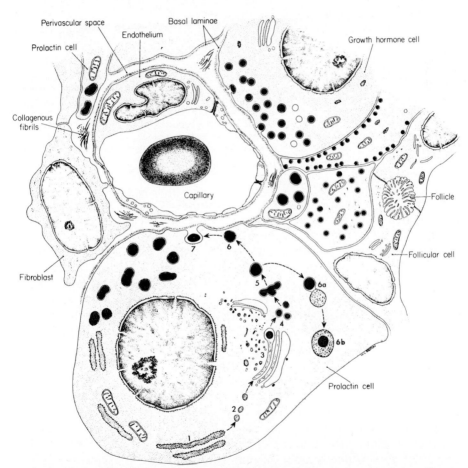

FIGURE 17. This diagram shows the ultrastructural relationship of secretory cells to a capillary in the rat anterior pituitary gland. Lower prolactin cell illustrates the steps in the secretory process. 1, Synthesis of polypeptides in endoplasmic reticulum. 2, Transport of polypeptide to Golgi system. 3, Condensation into granules in Golgi apparatus. 4, Liberation of membrane-enclosed granules from Golgi. 5, Coalescence of granules. 6, Movement of granules to peripheral plasmalemma. 7, Extrusion of granule by exocytosis. Intracellular disposal of secretion of lysosomes is shown by 6a and 6b. (From Baker, BL: *Functional cytology of the hypophysial pars intermedia.* In Greep, RO, and Astwood, EB (eds): *Handbook of Physiology, Section 7: Endocrinology, vol. 4, part 1.* American Physiological Society, Williams & Wilkins, Baltimore, 1974, with permission.)

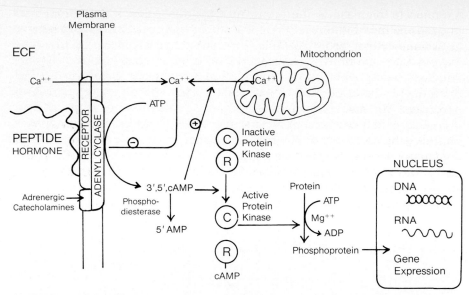

FIGURE 18. Proposed cellular mechanism through which a peptide hormone effector might activate gene expression of an endocrine cell. In model shown, binding of peptide to plasma membrane receptor activates adenylate cyclase, leading to formation of 3′, 5′-cyclic AMP and a cascade of reactions leading to conversion of inactive to active protein kinases; kinases then phosphorylate specific proteins. The presumed final active protein in this cascade of reactions is a phosphoprotein that interacts with regulatory sites on the gene, thereby activating gene transcription and expression. *C* and *R* refer to catalytic and cAMP-receptor subunits of protein kinase, respectively.

cell function is by way of the "phosphoinositol" mechanism, which is linked to calcium acting as a second messenger in cell activation. As outlined in Fig. 19, occupancy of the receptor by the releasing hormone leads to activation of a series of membrane-bound enzymes which break down phosphatidyl inositol (a phospholipid constituent of the membrane) through several intermediate steps leading ultimately to its reconstitution. This process is believed to open calcium channels in the membranes of the cell, both in the external plasma membrane and in the membrane of structures such as mitochondria which sequester calcium within the cell. The presence of free calcium within the cell activates many metabolic pathways and leads to increased hormone synthesis as well as release. In some cells, even those in which the phosphotidyl inositol (PI) pathway appears to be of major importance, activation of cyclic AMP can also occur. Work in this field is accumulating at a rapid rate, and concepts are changing rapidly, but at present it appears that the actions of TRH,[25,83] GnRH,[18,19] and dopamine are exerted mainly through the PI pathway, and those of GHRH,[12] CRH,[2] and VIP[87] are exerted mainly through the formation of cyclic AMP.

The role of calcium as second messenger is very important. Any mechanism that opens the calcium channel in cell membranes can activate cell secretion, and agents that inhibit calcium channels block secretion. A class of drugs called calcium ionophores that traverse the cell membrane can act like intracellular calcium to activate many cell processes.

Crucial to the release process in the anterior pituitary (as in other endocrine organs) is the translocation of preformed product in secretory granules to the plasma membrane, fusion of the granular membrane with the plasma membrane, and the ejection of the product by reverse pinocytosis (emiocytosis, exocytosis [Fig. 20]). The active translocation process is believed to involve the contraction of cellular filamentous processes (micro-tubules) which, like actin in muscle cells, are contracted in the presence of adenosine triphosphate (ATP), one of the intracellular products of cyclic AMP, and by calcium ions.

Although these comments have dealt with the mechanism of action of the releasing hormones on the anterior pituitary, it is important to recognize that many neuronal events are regulated similarly by the cyclic AMP or PI mechanism and that electrical depolarization activates neuronal function by permitting the entry into the neuron of free calcium. Neurotransmitters such as norepinephrine act primarily on membrane adenylate cyclase.

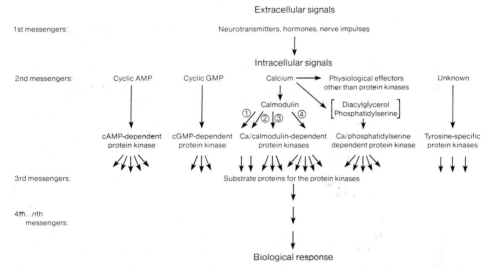

FIGURE 19. This is an illustration of the first and second messenger signals in the nervous system. Extracellular signals (first messengers) produce specific biologic responses in target cells via a series of intracellular messengers (second, third, and so forth, messengers). Second messengers in the brain include cyclic AMP, cyclic GMP, diacyglycerol, and calcium. Cyclic AMP and cyclic GMP produce most, and possibly all, of their second messenger actions through the activation of virtually one type of cyclic AMP-dependent protein kinase and one type of cyclic GMP-dependent protein kinase, respectively. The former enzyme exhibits a broad substrate specificity, and the latter, a more restricted specificity. Calcium exerts certain of its second messenger actions through the activation of calcium-dependent protein kinases and other of its actions through a variety of physiologic effectors other than protein kinases. Calcium activates protein kinases in conjunction with calmodulin or with diacylglycerol and phosphatidylserine. There are at least four types of calcium/calmodulin-dependent protein kinases in the brain: (a) phosphorylase kinase, which phosphorylates only glycogen phosphorylase (and possibly glycogen synthase); (b) myosin light chain kinase, which phosphorylates only myosin light chain; (c) calcium/calmodulin-dependent protein kinase I, which appears to phosphorylate several substrate proteins; and (d) calcium/calmodulin-dependent protein kinase II, which appears to phosphorylate numerous substrate proteins, as does the calcium/phosphatidylserine-dependent protein kinase. These various cyclic nucleotide-dependent and calcium-dependent protein kinases phosphorylate proteins specifically at serine and threonine residues. There is also a class of protein kinase that phosphorylates protein specifically at tyrosine residues (the tyrosine-specific protein kinases). The activation of individual protein kinases causes the phosphorylation of specific substrate proteins in target neurons. In some cases, these substrate proteins, or third messengers, may be the immediate effector for the biologic response. In other cases, they produce the biologic response indirectly through fourth, fifth, sixth, and so forth messengers. (From Hemmings, HC, Jr, Nairn, AC, Greengard, P: *Protein kinases and phosphoproteins in the nervous system: Neuropeptides in neurologic and psychiatric disease.* In Martin, JB, and Barchas, JD (eds): *Association for Research in Nervous and Mental Disease,* vol 64. Raven Press, New York, 1986, pp 47–70, with permission.)

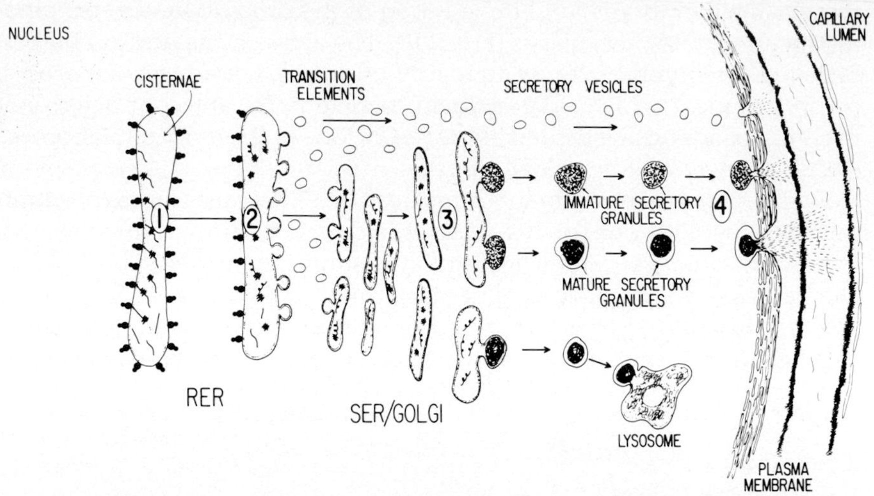

FIGURE 20. Schematic representation of subcellular organelles involved in transport and secretion of polypeptide hormones or other secreted proteins within a protein-secreting cell. RER = rough endoplasmic reticulum; SER = smooth endoplasmic reticulum; Golgi = Golgi complex. (1) Synthesis of proteins on polyribosomes attached to endoplasmic reticulum (RER), and vectorial discharge of proteins through membrane into cisterna. (2) Formation of shuttling vesicles (transition elements) from endoplasmic reticulum followed by their transport to and incorporation by Golgi complex. (3) Formation of secretory granules in Golgi complex. (4) Transport of secretory granules to plasma membrane, fusion with plasma membrane, and exocytosis resulting in release of granule content into extracellular space. Note that secretion may occur via transport of secretory vesicles and immature granules, as well as via mature granules. Some granules are taken up and hydrolyzed by lysomes (crinophagy). (From Habener, JF: *Hormone biosynthesis and secretion.* In Felig, P, et al (eds): *Endocrinology and Metabolism.* McGraw-Hill, New York, 1981, pp 29–59, with permission.)

EXTRAHYPOTHALAMIC REGULATION OF THE HYPOTHALAMIC-ADENOHYPOPHYSIAL SYSTEM

Neurosecretory neurons of the medial basal hypothalamus form the final common pathway for neuroendocrine regulation. Inputs from other regions of the hypothalamus and ascending and descending pathways from other brain regions converge upon these neurons to subserve neuroendocrine responses. Certain neuroendocrine reflexes are mediated over quite specific and well-defined anatomic pathways. For example, suckling stimulates breast receptors that signal via segmental nerves to the spinal cord, where impulses ascend to the midbrain and reach the hypothalamus via the medial forebrain bundle or the dorsal longitudinal bundle of Schütz. Input to the paraventricular nuclei stimulates release of oxytocin, vasopressin, ACTH, and prolactin.

With the exception of the olfactory radiation to the hypothalamus and the fibers comprising the retinohypothalamic tract (terminating principally in the suprachiasmatic nuclei), the hypothalamus receives few if any direct connections from generally recognized sensory pathways. Its most massive associations are with the limbic forebrain structures and the paramedial region of the mesencephalon. In addition to the pituitary-control system, the hypothalamus affects visceral motor function (i.e., parasympathetic and sympathetic outflow) by pathways through the reticular formation of the mesencephalon and lower brainstem. Of the inputs to the hypothalamus demonstrated to have an effect on anterior pituitary control, those containing the biogenic amines are of particular importance. These are discussed in detail in chapter 3.

The integrative functions of the hypothalamus in visceral and endocrine regulation, and in behavior, drive, affect, and consciousness arise in part from within the hypothalamus itself but to a greater extent from the interactions between the hypothalamus and the limbic lobe or limbic system.

> The limbic lobe as first described by Broca[15] consists of several brain regions distributed largely as a fringe (limbus) around the diencephalon, including cingulate and hippocampal gyri, amygdala, and adjacent cerebral cortex. Because of prominent anatomic relationships of these structures with the olfactory system and their large size in lower forms in which smell is important, it was believed for a long time that the limbic lobe (also called rhinencephalon) was concerned primarily with smell afferents and smell-related behavior. This restricted view of the limbic lobe was modified in the first few decades of the twentieth century as a result of increased anatomic knowledge and clinical observations of behavioral effects of lesions in these structures. In 1937, Papez proposed the existence of a "hypothalamic-anterior thalamic-cingulate cortex-hippocampal-fornix-hypothalamic circuit" that subserved certain aspects of emotion.[70] Deliberate production of lesions in the amygdaloid nuclei of the monkey was shown in the same year by Kluver and Bucy[51] to produce changes in visual and food discrimination and in sexuality, thus confirming the relationship of this structure to nonolfactory behavior.[64] Maclean in 1949 expanded the concept of the "limbic system" to that of the "visceral brain" as the integrator of emotional and vegetative information concerned with internal events of the organism.[64] The limbic system was defined anatomically in a much broader sense to include the interconnections of the limbic lobe with thalamic, hypothalamic, and midbrain regions.

The precise ways in which regions of the limbic system are integrated with the hypothalamus are areas of continued intensive investigation (see Bruesch,[16] Haymaker, Anderson, Nauta,[41] and Knigge and Silverman[52] for reviews).

ANATOMY OF THE LIMBIC SYSTEM

The limbic system as generally defined anatomically includes the medial part of the mesencephalic reticular formation (the so-called midbrain limbic system), hypothalamus, hippocampus, septum, amygdala, and cingulate, orbitofrontal, pyriform and entorhinal cortical areas (Fig. 21). The main pathway that connects these areas is the medial forebrain bundle, characterized by an admixture of cells and nerve fibers in a multineuronal, multisynaptic system.[57,89]

Hippocampus

The hippocampus has important direct anatomic connections with the hypothalamus. It has been implicated in modifying pituitary secretion of prolactin, growth hormone, ACTH, and the gonadotropins.

The principal efferent system of the hippocampus is the fornix, which, in addition to its major distribution to the mammillary bodies, has direct (monosynaptic) inputs to the arcuate and ventromedial hypothalamic nu-

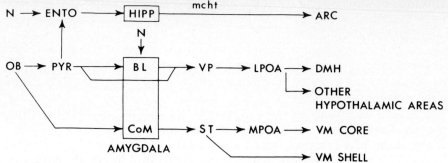

FIGURE 21. A schematic representation of some of the principal connections of the limbic system, indicating the main neocortical and olfactory afferents and the major pathways from the hippocampus and the amygdala to the hypothalamus. Abbreviations: ARC, arcuate nucleus; BL, basolateral nucleus; CoM, corticomedial nucleus; DMH, dorsomedial hypothalamic nucleus; ENTO, entorhinal area; HIPP, hippocampus; LPOA, lateral preoptic area; mcht, medial corticohypothalamic tract; MPOA, medial preoptic area; N, neocortex; OB, olfactory bulb; PYR, pyriform cortex; ST, stria terminalis; VM, ventromedial nucleus; VP, ventral amygdalofugal pathway. (From Raisman, G, and Field, PM: *Anatomical considerations relevant to the interpretation of neuroendocrine experiments.* In Martini, L, and Ganong, WF (eds): *Frontiers in Neuroendocrinology,* Oxford University Press, New York, 1971, with permission.)

clei. Electrophysiologic studies have shown that some of these inputs terminate directly on tuberoinfundibular neurons.

> One component of the fornix in the rat originates in the prosubiculum of the hippocampus and deviates medially at the level of the anterior commissure to form the medial corticohypothalamic tract. This group of fibers terminates in the anterior pole of the arcuate nucleus. The remainder of the fornix distributes to other hypothalamic and adjacent structures including the septum, the anterior thalamic nuclei, preoptic area, and periventricular zone of the hypothalamus, as well as the mammillary bodies. The exact distribution from the fornix to these nuclear groups varies considerably with different species.

Afferent connections to the hippocampus arise in the entorhinal cortex of the temporal lobe. This region in turn receives afferents from the olfactory system and the pyriform cortex. The septum is the origin of a cholinergic pathway that innervates the hippocampus.

Amygdala

The amygdala functions, in part, to determine emotionality. Animals with lesions of the amygdala show reduced reactivity to environmental changes and may consequently show a defect in acquisition of information. The extremes of emotion are lost. A wild animal shows increased tameness, even lethargy. Bilateral lesions of the amygdala also affect appetitive behavior, although the results are not consistent. Aphagia and adipsia, or excessive food intake, have been reported to follow amygdaloid lesions in experimental animals. In the Klüver-Bucy syndrome, abnormalities of appetitive behavior occur, characterized by loss of discrimination. Inedible objects are mouthed, and sexual hyperactivity may be evident, copulation occurring inappropriately (e.g., with inanimate objects). The lesions in these animals were extensive and included destruction of the amygdala and the adjacent medial temporal lobe. Similar clinical disturbances have been described in humans with bilateral temporal lobe lesions.

The amygdaloid complex is comprised of a number of subdivisions; it can be divided into basolateral and corticomedial nuclear groups. The basis of this division is both anatomic and phylogenetic. The corticomedial subdivisions are the most primitive, the basolateral groups appearing later in evolutionary development.

Anatomic studies suggest a functional distinction between these groups. The corticomedial nuclei send fibers through the stria terminalis to the septum, preoptic area, and the external border of the hypothalamic VMN. This efferent system is partly crossed so that bilateral inputs from each amygdala reach the hypothalamus. The primary efferents of the basolateral amygdala reach the lateral hypothalamus via a ventral amygdalofugal pathway. The precise anatomic termination of this pathway is in some doubt. Direct connections are described in the lateral and anterior hypothalamus. Presumably information from the basolateral amygdala is relayed to the medial hypothalamus via synaptic connections in the medial forebrain bundle or the anterior hypothalamus.

Electrophysiologic studies support a distinction between these two efferent amygaloid pathways. Neurons of the ventromedial nucleus are affected differently by stimuli applied to the stria terminalis or to the basolateral amygdala. Stimulation of the basolateral amygdala caused excitation of ventromedial hypothalamic neurons, whereas stimulation of the stria terminalis was inhibitory.[84]

The amygdala also receives afferent connections from the hypothalamus. The possibility should be considered that these recurrent connections function in part as a feedback modulation for neuroendocrine responses. Connections between the amygdala and ventromedial nucleus, for instance, may partake in the control of GH secretion. Both regions are reported to contain significant concentrations of somatostatin.

Septum

Rodents with lesions in the septal area exhibit rage reactions and hyperemotionality. This effect is less evident in cats and difficult to produce in monkeys. The septal area is also concerned with regulation of water intake. In higher animals, the septal area is smaller than other components of the limbic system. In man, the septum is small and limited to a few cells in the septum pellucidum and the medial cortex beneath the genu of the corpus callosum. Lesions in this area, such as those which may be produced by subarachnoid hemorrhage after rupture of an anterior communicating aneurysm, may produce remarkable disturbances in personality. Such patients frequently are belligerent, uncooperative, and emotionally unstable. This region, together with the adjacent nucleus basalis of Meynert, and other related nuclei (together called the substantia innominata) are now known to contain cholinergic cells which project to most of the forebrain, including the hippocampus and cerebral cortex which are profoundly abnormal in Alzheimer's disease.

Corticohypothalamic Inputs

The existence and potential significance of cortical inputs to the hypothalamus long have been debated. Several recent neuroanatomic and neurophysiologic studies indicate that direct connections do exist, but their functions remain obscure.

Limbic Midbrain Connections

There are important ascending inputs from the midbrain reticular formation and from midbrain nuclear groups that contain the cells of origin of the monoaminergic fiber systems (see chapter 3). Most of these inputs are relayed to the hypothalamus through the mammillary peduncle or the medial forebrain bundle. A midline periventricular system also ascends from the periaqueductal gray substance of the midbrain to become continuous with the periventricular gray of the third ventricle. This system is coextensive with the dorsal longitudinal fasciculus of Schütz, which carries fibers to and from the hypothalamus and brainstem.

As related to neuroendocrine regulation, the various hypothalamic and extrahypothalamic pathways are assumed to mediate (1) circadian rhythms in hormonal secretion; (2) stress-induced alterations in hormone secretion; (3) integration of neuroendocrine activity with autonomic nervous system responses; (4) neuroendocrine effects triggered by olfactory and peripheral sensory responses; and (5) elaboration of neurosecretomotor activation for regulation of organs such as the pancreas, pineal gland, and the renal juxtaglomerular apparatus. These aspects of neuroendocrine regulation are discussed in subsequent chapters on control of individual tropic hormones.

REFERENCES

1. ABE, H, ENGLER, D, MOLITCH, ME, BOLLINGER-GRUBER, REICHLIN, S: *Vasoactive intestinal peptide is a physiological mediator of prolactin release in the rat.* Endocrinology 116:1383–1390, 1985.
2. AGUILERA, G, HARWOOD, JP, WILSON, JX, ET AL: *Mechanisms of action of corticotropin-releasing factor and other regulations of corticotropin release in rat pituitary cells.* J Biol Chem 258:8039–8045, 1983.
3. AJIKA, K, HOKFELT, T: *Ultrastructural identification of catecholamine neurons in the hypothalamic periventricular-arcuate nucleus-median eminence complex with special reference to quantitative aspects.* Brain Res 57:97–117, 1973.
4. AMBACH, G, PALKOVITS, M: *The blood supply of the hypothalamus in the rat.* In MORGANE, PJ, PANSKEEP, J (EDS): *Handbook of the Hypothalamus,* vol 1. Dekker, New York, 1979, pp 267–378.
5. ANDERSON, E, AND HAYMAKER, W: *Breakthroughs in hypothalamic and pituitary research,* In SWAAB, DF, AND SCHADE, JP (EDS): *Progress in Brain Research,* vol. 41. Elsevier, New York, 1974, p 1.
6. ASCHNER, B: *Uber die Funktion de Hypophyse.* Pfleugers Arch Ges Physiol 146:1–146, 1909.
7. BEN-JONATHAN, N, MICAL, RS, PORTER, JC: *Transport of LRF from CSF to hypophysial portal and systemic blood and release of LH.* Endocrinology 95:18–25, 1974.
8. BERGLAND, RM, PAGE, RB: *Pituitary-brain vascular relations: A new paradigm.* Science 204:18–24, 1979.
9. BERGLAND, RM, PAGE, RB: *Can the pituitary secrete directly to the brain? (Affirmative anatomical evidence)* Endocrinology 102:1325–1338, 1978.
10. BLOCH, B, BRAZEAU, P, LING, N, BOHLEN, P, ESCH, F, WEHERENBERG, WB, BENOIT R, BLOOM, F, GUILLEMIN, R: *Immunohistochemical detection of growth hormone-releasing factor in brain.* Nature 301:607–608, 1983.

11. BOWERS, CY, SCHALLY, AV, ENGMANN, F, ET AL: *Porcine thyrotropin releasing hormone is (pyro)glu-his-pro(NH₂).* Endocrinology 86:1143–1153, 1970.

12. BRAZEAU, P, LING, N, ESCH, F, ET AL: *Somatocrinin (growth hormone-releasing factor) in vitro bioactivity: Ca⁺⁺ involvement, cAMP mediated action and additivity of effect with PGE₂.* Biochem Biophys Res Commun 109:588–594, 1982.

13. BRAZEAU, P, VALE, W, BURGUS, R, ET AL: *Hypothalamic polypeptide that inhibits the secretion of immunoreactive pituitary growth hormone.* Science 179:77–79, 1973.

14. BROADWELL, RD, OLIVER, C, BRIGHTMAN, MW: *Localization of neurophysin within the organelles associated with protein synthesis and packaging in the hypothalamo-neurohypophysial system: An immunocytochemical study.* Proc Natl Acad Sci USA 76:5999–6003, 1979.

15. BROCA, P: *Anatomie comparee des circonvulutions cerebrales. Le grand lobe limbique et la scissura limbique dans la serie des mammiferes.* Rev Anthrop Ser 21:385, 1878.

16. BRUESCH, SR: *Anatomy of the human hypothalamus.* In GIVENS, JR (ED): *The Hypothalamus.* Year Book Medical Publishers, Chicago, 1984, pp 1–16.

17. CANONICO, PL, AND MACLEOD, RM: *The role of phospholipids in hormonal secretory mechanisms.* In MÜLLER, EE, MACLEOD, RM (EDS): *Neuroendocrine Perspectives,* vol. 2. Elsevier, Amsterdam, 1983, 123–172.

18. CLAYTON, RM, CATT, KJ: *Gonadotropin-releasing hormone receptors: Characterization, physiological regulation, and relationship to reproductive function.* Endocrine Rev 2:186–209,1981.

19. CONN, RM, HAZUM, E: *Luteinizing hormone release and gonadotropin-release hormone (GnRH) receptor internalization: Independent actions of GnRH.* Endocrinology 109:2040–2045, 1981.

20. CONN, PM, MARIAN, J, MCMILLIAN, M, STERN, J, ROGERS, D, HAMBY, M, PENNA, A, GRANT, E: *Gonadotropin-releasing hormone action in the pituitary: A three step mechanism.* Endocrine Rev 2:174–185, 1981.

21. CONRAD, LCA, AND PFAFF, DW: *Efferents from medial basal forebrain and hypothalamus in the rat. II. An autoradiographic study of the anterior hypothalamus.* J Comp Neurol 169:221–261, 1976.

22. CROWLEY, WR, AND TERRY, LC: *Biochemical mapping of somatostatinergic systems in rat brain: Effects of periventricular hypothalamic and medial basal amygdaloid lesions on somatostatin-like immunoreactivity in discrete brain nuclei.* Brain Res 200:283–291, 1980.

23. DANIEL, PM, AND PRICHARD, MML: *Studies of the hypothalamus and the pituitary gland. With special reference to the effects of transection of the pituitary stalk.* Acta Endocrinol (Suppl) 80:1–216, 1975.

24. DE OLMOS, JS, AND INGRAM, WR: *The projection field of the stria terminalis in the rat brain. An experimental study.* J Comp Neurol 146:303–334, 1972.

25. DRUST, DS, MARTIN, TFJ: *Thyrotropin-releasing hormone rapidly and transiently stimulates cytosolic calcium-dependent protein phosphorylation in GH₃ pituitary cells.* J Biol Chem 257:7566–7573, 1982.

26. ERDHEIM, J: *Uber Hypophysenganggeschwulste and Hirncholesteratome.* Sitzber Akad Wien 113:537–726, 1904.

27. EVANS, HM: *Clinical manifestations of dysfunction of the anterior pituitary.* In AMERICAN MEDICAL ASSOCIATION: *Glandular Physiology and Therapy.* Chicago, 1935, p 7.

28. EVERETT, JW: *The mammalian hypothalmo-hypophysial system.* In JEFFCOATE, SL, AND HUTCHINSON, JSM, (EDS) *The Endocrine Hypothalamus.* Academic Press, London, 1978, pp 1–34.

29. FRIEDGOOD, HB: *Studies on the sympathetic nervous control of the anterior hypophysis with special reference to a neuro-humoral mechanism.* Symposium on Endocrine Glands. Harvard Tercentennial Celebration, 1936, reprinted in J Reprod Fertil 10:3–14, 1970.

30. FULTON, JF (ED): *Proceedings of the Association for Research in Nervous and Mental Disease.* Hafner Publishing, New York, 1940 (reprinted 1966).

31. GREEN, JD: *Comparative anatomy of hypophysis, with special reference to its blood supply and innervation.* Am J Anat 88:225–311, 1951.

32. GREEN, JD, AND HARRIS, GW: *Neurovascular link between neurophysis and adenohypophysis.* J Endocrinol 5:136–146, 1947.

33. GREEN, JD, AND HARRIS, GW: *Observation of the hypophysiol-portal vessels of the living rat.* J Physiol (Lond) 108:359–361, 1949.

34. GREEP, RO, AND ASTWOOD, EB (EDS): *Handbook of Physiology, Section 7: Endocrinology,* vol 4, parts 1 and 2. American Physiological Society. Williams & Wilkins, Baltimore, 1974.

35. GUBLER, U, MONAHAN, JJ, LOMEDICO, PT, ET AL: *Cloning and sequence analysis of cDNAs for the precursor of human growth hormone-releasing factor, somatocrinin.* Proc Natl Acad Sci USA 80:4311–4314, 1983.

36. GUILLEMIN, R: *Peptides in the brain: The new endocrinology of the neuron.* Science 202:390–402 (Nobel Lecture), 1978.

37. GUILLEMIN, R, BRAZEAU, P, BOHLEN, P, ET AL: *Growth hormone-releasing factor from a human pancreatic tumor that caused acromegaly.* Science 218:585–587, 1982.

38. HALPERN, J, AND HINKLE, PM: *Direct visualization of receptors for thyrotropin-releasing hormone with a fluorescein-labeled analog.* Proc Natl Acad Sci USA 78:587–591, 1981.

39. HARRIS, GW: *Neural control of pituitary gland.* Physiol Rev 28:139–179, 1948.
40. HARRIS, GW, AND JACOBSOHN, D: *Functional grafts of anterior pituitary gland.* Proc Roy Soc Ser B 139:273–276, 1952.
41. HAYMAKER, W, ANDERSON, E, NAUTA, WJH: *The Hypothalamus.* Charles C Thomas, Springfield, IL, 1969.
42. HEIMER, L, AND NAUTA, WJH: *The hypothalamic distribution of the stria terminalis in the rat.* Brain Res 13:284–297, 1969.
43. HERBERT, E, ROBERTS, J, PHILLIPS, M, ET AL: *Biosynthesis, processing and release of corticotropin, B-endorphin, and melanocyte-stimulating hormone in pituitary cell culture systems.* In MARTINI, L, GANONG F (EDS): *Frontiers in Neuroendocrinology,* vol. 6. Raven Press, New York, 1980, pp 67–102.
44. HÖKFELT, T, FAHRENKRUG, J, TATEMOTO, K, ET AL: *The PHI (PHI-27)/corticotropin-releasing factor/enkephalin immunoreactive hypothalamic neuron: Possible morphological basis for integrated control of prolactin, corticotropin, and growth hormone secretion.* Proc Natl Acad Sci USA 80:895–898, 1983.
45. HORVATH, E, AND KOVACS, K: *Pathology of the pituitary gland.* In EZRIN, C, HORVATH, E, KAUFMAN, B, KOVACS, K, WEISS, MH (EDS): *Pituitary Diseases.* CRC Press, Boca Raton, FL, 1980, pp 1–83.
46. HOUSSAY, BA, BIASOTTI, A, SAMMARTINO, R: *Modifications functionelles de l'hypophyse apres les lesions infundibulotuberiennes chez le crapaud.* C R Soc Biol 120:725, 1935.
47. ISHII, S: *Association of luteinizing hormone-releasing factor with granules separated from equine hypophyseal stalk.* Endocrinology 86:207–216, 1970.
48. ITOH, N, OBATA, K, YANAIHARA, N, ET AL: *Human preprovasoactive intestinal polypeptide contains a novel PHI-27-like peptide, PHM-27.* Nature 304:547–549, 1983.
49. JOSEPH, SA, AND KNIGGE, KN: *The endocrine hypothalamus: Recent anatomical studies.* In REICHLIN, S, BALDESSARINI, RJ, MARTIN, JB (EDS) *The Hypothalamus,* vol. 56:15–47. Raven Press, New York, 1979.
50. KASTIN, AJ, VIOSCA, S, SCHALLY, AV: *Regulation of melanocyte-stimulating hormone release.* In GREEP, RO, ASTWOOD, EB (EDS) *Handbook of Physiology, Section 7: Endocrinology,* vol 4, part 2. American Physiological Society, Williams & Wilkins, Baltimore, 1974, pp 551–562.
51. KLUVER, H, AND BUCY, P: *Preliminary analysis of functions of the temporal lobes in monkeys.* Arch Neurol Psychiat 42:979–1000, 1938.
52. KNIGGE, KM, AND SILVERMAN, A-J: *Anatomy of the endocrine hypothalamus.* In KNOBIL, E, SAWYER, WH (EDS): *Handbook of Physiology, Vol. 4, The Pituitary Gland, Part 1.* American Physiological Society, Washington, DC, 1974, pp 1–32.
53. KNIGGE, KM, SCOTT, DE, ET AL, (EDS) *Brain-Endocrine Interaction. Median Eminence: Structure and Function. I (International Symposium on Brain-Endocrine Interaction, Munich, 1971).* White Plains, NY, AJ Phiebig, S. Karger, Basel, 1972, Vol. II, 1975, Vol. III, 1978.
54. KNOBIL, E, SAWYER, WH (EDS): *The pituitary gland and its neuroendocrine control.* In GREEP, RO, ASTWOOD, EB (EDS): *Handbook of Physiology, Section 7: Endocrinology,* vol. IV, part 2. American Physiological Society. Williams & Wilkins, Baltimore, 1983.
55. KOVACS, K, AND HORVATH, E: *Pituitary tumors: Pathologic Aspects.* In TOLIS, G, LABRIE, F, MARTIN, JB, NAFTOLIN, F, (EDS): *Clinical Neuroendocrinology: A Pathophysiological Approach.* Raven Press, New York, 1977, pp 367–384.
56. KOVACS, K, AND HORVATH, E: *Pathology of pituitary adenomas.* In GIVENS, JR (ED): *Hormone Secreting Pituitary Tumors.* Yearbook Medical Publishers, Chicago, 1982, pp 97–119.
57. KRETTEICK, JE, AND PRICE, JL: *Amygdaloid projections to subcortical structures within the basal forebrain and brainstem in the rat and cat.* J Comp Neurol 178:225–254, 1978.
58. KRIEGER, DT. *Brain peptides: What, where and why?* Science 222:975–85, 1983.
59. KRIEGER, DT, AND LIOTTA, AS: *Pituitary hormones in brain: Where, how, and why?* Science 205:366–372, 1979.
60. KRIEGER, DT, AND MARTIN, JB: *Brain peptides.* N Engl J Med 304:876–885, 1981.
61. LECHAN, RM, LIN, HD, LING, N, JACKSON, IMD, JACOBSON, S, REICHLIN, S: *Distribution of immunoreactive growth hormone releasing factor $(1-44)NH_2$ in the tuberoinfundibular system of the rhesus monkey.* Brain Res 309:55–61, 1984.
62. LECHAN, RM, NESTLER, JL, JACOBSON, S, REICHLIN, S: *The hypothalamic tuberoinfundibular system of the rat as demonstrated by horseradish peroxidase (HRP) microiontophoresis.* Brain Res 195:13–27, 1980.
63. LECHAN, RM, NESTLER, JL, JACOBSON, S: *The tuberoinfundibular system of the rat as demonstrated by immunohistochemical localization of retrogradely transported wheat germ agglutinin (WGA) from the median eminence.* Brain Res 245:1–15, 1982.
64. MACLEAN, PD: *Influence of limbic cortex on hypothalamus.* In LEDERIS, K, AND COOPER, KE (EDS): *Recent Studies of Hypothalamic Function.* Karger, Basel, 1974, p 216.
65. MACLEOD, RM: *Regulation of prolactin secretion.* In MARTINI, L, GANONG, WF (EDS): *Frontiers in Neuroendocrinology,* vol 4. Raven Press, New York, 1976, pp 169–194.
66. MEZEY, E, AND PALKOVITS, M: *Two-way transport in the hypothalamohypophyseal system.* In

GANONG, WF, AND MARTINI, L (EDS): *Frontiers in Neuroendocrinology*, vol 7. Raven Press, New York, 1982, pp 1–29.

67. MOORE, KE, AND JOHNSTON, CA: *The median eminence: Aminergic control mechanisms.* In MULLER, EE, MACLEOD, RM (EDS): *Neuroendocrine Perspectives*, vol 1. Elsevier, Amsterdam, 1982, pp 551–562.

68. MOORE, RY: *Organization and function of a central nervous system circadian oscillator: The suprachiasmatic hypothalamic nucleus.* Fed Proc 42:2783–2789, 1983.

69. MOORE-EDE, MC: *The circadian timing system in mammals: Two pacemakers preside over many secondary oscillators.* Fed Proc 42:2802–2808, 1983.

70. NAUTA, WJH, AND HAYMAKER, W: *Hypothalamic nuclei and fiber connections.* In HAYMAKER W, ANDERSON, E, NAUTA, WJH (EDS): *The Hypothalamus*, Charles C Thomas, Springfield, IL, 1969, pp 136–209.

71. NEILL, JD: *Neuroendocrine regulation of prolactin secretion.* In MARTINI, L, AND GANONG, WF (EDS): *Frontiers in Neuroendocrinology*, vol 6. Raven Press, New York, 1980, pp 129–155.

72. NIKITOVITCH-WINER, M, AND EVERETT, JW: *Functional restitution of pituitary grafts re-transplanted from kidney to median eminence.* Endocrinology 63:916–930, 1958.

73. NIKOLICS, K, MASON, AJ, SZONYI, E, RAMACHANDRAN, J, SEEBURG, PH: *A prolactin-inhibiting factor within the precursor for human gonadotropin-releasing hormone.* Nature 316:511–517, 1985.

74. OLIVER, CRS, MICAL, RS, PORTER, JC: *Hypothalamic pituitary vasculature: Evidence for retrograde blood flow in the pituitary stalk.* Endocrinology 101:598–604, 1977.

75. PAGE, RB: *Directional pituitary blood flow: A microcinephotographic study.* Endocrinology 112:157–165, 1983.

76. PAGE, RB: *Pituitary blood flow.* Am J Physiol 243:E427–E442, 1982.

77. PAGE, RB, AND BERGLAND, RM: *The neurohypophyseal capillary bed. I. Anatomy and arterial supply.* Am J Anat 148:345–357, 1977.

78. PAGE, R, AND DOVY-HARTMAN, BJ: *Neurohemal contact in the internal zone of the rabbit median eminence.* J Comp Neurol 226:274–288, 1984.

79. PALKOVITS, M, KOBAYASHI, RM, BROWN, M, VALE, W: *Changes in hypothalamic, limbic and extrapyramidal somatostatin levels following various hypothalamic transections in rats.* Brain Res 195:499–505, 1980.

80. PELLETIER, G: *Immunohistochemical localization of hypothalamic hormones and other peptides in the central nervous system.* In COLLU, R, BARBEAU, A, ET AL (EDS): *The Central Nervous System Effects of Hypothalamic Hormones.* Raven Press, New York, 1979, pp 331–334.

81. PHILLIPS, HS, NIKOLICS, K, BRANTON, D, SEEBURG, PH: *Immunocytochemical localization in rat brain of a prolactin release-inhibiting sequence of gonadotropin-releasing prohormone.* Nature 316:542–545, 1985.

82. POPA, G, AND FIELDING, U: *A portal circulation from the pituitary to the hypothalamic region.* J Anat 65:88, 1930.

83. RECECCHI, MJ, AND GERSHENGORN, MC: *Thyroliberin stimulates rapid hydrolysis of phosphatidylinositol 4, 5-bisphosphate by a phosphodiesterase in rat mammotropic pituitary cells.* Biochem J 215:287–294, 1983.

84. RENAUD, LP: *Neurophysiology and neuropharmacology of medial hypothalamic neurons and their extrahypothalamic connections.* In MORGANE, PJ, PANSKEPP, J (EDS): *Handbook of the Hypothalamus*, vol 1. Dekker, New York, 1979, pp 593–693.

85. RETHELYI, M, AND HALASZ, B: *Origin of the nerve endings in the surface zone of the median eminence of the rat hypothalamus.* Exp Brain Res 11:145–158, 1970.

86. RIVIER, J, SPIESS, J, THORNER, M, VALE, W: *Characterization of a growth hormone releasing factor from a human pancreatic islet tumor.* Nature 300:276–278, 1982.

87. SAID, SI: *Vasoactive intestinal polypeptide: Current status.* Peptides 5:143–150, 1984.

88. SCHALLY, AV: *Aspects of hypothalamic regulation of the pituitary gland: Its implications for the control of reproductive processes* (Nobel Lecture). Science 202:18–28, 1978.

89. SHIBAHARA, S, MORIMOTO, Y, FURUTANI, Y, ET AL: *Isolation and sequence analysis of the human corticotropin-releasing factor precursor gene.* EMBO J 2:775–779, 1983.

90. SZENTAGOTHAI, J, FLERKO, B, MESS, B, HALASZ, B: *Hypothalamic control of anterior pituitary function*, ch 2. Akademai Kiado, Budapest, 1968, p 87.

91. VALE, W, RIVIER, C, BROWN, MR, ET AL: *Chemical and biological characterization of corticotropin releasing factor.* Rec Prog Horm Res 39:245–270, 1983.

92. VALE, W, SPIESS, J, RIVIER, C, ET AL: *Characterization of a 41-residue ovine hypothalamic peptide that stimulates secretion of corticotropin and beta-endorphin.* Science 213:1394–1397, 1981.

93. VAN DEN POL, AN, AND CASSIDY, JR: *The hypothalamic arcuate nucleus of rat—a quantitative Golgi analysis.* J Comp Neurol 204:65–98, 1982.

94. VALVERDE, C, CHIEFFO, V, REICHLIN, S: *Prolactin releasing factor in porcine and rat hypothalamic tissue.* Endocrinology 91:982–992, 1972.

95. WERNER, S, HULTING, AL, HOKFELT, T, ENEROTH, P, TATEMOTO, K, MUTT, V, MARODER, L,

WUNSCH, E: *Effect of the peptide PHI-27 on prolactin release in vitro.* Neuroendocrinology 37:476–478, 1983.

96. WIEGAND, SJ, AND PRICE, JLJ: *The cells of the afferent fibers to the median eminence of the rat.* J Comp Neurol 192:1–19, 1980.

97. WINGSTRAND, KG: *Microscopic anatomy, nerve supply and blood supply of the pars intermedia.* In HARRIS, GW, DONOVAN, BT (EDS): *The Pituitary Gland.* Butterworths, London, 1966, pp 1–27.

98. WISLOCKI, GB: *Vascular supply of hypophysis cerebri of rhesus monkey and man.* Res Publ Assoc Res Nerv Ment Dis 17:48–68, 1938.

99. WISLOCKI, GB, AND KING, LS: *Permeability of the hypophysis and hypothalamus to vital dyes, with study of hypophysial vascular supply.* Am J Anat 58:421–472, 1936.

100. WORTHINGTON, WC, JR: *Vascular responses in the pituitary stalk.* Endocrinology 66:19–31, 1960.

101. YASUDA, N, GREER, MA, AIZAWA, T: *Corticotropin-releasing factor.* Endocrine Rev 3:123–141, 1982.

102. ZABORSZKY, L, AND MAKARA, GB: *Intrahypothalamic connections: An electron microscopic study in the rat.* Exp Brain Res 34:201–215, 1979.

103. ZIMMERMAN, EA: *Localization of hypothalamic hormones by immunocytochemical techniques.* In MARTINI, L, AND GANONG, WF, (EDS): *Frontiers in Neuroendocrinology,* vol. 4. Raven Press, New York, 1976, pp 25–62.

Chapter 3

NEUROPHARMACOLOGY OF ANTERIOR PITUITARY REGULATION

Inasmuch as studies of sex function provided the first unequivocal evidence of neural control of the anterior pituitary, it is not surprising that the earliest attempts to identify chemical factors in the brain capable of affecting pituitary function also used endpoints of reproductive physiology. The first efforts to determine the effect of catecholamines on anterior pituitary function were those of Sawyer and coworkers[36] who in 1949 observed that ovulation followed infusion of epinephrine into the anterior pituitary of the rabbit. In 1956, Donovan and Harris[17] attempted to repeat this work, taking pains to use minimal amounts of epinephrine over prolonged periods of time in order to avoid the backtracking of injected material along the needle to the hypothalamus. When these precautions were taken, gonadotropins were not released by direct intrapituitary injections of epinephrine. It seemed likely, therefore, that the earlier experiments of Sawyer and colleagues had been due to hypothalamic stimulation. Vogt[40] then showed by bioassay methods that the hypothalamus contained large amounts of norepinephrine, and soon thereafter Carlsson and coworkers[7] demonstrated substantial concentrations of dopamine in the brain. These observations clearly indicated that the hypothalamus was rich in catecholamines, which might participate in regulation of the pituitary gland through effects mediated at the hypothalamic level.[22,23,25,35,39] Subsequent work has shown that pituitary function is regulated by a wide variety of neurotransmitters, including catecholamines (dopamine, norepinephrine, epinephrine), serotonin, acetylcholine, γ-aminobutyric acid (GABA), and a number of neuropeptides including the endogenous opioids. An important exception to the generalization that these agents act on the hypothalamus and not on the pituitary gland itself is dopamine, which in addition to acting centrally also acts to inhibit prolactin secretion by direct effects on pituitary lactotropes. Epinephrine and norepinephrine also act synergistically with corticotropin releasing hormone (CRH) on corticotropes.

The majority of monoaminergic neural cell bodies which synthesize the biogenic amines are located in the mesencephalon and lower brainstem[9] (Fig. 1A). Their axons ascend in the medial forebrain bundle to terminate in various forebrain structures including the hypothalamus, striatum, hippocampus, amygdala, and cortex. Terminals of these systems end directly on hypophysiotropic neurons and in the median eminence

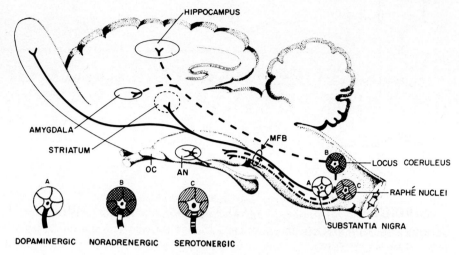

A.

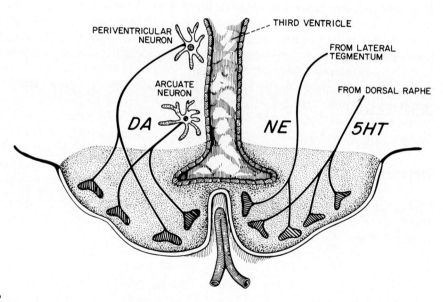

B.

FIGURE 1. *(A)* This is a simplified diagram to show the major distribution of the ascending monoaminergic pathways in mammalian brain. The principal source of all three major biogenic amines in the brain is nuclei in the brainstem. Locus coeruleus is the source of most noradrenergic-fibers; raphe nucleus, the source of most serotonin fibers; and substantia nigra, the source of most dopaminergic fibers. An important dopaminergic pathway arises in the arcuate nucleus of the hypothalamus and is the principal source of dopamine to the hypophysial circulation. Epineph-rinergic fibers arise from the region of the locus coeruleus in a pattern similar to that of norepineph-rine. (From Martin, JB, Reichlin, S, Brown, GM (eds): *Hypothalamic control of anterior pituitary secretion.* In *Clinical Endocrinology*, FA Davis, Philadelphia, 1977, pp 13–44). (*B*) This is a diagram-matic representation of biogenic aminergic terminations in the median eminence. Abbreviations: DA: dopamine, NE: norepinephrine; 5 HT: serotonin.

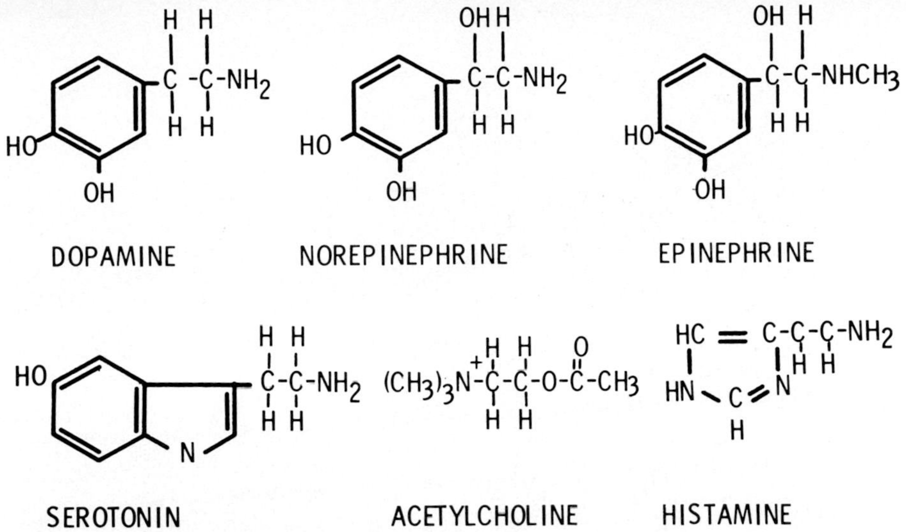

FIGURE 2. Structures of neurotransmitters which may be involved in hypophysiotropic hormone control are represented here.

(Fig. 1B), thereby providing an anatomic pathway by which noradrenergic impulses can act directly to modulate releasing factor secretion. The structures of the principal biogenic amines involved in regulation of anterior pituitary hormone secretion are shown in Figure 2.

ANATOMY AND PHARMACOLOGY OF BIOGENIC AMINERGIC PATHWAYS

AMINERGIC INNERVATION OF THE HYPOTHALAMUS

Dopamine (DA)

Dopamine (DA) in the hypothalamus is found in highest concentrations in the median eminence and arcuate nuclei, with smaller amounts in other regions (dorsomedial nucleus, ventromedial nucleus, periventricular nucleus, medial forebrain bundle).[30] Median eminence DA is present in a dense plexus of DA-containing terminals,[28,29] densest in the lateral third of the external lamina, where they account for one third of the axon terminals present.[1] A less dense band of DA-containing terminals is located in the medial part of the external lamina. DA-containing terminals, like the peptidergic terminals of the median eminence, do not make classical synapses with other terminals but instead appear to release DA into the extracellular space in the neurovascular contact zone of the stalk and median eminence. Dopamine thus can act on receptors located on nearby peptidergic terminals or diffuse into the adjacent capillaries of the portal circulation to act on the anterior pituitary gland.

The majority, and perhaps all, of the DA-containing terminals of the median eminence arise from cell bodies in the arcuate nucleus (ARC) to form the tuberinfundibular dopamine (TIDA) system (see Figs. 1B and 3).

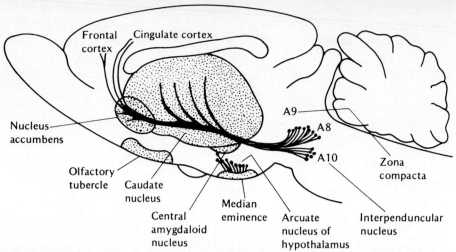

FIGURE 3. This is a schematic diagram indicating the distribution of the main central neuronal pathways containing dopamine. The stippled regions indicate the major nerve terminal areas. See text for details. The cell groups in this figure are named according to the nomenclature of Dahlstrom and Fuxe.[12]

Only 3 to 5 percent of the neurons of the ARC contain DA (A_{12} cell group of Dahlstrom and Fuxe[12]). Axon collaterals of TIDA neurons synapse in the ARC itself, as well as in the ventromedial nucleus (VMN) and the premammillary nuclei.[26]

There is convincing evidence that DA secreted by the TIDA neurons is the principal prolactin-inhibiting factor (see chapter 7). Activity of the TIDA cells is regulated physiologically by prolactin (PRL). This action of PRL, which has little or no effect on other brain DA systems, is an important mechanism in the feedback control of PRL secretion, whereby increased circulating levels of PRL stimulate increased DA secretion, which then acts to suppress PRL secretion. Decreased levels of PRL diminish DA output, tending to raise PRL levels. This is an example of a *positive feedback system* responsible for maintenance of inhibitory control of pituitary secretion. This system is also affected by drugs that alter synthesis and release of DA (such as alpha-methyl paratyrosine and reserpine), and by morphine, which inhibits the secretion of DA—thus accounting, at least in part, for the morphine-induced stimulation of PRL secretion.

DA-containing cell bodies are also located in the anterior periventricular region of the hypothalamus (the A_{14} cell group) (see Figure 1B). These cells may project to the preoptic area as well as to the median eminence.[13] Together with the DA-containing cells of the more rostral arcuate nucleus, A_{14} cells project axons to neural and intermediate lobes of the pituitary in those species with defined intermediate lobes. This complex has been termed *tuberohypophysial* by Moore and Johnston.[27] The DA nuclear groups A_{12} and A_{14} can be viewed as a single nucleus organized so that the most rostral cells project to the intermediate lobe and the next caudal group project to the neural lobe. In both lobes, axon terminals form a meshwork of fine fibers with varicose swellings located in proximity to pituicytes but without evident organized synapses. Dopamine terminals of the neurointermediate lobe, as well as those of the median eminence, lack a high affinity uptake system for DA.[2,14] This attribute, which is in contrast to other central dopaminergic systems (mesolimbic, mesocortical), means that they are not subject to presynaptic feedback inhibition by DA and, incidentally, that they are resistant to the neurotoxic effects of 6-OH-dopamine.[11]

> DA-containing neurons of the zone incerta (A_{13} cell group), give rise to the incerto-hypothalamic projection.[28] The cell bodies lie primarily in Forel's H_1 field; their axons pass forward in the dorsal part of the periventricular hypothalamus to the border of the hypothalamus and preoptic area (POA). The terminal projections have not been worked out completely, but the system is primarily intrahypothalamic. It supplies DA-containing terminals to the adjacent zone incerta, to the dorsomedial nucleus of hypothalamus, to periventricular hypothalamus, and perhaps to POA.

There is some question as to whether the DA-containing cells of the ventral midbrain contribute innervation to the hypothalamus. These cells located in the substantia nigra and the ventral tegmental area send axons rostralward in the median forebrain bundle (MFB) to supply the dopaminergic innervation of the forebrain, including the basal ganglia, limbic system, and cerebral cortex. It is possible that some fibers are given off by this system to the hypothalamus.

Norepinephrine (NE)

Norepinephrine (NE) is present in all hypothalamic nuclei but in a nonuniform distribution. The highest concentrations are in the paraventricular nucleus, the retrochiasmatic area, and in ventromedial and dorsomedial nuclei.[30] Concentrations of NE in the median eminence are moderate, about one fifth that of DA. Deafferentation of the medial basal hypothalamus produces an 80 percent fall in NE concentration in the median eminence, implying an origin for a majority of the NE in the median eminence from outside the medial basal hypothalamus.[5] More specific lesion studies indicate that the origin of the NE is from brainstem noradrenergic cell groups, the region of the lateral reticular nucleus of the medulla and of the locus coeruleus making the largest contributions (Fig. 4).[32] Most of the noradrenergic innervation of the hypothalamus is carried by the ventral bundle.[24]

Terminals and fibers positive for immunoreactive dopamine-beta-hydroxylase (the enzyme responsible for NE synthesis) are present in the median eminence primarily in the internal palisade zone, with only rare positive staining terminals found in the external lamina.[21] However, all hypothalamic nuclei contain noradrenergic fibers and terminals. This distribution supports the view that noradrenergic effects on anterior pituitary function are mediated by synapses on neurons within the hypothalamus, whereas DA exerts its effect primarily at the pituitary by being released into the portal circulation.

Epinephrine (Epi)

Epinephrine (Epi) and its synthetic enzyme, phenylethylamine-N-methyl transferase (PNMT), are found in the hypothalamus, but the overall content of Epi is only about 10 percent that of NE.[29]

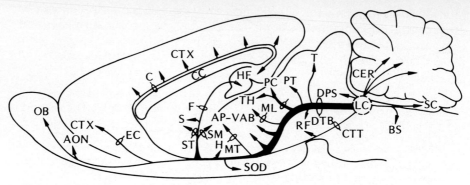

FIGURE 4. This is a diagram of the projections of the locus coeruleus viewed in the sagittal plane. See text for description. Abbreviations: AON, anterior olfactory nucleus; AP-VAB, ansa peduncularis-ventral amygdaloid bundle system; BS, brainstem nuclei; C, cingulum; CC, corpus callosum; CER, cerebellum; CTT, central tegmental tract; CTX, cerebral neocortex; DPS, dorsal periventricular system; DTB, dorsal catecholamine bundle; EC, external capsule; F, fornix; H, hypothalamus; HF, hippocampal formation; LC, locus coeruleus; ML, medial lemniscus; MT, mammillothalamic tract; OB, olfactory bulb; PC, posterior commissure; PT, pretectal area; RF, reticular formation; S, septal area; SC, spinal cord; ST, stria terminalis; T, tectum; TH, thalamus. (Diagram compiled by R. Y. Moore.[28])

The highest concentration is in the dorsomedial nucleus, paraventricular nucleus (PVN), the periventricular region, arcuate nucleus (ARC), and supraoptic nucleus (SON). By immunocytochemistry directed at PNMT, terminals are stained throughout the hypothalamus, but primarily in dorsomedial nucleus, ARC, the medial parvocellular division of PVN, the perifornical region, and the periventricular region.[25] There are few PNMT-containing terminals in the median eminence, and none have been seen in the external lamina.

All Epi-containing cell bodies of the brain are thought to be located in the medulla; however, deafferentation of the medial basal hypothalamus produces only about a 60 percent fall in Epi content, suggesting an intrinsic origin for many fibers.[29]

Serotonin

Serotonin (5-hydroxytryptamine, 5-HT) is found in many tissues throughout the body. About 90 percent is in enterochromaffin cells of the intestinal tract, and only 1 to 2 percent is present in the central nervous system (CNS) and pineal gland. This indolalkylamine is formed from the precursor tryptophan, an essential amino acid. The concentration of plasma tryptophan, as shown by Wurtman and Fernstrom,[42] determines the rate of synthesis of serotonin; plasma levels vary markedly with diet. In the neuron, tryptophan is converted by the enzyme tryptophan hydroxylase to 5-hydroxytryptophan, and thence to serotonin by the enzyme amino acid decarboxylase.

The serotonergic neural pathways in the CNS arise in the raphe nuclei of the lower pons and upper brainstem and are distributed to the forebrain and to the hypothalamus (Fig. 5).[9,33] A rich innervation of serotonergic fibers reaches the median eminence and the suprachiasmatic nucleus; the highest concentration of 5-HT within the hypothalamus is in the suprachiasmatic nuclei, suggesting a role for 5-HT in circadian rhythmicity.[34] The

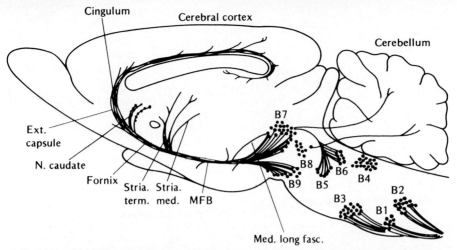

FIGURE 5. Schematic diagram illustrating the distribution of the main serotonin containing pathways in the rat central nervous system. B1 to B9 refer to brainstem nuclear groups. Abbrev. MFB-Medical forebrain bundle. (Modified after Breese, G, in Iversen, LL, Iversen, S, Snyder, SH (eds): *Handbook of Psychopharmacology,* vol. 1. Plenum, New York, 1975, p. 171.)

ARC and the basal and posterior regions of the hypothalamus are also rich in 5-HT; but only moderate levels are found in the median eminence.

> With the use of the Falck-Hillarp fluorescence histochemical method, and more refined recent improvements, nine separate cell clusters (labeled B_1 to B_9) have been identified in the mammalian brainstem.[10] All are situated in or near the midline raphe regions of the pons and the mesencephalon. The more rostral groups (B_7 to B_9) project to the diencephalon and telencephalon.

Hypothalamic deafferentation produces only a 60 percent fall in serotonin within the medial basal hypothalamus, suggesting a combination of intrinsic and extrinsic sources.[31] The intrinsic source is not known with certainty, but small clusters of neuronal perikarya fluorescent for serotonin are located within the hypothalamus.

Biosynthesis and Degradation of the Catecholamines

The metabolic pathways for synthesis of the catecholamines, dopamine, norepinephrine, and epinephrine are shown in Figure 6. Steps in the synthesis and secretory process have been outlined by Cooper, Bloom, and Roth[9] and Corrodi and coworkers,[10] whose descriptions are presented here in modified fashion.

Step 1: Uptake of Amino Acids into Aminergic Neurons

Tyrosine, an essential amino acid and precursor of DA, NE, and Epi, is transported actively into brain. Other large neutral amino acids compete with tyrosine for uptake into brain, but it is not known whether this is true for specific catecholaminergic neurons in brain. Fernstrom and Wurtman[18,42] reviewed in detail the possible role of tyrosine availability as a

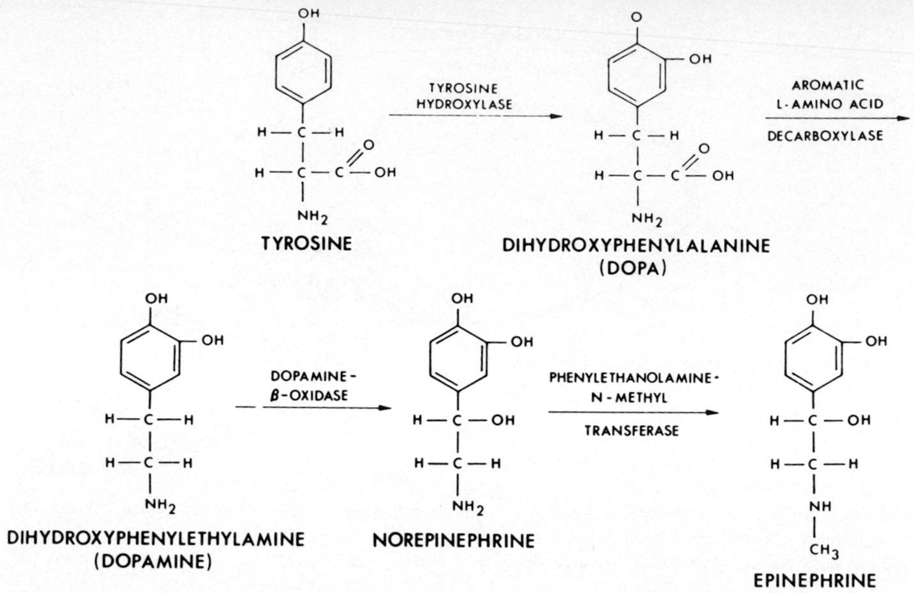

FIGURE 6. Represented here are metabolic pathways for synthesis of dopamine, norepinephrine, and epinephrine.

regulator of catecholamine synthesis, suggesting that variations in dietary intake may alter central neurotransmitter concentrations and function significantly. The amino acid L-dopa also is taken up actively by catecholaminergic neurons, and by virtue of its activity as a substrate, it increases synthesis and content of brain DA and NE.[8] This is the basis of its therapeutic action in Parkinson's disease and of its actions to stimulate GH secretion and to inhibit prolactin secretion.

Step 2: Enzymatic Synthesis

After its entry into cells, tyrosine is hydroxylated in a rate-limiting step by the synaptosomal enzyme tyrosine hydroxylase to form L-dihydroxy-phenylalanine (L-dopa).[41] Tyrosine hydroxylase has been purified, and its cofactors and kinetic properties have been studied in detail. The drug alpha-methylparatyrosine, an inhibitor of tyrosine hydroxylase, blocks L-dopa formation. L-dopa is decarboxylated by a nonspecific enzyme, L-aminodecarboxylase, to DA, which is in turn hydroxylated by the enzyme dopamine β-hydroxylase (DBH) to NE. Dopamine β-hydroxylase is localized to the secretory granule. Norepinephrine can be methylated to form epinephrine by phenylethanolamine N-methyltransferase (PNMT), an enzyme present in adrenal medulla, and as mentioned above, also in certain areas of the brain.

Step 3: Storage Phase

After their synthesis, NE and DA are stored in specific granules within nerve terminals, probably bound to ATP and other carrier substances (Figs. 7 and 8). Within the granule they are protected from degradation. Storage

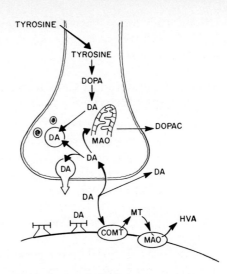

FIGURE 7. This is a schematic representation of a central dopaminergic synapse. See text for abbreviations. (Modified from Cooper, JC, Bloom, FE, and Roth, RH: *The Biochemical Basis of Neuropharmacology*, ed 5. Oxford University Press, New York, 1986.)

granules in peripheral sympathetic nerves are accessible to NE and DA when introduced into the systemic circulation because of active reuptake into axon terminals, but NE and DA do not readily cross the blood-brain barrier and therefore do not reach central monoaminergic neurons. Interference with the capacity to store amines in the granules of nerve endings (as by reserpine and tetrabenazine) leads to depletion of aminergic stores, both centrally and peripherally. The administration of either drug leads to a decrease in catecholamine storage in brain and peripheral autonomic tissues, an effect persisting for several days probably because the granules are damaged irreversibly.

Step 4: Release of Preformed Granules

Propagated action potentials in catecholaminergic neurons lead to neuronal depolarization and granule extrusion from the nerve endings by a calcium-dependent mechanism. Amphetamines act, at least in part, by

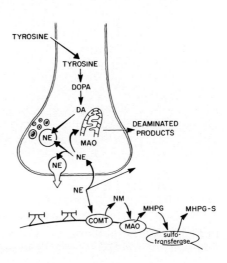

FIGURE 8. This is a schematic representation of a central noradrenergic synapse. See text for abbreviations. (Modified from Cooper, JC, Bloom, FE, and Roth, RH: *The Biochemical Basis of Neuropharmacology*, ed 5. Oxford University Press, New York, 1986.)

ANTERIOR PITUITARY REGULATION

53

stimulating the release of preformed NE and, in high doses, also DA. γ-Hydroxybutyrate blocks the release of DA by blocking propagation of action potentials.

Step 5: Interaction of Catecholamines with Receptors Located on the Postsynaptic Neuron

Specific binding sites for NE and DA are present on the postsynaptic cell body in catecholamine-responsive tissues such as fat cells and cardiac muscle. It is assumed that similar receptors are present on hypophysiotropic neurons. By analogy with peripheral autonomic pharmacology and the study of central nervous system control, it may be assumed that there are at least four classes of NE receptors on hypophysiotropic neurons, two corresponding to alpha-receptors (α_1 and α_2) and two others corresponding to beta-receptors (β_1 and β_2). α_2 receptors are predominantly—and perhaps exclusively—located on the presynaptic membrane, whereas α_1 receptors are located postsynaptically. Agents that duplicate the effects of the biogenic amines are called agonists, and agents that block agonist effects are called receptor-blockers or antagonists. Clonidine is an α_1 receptor agonist. Phenoxybenzamine and phentolamine act principally by blocking α_1-receptors and yohimbine and piperoxane by blocking α_2 receptors. These effects have not, however, been shown conclusively to be true in brain.

Dopamine receptors are probably also present on certain hypophysiotropic neurons.[9] Two types of dopamine receptors, called D_1 and D_2, have been described. D_1 receptors activate the adenylate cyclase system, whereas D_2 receptors are not coupled to this second messenger system. D_1 receptors are the predominant type in the striatum, and D_2 receptors are found in prolactin cells. From an analysis of pituitary control, it appears likely that some hypophysiotropic neurons may have more than one type of receptor. Dopamine receptor agonists include apomorphine, lergotrile mesylate, and bromocriptine. Because these classes of receptors have important potential therapeutic applications in endocrinology, neurology, and psychiatry, an enormous amount of investigative work is underway to develop new agonists and antagonists.

The nature of the DA receptor and aberrations in DA metabolism have become increasingly important areas of investigation in both basic research and clinical medicine. Parkinson's disease results from a deficiency in DA agonist effects in the caudate and putamen, and DA agonists such as L-dopa and bromocriptine can ameliorate many of the manifestations of this disorder. Dopamine agonists are also potent inhibitors of PRL secretion and stimulators of GH release.[19] Recently, other agonists such as lisuride and pergolide have been shown to be effective in the inhibition of PRL secretion. Dopamine-antagonist drugs include chlorpromazine, perphenazine, haloperidol, and pimozide.

Step 6: Reuptake Process

Following the release of preformed hormone, free neurotransmitter in the synaptic cleft that has not reacted with receptor is taken up into the presynaptic nerve ending where it is either destroyed (see below) or incorporated again into a storage granule. The reuptake process is the principal mechanism responsible for terminating the effects of postsynaptic nerve cell stimulation. A number of drugs increase NE and DA effects by blocking the reuptake process, thus making more neurotransmitter available at the postsynaptic receptor site. These include cocaine and the tricyclic antidepressants desipramine and amitriptyline. Amphetamine may also act in part by this mechanism.

Step 7: Degradation of Neurotransmitter

Norepinephrine bound to postsynaptic membranes, or free (nongranule-bound) in the presynaptic nerve ending, is vulnerable to destruction by the cytoplasmic enzyme monoamine oxidase (MAO) that converts NE to its aldehyde, 3,4-dihydroxymandelic acid (see Figure 8). This enzyme also affects DA, converting it to homovanillic acid (HVA) and dihydroxyphenylacetic acid. Increased noradrenergic activity results from administration of drugs such as pargyline, isocarboxazide, and tranylcypromine, which block MAO activity. By inhibition of the degrading enzyme, more neurotransmitter becomes available to the postsynaptic cells.

A second enzyme responsible for inactivating NE and DA is catechol-O-methyltransferase (COMT). The precise site at which this reaction takes place is unknown, but in brain, the metabolic products of the reaction find their way into the cerebrospinal fluid where measurements of them serve as an index of turnover. The principal products of DA are 3-methoxytyramine and HVA, and those of NE are normetanephrine (NM), 3-methoxy-4-hydroxyphenylglycol (MHPG), and its sulfate, MHPG-sulfate. The drug tropolone is believed to act as an inhibitor of COMT. Turnover of catecholamines in brain is influenced by various endocrine states.[3,4,16]

AXONAL TRANSPORT OF CATECHOLAMINES

Labeling and ligature experiments indicate that the protein-binding matrix of catecholaminergic storage granules is synthesized in the cell body and transported down the nerve by axoplasmic flow to its site in the nerve ending. Similarly, the enzymes for biosynthesis and degradation of the catecholamines are formed as proteins in the cell body and are transported to the axon terminal. The principal site of synthesis of the catecholamines, however, is in the terminal itself.

ACTIONS OF CATECHOLAMINES ON HYPOTHALAMIC-PITUITARY FUNCTION

As summarized in Table 1, a number of drugs that affect catecholamines also influence anterior pituitary hormone secretion. These drugs have been widely applied to the basic study of neuroendocrine control and have been used for clinical application to stimulate or to inhibit hormone secretion.

BIOSYNTHESIS AND DEGRADATION OF SEROTONIN

The metabolic steps in the biosynthesis of serotonin are illustrated in Figure 9.

TABLE 1. Actions of Pharmacologic Agents and Effects on Anterior Pituitary Secretion

Drug	Trade Name	Mechanisms of Action	Effects of Monoamines	Growth Hormone	Prolactin	Gonadotropins	TSH	ACTH
Precursors								
L-dopa	Larodopa	Increases substrate for DA and NE formation	Increases DA and NE levels in brain	↑	↓	↑	blocks TSH response to TRH	↑
Tryptophan and 5-hydroxytryptophan		Increases substrate for serotonin formation	Increases serotonin level in brain	↓	↑	↑	→ response to TRH	←
Receptor Agonists (Stimulators)								
Apomorphine Bromocriptine Clonidine	Parlodel Catapres	Stimulates DA receptors Stimulates α-adrenergic receptors	Mimics DA effects Mimics α-receptor effects	↑	↓	↑	↑	↑
Isoproterenol	Isuprel	Stimulates β-adrenergic receptors	Mimics β-receptor effects	↑	↓	↑	←	↑
Histamine		H$_1$ and H$_2$ receptor agonist		↓	↑	↑	←	←
GABA		GABA receptor agonist		↑	↑	←	↑	→
Receptor Blockers								
Pimozide Haloperidol Chlorpromazine	Haldol Largactil Thorazine	Blocks DA receptors (and NE receptors in large doses)	Prevents DA effects	↓	←	↓ blocks ovulation	↑	↑
Phentolamine Phenoxybenzamine	Rogitine Dibenzyline	α-adrenergic blocker	Blocks peripheral and central α-receptors	↓ GH responses*	↑	↓ pulsatile secretion	→	↓ response to insulin
Propranolol	Inderal	β-adrenergic blocker	Blocks peripheral and central β-receptors	↑ GH responses	↑	↑	↑	↑ response to insulin
Cyproheptadine Methysergide	Periactin Sansert	Serotonin receptor blocker	Blocks peripheral and central serotonin receptors	↓ GH responses* ↑ sleep release	stress and ↓ sleep release	↓	↑	↓ response to insulin
Atropine		Muscarinic cholinergic antagonist	Blocks muscarinic receptor	↓ GH response to GHRH	↑	↑	↑	↑ response to insulin hypoglycemia

Drug	Trade name	Action					
Methylscopolamine		Muscarinic acetylcholine receptor antagonist	↑+	↑	↑	↑	↑
Cimetidine	Tagamet	H$_2$ receptor antagonist	↓	↓	↑	↑	←
Enzyme Inhibitors							
α-methyl-p-tyrosine		Blocks formation of DA and NE	↓	↓ suckling response	blocks ovulation	→	←
Disulfram	Antabuse	Blocks DA-β-oxidase	↓		?	?	?
Fusaric acid				response →			
p-chlorophenylalanine		Blocks tryptophan hydroxylase	↓		?	?	?
Precursor Analogs							
α-methyldopa	Aldomet	Converted into methylated monoamine	?	↓	?	?	?
Presynaptic Storage Blockers							
Reserpine	Serpasil	Inhibits storage and reuptake of biogenic amines by granules	↓	↓	blocks ovulation‡	→	←
Tricyclic antidepressants							
Imipramine / Amitriptyline	Tofranil / Elavil	Blocks reuptake by nerve terminals; Depletes terminals of catecholamines and serotonin	↓ GH sleep response	↓	↑	↑	↑
Mixed Function							
Amphetamines		Releases biogenic amines, blocks reuptake; Increases NE turnover, increases availability of NE	↑	↓	?	?	←

Key: ↑ increases; ↓ decreases; → no effect; ? not tested
Data are based chiefly on work in rats, monkeys, and human beings. Inasmuch as there are species differences in effects of these agents, and all agents have not been tested in all three species, this table is incomplete and possibly inaccurate in some details.
*Data are conflicting; partially blocks insulin-induced GH release, but increases sleep release.
+Blocks GH secretion during sleep.
‡In rodents.

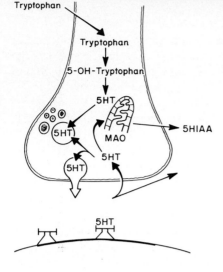

FIGURE 9. This is a schematic representation of a central serotonergic synapse. See text for abbreviations. (Modified from Cooper, JC, Bloom FE, and Roth, RH: *The Biochemical Basis of Neuropharmacology,* ed 5. Oxford University Press, New York, 1986.)

Step 1: Uptake of Tryptophan

Tryptophan, like other large neutral amino acids, is taken up actively by brain cells. Cellular concentration of the amino acid in brain depends upon dietary intake and varies rapidly within a few minutes to hours with changes in circulating levels in the blood. Uptake into brain is suppressed by excess amounts of other amino acids of the same class.

Step 2: Enzymatic Synthesis

Tryptophan is converted to 5-hydroxytryptophan by the enzyme tryptophan hydroxylase. The subsequent conversion to serotonin is accomplished by the enzyme L-aminodecarboxylase, which appears to be identical to that responsible for the synthesis of NE.[42] The conversion of tryptophan to 5-hydroxytryptophan can be blocked by p-chlorophenylalanine, and the conversion to serotonin can be blocked by disulfiram. In tissues, such as the pineal gland and the retina, serotonin is converted to melatonin, an indoleamine that is also present in the brain and which may function as a neurotransmitter. Serotonin also can be converted to N-acetylserotonin in cerebellum and brainstem; the function of this substance is unknown.

Step 3: Storage Phase

Serotonin, like NE and DA, is stored in granules in nerve endings, complexed with a protein carrier and adenosine triphosphate (ATP) (see Figure 9). The storage mechanism for serotonin is also similar to that of the catecholamines, because it is abolished by the same drugs, reserpine and tetrabenazine, which cause a depletion of serotonin.

Step 4: Release Phase

The control of the release process has not been completely established in the CNS, but results from other tissues suggest that release of storage granules at nerve terminals occurs in response to a propagated action potential.

Step 5: Interaction of Serotonin with Receptors Located on the Postsynaptic Membrane

Serotonin probably interacts with specific receptors on the postsynaptic membrane. A number of serotonin analogs may mimic serotonin-agonist functions, including quipazine and the hallucinogenic drug, lysergic acid (LSD). The latter appears to act, in part, by affecting autoreceptors on serotonin-producing raphe neurons, causing inhibition of cellular firing. Important serotonin antagonists that have been used widely for study of hypophysiotropic neuropharmacology are methysergide and cyproheptadine.[19] The specificity of these antagonists has not been established with certainty, particularly in the CNS.

Step 6: Reuptake Process

As with catecholamines, the action of the neurotransmitter is terminated by reuptake from the synaptic cleft into the presynaptic nerve ending. Drugs such as the tricyclic antidepressants, imipramine and amitriptyline, potentiate serotonin effects by inhibiting the reuptake process.

Step 7: Enzymatic Degradation

As with catecholamines, the enzyme monoamine oxidase (MAO) degrades free serotonin in the nerve ending. The product of this metabolism is 5-hydroxyindoleacetic acid (5-HIAA). Agents such as pargyline that interfere with MAO also potentiate serotonin effects.

EFFECTS OF SEROTONIN ON HYPOPHYSIOTROPIC NEURONS

Understanding the role of serotonergic neurons in anterior pituitary regulation is based largely on pharmacologic manipulations, all of which have inherent limitations. It is reasonable to postulate that serotonin receptors on certain classes of hypophysiotropic neurons activate release mechanisms analogous to those postulated for the catecholamine-dependent neurons. 5-Hydroxytryptophan administration, known to increase serotonin formation, is followed by the release of prolactin,[19,23] suggesting that there is an excitatory serotonergic pathway that regulates prolactin secretion. This hypothesis is confirmed by the finding that stress-induced prolactin release is blocked by methysergide, a serotonin antagonist. Suckling-induced prolactin release in the rat is also reported to be blocked by administration of parachlorophenylalanine, an inhibitor of serotonin synthesis. Electric stimulation of the raphe nucleus in the rat results in growth hormone release, and precursor administration of the serotonin precursor 5-hydroxytryptophan causes growth hormone release in man. A summary of drugs used clinically and in the experimental elucidation of serotonergic neurotransmitter control of hypophysiotropic function is presented in Table 1.[10,15,19,20]

CENTRAL HISTAMINERGIC PATHWAYS

Histamine is a normal brain constituent; approximately 50 percent is present in perivascular mast cells, and the remainder is thought to be in neurons, many of which are found in the hypothalamus. The highest concentrations are found in the median eminence.[6,37,38] A specific enzyme, histidine decarboxylase, is present in certain regions of the brain, including the hypothalamus, and acts on the precursor amino acid histidine to form histamine. Unilateral lesions in the lateral hypothalamus that interrupt the medial forebrain bundle cause depletion of histamine in the cortex, hippocampus, and hypothalamus on the same side. Histamine is also present in synaptosome preparations of cortex, and microiontophoresis onto single nerve cells causes excitation or, more rarely, depression of cellular activity. On the basis of these observations, Schwartz[37] has postulated that a histaminergic system exists in the brain analogous to the catecholaminergic and serotonergic systems and that histamine may act as a neurotransmitter.

Preliminary evidence suggests that both H_1 and H_2 receptors exist in the brain; H_2-sensitive adenylate cyclase has been partially characterized in hippocampus and cerebral cortex.[9] Agents that act on these receptors are reported to influence anterior pituitary hormone secretion (see Table 1).

ACETYLCHOLINE AND HYPOTHALAMIC-PITUITARY FUNCTION

The neurophysiologic functions of acetylcholine (Ach) have been the subject of study since the 1920s. Most of the strict criteria that have been established to define a bona fide neurotransmitter have been fulfilled by Ach at the neuromuscular junction, in autonomic ganglia, and at postganglionic parasympathetic nerve endings. Within the CNS, such definitive proof has been more difficult to establish, but studies of the cholinergic septo-hippocampal and habenulointerpeduncular tracts have given strong support to the idea that Ach functions as a true neurotransmitter. Much attention has been given to the nucleus basalis of Meynert and other nuclear groups comprising the substantia innominata as a major source of cholinergic input to the cerebral cortex and hippocampus. A loss of cells in this region of brain has been documented in Alzheimer's disease, thus explaining the reduced Ach found in the cortex in this disease. Although substantial amounts of Ach are found in the hypothalamus, including the median eminence, there are very few cell bodies found. This suggests that most Ach in the hypothalamus arises from cell bodies outside the region.

BIOSYNTHESIS AND ACTIONS OF ACETYLCHOLINE

Acetylcholine is synthesized from acetyl CoA and choline in a reaction catalyzed by the enzyme choline acetyltransferase (CAT). Ach is metabolized by acetylcholinesterase, an abundant and ubiquitous enzyme in brain. Ach acts on two types of receptors, muscarinic and nicotinic, and relatively specific agonists and antagonists have been developed for each. Nicotinic receptors are blocked by α-bungarotoxin, rabies virus, curare, and decamethonium; muscarinic receptors are blocked by atropine, scopolamine, and guinuclidinyl benzilate. Oxotremorine is also a muscarinic agent. Acetylcholinesterase is inhibited reversibly by physostigmine.

Many of the drugs that influence cholinergic functions in the periphery are ineffective in the brain because they fail to cross the blood-brain barrier at a significant rate. However, atropine, scopolamine, physostigmine, and diisopropyl phosphorofluorinate (DFP) do penetrate the CNS. Atropine and scopolamine cause a decrease in Ach in the brain by effects mediated on autoreceptors located on presynaptic sites. The administration of choline and lecithin (choline phosphoglyceride) causes an increase in brain Ach levels.

CHOLINERGIC PATHWAYS IN NEUROENDOCRINE REGULATION

Acetylcholine is present in the hypothalamus, and a few scattered cell bodies can be identified with antibodies to CAT.

There is evidence that cholinergic pathways are involved in pituitary regulation. The classic example of this is the neurohypophysial neuron, which is activated functionally and electrically by cholinergic drugs and is inactivated by anticholinergic agents (see chapter 4). With respect to anterior pituitary regulation, reflex ovulation in the rabbit is blocked by large doses of atropine, ACTH secretion is stimulated by a cholinergic system, and Ach also appears to facilitate GH and PRL secretion under some conditions. Ach has emerged as an unexpectedly important regulator of GH secretion. Stimuli to GH release such as the normal sleep-associated rise and injection of GHRH are not effective in subjects treated with atropine or other Ach blockers, although responses to hypoglycemia are unimpaired by these agents. Inasmuch as Ach has no direct effect on the anterior pituitary, it has been postulated that it must exert a tonic restraining influence on somatostatin secretion. Such an effect has been demonstrated *in vitro*. The effects of some of these agents on neuroendocrine regulation are summarized in Table 1.

AMINO ACID NEUROTRANSMITTERS

Of the amino acid neurotransmitters known to be abundant in the brain, only γ-aminobutyric acid (GABA) and glutamate have been studied in any detail with respect to neuroendocrine functions. γ-Aminobutyric acid is found is high concentration in the hypothalamus comparable with the high levels present in the globus pallidus and substantia nigra. It is abundant in the median eminence. It is synthesized from glutamic acid by the actions of the enzyme glutamic acid decarboxylase (GAD). Evidence has been marshalled that suggests a role of GABA in hypophysiotropic hormone release, in which it is active in release of somatostatin. Neuroendocrine studies in animals and man using drugs such as valproic acid and the benzodiazepines which affect GABA functions have shown effects on ACTH, GH, and PRL secretion. These are summarized in Table 1.

Glutamate has played a different role in neuroendocrine investigation. Administration to neonatal animals of large doses of monosodium glutamate (MSG, a common food additive) causes destruction of ARC neurons in rodents. This effect is believed to be due to interactions of glutamate with glutamate receptors contained on these cells. Such animals have a variety of neuroendocrine deficits that include hypothalamic hypogonadism and growth failure. Recent studies have shown that MSG-induced lesions lead to a marked depletion of GHRH in the hypothalamus and median eminence of rats, which is manifested physiologically by decreased pulsatile secretion of GH (see chapter 8).

A summary of drugs used clinically and in the experimental elucidation of neurotransmitter control of anterior pituitary hormone secretion is given in Table 1.

NEUROPEPTIDES

The extensive populations of hypothalamic neuropeptides that play a role in pituitary regulation are considered in chapter 18.

REFERENCES

1. AJIKA, K, AND HOKFELT, T: *Ultrastructural identification of catecholamine neurones in the hypothalamic periventricular-arcuate nucleus-median eminence complex with special reference to quantitative aspects.* Brain Res 57:97–117, 1973.
2. ANNUNZIATO, L, AND WEINER, RI: *Characteristics of dopamine uptake and 3,4-dihydroxyphenylacetic acid (DOPAC) formation in the dopaminergic terminals of the neurointermediate lobe of the pituitary gland.* Neuroendocrinology 31:8–12, 1980.
3. ANTON-TAY, F, PELHAM, RW, WURTMAN, RJ: *Increased turnover of ³H-norepinephrine in rat brain following castration or treatment with ovine follicle stimulating hormone.* Endocrinology 84:1489–1492, 1969.
4. ANTON-TAY, F, AND WURTMAN, RJ: *Norepinephrine: Turnover in rat brains after gonadectomy.* Science 159:1245, 1968.
5. BROWNSTEIN, MJ, PALKOVITS, M, TAPPAZ, ML, SAAVEDRA, JM, KIZER, JS: *Effect of surgical isolation of the hypothalamus on its neurotransmitter content.* Brain Res 117:287–295, 1976.
6. BROWNSTEIN, MJ, SAAVEDRA, JM, PALKOVITS, M, ET AL: *Histamine content of hypothalamic nuclei of the rat.* Brain Res 77:151–156, 1974.
7. CARLSSON, A, FALCK, B, HILLARP, NA: *Cellular localization of brain monoamines.* Acta Physiol Scand (Suppl)196:1–28, 1962.
8. CHALMERS, JP, BALDESSARINI, RJ, WURTMAN, RJ: *Effects of L-dopa on norepinephrine metabolism in the brain.* Proc Natl Acad Sci USA 68:662–666, 1971.
9. COOPER, JR, BLOOM, FE, ROTH, RH: *The Biochemical Basis of Neuropharmacology,* ed 5. Oxford University Press, New York, 1986.
10. CORRODI, H, FUXE, K, HOKFELT, T, ET AL: *Effect of ergot drugs on central catecholamine neurons: Evidence for a stimulation of central dopamine neurons.* J Pharm Pharmacol 25:409–412, 1973.
11. CUELLO, AC, SHOEMAKER, WJ, GANONG, WF: *Effect of 6-hydroxydopamine on hypothalamic norepinephrine and dopamine content, ultrastructure of the median eminence, and plasma corticosterone.* Brain Res 78:57–69, 1974.
12. DAHLSTROM, A, AND FUXE, K: *Evidence for the existence of monamine-containing neurons in the central nervous system. I. Demonstration of monamines in the cell bodies of brain stem neurons.* Acta Physiol Scand 62 (Suppl) 232:1–55, 1965.
13. DAY, TA, BLESSING, W, WILLOUGHBY, JO: *Noradrenergic and dopaminergic projections to the medial preoptic area of the rat. A combined horseradish peroxidase/catecholamine fluorescence study.* Brain Res 193:543–548, 1980.
14. DEMAREST, KT, MOORE, KE: *Lack of a high affinity transport system for dopamine in the median eminence and posterior pituitary.* Brain Res 171:545–551, 1979.
15. DE WIED, D, AND DE JONG, W: *Drug effects and hypothalamic anterior pituitary function.* Annu Rev Pharmacol 14:389–441, 1974.
16. DONOSO, AO, BISHOP, W, FAWCETT, CP, ET AL: *Effects of drugs that modify brain monoamine*

concentrations of plasma gonadotropin and prolactin levels in the rat. Endocrinology 89:774–784, 1971.

17. DONOVAN, BT, AND HARRIS, GW: *Adrenergic agents and the release of gonadotrophic hormone in the rabbit.* J Physiol (London) 132:577–585, 1956.
18. FERNSTROM, JD, AND WURTMAN, RJ: *Brain serotonin content: Physiological dependence on plasma tryptophan levels.* Science 173:149–152, 1971.
19. FROHMAN, LA: *Clinical neuropharmacology of hypothalamic releasing factors.* N Engl J Med 286:1391–7, 1972.
20. FROHMAN, LA, AND STACHURA, ME: *Neuropharmacologic control of neuroendocrine function in man.* Metabolism 24:211–234, 1975.
21. HOKFELT, T, ELDE, R, FUXE, K, JOHANSSON, O, LJUNGDAHL, A, GOLDSTEIN, M, LUFT, R, EFENDIC, S, NISSON, G, TERENIUS, L, GANTEN, D, JEFFCOATE, SL, REHFELD, J, SAID, S, MORA, M, POSSANI, L, TAPIA, R, TERAN, L, PALACIOS, R: *Aminergic and peptidergic pathways in the nervous system with special reference to the hypothalamus.* In REICHLIN, S, BALDESSARINI, RT, MARTIN, JB (EDS): *The Hypothalamus.* Raven Press, New York, 1978, pp. 69–136.
22. IMURA, H, NAKAI, Y, YOSHIMA, T: *Effect of 5-hydroxytryptophan on growth hormone and ACTH release in man.* J Clin Endocrinol Metab 35:204–206, 1973.
23. KATO, Y, ET AL: *Effect of 5-hydroxytryptophan (5-HTP) on plasma prolactin levels in man.* J Clin Endocrinol Metab 38:695–697, 1974.
24. KIZER, JS, MUTH, E, JACOBOWITZ, DM: *The effect of bilateral lesions of the ventral noradrenergic bundle on endocrine-induced changes of tyrosine hydroxylase in the rat median eminence.* Endocrinology 98:886–893, 1976.
25. LICHTENSTEIGER, W: *Cyclic variations of catecholamine content in hypothalamic nerve cells during the estrous cycle of the rat, with a concomitant study of the substantia nigra.* J Pharmacol Exp Ther 165:204–215, 1969.
26. MATSUMOTO, A, AND ARAI, Y: *Morphologic evidence for intranuclear circuits in the hypothalamic arcuate nucleus.* Exp Neurol 59:404–412, 1978.
27. MOORE, KE, AND JOHNSTON, CA: *The median eminence: Aminergic control mechanisms.* In MÜLLER, EE, AND MACLEOD, RM (EDS): *Neuroendocrine Perspectives.* Elsevier, Amsterdam, 1982, pp 23–42.
28. MOORE, RY, AND BLOOM, FE: *Central catecholamine neuron systems: Anatomy and physiology of the norepinephrine and epinephrine systems.* Annu Rev Neurosci 2:113–504, 1979.
29. PALKOVITS, M: *Catecholamines in the hypothalamus: An anatomical review.* Neuroendocrinology 33:123–128, 1981.
30. PALKOVITS, M, BROWNSTEIN, M, SAAVEDRA, JM, AXELROD, J: *Norepinephrine and dopamine content of hypothalamic nuclei of the rat.* Brain Res 77:137–149, 1974.
31. PALKOVITS, M, SAAVEDRA, JM, JACOBOWITZ, DM, KIZER, JS, ZABORSZKY, L, BROWNSTEIN, M: *Serotonergic innervation of the forebrain: Effect of lesions on serotonin and tryptophan hydroxylase levels.* Brain Res 130:121–134, 1977.
32. PALKOVITS, M, ZABORSKY, L, FEMINGER, A, MEZEY, E, FEKETE, MIK, HERMAN, JP, KANYICSKA, B, SZABO, D: *Noradrenergic innervation of the rat hypothalamus: Experimental biochemical and electron microscopic studies.* Brain Res 191:161–171, 1980.
33. SAAVEDRA, JM, PALKOVITS, M, BROWNSTEIN, MJ, ET AL: *Serotonin distribution in the nuclei of the rat hypothalamus and preoptic region.* Brain Res 77:157–165, 1974.
34. SAAVEDRA, JM, PALKOVITS, M, BROWNSTEIN, MJ, AXELROD, J: *Serotonin distribution in the nuclei of the rat hypothalamus and amygdaloid afferents in the stria terminalis.* Brain Res 149:223–228, 1978.
35. SAWYER, CH: *First Geoffrey Harris Memorial Lecture—Some recent developments in brain-pituitary ovarian physiology.* Neuroendocrinology 17:97–124, 1975.
36. SAWYER, CH, MARKEE, JE, TOWNSEND, BF: *Cholinergic and adrenergic components in neurohumoral control of release of LH in rabbits.* Endocrinology 44:18–37, 1949.
37. SCHWARTZ, JC: *Histamine as a transmitter in brain.* Life Sci 17:503–517, 1975.
38. SNYDER, SH, AND TAYLOR, KM: *Histamine in the brain: A neurotransmitter?* In SNYDER, S (ED): *Perspectives in Neuropharmacology.* Oxford University Press, New York, 1972, p 43.
39. VAN LOON, GR, ET AL: *Effect of intraventricular administration of adrenergic drugs on the adrenal venous 17-hydroxycorticosteroid response to surgical stress in the dog.* Neuroendocrinology 8:257, 1971.
40. VOGT, M: *Concentration of sympathin in different parts of central nervous system under normal conditions and after administration of drugs.* J Physiol Lond 123:451, 1954.
41. WEINER, N: *Regulation of norepinephrine biosynthesis.* Annu Rev Pharmacol 10:273–290, 1970.
42. WURTMAN, RJ, AND FERNSTROM, JD: *L-tryptophan, L-tyrosine, and the control of brain monoamine biosynthesis.* In SNYDER, SH (ED): *Perspectives in Neuropharmacology.* Oxford University Press, New York, 1972, p 143.

PART 2

Regulation of the Pituitary Gland: Basic and Clinical Aspects

Chapter 4

THE NEUROHYPOPHYSIS: PHYSIOLOGY AND DISORDERS OF SECRETION

Plasma osmolality and blood volume are among the most jealously guarded components of the internal milieu. Their constancy is maintained by central nervous system integrating mechanisms that regulate intake and excretion of water and salt. Most important of these mechanisms are

1. Neurohypophysial secretion of antidiuretic hormone (ADH, vasopressin), which controls free-water clearance of the kidney through its actions on tubular reabsorption of water.
2. Hypothalamic thirst mechanisms, which are regulated by peripheral blood volume receptors, by central osmoreceptors, and by angiotensin.
3. Renal secretion of renin (in part regulated by the sympathetic nervous system), which determines the blood level of angiotensin and in turn of aldosterone, the principal salt-regulating hormone system.
4. Cardiac and brain natriuretic factors.

This chapter deals with neuroendocrine control of salt and water balance, the function of the neurohypophysis in this regulation, and clinical disorders of the neurohypophysis. Also considered is oxytocin secretion, the second most important function of the neurohypophysis.

THE NEUROHYPOPHYSIS

Our understanding of the function of the neurohypophysis began with the work of two clinicians, Farini, assistant physician in the *Ospedale Civile*, Venice, and von den Velden, of the *Oberarzt* medical clinic in Dusseldorf, Germany* who separately and independently in 1913 came to realize from autopsy studies that diabetes insipidus was associated with hypothalamic destruction, postulated that this disorder was a deficiency state, and showed that injections of posterior pituitary extracts successfully controlled the excessive urination. Subsequently Starling and Verney[134] re-

---

*Cited in Reichlin.[100]

ported in 1924 that posterior pituitary extracts acted directly on the kidneys, and Verney later showed that infusion of hypertonic salt into the carotid artery could produce antidiuresis in the hydrated dog. Other important milestones in understanding the function of the neural lobe were the delineation of its neuroanatomy by Ranson and colleagues,[144] the discovery of the phenomenon of neurosecretion by Scharrer and his colleagues,[117] and the isolation and chemical characterization of the neurohypophysial peptides vasopressin (antidiuretic hormone, ADH) and oxytocin by Du Vigneaud and colleagues.[35,100,116]

Elucidation of the structure and function of the neurohypophysis has led the way to major advances in all aspects of the field of neuroendocrinology.[117] From neurohypophysial research has come the clinical-pathologic correlation of a clinical syndrome with a specific neural defect; the concepts of neurosecretion, axoplasmic transport, biosynthesis from prohormones; and regulation of neuroendocrine cells by neurotransmitters. Neurohypophysial hormones were the first neuropeptides to be isolated and synthesized and the first to be applied therapeutically (diabetes insipidus, delayed labor, postpartum hemorrhage). The first research efforts to devise clinically advantageous analogs began with the neurohypophysial peptides, and the first molecular explanation of the nature of an inherited defect of vasopressin has come from a study of the DNA sequence of the gene that codes for vasopressin in the Brattleboro rat, a species with congenital diabetes insipidus.[119]

ANATOMIC CONSIDERATIONS

The neural lobe of the pituitary (posterior pituitary) develops embryologically as a downgrowth from the ventral diencephalon and retains its neural connections and neural character in adult life.[17,65,141-143] Its principal components are the supraoptico-hypophysial and paraventricular-hypophysial nerve tracts which arise, respectively, from the supraoptic and paraventricular nuclei within the hypothalamus and descend through the infundibulum and neural stalk to terminate in the neural lobe (Fig. 1). The hormones vasopressin and oxytocin are synthesized in the hypothalamus, transported by axoplasmic flow, and released from the nerve terminals into the fenestrated capillaries of the neurohypophysis.[29,77]

Cells of origin of these tracts are relatively large (hence called magnocellular) and are consolidated into well-characterized groups situated in paired nuclei above the optic tract (supraoptic) and on each side of the ventricle (paraventricular)[8,13] (Fig. 2). A few cells of this system are distributed between the two nuclei, and some are also found in the paired suprachiasmatic nuclei[31,32] (Fig. 3). Most of the cell bodies in the supraoptic nucleus contain vasopressin, but some contain oxytocin.[102] A somewhat smaller percentage (but still the majority of stainable cells) in the paraventricular nucleus contain vasopressin. Cells contain either one peptide or the other.[103] This is also true for the respective prohormones (see below).

Although the principal projections of the magnocellular nuclei are to the neural lobe, vasopressin-containing nerve endings also terminate on the primary capillary plexus of the hypophysial-portal circulation.[9,93,140] From these anatomic observations and from direct measurements of vaso-

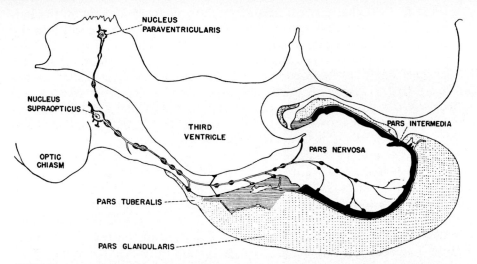

FIGURE 1. This is a diagram of the hypothalamic-neurohypophysial system in the dog. Axons of neurons in the supraoptic and paraventricular nuclei traverse the pituitary stalk to end in the posterior pituitary (pars nervosa). The dilated areas on the axon represent neurosecretory material (NSM). Electron microscopy indicates that the NSM is within the unmyelinated axons. (From Bargmann and Scharrer,[13] with permission.)

pressin in portal blood, it has been inferred that neurohypophysial neurons may have a role in anterior pituitary regulation, as well as in neural lobe secretion.[140,141] Indeed, recent work has shown that vasopressin synergizes with corticotropin-releasing hormone (CRH) to bring about stress-related ACTH release (see chapter 6). Corticotropin-releasing hormone and vasopressin are colocalized in some of the small cells (parvocellular group) of the paraventricular nucleus. Vasopressin also stimulates GH secretion (see chapter 8).

Vasopressin- and oxytocin-containing fibers arising in the paraventricular nucleus also are distributed to many other regions of the central nervous system, including the brainstem, spinal cord, hippocampus, and amygdala.[30,32,75,88,114,115,125,126,128–131,143] Within the spinal cord these fibers terminate on the cells of origin of the autonomic nervous system and hence can influence blood pressure; within the brainstem they end in the sensory nuclei of the vagal and glossopharyngeal nerves, which also receive information about blood pressure and blood volume. A few investigators have described vasopressin positive cells outside the hypothalamus located in the amygdala and locus coeruleus.[22] The central fibers of these "vasopressinergic" and "oxytocinergic" pathways function independently of those that innervate the neurohypophysis.[12] This has been shown by comparing changes in cerebrospinal fluid vasopressin with those of blood vasopressin. Central vasopressin levels show a circadian rhythm independent of the state of hydration.[94] In contrast, peripheral vasopressin levels, which reflect the secretion of the neurohypophysis, do not follow a circadian pattern and are related to blood volume and plasma osmolality (see below). Oxytocin in cerebrospinal fluid also follows a time-related pattern independent of blood levels.[5]

Although cell bodies of the supraoptic nucleus are large, the axons are small (0.1 to 0.3 in diameter), unmyelinated, and their conduction velocity (0.4 to 0.9 m/sec)

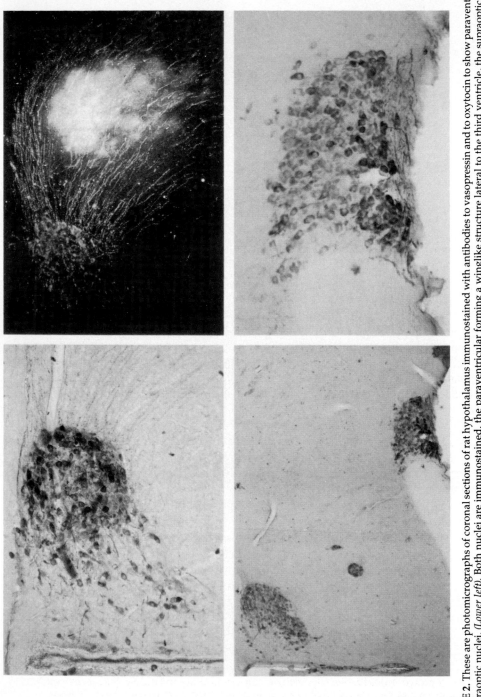

FIGURE 2. These are photomicrographs of coronal sections of rat hypothalamus immunostained with antibodies to vasopressin and to oxytocin to show paraventricular and supraoptic nuclei. (*Lower left*). Both nuclei are immunostained, the paraventricular forming a winglike structure lateral to the third ventricle, the supraoptic in this level appearing at the extreme lateral margin of the optic tract. (*Upper left*). Higher magnification of paraventricular nucleus. Vasopressin-staining neurons form a central core in the lateral magnocellular group rimmed by oxytocin-containing neurons. (*Lower right*). Higher magnification of the supraoptic nucleus vasopressin-containing neurons (staining darker) which are more concentrated in the ventral part of the nucleus at this level. (*Upper right*). Dark-field photomicrograph of paraventricular nucleus reacted only with monoclonal antibody specific to vasopressin. Numerous beaded axonal fibers project laterally from cell bodies through and around fornix, which shows here as a white mass in the lateral hypothalamus. (Photograph by Alfred T. Lamme, FBPA. From Zimmerman,[143] with permission.)

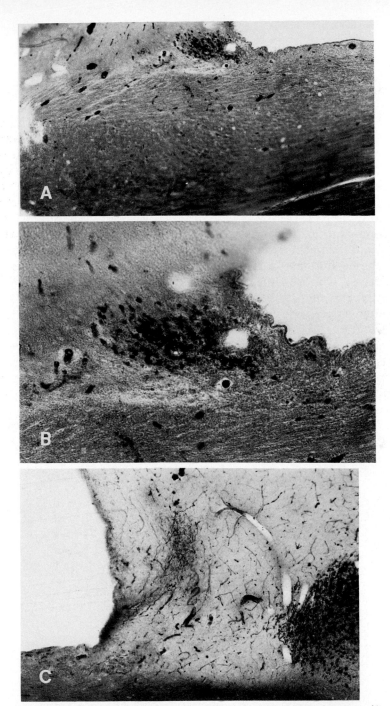

FIGURE 3. Presented here are VIP immunopositive cells in the suprachiasmatic region of human brain. *(A)* The suprachiasmatic region bordering the third ventricle in coronal section with a cluster of VIP containing neurons just dorsal to the optic chiasm. *(B)* These VIP positive cells are numerous and densely packed. Numerous immunopositive varicose processes and the bipolar character of these cells in a higher magnification. *(C)* Vasopressin immunopositive cells in the dorsal aspect of the human suprachiasmatic region. This cluster of cells and fibers is adjacent to the ependymal lining of the third ventricle and is distinct from the more lateral supraoptic nucleus with numerous vasopressin positive magnocellular neurons. (From Stopa et al,[154] with permission.)

estimated by antidromic stimulation is similar to that of unmyelinated peripheral nerve fibers of comparable size.

NEUROHYPOPHYSIAL HORMONES

One of the functions of the posterior pituitary was discovered first by Oliver and Schafer in 1895[91] when they injected extracts of bovine posterior lobe and demonstrated increases in blood pressure. These pressor effects, seen only with large doses of extract, now are regarded by most workers as being physiologically unimportant for blood pressure regulation. Over the succeeding 20 years, however, additional biologic effects of neurohypophysial extracts were defined, including antidiuretic, oxytocic (uterine-contracting), and milk-ejecting effects, the latter mediated by contraction of periacinar myoepithelial cells in the breast. Not until 1949 was the chemical nature of these substances identified by Du Vigneaud and associates, who isolated oxytocin and determined its structure.[35] Subsequently, between 1951 and 1953, these workers also elucidated the structure of vasopressin; Du Vigneaud was awarded a Nobel prize for these contributions. This landmark work established that the neurohypophysial hormones were small polypeptides, and were composed of nine amino acids. This paved the way for the structural elucidation of larger, more complex polypeptide hormones of the pituitary and of other glands. Du Vigneaud's studies were the model for the attack on the structure of the hypophysiotropic hormones of the hypothalamus. The chemistry and phylogenetic implications of neurohypophysial hormone structure have been studied in detail by Sawyer.[116] These hormones have also been the subject

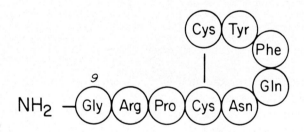

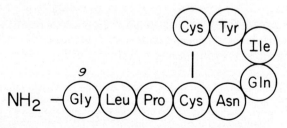

FIGURE 4. Shown here are the structures of vasopressin *(top)* and oxytocin *(bottom)*.

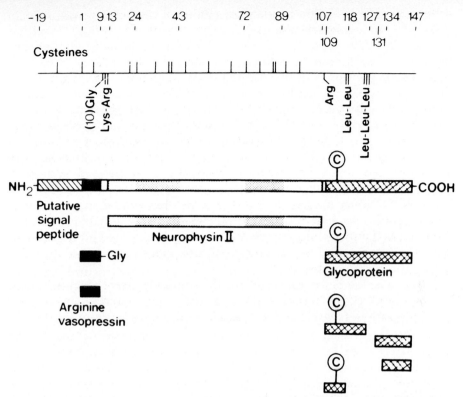

FIGURE 5. Illustrated here is the structure of the preprohormone for arginine vasopressin and neurophysin II. Sequence coding for arginine vasopressin is located immediately after the signal peptide, followed by sequence coding for neurophysin II. Following the neurophysin region is a glycoprotein segment. Top line illustrates amino acid number. Second line from top shows the crucial amino acid sequence at which posttranslational processing of the peptide takes place in secretory granules. Indication of glycine in position 10 is a characteristic extension in peptide hormones that contain a terminal amide. Glycine is exchanged for NH_2 during processing. Lys-Arg sequences at positions 11 and 12 are typical enzymatic cleavage sites, as is Arg in position 107.

In the neurohypophysial system, the entire prohormone is packaged in secretory granules, processed during axoplasmic transport, and vasopressin (nonapeptide) is secreted in equimolar amounts as neurophysin II. (From Land, et al,[74] with permission.)

of intense study of structure-activity relationships, molecular configuration, and molecular-receptor binding.

The structures of vasopressin and oxytocin are remarkably similar, differing by only two amino acids.[39] Both have a Cys-Cys bridge in the 1-6 position (Fig. 4). Vasopressin is found in all mammals and, with the exception of the pig, has identical amino acid sequences (arginine vasopressin); in swine, arginine in position 8 is replaced by lysine. In keeping with a common evolutionary origin of neurohypophysial nonapeptides is the finding that the large precursor prohormones share extensive structural homology[1,2,74,111] and that there is some degree of cross-over of biologic activity; vasopressin manifests slight oxytocic activity, and oxytocin, slight antidiuretic activity. Vasopressin and oxytocin are associated with distinct proteins, *neurophysins*, a part of their prohormones, termed propressophysin and prooxyphysin, respectively (Fig. 5).[20,21,46,47] The neurophysins are released simultaneously with their respective neurohypophysial peptide.[106,107,109,110] The two principal forms of neurophysin are immunologically distinct.[110,139] Factors regulating secretion of vasopressin and oxytocin therefore also regulate secretion of the respective neurophysin.[109,110] Other biologically active peptides and amines are found in the neurohypophysis, including somatostatin, thyrotropin-releasing hormone (TRH), corticotropin-releasing hormone, substance P, LHRH, dopamine, serotonin, histamine, and αMSH. Dynorphin, an opioid peptide, is contained in vasopressin neurons and, indeed, appears to be present in the same neurosecretory vesicles as vasopressin.[135,136] Corticotropin-releasing hormone has also been shown to colocalize with vasopressin in some secretory granules.

Oxytocin and its related neurophysin (neurophysin I), and vasopressin and its related neurophysin (neurophysin II) are synthesized as prohormones in the cell bodies of the supraoptic and paraventricular neurons[141,142] (Fig. 6). The prohormones are transported in membrane-bound vesicles through the axons to the neural lobe where they are stored until released. Processing of the prohormone to the secreted products vasopressin, oxytocin, and the two neurophysins takes place in the granules during the course of transport.

Nerve action potentials arising in the cell body are propagated along the axon and trigger hormone discharge (see Figure 6). The neurohypophysial hormones leave the cell together with neurophysin in fixed ratio.

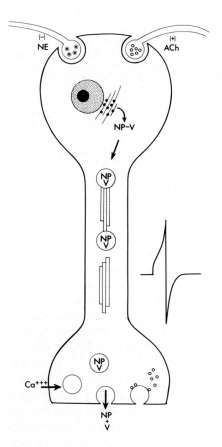

FIGURE 6. This schematic drawing of a vasopressin (ADH) secreting neuron shows synthesis, transport, and release of vasopressin and neurophysin. Neurophysin and vasopressin are synthesized in Golgi system and packaged into granules to be transported by axoplasmic flow to the nerve terminal. Axon terminal depolarization is followed by calcium uptake, union of granule membrane with cell membrane, and release of both neurophysin and vasopressin. The vasopressin neuron receives both noradrenergic (inhibitory) and cholinergic (excitatory) inputs. Abbreviations: NE, norepinephrine: ACh, acetylcholine; NP-V, neurophysin-vasopressin; Ca^{++}, calcium ions.

REGULATION OF ANTIDIURETIC HORMONE (ADH) SECRETION

In the early 1930s, Verney demonstrated the influence of hyperosmolar stimuli on antidiuresis by perfusing the carotid artery with hypertonic saline.[134] From these observations, he concluded that the brain was sensitive to alterations in osmolality. Verney localized the region of the brain critical for this antidiuretic effect to the anterior hypothalamus, in the region of the supraoptic and paraventricular nuclei.[134] As a consequence of Verney's work, the term *osmoreceptor* was applied to cells within the brain which monitor extracellular osmolality. Characteristically, such cells show alterations in electrical firing rates in association with osmotic stimuli. Verney pioneered in his delineation of neural control of osmotic balance, but his work was also important in the development of a strategy in neuroendocrine investigations. He showed that emotional factors were important in ADH regulation, thus pointing out, for the first time, the role of stress in neuroendocrine regulation. He also adapted the classic Sherringtonian approach of the neurologist to identify a neuroendocrine reflex analogous to a spinal reflex. This involves the identification of a receptor for afferent stimuli and a motor component effecting hormone secretion. Like Sherrington, Verney emphasized the use of selective neurologic ablations to identify neural pathways of neuroendocrine control. Now taken for granted, this approach has been used widely for studies of anterior as well as of posterior pituitary secretion.

The most important factors regulating vasopressin secretion are plasma osmolality and "effective" circulating blood volume[104,105] (Fig. 7) (Table 1). Blood pressure, nausea, and various forms of stress also influence vasopressin release.[61-64]

OSMOLALITY

Maintenance of normal blood water concentration is the major homeostatic function of the neurohypophysis. Blood osmolality is strictly controlled over a relatively narrow range ($\pm 1.8\%$). The mean setpoint of plasma osmolality for normal individuals is 280 mosmol/kg; vasopressin release is initiated when osmolality reaches 287 mosmol/kg, a value termed the osmotic threshold[81-83,100] (Fig. 8). Plasma ADH levels are approximately 2 pg/ml at this plasma osmolality. Above this value, vasopressin secretion increases rapidly and progressively with increasing plasma osmolality. Water loading inhibits vasopressin release. The exquisite sensitivity of the osmoreceptor-ADH-renal reflex can be demonstrated by combining radioimmunoassay measurements of ADH in blood with plasma osmolality.

> An increase of 1 percent in total body water causes a fall of 2.8 mosmol/kg H_2O, a decrease in ADH levels to 1 pg/ml, and a fall in urine osmolality from 500 to 250 mosmol/kg H_2O. An increase in total body water of 2 percent suppresses ADH maximally (<0.25 pg/ml). In the opposite direction, a 2 percent decrease in total body water will increase plasma osmolality by 2 percent (5.6 mosmol/kg). Plasma ADH will rise from 2 to 4 pg/ml, and urine will be maximally concentrated (>1,000 mosmol/kg).[120]

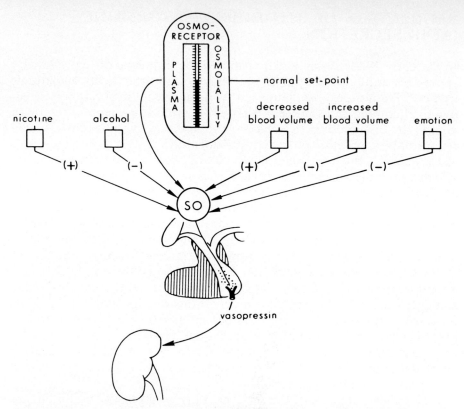

FIGURE 7. Control of ADH (vasopressin) release is illustrated here. The normal stimulus for ADH release is plasma osmolality higher than the normal setpoint, which is usually constant but may be altered in disease. ADH release also can be increased by severe decrease in blood volume or by administration of nicotine (or its absorption from tobacco smoking). ADH release can be decreased by reduction in plasma osmolality, increase in blood volume, or administration of alcohol. Generally, emotional stress results in decreased ADH release and hence produces polyuria. (From Ezrin, C, et al: *Systematic Endocrinology.* Harper & Row, New York, 1973, p 19, with permission.)

These observations on the extraordinary sensitivity of this regulatory system help explain the common occurrence of the syndrome of inappropriate ADH secretion (see below); minor irregularities of regulation may have profound effects on water retention, leading to hyponatremia.

This precise osmotic regulatory system operates through a hypothalamic osmoreceptor neuron system. A number of neurons in both supraoptic and paraventricular nuclei—including some that project directly to the neural lobe (hence are hormone-secreting)—show increased frequency of electrical discharge immediately following intracarotid injections of hypertonic saline.[65,120] This finding would suggest that supraopticohypophysial and paraventriculohypophysial neurons are intrinsically osmoreceptive. The possibility also exists, however, that another population of osmoreceptor cells may activate the vasopressin-secreting cells transsynaptically. Under some clinical conditions, osmoreceptor control of vasopressin secretion can be lost while thirst regulation is preserved, a finding that reinforces the suggestion that there is a distinct population of osmoreceptor cells. The neuronal nature of the osmoreceptive process remains obscure. Any os-

TABLE 1. Factors that Influence ADH Secretion in the Human Being

Physiologic (Appropriate)	Pathologic	Pharmacologic or Hormonal
Increase in ADH		
1. Upright position	1. Inappropriate ADH	1. Morphine
2. Decrease in blood	syndrome	2. Barbiturates
pressure	a. Hypothalamic disease	3. Carbamazepine
3. Hyperosmolality	b. Cerebral disease	4. Nicotine
4. Hypovolemia	c. Chest disease	5. Cholinergic drugs
5. Myocardial failure,	d. Tumors	(carbachol, methacholine)
edematous states with	e. Drugs (chlorpropamide,	6. ? Beta-adrenergic agents
hyponatremia	vincristine[52])	7. Angiotensin II
6. Emotional stress	f. Hypothyroidism	8. Clofibrate[44]
7. Elevated central		
temperature		
Decrease in ADH		
1. Recumbent position	1. Diabetes insipidus	1. Alcohol
2. Increase in blood pressure		2. Phenytoin
3. Hypoosmolality		3. ? Adrenergic agents
4. Increase in blood volume		4. Anticholinergic drugs
5. Decrease in central		
temperature		

Drugs that Facilitate ADH Action
1. Chlorpropamide[45]
2. Chlorthiazides
3. Adrenal cortical steroids

motically active particle (not only NaCl) that does not enter nerve cell bodies can stimulate vasopressin release.

VOLUME REGULATION

Hemorrhage or decreased blood volume owing to any cause, if sufficient in degree, is followed by release of vasopressin. The change in volume (as contrasted with the change in osmolality) has to be relatively large. For example, phlebotomy, which reduces blood volume by 6 to 9 percent, or assumption of the upright posture, which reduces central blood volume by 8 to 10 percent, has no effect on vasopressin release.[83,120] On the other hand, a change of blood volume of more than 10 percent, which can be produced by the combination of phlebotomy and assumption of the erect position, will bring about vasopressin release. Under usual conditions, plasma osmolality is the prime determinant of vasopressin secretion, but severe volume depletion can override the osmoreceptor control. With less severe degrees of volume change, osmotic control is precisely exerted, but there is a shift of "osmotic setpoint" so that a lower osmotic threshold is required to trigger vasopressin secretion in the volume-depleted animal.

GLUCOCORTICOIDS

Glucocorticoids also modulate the "setpoint" of neurohypophysial control. Adrenal deficiency raises it and thereby induces a relative increase in

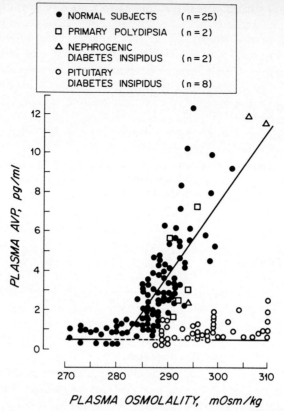

FIGURE 8. Shown here are relationships among plasma osmolality and plasma arginine vasopressin (AVP) in normal subjects (closed circles), and patients with primary polydipsia (open squares), nephrogenic diabetes insipidus (open triangles), and pituitary diabetes insipidus (open circles). See text for details. (From G. Robertson,[105] with permission.)

vasopressin secretion which may contribute to the lower serum sodium in patients with this disorder.[11] The basis of this effect appears to be due to modulation by steroids of vasopressin secretion which parallels corticotropin-releasing hormone (CRH) secretion. Glucocorticoid administration inhibits ADH release, and glucocorticoid deficiency increases it. Glucocorticoids directly regulate vasopressin gene expression presumably by acting on a specific regulatory gene sequence.

VOLUME CONTROL RECEPTORS

Receptors for volume control are located in the left atrium, in the baroreceptors of the carotid sinus, and perhaps elsewhere. Modest degrees of volume depletion, insufficient to lower blood pressure, activate the atrial receptors, and depletion sufficient to cause hypotension mobilizes baroreceptor reflexes. Because even high amounts of vasopressin are not associated with hypertension in the human being, it appears likely that the neurohypophysis has only a modest role in blood pressure regulation, although vasopressin plays a complex role in cardiovascular regulation under special conditions such as shock and volume depletion.[122]

Neural reflexes involved in volume and pressure control reach the brainstem by way of afferents of the glossopharyngeal and vagal nerves, which terminate in the brainstem, ascend through multisynaptic pathways, and ultimately impinge upon the nuclei of the neurohypophysial system. Presumably, the principal activating pathways are mediated mainly by cholinergic neurotransmitters, but other pathways could be involved in view of the wealth of potential neurotransmitters in the supraoptic nucleus.[33,34,76,115,135]

A novel additional endocrine function of the left atrium in blood volume control (separate from the reflex activation of the neurohypophysis) has been demonstrated recently. Several peptides with potent natriuretic activity (designated *atriopeptins*) have been isolated from atrial muscle of rat and human.[23,26–28,85,113,121] They have been postulated to be part of a homeostatic feedback loop for the regulation of intravascular volume (see below).

STRESS AND NAUSEA

The secretion of vasopressin is influenced by inputs from various parts of the "visceral brain" and the reticular activating system, regions involved in the maintenance of consciousness and in emotional expression. Nausea is accompanied by intense vasopressin release, presumably by reflex stimulation from the medullary vomiting center (area postrema).

When Verney began his studies of water regulation in the dog, he was struck by the marked effect of emotional stress on antidiuretic activity. It has been generally believed that humans and rats also release vasopressin in response to emotional stress, but Robertson[104,105] has shown by immunoassay methods that pain and other stresses incidental to physiologic experiments in the human rarely influence plasma vasopressin levels, nor does deliberately applied severe stress in rats. Nevertheless, the influence of "higher" neural centers on vasopressin secretion can be demonstrated by the experimental induction of diuresis or antidiuresis by hypnotic suggestion in man or by psychologic conditioning of dogs. Other examples of neurogenic disturbance in regulation of vasopressin secretion are the disturbed osmolar control of water excretion in patients with anorexia nervosa[50] and in some schizophrenics who have succeeded in overhydrating themselves to the point of water intoxication.[66]

Other stimuli can elicit vasopressin release in experimental animals. Endotoxin, a substance that induces fever and blood pressure changes by acting directly on hypothalamic thermoregulatory centers, causes release of vasopressin in rats.[68] This response, which may be triggered in part by changes in blood volume and blood pressure, may serve as a homeostatic mechanism to regulate temperature and cardiovascular responses.

MECHANISMS OF THIRST REGULATION

HYPOTHALAMIC MECHANISMS

It long has been recognized that either a decrease in blood volume or an increase in plasma osmolality arouses the sensation of thirst.[6,7,41–45,47,97]

Hypothalamic receptors for thirst sensation have been localized by studying the effects of lesions and of electrical, hyperosmotic, and pharmacologic stimulations.

Investigations by Stevenson and colleagues (see reviews in references 42 and 43) in 1949 showed that rats with lesions in the hypothalamic ventromedial nuclei increased their food intake and drank less. In these animals a combination of diabetes insipidus and decreased thirst led to a chronic state of dehydration manifested by hypernatremia. Subsequently, Andersson and McCann[6] showed that lesions restricted to the anterior hypothalamus (sparing the supraoptic nuclei and tracts) caused adipsia without either diabetes insipidus or disturbance in food intake. Results of more restricted lesions in the rat have indicated that a region exists in the lateral hypothalamus (within the medial forebrain bundle), destruction of which induces severe adipsia without aphagia. It is likely that lesions in the lateral hypothalamus cause adipsia because of interruption of pathways related to limbic system structures.

Several extrahypothalamic regions of the brain are important in the modulation of drinking.

Septal lesions in rats cause increased water intake. Regions of the hippocampal complex and of the amygdala also have been implicated in control of water intake; an excitatory "center" for drinking appears to exist in the anteroventral portion of the amygdala in some species. In the rat, bilateral lesions in this region cause a combination of aphagia and adipsia. Lesions of the amygdala in the dog also are reported to produce an adipsia-aphagia syndrome.

Drinking can be induced by intrahypothalamic microinjections of hypertonic saline, by electrical stimulation, or by artificial elevation of hypothalamic temperature. In the goat, Andersson and McCann[6] showed that intraventricular or intrahypothalamic infusions of a small volume (3 to 10 μl) of hypertonic saline (2 to 3 percent) elicited drinking. The region from which such responses were most consistently obtained was the perifornical area of the anterior hypothalamus. Similar results can be obtained with electrical stimulation. As will be noted below, these regions are rich in angiotensin II and atriopeptins, two classes of neuropeptides important in salt and water homeostasis.

Effective stimulation sites include the region between the anterior column of the fornix and the mammillothalamic tracts extending from dorsal to ventral hypothalamus. In the monkey, stimulation of extrahypothalamic sites, in particular the anterior gyrus and the substantia nigra, also have been effective in eliciting drinking.

Sites which induced eating have been clearly separated from those which cause drinking.

Local warming of the preoptic region of the hypothalamus also induces drinking, even in the water-replete animal. Local cooling has the opposite effect, in some instances causing instead an increase in food intake. Thus, increased environmental temperature may cause an increase in water intake by activation of both peripheral and central receptors, as well as by the osmotic effects of sensible and insensible water loss.

It has been proposed by Grossman[55] and Fitzsimmons[41] that the system for control of drinking has a specific neuropharmacologic basis. It was shown that the direct instillation of cholinergic substances into the hypothalamus of the rat led to increased drinking and that adrenergic substances elicited feeding behavior. Although carbachol-induced polydipsia is blocked by atropine, thirst secondary to hypovolemia or dehydration is not. A number of other noncholinergic phamacologic agents — such as barbiturates, chlordiazepoxide, and levorphanol — also may increase thirst, and thirst is inhibited by alcohol. These findings make it unlikely (as pointed out by Fitzsimmons) that there is precise neuropharmacologic coding for drinking behavior.

RELATION BETWEEN VASOPRESSIN SECRETION AND DRINKING BEHAVIOR

Drinking behavior, like vasopressin secretion, is regulated by plasma osmolality and circulating blood volume, is integrated by hypothalamic mechanisms, and is designed to maintain the constancy of the internal water milieu. The sensation of thirst (as contrasted with the sensation of dry mouth) results from an internally perceived signal arising from the hypothalamus. As with vasopressin secretion, thirst can be generated by severe hemorrhage or by inducing local hyperosmolality in the hypothalamus with hypertonic saline microinjections. The thirst mechanism is integrated with the vasopressin-controlling mechanism: Both are activated by hypothalamic osmoreceptors, and drinking behavior and vasopressin release can be activated neuropharmacologically by intrahypothalamic administration of acetylcholine analogs, thus suggesting that there may be a common neuromediator pathway for the two functions. Because the osmotic threshold for ADH release in human subjects is lower than that for increased drinking (287 versus 295 mosmol/liter), it would appear that conservation of water excretion is the first-line homeostatic mechanism to be mobilized in preservation of body water. The two functions can be dissociated in disease states, for example, in the syndrome of hyperosmotic hypodipsia in which vasopressin regulation is normal, but thirst is absent.[145,146,149]

It is clinically important to know that osmolar regulation is abnormal in the elderly. Several aspects are altered with age. The sensation of thirst is decreased, vasopressin secretion is increased, and renal response to vasopressin is blunted.[38,51] These abnormalities predispose the elderly to hyperosmolality and, if overhydrated, to inappropriate hypoosmolality. Based on work in aged rats, who also show excessive ADH release, it is suggested that aging causes the loss of a particular group of hippocampal cells normally inhibitory to vasopressin secretion.

ANGIOTENSIN AND THIRST

Angiotensin has an important regulatory function in drinking behavior, although there is less certainty about the role of the hypothalamic angiotensin II system in vasopressin regulation.[7,19] The biochemical components and enzyme systems for the formation of angiotensin-II-containing neurons have been demonstrated in the hypothalamus, as have angiotensin II binding sites.[95] Angiotensinogen mRNA also has been demonstrated in the brain.[89] Local injection of angiotensin II gives a dose-response-related stimulation of drinking behavior in the rat, and drinking by dehydrated rats is blocked by local administration of saralasin, an angiotensin II receptor antagonist. Central angiotensin receptors are also responsive to angiotensin II synthesized outside the brain, thus accounting at least in part for the severe thirst sometimes seen in renovascular hypertension and in hypovolemic shock. Circulating angiotensin II may gain entry to the perifornical organ in which the blood-brain barrier is absent. Angiotensin II applied directly to supraoptic neurosecretory neurons causes excitation.[86]

NEUROENDOCRINE CONTROL OF SODIUM EXCRETION

When sodium chloride is administered to a human (or dog or rat), the excretion of sodium ion by the kidney is adaptively increased, a response attributed to inhibition of aldosterone secretion, to redistribution of blood flow within the kidney, and possibly to "third factors," which serve as a natriuretic factor(s) to stimulate renal sodium loss.[98] Several candidate natriuretic hormones have been described. These include digitalis-like peptides—variously termed "endigin" (endogenous digitalis-like peptide), "endoxin" (endogenous digoxin-like peptide)—which possess either biodigitalis and/or immunodigitalis activity, and the "atriopeptins," peptides first extracted from the atria of the heart.

Endogenous Digitalis-like Compounds

The first endogenous digitalis-like activity was isolated from toad bladder on the basis of its effects in displacing ouabain in a binding assay and designated *endigin*.[37] Substances of this type also inhibit Na^+K^+-ATPase, and have been isolated from bovine and rat hypothalamic extracts and from the media of rat hypothalamic cells grown in tissue culture.[78] The chemical nature of this compound(s) is unknown.

> The factor described by Haupert and coworkers[58,59] was a low molecular weight basic nonpeptidic factor, and that of Akagawa et al[4] was also described as a low molecular weight fraction. In the studies of Alaghband-Zadeh et al,[3] of many tissues tested, only the hypothalamus contained this activity, and its physiologic relevance as a homeostatic mechanism was demonstrated by showing that the content of this material in blood and hypothalamus was increased markedly by high sodium diets. It has been speculated to contribute to the syndrome of preeclampsia.[16]

Yet another kind of circulating endogenous digitalis-like compound has been demonstrated using antisera directed against *digoxin*. This compound, termed *endoxin*, displaces ouabain from cell membrane receptors and, like digitalis alkaloids, inhibits membrane Na^+-K^+ ATPase, possesses potent natriuretic action, and stimulates the force of cardiac contraction.[124]

Circulating endogenous digoxin-like compounds appear to play a physiologic role in blood pressure maintainance.

> Administration of antidigoxin antisera lowered the blood pressure of rats made hypertensive by coarctation of the aorta and, to a lesser extent, that of normal animals,[67] but the effect is transient. Desoxycorticosterone (DOCA)-induced hypertension was also reduced by administration of antidigoxin antibody.[71] In both ex-

periments cited, control sera were without effect. Circulating levels of endoxin are elevated in hypertensive monkeys.[56]

Several clinical situations in which salt and water metabolism are abnormal are associated with changes in circulating levels of *endoxin.*

These include elevations in blood and amniotic fluid endoxin during hypertensive pregnancies[52,53] and elevated blood levels in preeclampsia,[16] renal failure,[52] salt loading[70] and primary hyperaldosteronism.[73] Assayed values were low or absent in patients with arterial hypotension and in edematous patients with primary aldosteronism.[73]

Taken together, these findings suggest that a digitalis-like factor is formed in the body and plays a role in blood pressure and salt homeostasis. It also may be involved in the pathogenesis of eclampsia. The source of this material is not clearly defined. It is found in extracts of the heart[49] and renal cortical tissue homogenates.[73] Its relationship to the hypothalamic material is not clearly defined.

Atriopeptins

The best characterized of the neuroendocrine factors that regulate sodium balance are the atrionatriuretic peptides (ANP, atrionatriuretic factor, ANF)[85,92,112,147] (Fig. 9). All are fragments of a common precursor prohormone varying in size from 24 to 33 amino acids in length, found in secretory granules in the cardiac atria of humans and rats. The prohormones for both species have been elucidated by molecular biologic methods, and they bear remarkable homology;[10,28,85,90] as a generalization, strict conservation of a protein structure among species is strongly suggestive that the function served by the compound is physiologically important.

In addition to promoting sodium excretion and diuresis, these compounds have other actions (Fig. 10). They are potent vasodilators (this may be the basis of the intrarenal action), antagonize the pressor effects of norepinephrine and angiotensin II, and inhibit the secretion of aldosterone through a direct action on the adrenal cortex. It has been hypothesized, therefore, that distention of the left atrium (a consequence of increased blood volume) brings about the release of atriopeptides, which promote diuresis and sodium excretion. Because left atrial distention long has been known to inhibit vasopressin release and hence to promote water loss, this theory provides a persuasive model describing the way in which blood volume can regulate water and salt excretion. The crucial bit of evidence that was required to validate this theory was the demonstration that atriopeptides circulate in blood and that their secretion is enhanced by salt loading. This has been demonstrated recently[132,147,148] (Fig. 11).

In severe cardiac failure, the concentration in blood of atrial natriuretic peptide is raised (Fig. 12), as it was in two patients who developed polyuria during an attack of paroxysmal supraventricular tachycardia. These observations indicate that ANP is a hormone and is secreted under appropriate hemodynamic situations. In volunteers administered ANP in amounts giving comparable blood levels, there was a two- to threefold increase in natriuresis and diuresis.[132]

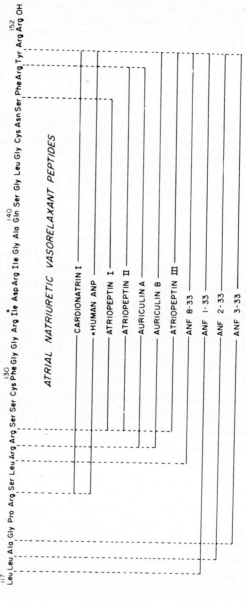

Met Gly Ser Phe Ser Ile Thr Lys

Gly Phe Phe Leu Phe Leu Ala Phe Trp Leu Pro Gly His Ile Gly Ala Asn Pro Val Tyr Ser Ala Val Ser Asn Thr Asp Leu Met Asp Phe Lys Asn Leu Asp

His Leu Glu Glu Lys Met Pro Val Glu Asp Glu Val Met Pro Pro Gln Ala Leu Ser Glu Gln Thr Asp Glu Ala Gly Ala Ala Leu Ser Ser Glu Val Pro

Pro Trp Thr Gly Glu Val Asn Pro Ser Gln Arg Asp Gly Gly Ala Leu Gly Arg Gly Pro Trp Asp Pro Ser Asp Arg Ser Ala Leu Leu Lys Ser Lys Leu Arg Ala

Leu Leu Ala Gly Pro Arg Ser Leu Arg Arg Ser Cys Phe Gly Gly Arg Ile Asp Arg Ile Gly Ala Gln Ser Gly Leu Gly Cys Asn Ser Phe Arg Tyr Arg Arg OH

ATRIAL NATRIURETIC VASORELAXANT PEPTIDES

CARDIONATRIN I

*HUMAN ANP

ATRIOPEPTIN I

ATRIOPEPTIN II

AURICULIN A

AURICULIN B

ATRIOPEPTIN III

ANF 8-33

ANF 1-33

ANF 2-33

ANF 3-33

* Ile₁₃₄ becomes Met in the human peptide

FIGURE 9. This is the predicted amino acid sequence for the precursor of atrial natriuretic peptide (*top*) and some atrial natriuretic peptides. (From Cole and Needleman,[26] with permission.)

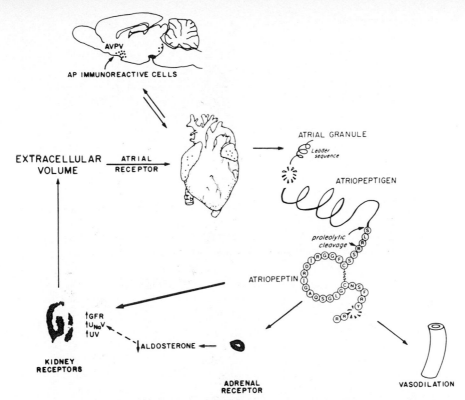

FIGURE 10. This is a diagram of the atriopeptin hormonal system. The prohormone atriopeptigen is stored in granules in atrial myocytes. Elevated vascular volume prompts release and or proteolytic cleavage, resulting in the discharge into the circulation of atriopeptin, which lowers vascular resistance, suppresses aldosterone production, and stimulates natriuresis and diuresis from the kidney. In addition, vascular volume expansion may stimulate the cerebral atriopeptin system that either may serve as a neuroregulatory substance or may provide an additional stimulus for cardiac atriopeptin release. Diminution of vascular volume provides negative feedback to both brain and cardiac receptors, and circulating atriopeptin levels fall. (From Cole and Needleman,[26] with permission.)

Although atriopeptides were first demonstrated in the heart, they have also been identified as neuropeptides by the finding of atriopeptide immunoreactive neurons in the brain.[113]

In the hypothalamus, atriopeptinergic fibers extend "from the periventricular nucleus into the medial preoptic area, the ventral and lateral parts of the bed nucleus of the stria terminalis, the lateral hypothalamic area, and the paraventricular and arcuate nuclei." A second set of fibers is found, "in the pons emerging from the periventricular gray matter of the fourth ventricle". . . and "innervate the dorsal and lateral divisions of the interpeduncular nucleus."[113] Cell bodies were heavily distributed in the anterioventral regions of the third ventricle, including periventricular, paraventricular, and preoptic areas, and in the pons, especially in the floor of the fourth ventricle.[113]

These localizations probably are significant in mediating central nervous system (CNS) regulation of the cardiovascular system. As noted above, lesions of the anterior third ventricle lead to decreased drinking, and local injections of sodium chloride increase drinking behavior.

It has been proposed that CNS atriopeptides interact with peripheral circulating atriopeptins in much the same way as do central and peripheral

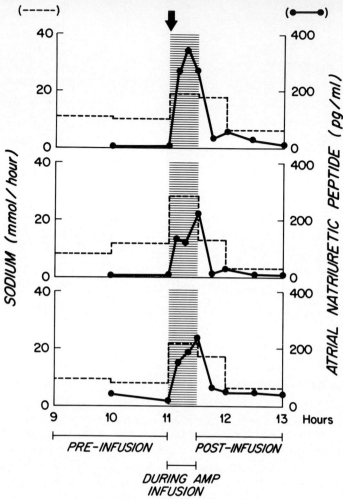

FIGURE 11. Plasma ANP concentration *(solid line)* and urine sodium excretion *(dotted line)* in three healthy volunteers in relation to ANP infusion are depicted. (From Tikkanen et al,[132] with permission.)

angiotensin II in blood pressure regulation, and central and peripheral cholecystokinin in regulation of satiety.

NEURAL CONTROL OF OXYTOCIN SECRETION

MILK LET-DOWN REFLEX

When a hungry infant begins to nurse from its mother's breast, it does not obtain milk immediately. Rather, milk appears at the nipple after a delay of one half minute or so. This response is termed "let-down."[18,24] The stimulus of suckling initiates a neurogenic reflex transmitted from afferent nerve endings in the nipple that is conducted through the spinal cord, midbrain, and finally hypothalamus, where it triggers release of oxytocin from the neurohypophysis. Oxytocin causes contraction of the myoepithelial cells that encircle mammary acini, thereby expelling milk into the nipple. In the

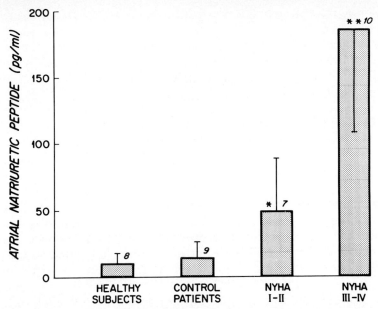

FIGURE 12. Shown here are plasma ANP concentrations (mean ± SD) in healthy subjects, control patients, and patients with congestive heart failure (CHF). (*p < 0.05 compared with control patients, **p < 0.01 compared with NYHA class I-II, and p < 0.001 compared with control patients.) (From Tikkanen et al,[132] with permission.)

absence of this reflex contraction, milk cannot be obtained even from a full breast. Nursing rats, for example, cannot obtain milk from mothers previously subjected to removal of the neural lobe but can do so after oxytocin injection. The milk let-down reflex is accompanied by changes in hypothalamic neuronal function and can be blocked by specific neural lesions and also by certain types of neural stimuli. In cows, let-down can be abolished by a strange or threatening environment, and similar blockade has been noted in stressed rabbits. Pain or fright inhibits milk let-down in the rabbit through adrenergic stimulation. In women, oxytocin release and milk let-down occur in response to suckling and frequently precede suckling, presumably a reflex conditioned by the crying of a hungry baby. Milk let-down can be inhibited by emotional stress and triggered by sexual excitement and orgasm. Oxytocin has been administered therapeutically to some women with failure to show normal milk let-down.

OXYTOCIN SECRETION IN RELATION TO LABOR

There is still considerable question about the importance of oxytocin in the initiation and maintenance of normal labor in the human.

Labor is said to be relatively normal in women with diabetes insipidus, even those in whom oxytocin deficiency can be demonstrated.[24] It has been postulated that oxytocin secreted by the fetus may initiate labor; stated teleologically, the fetus signals its readiness to be born by releasing oxytocin. Once labor has begun in normal women, maternal oxytocin secretion, which takes place in spurts, increases and reaches a maximum at the time of delivery. Reflexes arising from the contracting uterus, in turn, trigger oxytocin release, thus providing a powerful positive feedback control of the process of labor.

Vasopressin and oxytocin secretion are regulated independently. For example, in lactating women, ADH secretion can be achieved by hypertonic saline infusion without producing let-down, and the suckling stimulus induces let-down without antidiuresis.

NEUROPHARMACOLOGIC REGULATION OF VASOPRESSIN AND OXYTOCIN SECRETION

VASOPRESSIN REGULATION

Cholinergic and adrenergic inputs to the magnocellular neurons, cells of origin of the supraoptic and paraventricular tracts, influence cellular activity and mediate reflex control of secretion.[14,15,35,36,84] These effects are superimposed upon the direct osmotic and glucocorticoid regulation. Intravenous administration of acetylcholine or intrahypothalamic injection of acetylcholine or analogs cause inhibition of water diuresis in dogs,[96] a response dependent on an intact neurohypophysis. In parallel with the changes in ADH release are an increased firing rate of the supraoptic neurons.

In contrast, adrenergic drugs such as norepinephrine inhibit the release of ADH.[15,84] Systemic administration of epinephrine or norepinephrine acts predominantly through peripheral baroreceptor mechanisms, but central adrenergic mechanisms are also important because norepinephrine administered into the third ventricle also will inhibit ADH release.

Noradrenergic fibers terminate directly on cell bodies of the supraoptic and paraventricular nuclei[15] but not in the neural lobe. It is likely, therefore, that the effects of noradrenergic agents are mediated by direct actions on axosomatic synapses.

> Direct iontophoresis studies of these putative neurotransmitters upon cells of the supraoptic nuclei have provided additional evidence for their role in synaptic regulation of ADH secretion. Barker and coworkers, using antidromically identified neurosecretory cells in the cat, found that the monoamines dopamine, norepinephrine, and serotonin uniformly reduced the activity of these cells. The inibition of activity was blocked by α-adrenergic blocking agents. Acetylcholine, on the other hand, produced a dual effect. These workers postulated that supraoptic neurons may have both excitatory (nicotinic) and inhibitory (muscarinic) cholinergic receptors.[15]
>
> There is, however, contrary evidence supporting an excitatory influence of noradrenergic fibers on magnocellular neurons. Renaud and coworkers[101] have shown that stimulation of noradrenergic neurons in the brainstem (A_1 and A_2 groups) elicited excitation of magnocellar neurons identified by antidromic stimulation of neural lobe terminals. In vitro studies using hypothalamic tissue slices or perfused hypothalamic explants demonstrated similar excitatory effects. In the latter experiments, phenylephrine caused continuous firing of supraoptic neurons. Hence, the possibility exists that noradrenergic afferents to the supraoptic nuclei facilitate firing.

These experimental observations appear also to hold true in the human. Tobacco smoking releases vasopressin in response to nicotinic acid receptor stimulation. Secretion of vasopressin and electrophysiologic activation of supraoptic neurons also are modified by certain neuropeptides. Direct intrahypothalamic application of angiotensin II releases vasopressin and influences drinking behavior.[48] Neurohypophysial neurons also are stimulated by endogenous opioids (endorphins). The well-known antidiuretic action of morphine is due to the release of vasopressin, an effect that can be duplicated by the intracerebroventricular administration of β-endorphin. That the endorphins may be involved in regulation of vasopressin secretion is further supported by the observation that naloxone, an opiate antagonist, reverses neurogenically inappropriate ADH secretion in some cases.

Other drugs exert important effects on ADH secretion. Alcohol strongly inhibits ADH release, both decreasing basal levels and preventing normal ADH responses to stimuli such as reduced blood volume. Phenytoin also inhibits ADH release transiently. On the other hand, ADH release is stimulated by morphine, barbiturates, and other hypnotics, and these agents can cause significant antidiuresis. From a practical point of view, drug-induced ADH release leads to impaired water excretion and may be responsible in part for water intoxication in hospitalized patients given intravenous fluids. Pain and stress, which also stimulate ADH secretion, can intensify the defect in water clearance. These effects are more striking in the elderly.

Oxytocin Regulation

Acetylcholine also stimulates oxytocin secretion. It is likely that the stress-induced inhibition of the milk let-down reflex, well known from both animal husbandry and human nursing experience, is due to α-adrenergic inhibition of oxytocin release. The same kind of reaction may be responsible for stress-induced diuresis.

ELECTROPHYSIOLOGY OF NEUROHYPOPHYSIAL NEURONS

Release of ADH and oxytocin from the neurohypophysis is initiated by depolarization of axon terminals of neurosecretory neurons of the hypothalamic-neurohypophysial system. Increased rates of neuronal firing result in increased hormone release. Electrophysiologic responses of these neurons have been studied extensively and clarify the relation of the osmoreceptor function to hormone secretion.

The spontaneous discharge rate of hypothalamic neurosecretory cells is slow, usually less than one discharge per second.[14,34] Changes in cellular firing rates are found in the supraoptic nucleus following intravenous administration of hypertonic saline. The cells possess resting transmembrane potentials of -50 to -80 mV, and both excitatory and inhibitory postsynaptic potentials have been identified in these cells. By a combination of single-unit recording and antidromic stimulation, it can be shown that not all osmoreceptive cells are antidromically excitable. These findings suggest that at least some cells sensitive to osmotic changes are separate from the large neurosecretory cells and perhaps function as interneurons. Conversely, not all antidromically excitable cells are influenced by osmotic changes. Osmoreceptor cells also have been identified in other regions of the brain and in the spinal cord.

Neuroendocrine cells in the supraoptic nucleus of the monkey show excitatory-inhibitory sequences following activation.[61,62,87] A *recurrent collateral inhibitory* mechanism analogous to that involving the Renshaw cell in the spinal cord is suggested by these findings. It may be postulated that this mechanism functions to prevent excessive discharges from such cells. Disorders of the inhibitory impulse conceivably could account for the inappropriate antidiuretic hormone secretion which occurs in certain brain diseases.

SUPRAHYPOTHALAMIC REGULATION OF ADH SECRETION

Animals with hypothalamic islands are capable of maintaining normal water balance, indicating that the necessary components for basal fluid regulation reside within this region of the brain. In addition, these nuclei receive a rich innervation of bioaminergic and cholinergic neurons from the limbic system and brainstem. Pain and emotional stress bring about a rapid release of ADH accompanied by antidiuresis. Extrahypothalamic projections have been well characterized.

> Electric stimulation of either the medial or the basolateral nuclei of the amygdala causes ADH release in the rhesus monkey, as indicated by an abrupt decrease in water secretion.[60] Similarly, stimulation of limbic midbrain areas, including the ventral tegmental area of Tsai, the periaqueductal gray matter, and the midbrain reticular formation, are effective in inducing antidiuretic responses in unanesthetized monkeys.[137] Responses to stimulation of the thalamus, tectum, and pyramidal tract are negative. Many of these same limbic-hypothalamic-midbrain areas also mediate drinking responses following osmotic, electric, or cholinergic stimuli.
>
> Neurosecretory cells in both the supraoptic and paraventricular nuclei can be excited by single-pulse-stimulations of widespread areas of the brain including the septum, the midbrain reticular formation and central gray matter, the anterior commissure, and the hippocampus.[137] Such excitations are frequently followed by a prolonged inhibitory period, lasting as long as 500 msec, after application of a single pulse. These effects are clinically relevant because excessive ADH secretion occurs in association with a variety of intracranial disease processes, many of which are not restricted to hypothalamic centers.

NEUROLOGIC DISORDERS OF WATER AND SALT REGULATION

The major neurologic disorders of water and salt balance are diabetes insipidus (ADH deficiency), compulsive water drinking, hypodipsia, essential hypernatremia, and inappropriate ADH secretion.

DIABETES INSIPIDUS (DI)

Diabetes insipidus (DI) is a disorder of excessive renal water loss caused by ADH deficiency. The condition may be congenital or acquired. A somewhat similar clinical picture may be produced by *nephrogenic* diabetes insipidus, either a congenital disorder in which the renal tubules are insensitive to ADH or an acquired disease of the renal tubules. Lithium administration, for example, which blocks vasopressin effects on the kidney, leads to mild nephrogenic DI.

Reduction in ADH secretion sufficient to interfere with normal renal water-conservation mechanisms is normally accompanied by appropriate increased water intake (polydipsia). If central thirst mechanisms also are disordered, the failure to compensate with increased water intake results in further dehydration and, in severe cases, death. The polydipsia of diabetes insipidus is appropriate, that is, it is a corrective mechanism to maintain water balance. Patients with diabetes insipidus may occasionally present with abnormal stimulation of central thirst mechanisms early in the course of the disorder; the clinical picture of compulsive water drinking may, for example, herald the onset of a hypothalamic tumor. Primary polydipsia may also occur in sarcoidosis of the hypothalamus with abnormalities of thirst (see below).

Etiology

The main causes of diabetes insipidus are summarized in Table 2.

Familial or congenital diabetes insipidus is an exceedingly rare disorder that occurs in infancy or childhood and affects either sex.[54] A few cases have been autopsied, and these show failure of development of the supraoptic neurons; the paraventricular neurons may also be involved, and the posterior pituitary is reduced in size.[54] Congenital diabetes insipidus must be distinguished from the superficially similar congenital *nephrogenic diabetes insipidus,* owing to an inherited defect in renal tubule responsiveness to ADH. The latter condition is mainly a disease of young men or boys.

Idiopathic diabetes insipidus is a far more common cause of ADH deficiency, comprising 25 to 50 percent of the cases of acquired disease. It may occur at any age in either sex. Absence of other clinical signs of hypothalamic destruction or of disturbance in other pituitary functions and failure to develop other hypothalamic abnormalities over prolonged periods of time indicate that the disease is restricted to the hypothalamic-neurohypophysial axis. Its cause is unknown, but several cases with antibodies reacting with supraoptic neurons have been described suggesting that autoimmune mechanisms directed against the hypothalamic-neurohypophysial system may be a cause of idiopathic DI.[118] Idiopathic DI is almost always permanent, but a case that spontaneously remitted has been reported.[81] If autoimmunity can be a cause, it is theoretically conceivable that immunosuppression therapy might be useful in some cases.

Posttraumatic diabetes insipidus is brought about by crushing or tearing of the upper stalk and infundibulum. Following severe head injury the acutely decelerating brain produces a *contre-coup* compression of the stalk against the sharp edge of the diaphragma sella. This form of the disease

TABLE 2. Principal Causes of Diabetes Insipidus

1. Familial or congenital
2. Idiopathic
3. Post-traumatic—basal skull fractures
4. Neoplastic—primary or secondary, including leukemia and lymphoma
5. Histiocytosis X
6. Granulomatous disease (sarcoidosis, tuberculosis, meningovascular syphilis)
7. Vascular lesions
8. Infections—pyogenic meningitis
9. Postneurosurgical

may be temporary or permanent. Some patients follow a water-balance pattern like that seen following experimental stalk-section of the cat. A similar pattern is observed in some humans subjected to pituitary or hypothalamic surgery. The classic three-stage response begins with acute severe DI owing to damage to the neural mechanism controlling ADH release. As the neurohypophysis degenerates and releases ADH into the blood, the DI pattern abates, predisposing to hyponatremia; the third stage, permanent DI, follows. Other patients show a relatively delayed permanent DI, and in still others, the somewhat delayed DI is followed after a long period by resumption of normal water balance. For this reason, in posttraumatic (and postsurgical) cases it is important to reevaluate the status of DI periodically for as long as two years. Recovery taking as long as 10 years posttrauma has been reported.

Neurohypophysial tumors may cause DI. *Metastatic* tumors are the most important (see below). The most common *primary* tumor of the neurohypophysis is the *granular cell tumor*, also called choristoma, granular myoblastoma, or tumorette.[72] These have been noted in 1 to 8 percent of unselected autopsies, the smaller estimates owing to the fact that most are very small and would be missed unless serial sections are taken.

> As outlined by Kovacs,[72]
>
> "the majority of granular cell tumors remain asymptomatic and are found incidentally at autopsy. Occasionally, however, they exhibit more rapid growth and may reach a large size, producing headache, visual disturbances, adenohypophysial insufficiency, and diabetes insipidus. In exceptional cases, owing either to elevation of intracranial pressure or to cranial neuropathy, surgical removal of the tumor becomes necessary."
>
> The cellular origin of these tumors is unknown; most evidence points to the glia cell as the source of the cells.

Other rare primary neurohypophysial tumors are infundibuloma, hamartoma, glioma, and astrocytoma. Rarely hamartomas can secrete physiologically significant amounts of a releasing hormone, including luteinizing hormone releasing hormone, corticotropin releasing hormone, and growth hormone releasing hormone to produce precocious puberty, Cushing's disease, and acromegaly, respectively (see chapters 6,8,9). If large enough and critically located, any of these tumors can cause diabetes insipidus.[72]

Metastatic neoplasms and granulomas may also cause DI. Direct destruction of the posterior pituitary is rarely the cause, because diabetes insipidus usually does not occur in pituitary disease unless the basal hypothalamus or upper stalk is damaged. This feature is due to the anatomic fact that some axons of the supraoptic-hypophysial tract terminate on blood vessels high in the stalk or in the median eminence. Moreover, fibers of the neurohypophysial system show some capacity for regeneration; following hypophysectomy in the sheep, rat, or goat, a vestigial but nevertheless functional neural lobe regenerates as a stump and re-establishes a neurovascular anastomosis.[72] When neoplastic or inflammatory conditions cause DI, they usually do so by destruction in the upper stalk and in the median eminence where the neurohypophysial neurons streaming into the neural lobe converge in a superficial position. At this point they are extremely vulnerable to destruction by relatively circumscribed lesions (which may

REGULATION OF THE PITUITARY GLAND

not be apparent by conventional neuroradiologic methods). Tumor infiltration and granulomatous basilar meningitis invade the hypothalamus by way of the vascular mantle of the infundibulum. The DI of suprasellar tumors also comes about mainly through damage in the infundibular region and upper stalk.

Sarcoidosis is the most common of the granulomatous causes of DI (see chapter 17), but tuberculosis, syphilis, and cryptococcosis also have been observed. Histiocytosis X (eosinophillic granuloma) is an important cause of diabetes insipidus, especially in the young (see chapter 17). Almost any tumor metastatic to the brain may lodge in the infundibulum or upper stalk and cause DI; carcinoma of the lung is notorious in this regard. According to Kovacs,[72] metastases to the neurohypophysis are not rare (1 to 3 percent or more) and are more frequent than those to the anterior lobe. Carcinoma of the bronchus, breast, colon, prostate, malignant melanoma, sarcoma, lymphoma, Hodgkin's disease, and leukemia all have been described.

Vascular lesions may cause DI in several ways. Aneurysm of the circle of Willis, most commonly of the anterior communicating artery, may cause infundibular damage as well as anterior pituitary deficiency. Postpartum pituitary necrosis (Sheehan's syndrome) occasionally causes DI in addition to anterior lobe deficiency, presumably through vascular damage to the upper stalk. Rupture of aneurysms of the anterior circle of Willis may damage the supraoptic nuclei or the infundibulum as an acute event.

Neurosurgical intervention is one of the most common causes of DI.[99] This may come about inadvertently or by necessity in the removal of tumors of the hypothalamus or pituitary. Surgical stalk section also has been used in the past as an alternative to the more difficult hypophysectomy in the treatment of carcinoma of the breast and other endocrine-dependent tumors and for the management of rapidly progressive diabetic retinopathy. The occurrence of DI depends on the stalk section level; for reasons listed above, high section causes ADH deficiency and low section generally does not.

Hypotensive encephalopathy following shock caused by trauma, hemorrhage, drug reactions, heroin overdose, and diabetic ketoacidosis can lead to anoxic encephalopathy and acute DI. The onset is usually after 24 to 48 hours but has been noted as soon as 3 hours after injury. Profound brain damage including brain death is typically present; presumably DI in these cases is due to anoxic damage to the supraoptic neurohypophysial system. It is obviously important that the attending physician recognize this complication. Diabetes insipidus in this setting has a grave prognosis. We are not aware of any individual with this syndrome who has survived.

Diagnosis

The diagnosis of DI must be considered in patients who pass large amounts of low-osmolality urine. Nocturia and excessive thirst at night are almost always present; these features may help distinguish true polydipsia owing to excessive water loss from psychogenic polydipsia. If thirst mechanisms are intact, neither dehydration nor hypovolemia will develop, although most patients usually fall slightly behind in fluid replacement, as shown by a modest (but usually not diagnostically useful) elevation in plasma osmolality.

However, if DI is accompanied by a defect in thirst sensation, the results may be catastrophic (see below). The accompanying hypovolemia, hyperosmolality, and dehydration may lead to fever, hyperpnea, stupor, coma, and death. Dehydration may not be clinically striking, and normal skin turgor is often preserved even in severe water depletion.

The diagnosis of DI requires two elements: proof that stimuli to water conservation are ineffective in bringing about decreased urine volume and increased urine concentration and proof that the kidney is capable of responding to ADH. Because the diagnosis of DI usually means that the patient will be treated for life with replacement medications, it is essential that there be no question about the diagnosis. Normally, plasma osmolality ranges from 280 to 285 mosmol/liter. Many patients with DI have slightly elevated plasma osmolality when given free access to drinking water, but patients with compulsive water drinking tend to have low normal plasma osmolality. Proof that the kidney can respond to exogenous hormone is demonstrated by the subcutaneous injection of vasopressin (Pitressin, 5 pressor units) or desamino, D-arginine vasopressin (DDAVP, Desmopressin), which should bring about a marked decrease in urine volume and an increase in urinary osmolality to at least 300 to 500 mosmol/liter (specific gravity greater than 1.011). Vasopressin is usually well tolerated, but it does have pressor and coronary vasoconstrictor properties and should not be administered in full dosage to patients with known heart disease or hypertension. Instead, DDAVP, a synthetic analog with virtually no cardiovascular effects, should be used. This is available either for parenteral or nasal use (see below for mode of administration). The second reservation about the use of ADH (or DDAVP) as a diagnostic aid is that patients with long-standing compulsive water drinking may show only modest responses to the hormone. They may in fact mimic patients with intrinsic renal disease. Therefore, it may be necessary to reduce excess water intake for several days in order to clarify the diagnosis. If the patient still fails to respond to exogenous ADH, intrinsic renal disease of some type is probably present.

The simplest way to determine the ability to conserve water is a 6- to 8-hour dehydration test. The patient must be observed very closely and not permitted to lose more than 3 percent of body weight, because water deficiency can lead to severe mental disturbance, fever, and profound prostration. In normal individuals, 6 to 8 hours without water intake will produce an increase in urine osmolality equal to that of plasma or up to twice that value (urine specific gravity greater than 1.015) with no change in plasma osmolality. In DI, urine volume remains high and concentration low, and the administration of vasopressin or DDAVP will increase urine osmolality. However, when severely dehydrated, patients with DI may show a modest increase in urine concentration and a decline in urinary volume owing to severe decreased renal plasma flow secondary to blood volume contraction. The compulsive water drinker poses a major diagnostic problem, and it may be necessary to extend the dehydration period for as long as 18 hours, by which time compulsive water drinkers are almost always able to concentrate their urine. One must be cautious in diagnosing compulsive water drinking because cases of primary hypothalamic polydipsia caused by hypothalamic lesions have been described. In a recent report of sarcoidosis affecting the hypothalamic-pituitary axis, primary polydipsia occurred in one third of cases.[127]

A detailed diagnostic approach to patients with polyuria has been outlined by Moses.[83] He advocates withholding fluids during the day, "usually from about 6 a.m. until the osmolality of successive hourly urine samples increases by less than 30 mosmol/kg, indicating that a plateau of urine concentration has been reached. When the plateau is reached, a blood sample is obtained for osmolality and the patient is given aqueous Pitressin, 5U by subcutaneous injection. Urine is collected at 1/2 hour and 1 hour after this injection for osmolality measurement. Body weights should be recorded at the beginning and end of the dehydration period to determine the percentage of weight loss."

> *Normal* individuals so tested will show urinary osmolality of 800 to 1400 mosmol/kg. Values fall slightly or rise less than 9 percent after Pitressin administration. These results indicate that endogenous vasopressin has produced a maximum or near maximum concentrating effect on the kidney.
>
> In patients with *severe DI*, urine osmolality remains low, below that of the plasma, and increases by more than 50 percent after administration of Pitressin.
>
> Patients with *mild DI* may be able to concentrate their urine to values above that of plasma, but unlike well or chronically ill individuals, they will show responses to Pitressin greater than 9 percent. Chronically sick or malnourished individuals normally may not be able to concentrate urine to more than 450 to 800 mosmol/kg, but, like well persons, they do not increase their values by more than 9 percent after Pitressin.
>
> Patients with *nephrogenic DI* rarely increase their urine osmolality above that of plasma and show a subnormal (<50 percent) or no rise after Pitressin injection.
>
> Patients with *primary polydipsia (compulsive water drinkers)* may not show an increase in plasma osmolality after even 6 hours of dehydration. This observation might, on casual inspection, appear to indicate the presence of DI, but the normal or low plasma osmolality at that time is indicative that the patients may still be overhydrated and may need a longer period of dehydration.

Moses points out that even with the use of these criteria, approximately 5 percent of cases cannot be definitively classified, the groups of greatest question being mild DI versus compulsive water drinking.

Radioimmunoassays for ADH show that ADH is usually low or undetectable in plasma of patients with DI. Robertson and coworkers found reduced levels of ADH of 0.8 ± 0.3 pg/ml in patients with DI, compared with 2.7 ± 1.4 pg/ml in normal patients. These patients did not show a normal secretory response to fluid restriction.

A number of other tests for DI have been reported in the literature. These include the hypertonic saline infusion test (Hickey-Hare or Carter-Robbins test), a procedure that increases blood solute concentration, and the nicotine test, which stimulates acetylcholine receptors on the supraoptic neurons. The former test is not superior to the dehydration procedure and, although it is quicker, requires more effort on the part of patient and doctor. Nicotine (which can be supplied by smoking one or two cigarettes quickly) stimulates ADH release in normal persons but not in DI patients.

Sensitive tests for plasma vasopressin by radioimmunoassay are not widely available but can be very helpful.

Management

Chronic Mild DI. In patients with partial or incomplete DI who are capable of normal regulation of water intake, an effort should be made to control polyuria by means of either chlorpropamide 100 to 200 mg per day or hydrochlorthiazide 50 to 100 mg per day. These agents synergize with residual endogenous ADH at the level of the renal tubule and may provide a useful amount of control using relatively simple (and inexpensive) oral medications. However, these drugs, rarely, may cause severe water retention and hyponatremia even in partial DI; chlorpropamide normally is used to treat diabetes mellitus; it can cause hypoglycemia. If the oral agents are not effective, one of the forms of ADH therapy is indicated.

Severe DI. Several forms of ADH therapy have been used; aqueous vasopressin, vasopressin tannate in oil, synthetic lysine vasopressin nasal spray, vasopressin snuff, and DDAVP. The last-named compound, a synthetic long-acting analog of arginine vasopressin, is the best form of therapy.

Aqueous vasopressin (Pitressin) was originally introduced as a partially purified extract of bovine neurohypophyses, standardized by bioassay. Currently, synthetic vasopressin is dispensed. Because its effect after subcutaneous injection is short-lived (2 hours or less), it is used mainly as a diagnostic aid in differentiating central from renal polyuria and as treatment for the acute DI that develops after brain surgery or head trauma. In the latter cases, the neurosurgeon may be reluctant to use longer-acting vasopressin tannate in oil for fear of inducing cerebral edema.

Vasopressin tannate in oil (Pitressin tannate, 5 U/ml) is a tannic acid salt of vasopressin suspended in oil. Antidiuretic action lasts 6 to 72 hours after administration of 0.1 to 1.0 ml intramuscularly. In starting therapy it is advisable to begin with lower doses (0.3 ml or less) and adjust the amount and the timing of subsequent doses according to the response. DDAVP is a more satisfactory drug, but Pitressin tannate in oil is less expensive. Most patients prefer DDAVP therapy which has fewer side effects and lacks cardiac effects in the doses used. Several important practical precautions in its use must be observed.

> 1. The ampuls containing vasopressin tannate must be shaken thoroughly to ensure complete suspension. Failure to respond is almost always due to faulty mixing or faulty injection techniques. Suspension is easier if the ampul is first warmed. The ampuls should not be stored upside down, because the active compound will then settle in the tip and may be discarded inadvertently when the ampul is opened.
>
> 2. If the patient does not require the full 1.0 ml dose, the remaining amount can be stored safety in a disposable plastic syringe until the next injection.
>
> 3. Successive doses of vasopressin tannate in oil usually are given before the previous dose has worn off completely. Consequently, unless care is taken, patients may show excessive water retention and the syndrome of inappropriate ADH secretion (see below). Plasma sodium or osmolality should be monitored from time to time. An easy way to detect excessive water retention is by daily standardized weighings. Weight gain of 2 to 4 pounds in a day may indicate excessive ADH action. In patients with long-standing ADH deficiency, the renal tubule may become relatively insensitive to exogenous hormone and initially may require larger doses than will be needed later.

Allergic reactions to older preparations of vasopressin occurred because they were derived from animal sources and were contaminated with trace amounts of bovine tissue proteins, neurophysins, anterior pituitary hormones, and somatostatin. In addition to hives, and even anaphylactic reactions, antibodies to GH, ACTH, and prolactin may be detected in patients under treatment. This immune response does not have important physiologic effects but may cause spurious radioimmunoassay values because the antibodies interfere with the radioimmunoassay. The use of synthetic vasopressin and analogs will obviate these problems.

Lysine 8-vasopressin (DIAPID), available in a nasal spray form containing 50 U/ml, provides fair control of DI in most patients but must be taken every 3 to 4 hours. It does not control symptoms in all patients with severe DI, but it is useful in conjunction with other treatment even in cases in which it is not the sole therapy. A few patients show nasal irritation, but most do not. Nasal spray has supplanted the use of *vasopressin snuff*, which has the same limitations of duration of action but, in addition, as a crude compound is more likely to cause local sensitization.

DDAVP, a synthetic analog of arginine vasopressin, can be taken by nasal insufflation and is now the treatment of choice for DI.[108] The analog is relatively resistant to degradation in plasma and has prolonged action; most patients are controlled with one or two insufflations a day. The proper dose is determined by a series of preliminary test doses. Unfortunately, it is approximately three to four times as costly as Pitressin tannate. A detailed approach to therapy has been outlined by Cobb[25] and is summarized below.

> Treatment can be started at home by establishing, as the first objective, a dose taken at bedtime that allows the patient to sleep uninterrupted by the need to urinate. We begin with 2.5 μg (administered intranasally by special tube [see package insert]) and increase by 2.5 μg increments until this objective is reached. While determining the optimal nighttime dose we instruct the patients to take the same or a smaller dose during the day, although we ask them first to wait until the effect of the previous night's dose has worn off, so an approximation of its duration of effect can be made. When the evening dose has been determined the daytime dose is then taken shortly before the evening dose loses its effect, and it is adjusted to provide satisfactory control of polyuria throughout the day. If it becomes necessary to raise the daytime dose to more than 1.5-2 times the bedtime dose, a more frequent administration schedule should be considered. As a practical matter, once a dose that provides 8 or more hours of good control has been determined, attempts to prolong the duration of antidiuresis by increasing the size of a single dose may result in a much greater daily consumption of DDAVP than the use of smaller, divided doses.

In some patients increasing amounts of drugs must be given. Side effects are rare.

CENTRAL "ESSENTIAL" HYPERNATREMIA

In some cases of partial DI, a compensatory intermediate homeostatic state develops, characterized by chronic hypernatremia, mild dehydration, and hypovolemia in which net water balance is adequate because ADH secretion is driven by the hypovolemic state. In isolated descriptions of such cases, the diagnosis had been "essential hypernatremia." In some instances, hypernatremia and hyperosmolarity persist chronically for many months or years. The possibility exists that in such cases the regulatory osmoreceptor center(s) in the hypothalamus operates at a new "setpoint." Serum sodium levels as high as 170 to 190 mEq/liter may occur without significant symptoms. Robertson[105] challenges the concept of altered set-point, suggesting rather that the syndrome results from the combination of defective thirst mechanisms and variable degrees of ADH deficiency.

The adipsia enables the patient to maintain chronically a level of hypertonic dehydration sufficient to force the release of vasopressin in subnormal but physiologically adequate amounts. This observation "graphically demonstrates that the volume of urine excreted by a given patient is as much a function of the set or sensitivity of his thirst mechanism as of the amount of vasopressin he is able to secrete."

> Patients with combined defects in ADH and thirst regulation may present other confusing clinical syndromes. In one such patient reported by Robertson[105] who had no radiologic abnormality but did have a history of surgery to ligate the anterior communicating artery, plasma vasopressin behaved abnormally during rehydration. After an initial slight decline associated with correction of his hypotension, it fluctuated in an apparently random manner which bore no relationship to the decline in plasma osmolality. In fact, even when the patient became hyponatremic as a result of accidental overhydration, vasopressin continued to circulate at concentrations between 1 and 3 pg/ml, a "resetting" of the osmoreceptor level sufficient to maintain an antidiuresis. In this respect he resembled a patient with type I SIADH (see below). Lacking the ability either to stimulate thirst or to suppress vasopressin, the patient had no protection against large changes in water balance in either direction. Consequently, he continuously exhibited wide swings in serum sodium ranging from 120 to 170 mEq/liter. Even a brief exposure to the problems involved in managing such a patient leaves the physician with a healthy respect for the unobtrusive but highly effective way in which nature normally regulates this important physiologic variable.

Findings from studies of such patients permit several conclusions about the function of the hypothalamic-neurohypophysial unit in humans. First, it is apparent that vasopressin secretion can occur normally in the absence of normal thirst. Therefore, the osmoreceptors that drive central thirst are separable from those that regulate vasopressin secretion. Second, vasopressin secretion can be induced in patients with defective osmoreceptor control of vasopressin by changes in blood volume or by pharmacologic stimuli. Therefore, it can be inferred that defects in osmoreceptor control of vasopressin secretion can occur without destruction of the vasopressin neurohypophysial system.

SYNDROME OF INAPPROPRIATE SECRETION OF ADH (SIADH, SCHWARTZ-BARTTER SYNDROME)

Dilutional hyponatremia owing to excessive water retention is a common disorder seen in many different clinical states, including abnormalities of neural control of the neurohypophysis and ectopic secretion of ADH by tumors (Table 3). Because the syndrome closely resembles that produced experimentally by prolonged administration of ADH, it was named the syndrome of inappropriate ADH secretion (SIADH) by Schwartz and Bartter,[123] a diagnosis confirmed by the demonstration that plasma ADH is inappropriately high for the degree of plasma hypoosmolality present (Fig.

TABLE 3. Causes of Inappropriate ADH Secretion

   I. Central hypersecretion of ADH
       A. Hypothalamic disorders
           1. Trauma
           2. Surgery
           3. Metabolic encephalapathy
           4. Acute intermittent porphyria
           5. Myxedema
           6. Subarachnoid hemorrhage
           7. Vascular lesions
       B. Suprahypothalamic disorders
           1. Cerebral infarcts
           2. Subdural hematoma
           3. Infections, meningitis (tuberculosis)
  II. Peripheral hypersecretion
       A. Excessive stimulation in recumbent posture (coma)
 III. Excessive production from nonhypothalamic sites (ectopic ADH)
       A. Pulmonary infections — TB
       B. Tumors — lung, etc.
  IV. Drugs
           1. Vincristine
           2. Chlorpropamide
           3. Chlorthiazide
           4. Cyclophosphamide
           5. Carbamazepine
           6. Clofibrate
           7. Chlorpromazine

13). In SIADH of the idiopathic or neurogenic type, ADH levels are usually only slightly elevated above normal, but there is a failure to suppress further secretion in the face of the hypoosmolar state. This implies a functional derangement of osmoreceptor-ADH control. In patients with ADH-secreting neoplasm, plasma levels of ADH are commonly very high, reaching 10 to 100 times those in normal subjects. In one patient with vincristine neurotoxicity, ADH levels were also markedly elevated.

Although the thirst sensation is regulated in part by plasma osmolality, most individuals continue to ingest water even in the face of low serum osmolality and increased effective blood volume. Persistent water intake together with excessive ADH leads to the critical disturbance in this syndrome which is the retention of excessive body water.

Etiology

The main causes of inappropriate secretion of ADH are summarized in Table 3. The syndrome may be caused by

1. excessive release of ADH from the neurohypophysial system, secondary to suprahypothalamic brain disease
2. hypothalamic disturbances caused by local processes which lead to damage and "leakage" of ADH from the supraoptic neurons
3. abnormal reflex ADH release owing to persistent drive from baroreceptors or volume receptors, secondary to diseases in the chest or heart or to prolonged recumbent posture

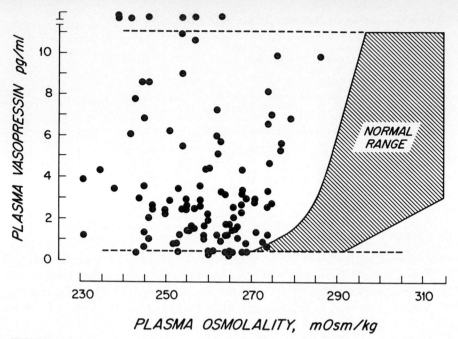

FIGURE 13. Plasma vasopressin as a function of plasma osmolality in 106 patients with clinical SIADH is illustrated here.

4. ectopic production of ADH by inflammatory or neoplastic tissue
5. drug administration

The first and fourth causes are the most common causes of the syndrome.

Suprahypothalamic Brain Disease. Acute subarachnoid hemorrhage, concussion, transfrontal lobotomy, craniotomy, subdural hematoma, and brain tumors are among the common central causes of inappropriate ADH secretion. The localization of the disturbance is not specific. Also seen as causes of the syndrome are cerebral infarction, brain abscess, and meningitis. Rarely, the disorder occurs in diffuse brain disease owing to encephalitis, metabolic encephalopathy, and disseminated microvascular disease. The enormous variety of lesions capable of causing excessive ADH secretion and their lack of anatomic specificity have not been explained. An earlier view that the suprahypothalamic brain exerts a predominantly inhibitory effect on basal ADH secretion, and that hypersecretion in this syndrome is due to "denervation" hyperactivity, has not been supported by experimental studies. Selective inhibitory pathways from the limbic system cortex or brainstem may be responsible for some cases of inappropriate ADH secretion, but there is no evidence to support or to disprove this possibility. Animals prepared with "hypothalamic islands," in which the supraoptic nuclei or the medial basal hypothalamus has been separated from the overlying brain, maintain water balance in response to osmotic stimuli much as do intact animals.

One potential pathogenetic feature common to many cases of inappropriate ADH secretion is stupor or coma. It has been proposed that in patients with a variety of brain disturbances, a prolonged stay in the supine position may lead to ADH hypersecretion through aberrant or "inappropriate" stimulation of peripheral baroreceptors.

Ectopic Humoral Syndromes. The other major cause of inappropriate ADH secretion is the ectopic production of the hormone by certain types of malignant tumor. The most common variety causing the syndrome is oat cell tumor of lung, which may present clinically with little or no evidence of thoracic disease. In a few cases, ADH has been isolated from the tumor itself, together with the prohormone neurophysin. Electron micrographs of the tumor cells show secretory granules resembling those found in neural lobe axon terminals.

Drugs. Patients experiencing severe stress, particularly in the immediate postoperative period, or who are treated with a variety of pain-relieving or tranquilizing drugs (see Table 3) may also show inappropriate ADH secretion. This possibility should be borne in mind in patients with unexplained hyponatremia. Aged individuals are especially vulnerable to this complication.[51]

Recently, attention has been drawn to a particular form of the syndrome of inappropriate ADH secretion caused by drugs such as chlorpropamide,[80] an oral hypoglycemic agent, and chlorthiazide, a diuretic that potentiates the action of ADH at the level of the renal tubule. These agents (accidentally discovered to have therapeutic benefit in DI) facilitate effects of ADH at the renal level in patients with minimal ADH secretion. They also may cause hyponatremia in both normal individuals and in patients with DI.

Vincristine, a cancer chemotherapeutic agent, also may cause the disorder,[103] as may clofibrate[79] and carbamazepine.[69]

Pathophysiology of SIADH

Plasma vasopressin levels are inappropriately high for the level of serum osmolality (see Figure 13). As defined by plasma responses of ADH to infusion of hypertonic saline, Robertson[104] defined four types of vasopressin regulatory abnormalities in patients with SIADH (Table 4).

Clinical Manifestations

Neurologic manifestations of inappropriate ADH secretion are identical to those of water intoxication and correlate to some extent with the degree of hyponatremia. Associated brain disturbance — for example, Alzheimer's disease — hypoxemia, or anemia may interact with hypoosmolality to modify the neurologic picture. Symptoms do not usually occur until serum sodium levels fall below 120 to 125 mEq/liter. Early symptoms are anorexia, nausea, vomiting, lethargy, and irritability. Subtle personality changes, inattentiveness, and forgetfulness may progress to paranoia and delusions. With a further fall in serum sodium to 100 to 110 mEq/liter, the neurologic disturbance becomes even more severe and includes stupor,

TABLE 4. Types of SIADH (Modified from Robertson)[104]

TYPE   I. Infusion of hypertonic saline is associated with large and erratic fluctuations in plasma vasopressin that bear no relationship to the rise in plasma osmolality. The findings suggest that vasopressin secretion is completely uncoupled from osmoreceptor control or that secretion was responding to some periodic nonosmotic stimulus. Patients falling into this category include those with acute respiratory failure, bronchogenic carcinoma, pulmonary tuberculosis, schizophrenia, and rheumatoid arthritis. This abnormality is common in severe anorexia nervosa and may be a consequence of severe inanition.

TYPE   II. Vasopressin responses to osmotic stimuli show a linear response, but the intercept or threshold is inappropriately low. In one patient, a plasma osmolality of 253 mosmol/kg elicited vasopressin secretion. This pattern appears to reflect a resetting of the osmoreceptors. Clinical associations include bronchogenic carcinoma, cerebrovascular disease, tuberculosis, acute respiratory disease, and carcinoma of the pharynx. The pathophysiologic basis of this osmoreceptor change is unknown.

TYPE   III. Plasma vasopressin levels are elevated in the hyponatremic state but are responsive to changes in plasma osmolality at a normal threshold (280–285 mosmol/kg). Its pathogenesis is uncertain but appears to be due to constant, nonsuppressible "leak" of vasopressin despite otherwise normal osmoregulatory functions. This type is reported in central nervous system disease, lung tumors, and pulmonary tuberculosis.

TYPE   IV. Osmoregulation seems to be completely normal, despite inability to secrete a water load. Thus vasopressin secretion is appropriately suppressed in the hypoosmolar state and responds at normal threshold. It appears that these patients have a change in renal sensitivity to vasopressin or secrete other substances that affect urinary sodium and water excretion. This type is the least common and occurred in patients with bronchogenic carcinoma and diabetes mellitus.

coma, and intractable generalized seizures which are usually refractory to treatment with anticonvulsants.

Attempts have been made to define experimentally the neurologic basis for dysmentation in the syndrome of inappropriate ADH secretion, but the results are somewhat conflicting. Severe hyponatremia (and water intoxication) is not associated with significant increase in intracranial pressure, that is, cerebral edema is not present. Cerebrospinal fluid (CSF) pressure is normal. Dila and Pappius[148] found in rats in which water intoxication was induced by exogenous ADH administration that loss of potassium occurred from cerebral tissues (and from muscle), and they postulated that this loss may contribute to the symptoms. In contrast, the sodium content was less markedly decreased. Rymer and Fishman[150] confirmed these findings in the rat but found that these metabolic derangements persisted for a time after neurologic recovery. They speculated that the potassium defect in brain is in fact protective, minimizing brain swelling. They concluded that the critical factor in the level of consciousness was the level of brain water, not sodium or potassium levels. Although these observations received different interpretations by the two teams of investigators, both show that cerebral swelling is not a significant factor in the disorder. Administration of corticosteroids has no beneficial or adverse effect on the condition.

The combination of excess water retention and excess water intake leads to expansion of the extracellular fluid volume and increases in renal plasma flow, glomerular filtration rate, and sodium load in the glomerular filtrate. The apparently paradoxic situation arises in which urine sodium excretion is high in the face of low plasma sodium concentration, and patients excrete a hyperosmolar urine with sodium concentration higher than that of plasma. Water administration does not cause water diuresis in SIADH, whereas salt diuresis occurs after salt loading. The syndrome reverses relatively rapidly with water restriction. Most patients continue to drink water (a few complain of thirst) and may steal water even in the presence of severe hyponatremia.

Diagnosis and Management

Because hyponatremia may be a sign of sodium depletion (such as that seen after prolonged vomiting or in adrenal insufficiency) the clinician is commonly faced with the differential diagnosis of disorders that require distinctly different treatments. In inappropriate ADH secretion, salt administration does not raise plasma sodium levels (except transiently), and adrenal mineralocorticoids are without effect. In this syndrome blood volume is normal, signs of peripheral circulation are normal (normal pulse and blood pressure), renal clearance is normal, and plasma blood urea nitrogen (BUN) and creatinine as a consequence are also normal, or even lower than normal. In sharp contrast, hyponatremia owing to sodium depletion is accompanied by contraction of blood volume (low blood pressure, tachycardia), decreased renal blood flow, and renal retention of BUN and creatinine (prerenal azotemia). Occasionally mixed types of the disease are observed—especially in patients on diuretics.

In SIADH, the cornerstone of treatment is strict water restriction (400 to 600 ml per day). This regimen, which is both diagnostic and therapeutic, is all that is needed in most cases. If serious brain disturbance demands urgent treatment, administration of hypertonic sodium chloride (3 to 5 percent) is indicated.[57] Unless water intake is simultaneously restricted, the salt load will be quickly excreted (see below). In contrast, the treatment for sodium depletion is the administration of isotonic or slightly hypertonic sodium chloride solution; if adrenal cortical deficiency is present, glucocorticoids and mineralocorticoids are required. When the diagnosis is in doubt, the patient should be given slightly hypertonic sodium chloride intravenously, with or without cortisol, because this treatment is lifesaving in depleted patients and will usually have no detrimental (or beneficial) effect on patients with inappropriate ADH. Hyponatremia can have permanent neurologic effects, especially if it develops rapidly. Arieff and Guisado[151] have stated that a rapid drop to sodium concentrations of 125 meq/liter caused a mortality of 50 percent. Moreover, rapid correction of hyponatremia can induce cerebral demyelination. Central pontine demyelination and extensive lesions in the white matter of the centrum semiovale are described.[40]

Several investigators have advocated the use of furosemide for rapid correction of hyponatremia. This may be important in congestive heart failure caused by the fluid overload. Furosemide usually causes a diuresis sufficient to reduce cardiac overload. When furosemide is given, careful attention must be paid to correction of potassium and other electrolyte losses induced by the diuretic. Once the hyponatremia has been corrected, careful adherence to a regimen of fluid restriction is important to prevent recurrence of water intoxication. Treatment should then be directed at the underlying problem if at all possible.

> Replacement with intravenous NaCl in severe cases must be done cautiously because vigorous and rapid correction of severe hyponatremia has been incriminated in the pathogenesis of central pontine myelinolysis (CPM) and related brainstem, cerebellar, and cerebral syndromes.[152] Ayus[153] emphasized the risks of persistent severe hyponatremia and recommended the following therapeutic guidelines: serum sodium above 120 mEq/liter does not require immediate correction. If sodium is greater than 105 mEq/liter, it can be safely corrected to a level of 125–130 mEq/liter at a rate of administration of sodium of 2 mEq/hour. If serum sodium is less than 105 mEq/liter, it is corrected by 20 mEq/liter at a rate of 2 mEq/hour and then permitted to return slowly to normal.

As outlined by Hou,[66] several drugs have a more specific effect in treatment of the disorder. Lithium interferes with vasopressin action on the kidney, and treatment to achieve serum levels of 0.3 to 0.6 mEq/liter is often effective; these are below the usual therapeutic range for treatment of depression. A more effective drug in SIADH is desmocycline, a tetracycline-like antibiotic. Doses of 600 to 1200 mg/day are usually effective. Onset of effect is within 5 days, and the drug acts for up to 10 days after it has been stopped. Patients should avoid sunlight exposure (desmocycline is a photosensitizer), and the drug can cause renal damage. Naloxone has been successfully used in a few patients with neurogenic SIADH, as has phenytoin.

REFERENCES

1. ACHER, R: *Chemistry of neurohypophysial hormones: An example of molecular evolution.* In *The Pituitary Gland and Its Neuroendocrine Control,* Part I, Washington, DC. American Physiological Society, pp 119–130, 1974.
2. ACHER, R: *Principles of evolution: The neural hierarchymodes.* In KRIEGER, DT, BROWNSTEIN, MJ, MARTIN, JB (EDS): *Brain Peptides.* John Wiley & Sons, New York, 1983, pp 135–164.
3. AKAGAWA, K, HARA, N, TSUKADA, Y: *Partial purification and properties of the inhibitors of Na, K-ATPase and ouabain-binding in bovine central nervous system.* J Neurochem 42:775–780, 1984.
4. ALAGHBAND-ZADEH, J, FENTON, S, HANCOCK, K, ET AL: *Evidence that the hypothalamus may be a source of a circulating Na+K+-ATPase inhibitor.* J Endocrinol 98:221–226, 1983.
5. AMICO, JA, TENICELA, R, JOHNSTON, J, ET AL: *A time dependent peak of oxytocin exists in the cerebrospinal fluid but not in the plasma of humans.* J Clin Endocrinol Metab 57:947–951, 1982.
6. ANDERSSON, B, AND McCANN, SM: *Drinking, antidiuresis and milk ejection from electrical stimulation within the hypothalamus of the goat.* Acta Physiol Scand 35:191–197, 1955.
7. ANDERSSON, B, AND WESTBYE, O: *Synergistic action of sodium and angiotensin on brain mechanisms controlling water and salt balance.* Nature 228:75, 1970.
8. ANTUNES, JL, AND ZIMMERMAN, EA: *The hypothalamic magnocellular system of the rhesus monkey: An immunocytochemical study.* J Comp Neurol 181:539–566, 1978.
9. ANTUNES, JL, CARMEL, PW, ZIMMERMAN, EA: *Projection from the paraventricular nucleus to the zona externa of the median eminence of the rhesus monkey: An immunohistochemical study.* Brain Res 137:1–10, 1977.
10. ATLAS, SA, KLEINERT, HD, CAMARGO, MJ, JANUSZEWICZ, A, SEALEY, JE, LARAGH, JH, SCHILLING, JW, LEWICKI, JA, JOHNSON, LK, MAACK, T: *Purification, sequencing and synthesis of natriuretic and vasoactive rat atrial peptide.* Nature 309:717–719, 1984.
11. AUBRY, RH, NANKIN, HR, MOSES, AM, ET AL: *Measurement of the osmotic threshold for vaso-*

pressin release in human subjects, and its modification by cortisol. J Clin Endocrinol Metab 25:1481–1492, 1965.

12. AUDIBERT, A, MOEGLEN, JM, LANCRANJAN, I: *Central effects of vasopressin in man.* Int J Neurol 14:162–174, 1980.

13. BARGMANN, W, AND SCHARRER, E: *The site of origin of the hormones of the posterior pituitary.* Am Sci 38:255–259, 1951.

14. BARKER, JL, CRAYTON, JW, NICOLL, RA: *Antidromic and orthodromic responses to paraventricular and supraoptic neurosecretory cells.* Brain Res 33:353–366, 1971.

15. BARKER, JL, CRAYTON, JW, NICOLL, RA: *Noradrenaline and acetylcholine responses of supraoptic neurosecretory cells.* J Physiol (Lond) 218:19–32, 1971.

16. BEYERS, AD, ODENDAAL, HJ, SPRUYT, LL, PARKIN, DP: *The possible role of endogenous digitalis-like substance in the causation of pre-eclampsia.* Afr Med J 65:883–885, 1984.

17. BISSET, GW, CLARK, BJ, ERRINGTON, ML: *The hypothalamic neurosecretory pathways for the release of oxytocin and vasopressin in the cat.* J Physiol (Lond) 217:111–131, 1971.

18. BISSETT, GW: *Milk ejection.* In KNOBIL, E, AND SAWYER, WH (EDS): *Handbook of Physiology, section 7, vol. 4. The pituitary gland and its neuroendocrine control, part 1.* American Physiological Society, Washington DC, 1974, pp 493–520.

19. BRODY, MJ, AND JOHNSON, AK: *Role of the anterioventral third ventricle region in fluid and electrolyte balance, arterial pressure regulation and hypertension.* In MARTINI, L, AND GANONG, WF (EDS): *Frontiers in Neuroendocrinology.* Raven Press, New York, 1980, pp 249–292.

20. BROWNSTEIN, MJ, RUSSELL, JT, GAINER, H: *Synthesis, transport, and release of posterior pituitary hormones.* Science 207:373–378, 1980.

21. BROWNSTEIN, MJ, RUSSELL, JT, GAINER, H: *Biosynthesis of posterior pituitary hormones.* In GANONG, WF, AND MARTINI, L (EDS): *Frontiers in Neuroendocrinology,* vol. 7, Raven Press, New York, 1982, pp 31–43.

22. CAFFE, AR, AND VAN LEEUWEN, FW: *Vasopressin-immunoreactive cells in the dorsomedial hypothalamic region, medial amygdaloid nucleus and locus coeruleus of the rat.* Cell Tis Res 233:23–33, 1983.

23. CAMPBELL, WB, AND NEEDLEMAN, P: *Inhibition of aldosterone biosynthesis by atriopeptins in rat adrenal cells.* Circ Res 57:113–118, 1985.

24. CHARD, T: *Oxytocin.* In MARTINI, L, AND BESSER, GM (EDS): *Clinical neuroendocrinology.* Academic Press, New York, 1977, pp 569–583.

25. COBB, WE: *Management of neurogenic diabetes insipidus with DAVP and other agents.* In REICHLIN, S (ED): *The Neurohypophysis.* Plenum, New York, 1984, pp 139–164.

26. COLE, BR, AND NEEDLEMAN, P: *Atriopeptins: Volume regulatory hormones.* Clin Res 33:389–394, 1985.

27. CURRIE, MG, GELLER, DM, COLE, BR, ET AL: *Bioactive cardiac substances: Potent vasorelaxant activity in mammalian atria.* Science 221:71–73, 1983.

28. CURRIE, MG, GELLER, DM, COLE, BR, ET AL: *Proteolytic activation of a bioactive cardiac peptide by in vitro trypsin cleavage.* Proc Natl Acad Sci USA 81:1230–1233, 1984.

29. DANIEL, PM, AND PRICHARD, MML: *The human hypothalamus and pituitary stalk after hypophysectomy or pituitary stalk section.* Brain 95:813–824, 1972.

30. DEVRIES, GJ, AND BUIJS, RM: *The origin of the vasopressinergic and oxytocinergic innervation of the rat brain with special reference to the laternal septum.* Brain Res 273:307–317, 1983.

31. DIERICKX, K, AND VANDESANDE, F: *Immunocytochemical demonstration of separate vasopressin-neurophysin and oxytocin-neurophysin neurons in the human hypothalamus.* Cell Tiss Res 196:203–212, 1979.

32. DIERICKX, K: *Immunocytochemical localization of the vertebrate nonapeptide neurohypophyseal hormones and neurophysins.* Int Rev Cytol 62:119–185, 1980.

33. DI FIGLIA, M, AND ARONIN, N: *Immunoreactive leu-enkephalin in the monkey hypothalamus including observations on its ultrastructural localization in the paraventricular nucleus.* J Comp Neurol 225:313–326, 1984.

34. DREIFUSS, JJ, AND KELLY, JS: *The activity of identified supraoptic neurones and their response to acetylcholine applied by iontophoresis.* J Physiol 220:105–118, 1972.

35. DU VIGNEAUD, V: *Hormones of the posterior pituitary gland: Oxytocin and vasopressin.* Harvey Lectures, Sec. 50:1, 1954–1955.

36. DYBALL, RE, AND PATERSON, AT: *Neurohypophysial hormones and brain function: The neurohypophysiological effects of oxytocin and vasopressin.* Pharmacol Ther 20:419–436, 1983.

37. *Endogenous foxglove* (editorial) Lancet 2:1463–1464, 1983.

38. [Editorial.] Lancet, Nov 23, 1984, pp 1017–1019.

39. EDWARDS, CRW: *Vasopressin.* In MARTINI, L, AND BESSER, GM (EDS): *Clinical Neuroendocrinology.* Academic Press, New York, 1977, pp 527–567.

40. FINLAYSON, MH, SNIDER, S, OLIVA, LA, GAULT, MH: *Cerebral and pontine myelinolysis: Two cases with fluid and electrolyte imbalance and hypotension.* J Neurol Sci 18:399–409, 1973.

41. FITZSIMMONS, JT: *Thirst.* Physiol Rev 52:468, 1972.

42. FITZSIMMONS, JT: *Some historical perspectives in the physiology of thirst.* In EPSTEIN, AN, KISSILEFF, HR, STELLAR, E (EDS): *The Neurophysiology of Thirst.* VH Winston & Sons, Washington, 1973, pp 3–33.

43. FITZSIMMONS, JT: *Endocrine mechanisms in the control of water intake.* In MORGENSON, GJ, AND CALARESU, FR (EDS): *Neural integration of physiological mechanisms and behavior.* University of Toronto Press, Toronto, 1975, pp 226.

44. FITZSIMMONS, JT, EPSTEIN, AN, ET AL: *The peptide specificity of receptors for angiotensin-induced thrist.* In BUCKLEY, JP, AND FERRARIO, CW (EDS): *Central actions of angiotensin and related hormones.* Plenum, New York, 1977, pp 405–415.

45. FITZSIMMONS, JT: *Endocrine mechanisms in the control of water intake.* In MOGENSON, GJ, AND CALARESU, FR (EDS): *Neural Integration of Physiological Mechanisms and Behavior.* University of Toronto Press, Toronto, 1975, p 226.

46. GAINER, H: *Peptides in neurobiology.* Plenum, New York, 1977.

47. GAINER, H: *Biosynthesis of vasopressin and neurophysin.* In REICHLIN, S (ED): *The Neurohypophysis.* Plenum, New York, 1984.

48. GANTEN, D, FUXE, K, PHILLIPS, MI, ET AL: *The brain isorenin-angiotensin system: Biochemistry, localization, and possible role in drinking and blood pressure regulation.* In MARTINI, L, AND GANONG, WF (EDS): *Frontiers in Neuroendocrinology,* vol 5. Raven Press, New York, 1978, pp 61–100.

49. GODFRAIND, T, DEPOVER, A, CASTANEDA HERNANDEZ, G, ET AL: *Cardiodigin: Endogenous digitalis-like material from mammalian heat.* Arch Int Pharmacodyn Ther 258:165–167, 1982.

50. GOLD, PW, KAYE, W, ROBERTSON, GL, ET AL: *Abnormalities in plasma and cerebrospinal fluid arginine vasopressin in patients with anorexia nervosa.* N Engl J Med 308:1117–1123, 1983.

51. GOLDSTEIN, CS, BRAUNSTEIN, S, GOLDFARB, S: *Idiopathic syndrome of inappropriate antidiuretic hormone secretion possibly related to advanced age.* Ann Int Med 99:185–188, 1983.

52. GRAVES, SW, BROWN, B, VALDES, R: *An endogenous digoxin-like substance in patients with renal impairment.* Ann Int Med 99:604–608, 1983.

53. GRAVES, SW, AND WILLIAMS, GH: *An endogenous ouabain-like factor associated with hypertensive pregnant women.* J Clin Endocrinol Metab 59:1070–1074, 1984.

54. GREEN, JR, BUCHAN, GC, ET AL: *Hereditary and idiopathic types of diabetes insipidus.* Brain 90:707–714, 1967.

55. GROSSMAN, SP: *Eating or drinking elicited by direct adrenergic or cholinergic stimulation of hypothalamus.* Science 132:301–302, 1960.

56. GRUBER, KA, RUDEL, LL, BULLOCK, BC: *Increased circulating levels of an endogenous digoxin-like factor in hypertensive monkeys.* Hypertension 4:348–354, 1982.

57. HANTMAN, D, ET AL: *Rapid correction of hyponatremia in the syndrome of inappropriate secretion of antidiuretic hormone. An alternative treatment to hypertonic saline.* Ann Int Med 78:870–875, 1973.

58. HAUPERT, GT, JR, CARILLI, CT, CANTLEY, LC: *Hypothalamic sodium-transport inhibitor is a high-affinity reversible inhibitor of Na^+-K^+-ATPase.* Am J Physiol 247:919–924, 1984.

59. HAUPERT, GT, AND SANCHO, JM: *Sodium transport inhibitor from bovine hypothalamus.* Proc Natl Acad Sci 76:4658–4660, 1979.

60. HAYWARD, JN: *The amygdaloid nuclear complex and mechanisms of release of vasopressin from the neurohypophysis.* In ELEFTHERIOUS, BE (ED): *Neurobiology of the Amygdala.* Plenum, New York, 1972, p 685.

61. HAYWARD, JN, AND JENNINGS, DP: *Activity of magnocellular neuroendocrine cells in the hypothalamus of unanesthetized monkeys. I. Functional cell types and their anatomical distribution in the supraoptic nucleus and the internuclear one.* J Physiol 232:515–543, 1973.

62. HAYWARD, JN, AND JENNINGS, DP: *Activity of magnocellular neuroendocrine cells in the hypothalamus of unanesthetized monkeys. II. Osmosensitivity of functional cell types in the supraoptic nucleus and the internuclear zone.* J Physiol 232:545, 1973.

63. HAYWARD, JN: *Physiological and morphological identification of hypothalamic magnocellular neuroendocrine cells in goldfish preoptic nucleus.* J Physiol 239:103–124, 1974.

64. HAYWARD, JN, AND JENNINGS, DP: *Influence of sleep walking and nociceptor-induced behavior on the activity of supraoptic neurons in the hypothalamus of the monkey.* Brain Res 57:461–466, 1973.

65. HAYWARD, JN: *Neural control of the posterior pituitary.* Ann Rev Physiol 37:191, 1975.

66. HOU, S: *Syndrome of inappropriate antidiuretic hormone secretion.* In REICHLIN, S (ED): *The neurohypophysis.* Plenum, New York, 1984, pp 165–189.

67. HUANG, CT, AND SMITH, RM: *Lowering the blood pressure in chronic aortic coarctate hypertensive rats with anti-digoxin antiserum.* Life Sci 35:115–118, 1984.

68. KASTING, NW, CARR, DB, MARTIN, JB, BLUME, H, BERGLAND, R: *Changes in cerebrospinal fluid and plasma vasopressin in the febrile sheep.* Can J Physiol Pharmacol 61:427–431, 1983.

69. KIMURA, T, MATSUI, K, SATO, T, ET AL: *Mechanism of carbamazepine (Tegretol)-induced antidiuresis: Evidence for release of antidiuretic hormone and impaired excretion of a water load.* J Clin Endocrinol Metab 38:356–362, 1974.

70. KINGMULLER, D, WEILER, E, KRAMER, HJ: *Digoxin-like natriuretic activity in the urine of salt loaded healthy subjects.* Klin-Wochenschr. 60:1249–1253, 1982.

71. KOJIMA, I, YOSHIHARA, S, OGATA, E: *Involvement of endogenous digitalis-like substance in genesis of deoxycorticosterone-salt hypertension.* Life Sci 30:1775–1781, 1982.

72. KOVACS, K: *Pathology of the neurohypophysis.* In REICHLIN, S (ED): *The Neurohypophysis.* Plenum, New York, 1984.

73. KRAMER, HJ: *Natriuretic hormone—a circulating inhibitor of sodium-and potassium-activated adenosine trihosphatase. Its potential role in body fluid and blood pressure regulation.* Klin Wochenschr 59:1225–1230, 1980.

74. LAND, H, SCHULTZ, G, SCHMALE, H, RICHTER, D: *Nucleotide sequence of cloned cDNA encoding bovine arginine vasopressin-neurophysin II precursor.* Nature 295:299–303, 1982.

75. LANG, RE, HEIL, J, GANTEN, D, HERMANN, K, RASCHER, W, UNGER, T: *Effects of lesions in the paraventricular nucleus of the hypothalamus on vasopressin and oxytocin contents in brainstem and spinal cord of rat.* Brain Res 260:326–329, 1983.

76. LINDVALL, O, BJORKLUND, A, SKAGERBERG, G: *Selective histochemical demonstration of dopamine terminal systems in rat di-and telencephalon: New evidence for dopaminergic innervation of hypothalamic neurosecretory nuclei.* Brain Res 306:19–30, 1984.

77. MARTINI, L: *Neurohypophysis and anterior pituitary activity.* In HARRIS, GW, AND DONOVAN, BT (EDS): *The pituitary gland,* vol 3. University of California Press, Berkeley, 1966, p 535.

78. MORGAN, K, FOORD, SM, SPURLOCK, G, ET AL: *Release of an active sodium transport inhibitor (ASTI) from rat hypothalamic cells in culture.* Endocrinology 115:1642–1644, 1984.

79. MOSES, AM, HOWANITZ, J, GIEMERT, M VAN, MILLER, M: *Clofibrate-induced antidiuresis.* J Clin Invest 52:535–542, 1973.

80. MOSES, AM, NUMANN, P, MILLER, M: *Mechanisms of chlorpropamide-induced antiduresis in man: Evidence for release of ADH and enhancement of peripheral action.* Metabolism 22:59–66, 1973.

81. MOSES, AM: *Diabetes insipidus and ADH regulation.* In KRIEGER, DT, AND HUGHES, JC (EDS): *Neuroendocrinology.* Sinauer Associates, Sunderland, MA, 1980, pp 141–148.

82. MOSES, AM: *Longstanding postraumatic diabetes insipidus.* Medical Grand Rounds. 2:117–128, 1983.

83. MOSES, AM: *Clinical and laboratory features of central and nephrogenic-diabetes insipidus and primary polydipsia.* In REICHLIN, S (ED): *The Neurohypophysis.* Plenum, New York, 1984, pp 115–138.

84. MOSS, RL, DYBALL, REJ, CROSS, BA: *Responses of antidromically identified supraoptic and paraventricular units to acetylcholine, noradrenaline and glutamate applied iontophoretically.* Brain Res 35:573–575, 1971.

85. NEEDLEMAN, P, ADANS, SP, COLE, BR, ET AL: *Atriopeptins: Cardiac hormones.* Hypertension 7:469–482, 1985.

86. NICOLL, RA, AND BARKER, JL: *Excitation of supraoptic neurosecretory cells by angiotensin II.* Nature (New Biol) 233:172–174, 1971.

87. NICOLL, RA, AND BARKER, JL: *The pharmacology of recurrent inhibition in the supraoptic neurosecretory system.* Brain Res 35:501–511, 1971.

88. NILAVER, G, ZIMMERMAN, EA, WILKINS, J, ET AL: *Magnocellular hypothalamic projections to the lower brainstem and spinal cord of the rat. Immunocytochemical evidence for predominance of the oxytocin-neurophysin system compared to the vasopressin-neurophysin system.* Neuroendocrinology 30:150–158, 1980.

89. OHKUBO, H, KAGEYAMA, R, UJIHARA, M, ET AL: *Cloning and sequence analysis of cDNA for rat angiotensinogen.* Proc Natl Acad Sci USA 80:2000–2196, 1983.

90. OIKAWA, S, IMAI, M, UENO, A, TANAKA, AS, ET AL: *Cloning and sequence analysis of cDNA encoding a precursor for human atrial natriuretic polypeptide.* Nature 309:724–726, 1984.

91. OLIVER, G, AND SCHAFER, EA: *On the physiological action of extracts of pituitary body and certain other glandular organs.* J Physiol (Lond) 18:277, 1895.

92. PALLUK, R, GAIDA, W, HOEFKE, W: *Minireview, Atrial natriuretic factor.* Life Sci 36:1415–1425, 1985.

93. PARRY, HB, AND LIVETT, BG: *A new hypothalmic pathway to the median eminence containing neurophysin and its hypertrophy in sheep with natural scrapie.* Nature 242:63–65, 1973.

94. PERLOW, MJ, REPPERT, SM, ARTMAN, HA, ET AL: *Oxytocin, vasopressin, and estrogen-stimulated neurophysin: Daily patterns of concentration in cerebrospinal fluid.* Science 216:1416–1418, 1982.

95. PHILLIPS, MI, AND FELIX, D: *Specific angiotensin II receptive neurons in the cat subfornical organ.* Brain Res 109:531–540, 1986.

96. PICKFORD, M: *Inhibitory effect of acetylcholine on water diuresis in dog, and its pituitary transmission.* J Physiol (Lond) 95:226, 1939.

97. RAMSAY, DJ: *Effects of circulating angiotensin II use on the brain.* In MARTINI, L, AND GANONG, F (EDS): *Frontiers in Neuroendocrinology,* vol 7, Raven Press, New York, pp 263–285, 1982.

98. RAMSAY, DJ, AND GANONG, WF: *CNS regulation of salt and water balance.* In KRIEGER, DT, AND

HUGHES, JC (EDS): *Neuroendocrinology.* Sinaue Associates, Sunderland, MA, pp 123–130, 1980.

99. RANDALL, RV, CLARK, EC, DODGE, HW, ET AL: *Polyuria after operation for tumors in the region of the hypophysis and hypothalamus.* J Clin Endocrinol Metab 20:1614–1621, 1960.

100. REICHLIN, S (ED): *The Neurohypophysis.* Plenum, New York, 1984.

101. RENAUD, LP, DAY, TA, RANDLE, JCR, BOURQUE, CW: *In vivo and in vitro electrophysiological evidence that central noradrenergic pathways enhance the activity of hypothalamic vasopressinergic neurosecretory cells.* In SCHRIER, R (ED): *Water balance and antidiuretic hormone.* Raven Press, New York, 1984.

102. RHODES, CH, MORELL, JI, PFAFF, DW: *Immunohistochemical analysis of magnocellular elements in rat hypothalamus: Distribution and numbers of cells containing neuophysin, oxytocin, and vasopressin.* J Comp Neurol 198:45–64, 1981.

103. ROBERTSON, GL, BHOOPALAM, N, ZELKOWITZ, LJ: *Vincristine neurotoxicity and abnormal secretion of antidiuretic hormone.* Arch Int Med 132:717, 1973.

104. ROBERTSON, GL: *Physiopathology of ADH secretion.* In TOLIS, G, LABRIE, F, MARTIN, JB, NAFTOLIN, F (EDS): *Clinical neuroendocrinology: A pathophysiological approach.* Raven Press, New York, 1979, pp 247–260.

105. ROBERTSON, GL: *Diseases of the posterior pituitary in endocrinology and metabolism.* In FELIG, P, BAXTER, JD, BROADUS, AE, FROHMAN, LA: McGraw-Hill, New York, 1981, pp 251–280.

106. ROBINSON, AG, ARCHER, DF, TOLSTOL, LF: *Neurophysin in women during oxytocin-related events.* J Clin Endocrinol Metab 37:645, 1973.

107. ROBINSON, AG, AND FRANTZ, AG: *Radioimmunoassay of posterior pituitary peptides: A review.* Metabolism 22:1047, 1973.

108. ROBINSON, AG: *DDAVP in the treatment of central diabetes insipidus.* N Engl J Med 294:507–511, 1976.

109. ROBINSON, AG: *Neurophysins.* In MARTINI, L, AND BESSER, GM (EDS): *Clinical neuroendocrinology.* Academic Press, New York, 1977, pp 585–602.

110. ROBINSON, AG: *The contribution of measured secretion of neurophysins to our understanding of neurohypophysical function.* In REICHLIN, S (ED): *The Neurohypophysis.* Plenum, New York, 1984.

111. RUPPERT, S, SCHERER, G, SCHUTZ, G: *Recent gene conversion involving bovine vasopressin and oxytocin precursor genes suggested by nucleotide sequence.* Nature 308:554–557, 1984.

112. SAGNELLA, GA, AND MACGREGOR, GA: *Cardiac peptides and the control of sodium excretion.* Nature 309:666–667, 1984.

113. SAPER, CB, STANDAERT, DG, CURRIE, MG, SCHWARTZ, D, GELLER, DM, NEEDLEMAN, P: *Atriopeptin. Immunoreactive neurons in the brain: Presence in cardiovascular regulatory areas.* Science 227:1047–1049, 1983.

114. SAWCHENKO, PE, AND SWANSON, LW: *Immunohistochemical identification of neurons in the paraventricular nucleus of the hypothalamus that project to the medulla or to the spinal cord in the rat.* J Comp Neurol 205:260–272, 1982.

115. SAWCHENKO, PE, SWANSON, LW, STEINBUSCH, HWM, VERHOFSTAD, AAJ: *The distribution and cells of origin of serotonergic inputs to the paraventricular and supraoptic nuclei of the rat.* Brain Res. 277:355–360, 1983.

116. SAWYER, WH: *The mammalian antidiuretic response.* In GREEP, RO, AND ASTWOOD, BE (EDS): *Handbook of Physiology, Sect. VII, Endocrinology,* vol 4, part 1. American Physiology Society, Williams & Wilkins, Baltimore, 1974, p 443.

117. SCHARRER, E: *Principles of neuroendocrine integration.* Res Publ Assoc Res Nerv Ment Dis 43:1, 1966.

118. SCHERBAUM, WA, AND BOTTAZZO, GF: *Autoantibodies to vasopressin cells in idiopathic diabetes insipidus: Evidence for an autoimmune variant.* Lancet 23:897–901, 1983

119. SCHMALE, H, AND RICHTER, D: *Single base deletion in the vasopressin gene is the cause of diabetes insipidus in Brattleboro rats.* Nature 308:705–709, 1984.

120. SCHRIER, RW, BERL, T, ANDERSON, RJ: *Osmotic and non-osmotic control of vasopressin release.* Am J Physiol 236:F321–F332, 1979.

121. SCHWARTZ, D, GELLER, DM, MANNING, PT, ET AL: *SER-LEU-ARG-ARG-atriopeptin III is the major circulating form of atrial peptide.* Science 229:397–400, 1985.

122. SHARE, L (ED): *Vasopressin and cardiovascular regulation.* Symposium FAEB 43:78–106, 1984.

123. SCHWARTZ, WB, AND BARTTER, FC: *The syndrome of inappropriate secretion of antidiuretic hormone.* Am J Med 42:790, 1967.

124. SHIMONI, Y, GOTSMAN, M, DEUTSCH, J, KACHALSKY, S, LICHTSTEIN, D: *Endogenous ouabain-like compound increases heart muscle contractility.* Nature 307:369–371, 1984.

125. SOFRONIEW, MV, AND SCHRELL, U: *Evidence for a direct projection from oxytocin and vasopressin neurons in the hypothalamic paraventricular nucleus to the medulla oblongata: Immunohistochemical visualization of both the horseradish peroxidase transported and the peptide produced by the same neurons.* Neurosci Lett 22:211–217, 1981.

REGULATION OF THE PITUITARY GLAND

126. SOFRONIEW, MV, AND WEINDL, A: *Extrahypothalamic neurophysin-containing perikarya, fiber pathways and clusters, in the rat brain.* Endocrinology 102:334–337, 1978.

127. STUART, CA, NEELON, FA, LEBOVITZ, HE: *Disordered control of thirst in hypothalamic-pituitary sarcoidosis.* N Engl J Med 303:1078–1082, 1980.

128. SWANSON, LW, AND KUYPERS, HGJM: *The paraventricular nucleus of the hypothalamus; Cytoarchitectonic subdivisions and organization of projections to the pituitary, dorsal vagal complex, and spinal cord as demonstrated by retrograde fluorescence double-label methods.* J Comp Neurol 194:555–570, 1980.

129. SWANSON, LW, AND McKELLAR, S: *The distribution of oxytocin- and neurophysin-stained fibers in the spinal cord of the rat and monkey.* J Comp Neurol 188:87–106, 1979.

130. SWANSON, LW, SAWCHENKO, PE, WEIGAND, SJ, PRICE, JL: *Separate neurons in the paraventricular nucleus project to the median eminence and to the medulla or spinal cord.* Brain Res 198:190–195, 1980.

131. SWANSON, LW, AND SAWCHENKO, PE: *Hypothalamic integration: Organization of the paraventricular and supraoptic nuclei.* Annu Rev Neurosci 6:269–324, 1983.

132. TIKKANEN, I, METSARINNE, K, FYHRQUIST, F, LEIDENIUS, R: *Plasma atrial natriuretic peptide in cardiac disease and during infusion in healthy volunteers.* Lancet II:66–69, 1985.

133. VAN WIERMSMA GREIDANUS, TB, VAN RAEE, JM, DE WIED, D: *Vasopressin and memory.* Pharmacol Ther 20:437–458, 1983.

134. VERNEY, EB: *The antidiuretic hormone and the factors which determine its release.* Proc Roy Soc (Ser) B 135:25, 1947.

135. WATSON, SJ, AKIL, H, FISCHLI, W, GOLDSTEIN, A, ZIMMERMAN, E, NILOVER, G, VAN WIMMERSMA, TB: *Dynorphin and vasopressin: Common localization in magnocellular neurons.* Science 216:85–88, 1982.

136. WHITNALL, MH, GAINER, H, COX, BM, ET AL: *Dynorphin-A-(1-8) is containing within vasopressin neurosecretory vesicles in rat pituitary.* Science 222:1137–1139, 1983.

137. WOODS, WH, HOLLAND, RC, POWELL, EW: *Connections of cerebral structures functioning in neurohypophysial hormone release.* Brain Res 12:26, 1969.

138. YAMADA, M, GREENBERG, B, JOHNSON, L, ET AL: *Cloning and sequence analysis of the cDNA for the rat atrial natriuretic factor precursor.* Nature 309:719–722, 1984.

139. ZIMMERMAN, EA, HSU, KC, ROBINSON, AG, ET AL: *Studies of neurophysin secreting neurons with immunoperoxidase techniques employing antibody to bovine neurophysin. I. Light microscopic findings in monkey and bovine tissues.* Endocrinology 92:931–940, 1973.

140. ZIMMERMAN, EA, CARMEC, PW, HUSAIN, MK, ET AL: *Vasopressin and neurophysin: High concentrations in monkey hypophyseal portal blood.* Science 182:925–927, 1973.

141. ZIMMERMAN, EA: *Localization of hormone secreting pathways in the brain by immunocytochemical techniques.* In MARTINI, L, AND GANONG, WF (EDS): *Frontiers in Neuroendocrinology,* vol. 4. Raven Press, New York, 1976, pp 24–62.

142. ZIMMERMAN, EA, AND NILAVER, G: *The organization of neurosecretory pathways to the hypophysial portal system.* In CAMANNI, F, MÜLLER, EE, (EDS): *Pituitary hyperfunction: Physiopathology and Clinical Aspects.* Raven Press, New York, 1984, pp 1–25.

143. ZIMMERMAN, EA, HOU-YU, A, NILAVER, G, ET AL: *Anatomy of pituitary and extrapituitary vasopressin secretory systems.* In REICHLIN, S (ED): *The Neurohypophysis.* Plenum, New York, 1984, pp 5–34.

144. RANSON, SW: *Some functions of the hypothalamus.* Harvey Lect 32:92–128, 1937.

145. ROBERTSON, GL, AYEINENA, P, ZERBE, RL: *Neurogenic disorders of osmoregulation.* Am J Med 72:339–353, 1982.

146. ROBERTSON, GL, AND BERL, T: *Water metabolism.* In BRENNER, BM, AND RECTOR, FE, JR (EDS): *The Kidney,* ed 3. WB Saunders, Philadelphia, 1985, pp 385–432.

147. RAINE, ABG, ERNE, P, BÜRGISSER, B, MÜLLER, FB, BOLLI, P, BURKART, A, BÜHLER, FR: *Atrial natriuretic peptide and atrial pressure in patients with congestive heart failure.* N Engl J Med 315:533–537, 1986.

148. DILA, CJ, AND PAPPIUS, HM: *Cerebral water and electrolytes.* Arch Neurol 26:85–90, 1972.

149. HAMMOND, DN, MOLL, GW, ROBERTSON, GL, CHELMICKA-SCHORR, E: *Hypodipsic hypernatremia with normal osmoregulation of vasopressin.* N Engl J Med 315:433–436, 1986.

150. RYMER, MM, AND FISHMAN, FA: *Protective adaptation of brain to water intoxication.* Arch Neurol 28:49–57, 1973.

151. ARIEFF, AI, AND GUISADO, R: *Effects on the central nervous system of hypernatremia and hypernatremic states.* Kidney Int 10:104–116, 1976.

152. LAURENO, R: *Central pontine myelinolysis following rapid correction of hypernatremia.* Ann Neurol 13:232–239, 1983.

153. AYUS, JC, ET AL: *Changing concepts in treatment of severe symptomatic hyponatremia.* Am J Med 78:897–906, 1985.

154. STOPA, E, ET AL: *Human brain contains vasopressin and vasoactive intestinal polypeptide neuronal subpopulations in the suprachiasmatic region.* Brain Res 297:159–163, 1984.

Chapter 5

REGULATION OF TSH SECRETION AND ITS DISORDERS

The pituitary-thyroid axis has served neuroendocrinology as the example par excellence of a negative-feedback self-regulatory system.[85,161] This regulation is achieved by the interaction of three groups of hormones: hypothalamic, pituitary, and thyroid. Hypothalamic hormones are thyrotropin-releasing hormone (TRH), which stimulates the synthesis and release of thyrotropin (thyroid-stimulating hormone, TSH); somatostatin, which inhibits TSH secretion; and dopamine, which is also inhibitory. Thyroid-stimulating hormone, in turn, activates iodide uptake, hormonogenesis, and release of the thyroid hormones thyroxine (T_4) and triiodothyronine (T_3). The circulating thyroid hormones exert negative feedback effects on the pituitary to regulate TSH secretion (Fig. 1). In addition, metabolic conversion of T_4 to the more active T_3 takes place in both the pituitary gland and the hypothalamus.

Although this model describes most of the regulatory factors in pituitary-thyroid function, other mechanisms influence the rate of TSH secretion. These include the physical state of thyroid hormones in the blood and the peripheral degradation of TSH, of thyroid hormones, and of TRH. This chapter outlines these mechanisms of control and describes the disorders of TSH secretion in man. A number of reviews document progress in this area.[25,90,93,97,117,137,144,161,163,165,168,184] Abbreviations used are listed below:

TSH   thyroid-stimulating hormone

T_4 thyroxine (3,5,3′,5′-tetraiodothyronine)

T_3 triiodothyronine (3,5,3′-triiodothyronine)

rT_3 reverse T_3 (3,3′,5′-triiodothyronine)

TRH   thyrotropin-releasing hormone

THYROTROPIN

CHEMISTRY

Human pituitary TSH is a glycoprotein of molecular weight 28,000 daltons, secreted by a specific type of basophilic cells of the anterior pituitary gland

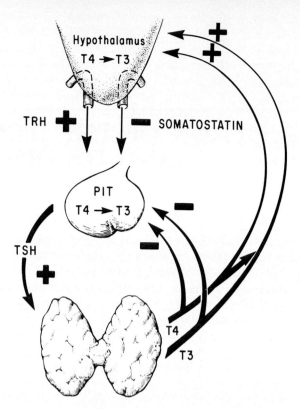

FIGURE 1. This is a diagram of regulation of the hypothalamic-pituitary-thyroid axis. Pituitary TSH secretion is stimulated by TRH and inhibited by somatostatin. The release of the hypothalamic hormones from peptidergic neurons are in turn regulated by bioaminergic neurons. Higher brain centers are involved in relay of stress- and temperature-mediated influences on hypothalamic centers. Thyroid hormones (T_3, T_4) feed back predominantly at the pituitary level but may have effects on hypothalamus. Estrogen facilitates, and growth hormone and glucocorticoids inhibit, pituitary responsiveness to TRH. The dopamine inhibitory component (conveyed by the tuberoinfundibular system) is not illustrated on this figure.

(thyrotrope cells). About 5 percent of adenohypophysial cells are thyrotropes.

TSH consists of two chemical subunits, α and β. The α-subunit, identical to and interchangeable with the α subunit of LH and FSH, is devoid of biologic activity. Determinants of the immunologic and biologic actions of TSH are located in the β-subunit. Circulating TSH is identical to pituitary TSH; small amounts of the β-subunit also are normally secreted into the blood. The TSH molecule contains approximately 16 percent carbohydrate, consisting of three oligosaccharide moieties attached to the peptide by asparagine residues.

The biosynthesis of TSH has been studied in some detail. Subunits of TSH are translated on ribosomes by separate RNAs regulated by genes located on different chromosomes. The subunits are then glycosylated, and disulfide bridges (five in the α-subunit, and six in the β-subunit) are formed. The glycosylated α- and β-subunits are linked and then folded into stable active dimers which are stored in secretory granules for release.[34]

Thyroid-stimulating hormone synthesis and release are stimulated by TRH and inhibited by thyroid hormones. Normal serum levels of TSH in man are less than 8 μU/ml. Thyroid-stimulating hormone circulates unbound in the blood and has a half-life of 50 to 60 minutes. Approximately 10 to 30 percent of total pituitary TSH content is secreted daily.[77]

Circulating TSH is not homogeneous; at least three forms are found, including native TSH, a larger prohormone, and the α-subunit. Circulating levels of the β-subunit may be increased in patients with hypothyroidism and in patients with TSH-secreting tumors.[176] Elevated blood levels of the α-subunit can be found in patients with thyrotropic or gonadotropic[176] tumors.

SECRETORY PATTERN

Thyroid-stimulating hormone is secreted in pulses; highest levels are usually observed during the morning hours from 4 to 8 AM (Fig. 2).[25]

Serum TSH levels rise transiently in the infant immediately after birth, a peak occurring within the first half hour of life.[56] Thyroid-stimulating hormone levels return to baseline adult values within 48 to 72 hours.

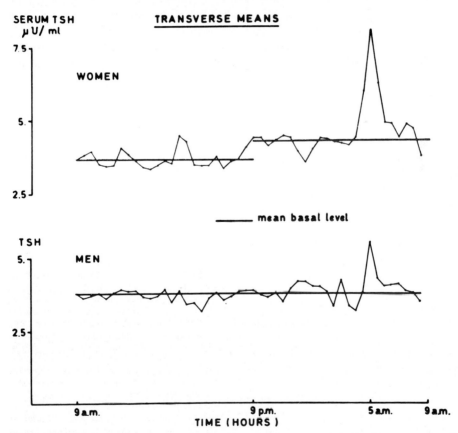

FIGURE 2. Shown here are mean basal levels of plasma TSH throughout the day in women and men. Concentration in blood rises during the night, reaching highest levels in morning hours before awaking. (From Vanhaelst, L, et al: *Circadian variations of serum thyrotropin levels in man.* J Clin Endocrinol Metab 35:479, 1972, with permission.)

PITUITARY-THYROID FEEDBACK

Administration of increasing doses of T_4 to hypothyroid individuals produces a graded suppression of plasma TSH levels. Thyroid hormone concentration in the blood can be viewed as the "controlled variable" in a servosystem. The normal setpoint of pituitary-thyroid function is the resting concentration of plasma thyroid hormone maintained by a specific concentration of TSH (Fig. 3). The secretion of TSH is inversely regulated by the concentration of thyroid hormones in such a way that deviations from the control setpoint lead to appropriate changes in the rate of TSH secretion.[170] Inhibition of TSH secretion follows 15 to 45 minutes after T_3 or T_4 administration.

The pituitary setpoint, or level at which TSH secretion is maintained, is determined by the amounts of TRH, somatostatin, and dopamine secreted by the hypothalamus. The TSH-releasing effects of hypothalamic TRH are immediate; increases in plasma TSH levels follow intravenous (IV) administration of TRH within 2 minutes.[25,58,72,73,76,77,90,193] The effects of TRH administration can be blocked by pretreatment with either T_3 or T_4[193] (Fig. 4). Moderate inhibition, however, can be overcome by subsequent administration of larger doses of TRH. These studies indicate that competitive interaction exists at the pituitary level between TRH and thyroid hormones to determine TSH secretion. TRH stimulation of TSH release does not depend on new protein synthesis, whereas T_3- and T_4-induced inhibitory effects on the pituitary gland do require new protein synthesis. This finding

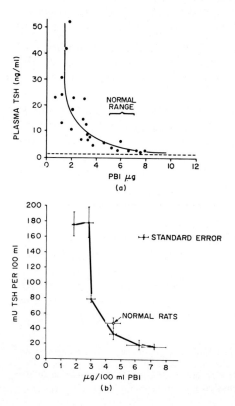

FIGURE 3. Illustrated here is the relationship of plasma TSH to plasma thyroid hormone levels in the human (a) and rat (b). Studies in humans were carried out by replacing six myxedematous patients with successive increments of thyroxine (T_4) at approximately 10-day intervals. Each point represents simultaneous measurement of plasma T_4 and plasma TSH at various times. The studies in rats were done by treating thyroidectomized rats with various doses of thyroxine for two weeks. In other studies using this approach, TSH is seen to be a function of the log of T_4. [(a) is from Reichlin and Utiger,[170] with permission. (b) is from Reichlin, S, et al: *Measurement of TSH in plasma and pituitary of the rat by a radioimmunoassay utilizing bovine TSH: Effect of thyroidectomy on thyroxine replacement.* Endocrinology 87:1022, 1970, with permission.]

REGULATION OF THE PITUITARY GLAND

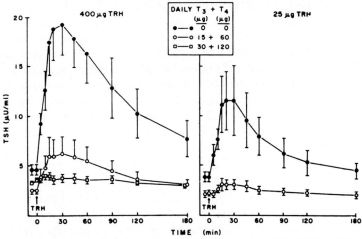

FIGURE 4. Illustrated here are plasma TSH responses to two doses of TRH (400 μg left and 25 μg right) in normal subjects before and after oral administration of small doses of T_3 and T_4. Administration of 15 μg T_3 and 60 μg T_4 for 2 weeks markedly suppressed the TSH response to TRH. (From Snyder, and Utiger,[195] with permission.)

has led a few to postulate that thyroid hormone causes the thyrotrope to produce an inhibitory protein that subsequently interferes with the TSH-releasing effects of TRH. Thyroid hormones bind to nuclear receptors in the thyrotrope. T_3 binds to this nuclear receptor about 10 times more avidly than T_4, making T_3 a more effective suppressor of TSH. After T_4 is transported into anterior pituitary cells, it is rapidly monodeiodinated to T_3.[117] Whether thyroid hormones also regulate TSH levels by effects on hypothalamic TRH secretion is unclear. Intrahypothalamic injections of thyroid hormones cause suppression of TSH secretion in experimental animals, but the possibility that these hormones may reach the anterior pituitary via the portal system has not been excluded, and they may act by stimulating somatostatin secretion.[12]

The remarkable sensitivity of the thyroid hormone feedback system to small changes in plasma levels of thyroid hormones is well documented. Daily administration to normal human volunteers of small doses of T_3 and T_4 (15 μg T_3 and 60 μg T_4 daily for 2 weeks) substantially reduced plasma TSH responses to intravenous TRH, without measurable increase in plasma T_3 or T_4 levels (see Figure 4).[195] These data suggest that the setpoint of control between TRH and thyroid hormones is exquisitely sensitive to thyroid hormone feedback effects within the physiologic range. This delicate setting can be overcome by high doses of TRH. A mild state of hyperthyroxinemia can be maintained for many weeks or months by infusion of high doses of TRH.[105] Increases in plasma T_3 and T_4 levels, as occur in hyperthyroidism, result in refractoriness of the pituitary gland to TRH administration. Even subclinical hyperthyroidism can reduce responsiveness to TRH.

THYROID HORMONE SECRETION

Although thyroid hormones are secreted principally as T_4 with a small amount of T_3, most thyroid hormone tissue activity comes from T_3, formed in peripheral tissues from T_4 by enzymatic degradation. Most T_3 is formed in the liver and kidney. Some T_4 is monodeiodinated to 3,3',5'-triiodothyronine, which is denoted "reverse T_3" and is biologically inactive. The conversion of T_4 to T_3 occurs very rapidly in the pituitary thyrotrope and in the brain, a mechanism that is considered to be important in the feedback regulation of TSH and perhaps TRH secretion. T_4 to T_3 conversion rate, and the activity of the several monodeiodinase enzymes in brain, pituitary gland, and elsewhere are regulated by thyroid state.[104]

Circulating T_3 is more available to cells than T_4 because it is less firmly bound by plasma proteins. T_3 is also more potent than T_4, probably because of its greater avidity for nuclear receptor binding. T_4 must be given at a dose ten times that of T_3 to suppress TSH secretion. An accurate assessment of thyroid state in a patient requires measurement of both plasma T_4 and T_3 and of TSH. The importance of measuring all three substances can be emphasized by a consideration of the hormonal changes that occur in varying degrees of thyroid failure.[117]

> In mild hypothyroidism, T_4 levels are depressed, T_3 levels remain normal and plasma TSH levels are slightly elevated. The TSH response to TRH is slightly increased. In patients with a moderate to severe degree of hypothyroidism (T_4 levels of 4 to 6 μg/dl), T_3 levels often remain within the normal range, TSH levels are increased further and the TRH stimulation test shows an increasingly exaggerated response. Only with extreme hypothyroidism (T_4 less than 2 μg/dl) do the T_3 levels show a decline to approximately 40 percent of normal.

These results suggest that circulating T_4, not T_3, is the principal regulator of TSH secretion, although, as noted above, T_4 acts at the pituitary level mainly via transformation to T_3.

NEURAL REGULATION OF TSH SECRETION

HYPOTHALAMIC CONTROL

Hypothalamic input is essential to normal pituitary-thyroid function. Because disconnection of the pituitary gland from the hypothalamus by stalk section or transplantation decreases pituitary TSH secretion and results in hypothyroidism, it can be concluded that the hypothalamus tonically drives TSH secretion under basal conditions. Nearly normal TSH secretion continues in animals in which a hypothalamic island has been prepared by surgical isolation methods, indicating that only the hypophysiotropic area is essential for maintaining basal secretion.[71] However, cold-induced thyroid activation is blocked in the deafferented preparation, indicating that there is control by remote brain sites as well.

Effects of Hypothalamic Ablation

Lesions placed in the vicinity of the paraventricular nuclei of the rat result in marked decrease in pituitary-thyroid function without major effects on regulation of other pituitary hormones.[135] Although TSH levels are reduced in such animals, the system remains capable of a compensatory increase in TSH secretion following thyroidectomy. Rats with hypothalamic lesions are also more sensitive than are intact controls to the feedback effects of small doses of T_4.[135,136,169] These studies suggest that anterior hypothalamic lesions lower basal TRH secretion and modify, but do not prevent, qualitatively normal secretory responses to alterations in plasma thyroid hormone levels. The hypothalamus thus acts to determine the sensitivity of the pituitary gland to feedback inhibition, presumably by regulating the quantity of TRH that reaches the pituitary gland.

Additional evidence for the importance of the anterior hypothalamic-paraventricular region in TSH control has been shown by the effects of anterior hypothalamic lesions that separate this region from the arcuate nucleus-median eminence area. Such cuts cause an increase in TSH secretion secondary to somatostatin depletion.[208]

Electrical stimulation also has demonstrated sites of TSH regulation.

Plasma TSH levels rise within 5 minutes after hypothalamic stimulation in pentobarbital-anesthetized rats (Fig. 5).[137] The area from which positive responses can be obtained include the anterior hypothalamus and preoptic area; the paraventricular nuclei; and the dorsomedial, ventromedial, and arcuate nuclei (Fig. 6). The largest responses occur with stimulation of the anterior hypothalamus in the vicinity of the paraventricular nuclei. Stimulation of the lateral hypothalamus, thalamus, and mammillary bodies is ineffective. The time course of TSH release induced by electrical stimulation resembles that occurring after intravenous administration of synthetic TRH. In addition, either electrically-induced or TRH-induced TSH release is blocked by pretreatment with T_4 (see Figure 5).[137]

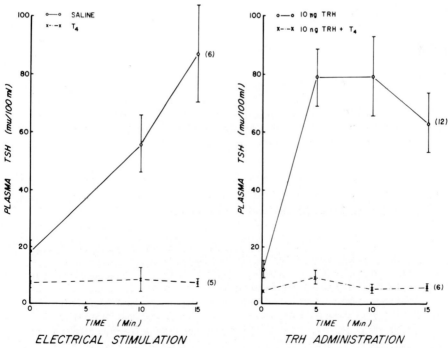

FIGURE 5. Shown here are plasma TSH responses to electrical stimulation (left) and TRH administration (right). Both responses are blocked by prior administration of T_4. (From Martin and Reichlin,[137] with permission.)

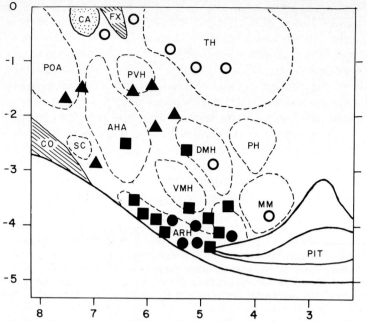

FIGURE 6. Shown here are hypothalamic sites that induced release of TSH after electric stimulation. Solid symbols indicate positive, and open circles negative, responses. The distribution of positive stimulation sites corresponds closely to distribution of TRH (see Figure 5). (From Martin and Reichlin,[137] with permission.)

These results obtained by electrical stimulation correspond to the anatomic distribution of TRH as determined by immunohistochemistry (see below).

Bioassayable TRH activity appears in the portal blood after electrical stimulation of the anterior hypothalamus. Prior T_4 administration had no effect on this response, indicating that the inhibitory action of T_4 is directly on the pituitary gland.[217] However, the direct thyroid hormone effects in regulating TRH secretion have not been characterized adequately.

Thyrotropin-releasing hormone-containing areas of the hypothalamus have been analyzed in detail by immunoassay of microdissected material (Fig. 7),[24] and immunohistochemistry (Fig. 8).

Thyrotropin-releasing hormone is found throughout the classically defined hypophysiotropic area, with the greatest concentrations in the periventricular area. Little is found in the mammillary nucleus, and modest amounts in the medial preoptic area. By immunohistochemical methods the highest concentration is seen to be present in nerve terminals of median eminence; nerve cells of origin containing TRH are located mainly in the anterior periventricular nucleus and the paraventricular nucleus[81,102,118,165] (see Figure 8). Anatomic and electrophysiologic studies support the concept that tuberohypophysial neurons are located over this entire region, although restricted to the medial zone which extends 1.0 to 1.5 mm on either side of the third ventricle (see chapter 2). The extrahypothalamic distribution of TRH and its functional significance are discussed below.

　　　　　　　　　　REGULATION OF THE PITUITARY GLAND

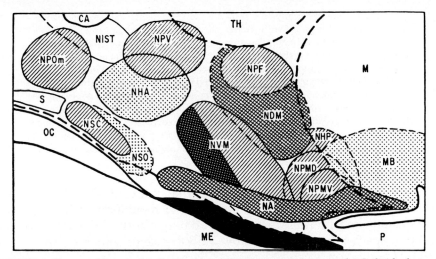

FIGURE 7. Illustrated here is the distribution of TRH in hypothalamic nuclei. Individual punch biopsies of frozen sections (300 μ) of hypothalamus were assayed for TRH content by radioimmunoassay. TRH is widely distributed throughout hypothalamus. Greatest concentrations are shown in black, moderate in diagonal lines and cross-hatch, and least in stippled areas. (From Brownstein,[24] with permission.)

Function of Somatostatin in TSH Regulation

A number of stressful stimuli in the rat cause a rapid reduction in plasma TSH levels,[40,161] a fall similar to that observed in growth hormone (GH) in this species.[185] It has been shown convincingly that TSH inhibition is independent of the pituitary-adrenal system.[42,185]

Several observations indicate that the hypothalamus exerts a direct inhibitory effect on TSH release through somatostatin.

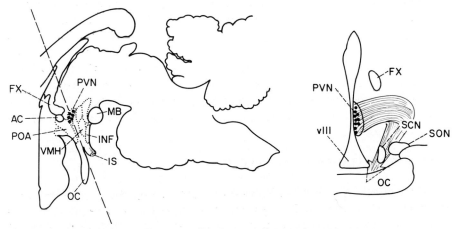

FIGURE 8. Illustrated here is the anatomic distribution of TRH-containing neuronal elements in the human hypothalamus. (From Riskind, P, and Martin, JB: *Functional anatomy of the hypothalamic-anterior pituitary complex.* In DeGroot, L (ed): *Endocrinology,* ed 2. Grune & Stratton, Orlando [in press].)

Somatostatin has clearly been shown to inhibit pituitary TSH secretion. This is true for pituitary cells grown in culture, and for *in vivo* studies in rat and man. Somatostatin infusions in humans suppress TSH levels in hypothyroid patients[126] and block TRH-induced stimulation of TSH secretion.[189,214] The administration of somatostatin antisera *in vivo* results in an increase in basal[7,65] and in TRH[8]-stimulated TSH levels. Hypothalamic lesions placed in the anterior periventricular nuclei to destroy somatostatin cell bodies cause depletion of levels of the peptide in the median eminence which is accompanied by a long-term elevation in blood TSH levels.[208] Hypothalamic somatostatin content is decreased in hypothyroid rats and is restored to normal with T_3 treatment.[12] Exposure of hypothalamic fragments to T_4 stimulates somatostatin secretion.[12] Somatostatin inhibits TRH release from hypothalamic fragments.[80]

It is probable that there is a dual hypothalamic control for TSH regulation similar to that for prolactin and for GH regulation. It is likely that somatostatin is responsible for stress inhibition of both TSH and GH in rats, and that species differ in the relative importance of somatostatin in TSH and GH regulation.

Function of Dopamine in TSH Regulation

Dopamine also exerts a physiologic inhibitory effect on TSH secretion in man.[184] Intravenous dopamine administration lowers TSH levels in normal and hypothyroid subjects and decreases the TSH response to TRH. Dopaminergic agonists such as bromocriptine inhibit TSH secretion in normal human beings, whereas dopaminergic antagonists such as metaclopramide and domperidone increase TSH. Dopamine exerts inhibitory effects on TSH secretion from anterior pituitary cells *in vitro* at concentrations of 10^{-7} M, consistent with the known levels of the biogenic amine measured in the pituitary portal blood. Bromocriptine also inhibits TSH release from TSH hypersecretion owing to defective feedback inhibition.[176]

Other Hormones in TSH Regulation

Other hormones also influence TSH secretion. The C-terminal octapeptide of cholecystokinin is reported to lower basal TSH secretion and to blunt TRH-stimulated TSH secretion in man. It remains to be determined whether this has any physiologic significance. Glucocorticoids exert multiple effects on the hypothalamic-pituitary-thyroid axis.[25] Pharmacologic doses inhibit basal TSH secretion and prevent the TSH response to TRH. Gonadal steroids also affect TSH secretion. The TSH response to TRH is greater in women than in men; estrogens facilitate TSH secretion in the human being.[25]

EXTRAHYPOTHALAMIC CONTROL

Considering the number of observations concerning the role of extrahypothalamic structures in GH, ACTH, and gonadotropin regulation, it is somewhat surprising that so little data are available with respect to the function of these structures in TSH control. Although the medial basal hypothalamus appears capable of maintaining basal TSH secretion, phasic release of TSH—such as occurs in diurnal or circadian rhythms, stress-induced inhibition, and cold-induced release — are probably mediated via extrahypothalamic structures and inputs.

> Physiologic studies (ablation and stimulation) have implicated the habenula,[205] basal ganglia,[33,134] and limbic system (septum, hippocampus, amygdala)[33,127] as possibly influencing pituitary-thyroid activity. The paraventricular nucleus in which TRH neurons are located receives a rich innervation from the locus coeruleus, midbrain raphe, preoptic nucleus, bed nuclei of the stria terminalis, solitary nucleus (afferent nucleus of the vagus nerve), and most — it not all — other hypothalamic nuclei, including the suprachiasmatic, the mediator of circadian rhythms.[118] Through these extensive projections, it is likely that virtually any part of the neuroaxis can influence TRH secretion.

The *pineal gland* has been implicated in thyroid regulation, but findings are contradictory. Melatonin reportedly inhibits pituitary-thyroid function,[171] but at least two studies showed that pinealectomy was without effect on the thyroid.[20,179]

ENVIRONMENTAL FACTORS THAT AFFECT TSH SECRETION

COLD

In most mammals, exposure to cold is followed by thyroid activation. For example, a modest decline in ambient temperature usually causes a prompt, transient, increase in plasma TSH in the rat and in the human newborn.[56] The effect in newborns may be due in part to peripheral circulatory adjustments,[57] but cold-receptor reflexes also appear to play a role in the response. Chronic exposure to cold is followed in most species by thyroid hypertrophy and increased secretion of thyroid hormones. In adult humans, however, it has been extremely difficult to demonstrate cold-induced thyroid activation.

Although it has been demonstrated clearly that pituitary-thyroid function is essential for survival at lowered environmental temperatures in many species, including man, acute release of TSH is probably not an important homeostatic factor.

Acute Cold Exposure

Acute cold-exposure–induced TSH release is triggered by peripheral cold receptors.[168] Thyroid-stimulating hormone release also can be induced in animals by the lowering of core temperature, indicating that inputs from either peripheral or central thermoreceptors may trigger TSH secretion,[5,160] but apparently not in man.[12]

The TSH response to cold is dependent on an intact hypothalamic-pituitary axis; the response is blocked by lesions in the preoptic area or by pretreatment with antibodies to TRH (in the rat).[168] α-Adrenergic blockade also inhibits the TSH response to cold, suggesting that the response is mediated by *central* noradrenergic fibers.[109] *Peripheral* noradrenergic stimulation of brown fat metabolism is the greatest source of cold-induced chemical heat production (in rats).[224] Other adaptive responses to cold exposure, including peripheral vasoconstriction, are also mediated by the peripheral sympathetic nervous system.

Chronic Cold Exposure

There is much less certainty concerning the primary role of the hypothalamic-pituitary-thyroid system in homeostatic responses to prolonged exposure to cold. The bulk of experiments performed in a number of species, including man, have in general failed to show any change in plasma T_4.[168]

> Serum protein bound iodine (PBI) was said to be elevated in residents of Montreal in the wintertime. It has been demonstrated in the rat that TSH and thyroid gland secretion are increased during prolonged exposure to cold, despite low or normal plasma T_4. This response has been attributed to increased utilization, excretion, or degradation of T_4 as part of metabolic adaptation to cold, which includes increased food intake, and it has been proposed that it may be entirely secondary to a decrease in negative-feedback effects on TSH secretion resulting from falling plasma thyroid hormone levels.[168]

The pituitary-thyroid component of adaptation to chronic cold is but one aspect of the larger homeostatic question as to how the thyroid hormones interact with the catecholamines in the regulation of thermogenesis. In the process of adaptation to chronic exposure to cold, activation of nonshivering thermogenesis plays a significant role. Increased heat production in cold-adapted human beings and animals is mainly related to increased catecholamine secretion by both adrenal medulla and noradrenergic sympathetic nerve endings. At the target-tissue level, thyroid hormones probably interact to regulate oxygen consumption and heat production. Thyroidectomy leads to a decreased tissue response to catecholamines, and thyroxine increases catecholamine receptors. These effects fit well the hypothesis of an integrated thyroid-catecholamine mechanism for heat production; increased catecholamine secretion in this instance serving as a compensation for thyroid insufficiency. Conversely, animals deprived of sympathetic-adrenal medullary function by a combination of immunosympathectomy and adrenal demedullation show a greater increase in thyroid function after chronic exposure to cold than do normal animals. Noradrenergic effects likely are exerted through activation of lipolysis of brown fat, an exothermic process.[224]

> There is a higher plasma concentration of T_3 (but not of T_4) in cold-exposed animals. Because T_3 is more active than T_4, increased effective thyroid hormone action is likely after exposure to cold.[25] The rate of peripheral conversion of T_4 to T_3 is increased in cold-adapted animals. T_4 disappears from the circulation more rapidly in normal cold-adapted animals than in normal cold-exposed animals, and exposure to cold leads to increase in concentration of T_3-binding proteins in a number of parenchymal tissues, including kidney and liver. Brown fat is rich in enzymes that convert T_4 to T_3. Inasmuch as cold adaptation is attributable to activation of brown fat, it is possible that cold effects are mediated through this tissue.
> Final proof of hypothalamic-activated TSH release during chronic TRH exposure to cold requires demonstration that TRH synthesis and secretion are enhanced. Increased TRH levels in median eminence interstitial fluid has been demonstrated in cold-exposed rats,[6] and cold-induced TSH release is blocked by anti-TRH-antibody.[168]

REGULATION OF THE PITUITARY GLAND

Stress

Several generations of investigators have concerned themselves with the effects of stress and medical disease on pituitary-thyroid function. This interest began with the earliest descriptions of what is now recognized as thyrotoxicosis "frozen fright" and the supposition, popular at the turn of the century, that this disease was a neurotic disorder. When it was finally shown that Graves' disease is due to the presence of circulating autoantibodies directed against the TSH receptor and that blood levels of TSH are almost always low or absent in this condition, it became evident that hypothalamic-induced TSH hypersecretion could not be the etiologic factor. Interest in the psychosomatic aspects of Graves' disease has now shifted mainly to the possible role of the nervous system in immune modulation, but concern with stress and the thyroid has persisted because modern techniques have shown that abnormalities in thyroid function are common in patients with chronic illnesses that do not directly involve the thyroid. Furthermore, thyroidal changes that sometimes occur in patients with depression and paranoid schizophrenia suggest that psychic factors *can* modify pituitary-thyroid activity.

In experimental animals, virtually all stressful procedures such as starvation, pain, restraint, chemical toxins, and infection lead to *suppression* of thyroid activity.[40,144,161] This is reflected in low blood thyroid hormone and low TSH levels and decreased thyroid gland activity. In the human being, the same response probably also occurs, but it is much more difficult to ascertain because sick people often develop abnormalities in peripheral metabolism and the physical form of the circulating thyroid hormones. The most comon of these abnormalities is termed the *sick euthyroid syndrome.* This topic is reviewed by Engler and Burger[47] and Wartofsky and Burman.[213]

Patients with this syndrome have low blood T_3 levels and, if sufficiently sick, may also show low T_4 (Fig. 9). The main cause of the low blood T_3 is a defect in the mechanism of peripheral conversion of T_4 to T_3, which takes place mainly in the liver. The production rate of T_3 is reduced. Starvation accompanying severe illness may be the most important factor, inasmuch as food restriction alone is sufficient to inhibit T_4 deiodination and to reduce T_3; restoration of carbohydrate to starved individuals reverses the defect, and maintenance of adequate nutrition in severely septic patients prevents the low T_3.[175] In the face of decreased T_4 to T_3 conversion, there is usually an increase in the concentration of reverse T_3 (rT_3) the other product of T_4 metabolism. Starved patients also have reduced pituitary TSH responses to TRH.[17]

In sick euthyroid patients, blood T_4 and T_4 production rate are usually normal or slightly reduced. However, the *free* T_4 level can be elevated significantly, owing mainly to the appearance in blood of a factor, presumably a protein, which displaces T_4 from circulating binding hormones.

Extremely sick patients are likely to have low T_4 blood levels. The free T_4 is markedly elevated, metabolic clearance of hormone markedly accelerated, and total hormone production low normal or low. The marked increase in free T_4 may be the main reason for the fast clearance of hormone from the blood, but increased degradation is also possible because it has been shown that activated circulating leukocytes degrade T_4 briskly.

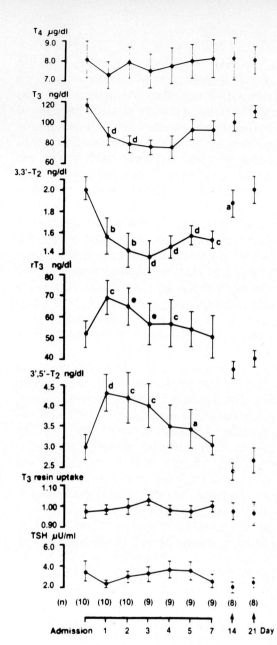

FIGURE 9. Illustrated here are variations in serum T_3, rT_3, 3,3'-diiodothyronine, and 3',5'-diiodothyronine induced by acute myocardial infarction and propranalol. (From Faber J, Kirkegaard C, Lumholtz IB, Siersbaek-Nielson K, Friis T: Acta Endocrinol (Copenh) 94:341, 1980.)

As the name implies, sick euthyroid individuals have no evidence of hypothyroidism despite low blood hormone levels, but evaluation of true thyroid state in very sick people is admittedly difficult, and the clinical differentiation from hypothyroidism can be challenging. Thyrotropin-releasing hormone tests show generally normal or slightly reduced responses.

In attempting to determine whether these patients are truly hypothyroid, a crucial question is whether the normal TSH values observed in such cases is inappropriately low in relation to the low circulating thyroid hormone levels. The introduction of sensitive TSH immunoassays which dif-

REGULATION OF THE PITUITARY GLAND

ferentiate within the normal range now show that TSH values are significantly reduced in sick euthyroids and hence are inappropriately low.[215]
One interpretation, therefore, is that TSH secretion is suppressed and that
the human being behaves like other stressed animals in showing reduced
pituitary-thyroid function. An alternative interpretation is that the high
free T_4 leads to appropriate tissue levels owing to more ready access to the
diffusible T_4 to tissues. In an attempt to resolve this question, measurements of tissue T_3 and T_4 levels have been undertaken. In one series of
studies, tissue T_3 levels were markedly reduced in sick euthyroids, but
tissue T_4 concentrations were normal or elevated.[167] A more recent study
shows that both T_3 and T_4 tissue concentrations are reduced in sick
euthyroids.[229]

Serum T_4 also can be elevated in nonthyroidal disease. During the first
few days of hospitalization, paranoid schizophrenics may show high T_4,[201]
and elevation of T_4 can be produced in monkeys and human beings by large
doses of amphetamines. It also can occur as a transient change in acute
myocardial infarction.[144] It would be reasonable to conclude that these
circumstances stimulate the pituitary-thyroid axis were it not for the fact
that plasma T_3 is usually normal in these patients. Hence, alternative interpretations have been offered, including mobilization of tissue stores of T_4
from the liver.

Slight elevations of T_4 and T_3 also have been reported in several, but
not all, studies of depressed patients. One interpretation of these findings is
that in some individuals depression leads to a mild increase in pituitary-
thyroid function.[124] These speculations are given some credence by the
finding that patients treated chronically with high doses of TRH develop
mild increases in plasma T_3, T_4, and TSH and become subnormally responsive to exogenous test doses of TRH.[105]

The relevance of these observations for psychoneuroendocrinology
lies in the possible role of central neurotransmitter abnormalities in the
pathogenesis of high or low thyroid functional states.

> For completeness it should be mentioned that the "high T_4" syndrome men-
> tioned in the literature refers to patients with high T_4 and normal T_3 owing to
> thyrotoxicosis, a situation that occurs in individuals who are also too sick from an
> associated illness (such as pneumonia) to convert T_4 to T_3 normally.

STEROID HORMONES AND GROWTH HORMONE EFFECTS ON TSH SECRETION

A number of hormones other than those of the thyroid interact with the
secretion of TSH in the human being.

Glucocorticoids

Perhaps the most important nonthyroidal hormones involved in TSH regulation are the glucocorticoids.[25] The earlier literature dealing with the effects of the adrenal cortex on thyroid function indicates that most aspects of
pituitary-thyroid secretion are inhibited by adrenal corticoids. For example,
many patients with Cushing's disease have a blunted TSH response to TRH

and slightly low T_4 levels. Brief or chronic exposure to excessively high levels of cortisol inhibits TSH secretion in the human being. The residual pituitary-thyroid activity observed in patients maximally suppressed with exogenous T_3 is further reduced by treatment with high doses of corticoids. Corticoids apparently act at two loci in bringing about this response. They appear to reduce the sensitivity of the pituitary gland to TRH, presumably by acting at the pituitary level, and probably act to reduce the secretion of TRH, as indicated in a few experiments by the finding of unchanged pituitary sensitivity to TRH in cortisol-suppressed glands. Glucocorticoids also inhibit conversion of T_4 to T_3.

It is important to note that stress-induced TRH suppression is not mediated by concomitant activation of adrenocorticotropin hormone-adrenal secretion, inasmuch as it is observed even in adrenalectomized animals maintained on a constant dose of glucocorticoid.[161]

Estrogenic Hormones

The high incidence of thyroid disease in women as compared with that in men (4:1 for multinodular goiter, 7:1 for Graves' disease, 9:1 for myxedema) has provoked inquiry as to differences in TSH secretory dynamics in relation to sex-hormone status. The early literature is complex and contradictory. This is partly because, in the widely studied rodent model, the estrogen doses usually administered cause inanition with secondary effects on thyroid function. Basal levels of TSH measured by immunoassay do not differ among men, women, and prepubertal children.[77] But the pituitary TSH secretory response to exogenous TRH is greater in women than in men.[73] This effect may be due to estrogen sensitization, inasmuch as pituitary responsiveness is greatest in that phase (late follicular) of the menstrual cycle associated with the highest levels of estradiol,[185] and the response of the pituitary gland in men is enhanced by prior treatment with estrogenic hormone. This is probably due to a direct effect of estrogen on thyrotrope cells analogous to the sensitizing effects on the LH-, growth hormone-, and prolactin-releasing effects of releasing factors. Estrogen effects on the pituitary gland are not necessarily related to the increased incidence of thyroid disorder in women.

Growth Hormone

Synthesis and secretion of GH are affected markedly by thyroid hormones, particularly in hypothyroidism. Contrariwise, GH also modifies the secretion of TSH. In patients with isolated GH deficiency, the administration of GH can cause hypothyroidism.[123,155,178] This effect is due to a decreased pituitary TSH responsiveness to TRH. This phenomenon may be partly responsible for the reduced TSH secretory responses to TRH observed in patients with acromegaly. It has been postulated that the functional GH state of hypopituitary patients determines the magnitude of TSH response.[35] To explain this finding it has been proposed that GH administration may bring about the release of somatostatin by a short-loop feedback mechanism which in turn inhibits pituitary responsiveness to TRH.

DRUGS

Many drugs influence pituitary-thyroid function, most by altering peripheral metabolism of thyroid hormone or by changing the thyroid-hormone-binding characteristics of plasma proteins.[87,225] Secondary changes then occur through activation of normal pituitary-thyroid feedback control. Examples of such phenomena are seen after treatment with phenobarbital, phenytoin, or chlorpromazine, drugs that induce microsomal changes in the liver leading to an increase in the rate of breakdown of T_4. Phenytoin, aspirin, and 2,3-dinitrophenol compete with T_4 for binding to plasma protein. Compensatory decrease in TSH secretion is then required to maintain constancy of the free thyroid hormone level. The conversion of T_4 to T_3 in peripheral tissue is partially blocked by propylthiouracil, but not by other thiouralenes, by effects on tissue monodeiodinase. Amiodarone, iopanic acid, glucocorticoids, and propranalol (but not other β blockers) inhibit T_4 to T_3 conversion, an effect of potential value in the treatment of thyrotoxic crisis. Under carefully controlled conditions in hypothyroid patients maintained on constant T_4 replacement, lowering of plasma T_3 by blockade of conversion of T_4 to T_3 increases TSH secretory response to TRH.

Most drugs that alter pituitary-thyroid function do so by changing elements in the peripheral control system, as noted above, but a few may act more directly on hypothalamic TSH control. In addition to its peripheral effects which cause a decrease in free T_4 concentrations, phenytoin may cause a depression in TSH secretion. The site of action of phenytoin in this response is unknown. In human beings, morphine also is reported to increase slightly TSH secretion, but endogenous opioids do not appear to be important in TSH regulation.[70] In experimental animals, phenobarbital in anesthetic doses will cause a lowering of plasma TSH, a response attributed to interference with the central monoaminergic control of TRH secretion (see below).

THYROTROPIN-RELEASING HORMONE (TRH)

As the first of the hypothalamic hormones to be chemically identified, synthesized, and administered to the human being, thyrotropin-releasing hormone (TRH) was a landmark in neuroendocrinology, which in a sense, legitimized the entire field. That a thyrotropin-hormone-releasing hormone existed was predicted by the experiments of Harris and collaborators in the early 1950s. Early studies by Shibasawa and collaborators, Yamazaki and Guillemin, Reichlin, Schally and collaborators, and Schreiber led to the proof that the hypothalamus contained materials capable of releasing TSH from the pituitary gland and that the effect was blocked by the administration of thyroid hormone.[161,181] Burgus[26] and Bowers[19] and their respective colleagues finally identified this material. The small amount of bioactive material available, even after the extraction of literally hundreds of thousands of hypothalamic fragments—plus the unique structure of the compound—led to a number of false starts; but finally the compound was found to be a tripeptide, pyroglutamyl-histidyl-proline-amide of molecular weight 362 (see chapter 2).

The process by which the structure of TRH was elucidated and its histori-cal setting had a crucial impact on the development of neuropeptide research.[19,27,156,181,212] Efforts to isolate TRH beginning in the early 1960s had led by 1968 to the appreciation that relatively pure TRH preparations contained only three amino acids — glutamine (glutamic acid), histidine, proline — and that the molecule was "protected" by unreactive groups. However, synthetic tripeptides consisting of all possible combinations of these amino acids were devoid of biological activity. During chemical efforts to modify the molecule by acetylation, the terminal glutamic acid of Glu-His-Pro was inadvertently cyclized. This compound possessed some activity, but not as much as the native compound. Addition of an amide group to the carboxyl terminus of pyroGlu-His-Pro led to a compound with activity equal to the native compound. The identity of naturally occurring TRH with the synthetic pyro-Glu-His-Pro-NH$_2$ was then proved by mass spectroscopy.

It is an ironic historical footnote that had TRH not been as small as a tripeptide, it could not have been structurally characterized by this "itera-tive process." Had it not been characterized chemically at the time of the most intense effort at isolation, it is likely that national funding for this type of work would have been terminated and that the later achievements of isolation of LHRH (10 amino acids), somatostatin (14 amino acids), CRH (41 amino acids), and growth hormone-releasing hormone (GHRH) (44 amino acids) would not have been accomplished, or at least would have been postponed for decades.[212]

The synthetic material has been shown to have all the biologic and chemical characteristics of the native material. Synthetic TRH now is widely available for both experimental and clinical use. Thyrotropin-re-leasing hormone has been shown to be active in every mammalian species to which it has been administered.

Chemistry and Structure-Activity Relationships

A number of TRH analogs have been synthesized in an effort to delineate the structural requirements for activity and to devise a molecule that would be either longer acting or block TRH effects. The presence of both the pyroglutamic acid terminus and the terminal amide is crucial to the activity of the compound.

As summarized by Wilber,[218] "the central histidine residue is a critical determinant of TRH activity. The TRH distereoisomeric analogue, in which the histidine residue is optically reversed to the D form, has only 3 percent of the native potency, and photooxidation of the imidazole ring abolished TRH activity completely." Several TRH analogs have greater activity. These include methylation on the 3 position of histidine (eightfold) and methylation or dimethylation of the proline (up to 100 times the native activity). The latter compounds have a higher ratio of CNS to pituitary effects. Many TRH analogs have been synthesized and tested.[59,139]

Biosynthesis of TRH

The earliest studies of TRH biosynthesis suggested that this peptide was formed by a nonribosomal enzymatic mechanism similar to that of the tripeptide glutathione.[169,227] Subsequent work failed to confirm this view;[162,226] most recently, convincing data have shown that TRH is formed, as in the case of other neuropeptides, by processing of a large prohormone. Extracts of frog brain (a rich source of TRH) contain a macromolecule that could be converted to TRH by serial treatment with enzymes.[182] The structures of proTRH in the frog have been deduced by recombinant analysis of mRNA[174] extracted from frog skin, a tissue that contains a relatively large amount of TRH[95] (Fig. 10). In the sequence identified, there are four repeats each coding for TRH, but the entire molecule was not sequenced. Rat hypothalamic proTRH has been fully elucidated.[121]

> The synthesized TRH includes the sequence Glu-His-Pro-Gly. Conversion of this fragment is carried out by well-characterized ribosomal and granular enzymes that cleave this sequence, cyclize the terminal glutamic acid to pyroglutamic acid, and exchange Gly for an NH_2 group.

TRH was the first of the hypophysiotropic peptides to be characterized chemically; its molecular biology the last to be elucidated.

METABOLIC DEGRADATION OF TRH

TRH is subject to rapid enzymatic breakdown in tissues and body fluids, a process that leads to the formation of several fragments (Fig. 11), some of which are active.[90,144,153]

> One such is the cyclized metabolite, histidyl-proline-diketopiperazine (His-Pro-DKP). His-Pro-DKP is pharmacologically active in antagonizing ethanol narcosis and elevating cerebellar cyclic guanosine monophosphate levels. Perhaps more importantly, it has been reported to possess prolactin-inhibitory factor activity, whereas TRH promotes prolactin release, but not all workers confirm this claim. Several observations suggest that His-Pro-DKP also may arise in brain by synthetic

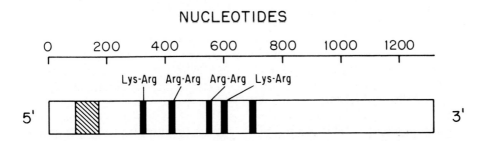

FIGURE 10. Sequence of the preprohormone of mammalian TRH. It contains 5 repeating sequences corresponding to the sequence Lys-Arg-Gln-His-Pro-Gly. Lys-Arg are basic amino acids that form a cleavage site in the prohormone. Gly is exchanged for NH_2 in posttranslational processing. (From Lechan et al,[121] with permission.)

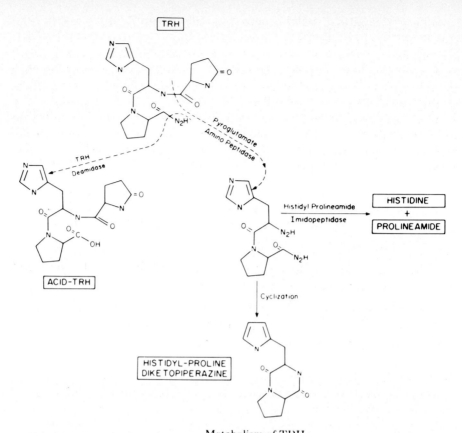

Metabolism of TRH.

FIGURE 11. Shown here are the metabolic degradative pathways of TRH in the central nervous system. The peptide is metabolized to the acid form by a deamidase, and it is also metabolized to a dipeptide (histidylproline) by pyroglutamate aminopeptidase. The resulting dipeptide spontaneously cyclizes to form histidyl-proline diketopiperazine. This compound possesses a number of physiologic activities in neural and pituitary tissue (see text). (From Morley,[144] with permission.)

pathways other than by TRH degradation. Concentration of TRH and His-Pro-DKP show wide variations, both anatomically and embryologically.[116] Thyroid-stimulating hormone has been shown to enhance the formation of His-Pro-DKP, which may provide a means by which the pituitary gland can "feedback" on the hypothalamus to regulate its own function. The deamidated form of TRH (the TRH-free acid) is present in low concentrations in the rat brain, and TRH (but not DKP) disappears from the spinal cord when the raphe nuclei are destroyed.[119]

Extrahypothalamic Distribution

Over 70 percent of total brain TRH is found outside the hypothalamus. Networks of TRH-staining nerve terminals can be observed within motor nuclei of the brainstem and on anterior horn motoneurons of the spinal cord. A bulbospinal TRH pathway with terminals ending in the region of the nucleus tractus solitarius and in the intermediolateral cell column has been described.[120] These observations suggest that TRH may function as a central regulator of the autonomic nervous system. Thyrotropin-releasing hormone receptors in spinal cord are most dense in the dorsal horn, with lesser concentration in the intermediolateral and ventral horn regions.[131]

The pineal gland of the sheep, cow, and pig are said to contain large quantities of TRH, but only low levels are found in the rat pineal gland. After lesions of the "thyrotropic" area of the hypothalamus, there is slight to no reduction in cerebral cortical TRH concentration, suggesting that most (though not necessarily all) of the TRH in extrahypothalamic brain is not synthesized in the hypothalamus.

Thyrotropin-releasing hormone is present in the extrahypothalamic brain of the human fetus and is easily detectable in adult brains, where it appears to be stable postmortem. Thyrotropin-releasing hormone content is reported to be increased in the basal ganglia of patients dying of Huntington's disease (see chapter 18). Substance P and TRH have been shown to coexist in certain cells of the brainstem raphe nuclei with serotonin, together forming a mixed innervation of the cord.[102] It is also distributed in certain peripheral nerves, including the vagal motor fibers, and in epithelial cells of the gut and pancreas.[143]

PHYLOGENETIC DISTRIBUTION

Thyrotropin-releasing hormone is found in all vertebrate species, in all prevertebrates, including the amphioxus, and in an invertebrate, the snail.[92,93,95]

Thyrotropin-releasing hormone has been found in the hypothalamus of chicks, snakes, frogs, tadpoles, and salmon, the values being particularly high in amphibia; the concentration in frogs was 3,620 pg/mg tissue, as compared with that in whole rat hypothalamus, which contains 280 pg/mg (Table 1). Substantial amounts of TRH are found in the neurohypophyses of rats and chickens, and the "pituitary complex" of lower vertebrates such as snakes and frogs, believed to be analogous to the median eminence or neurohypophysis, contains large concentrations of TRH. In the larval lamprey, the pituitary gland contains at least 700 pg/mg, as compared with the whole brain tissue which contains 39 pg/mg. That this material is identical with pyro Glu-His-Pro NH_2 is made evident by identical inhibition curves in immunoassay and by the demonstration of biologic TSH-releasing activity in material extracted from frog and salamander brains. As noted above, the sequence of proTRH was deduced using frog skin mRNA. Thyrotropin-releasing hormone is present in high concentration in frog skin, where it is found in neuroectodermal-derived glands. It is released from the skin by α-adrenergic stimuli. Immunoreactive TRH has even been found in plants. Thyrotropin-releasing hormone is colocalized with serotonin in frog skin poison glands. Interestingly, TRH is also colocalized with serotonin in midbrain raphe nuclei of mammals separated in evolution from amphibia by hundreds of millions of years.

TABLE 1. Distribution of TRH in Brain Areas of Several Species

Species	Hypothalamus (pg/mg)	Cortex (pg/mg)	Brain Stem (pg/mg)
Rat	280	2	5
Chicken	41	2	9
Snake	564	338	283
Tadpole	947	447	303
Human	300		

(Adapted from Jackson, IMD and Reichlin, S.[95])

The functional significance of TRH in lower forms is a matter of conjecture. It is found in the lamprey, which is believed to lack TSH, in the amphioxus, which has no pituitary gland, and in ganglia of the snail, which lacks any endocrine systems homologous with the vertebrate. It has been proposed by Jackson and Reichlin[95] that TRH is a primitive molecule, which has been "co-opted" by the pituitary gland for TSH secretory control. Thus, like many other neuropeptides, TRH is present in very primitive forms and is adapted for specialized functions in higher animals. The function of hypothalamic TRH is now well known in mammals, and it is also capable of stimulating TSH release in birds. However, in poikilotherms there is no evidence that TRH is a TSH-stimulating substance. Thyrotropin-releasing hormone does not induce metamorphosis in frog tadpoles (which are sensitive to TSH or T_4), nor in the Mexican axolotl, and it does not stimulate thyroid function in the lungfish.[91]

METABOLISM

The estimated half-life of circulating TRH in human beings is less than 2 minutes. Approximately 15 percent of injected TRH is rapidly excreted unchanged in the urine. It is rapidly inactivated in plasma by one or more heat-labile enzymes capable of splitting NH_2 from the terminal amide or breaking the peptide bonds of the molecule.

MECHANISMS OF ACTION

Thyrotropin-releasing hormone is effective when administered parenterally and is much less active when given orally. The effects of intravenous TRH are rapid, increases in plasma TSH levels occurring within 1 to 2 minutes in both human beings and animals (Fig. 12).[58,72,73] This is in con-

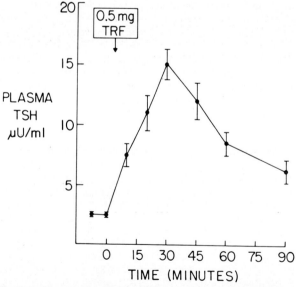

FIGURE 12. Illustrated here is the plasma TSH response to 0.5 mg TRF in normal subjects. The peak of the response occurs at 30 minutes (see also Figure 5). (From Fleischer,[56] with permission.)

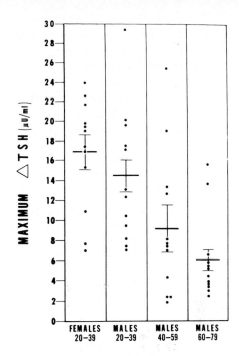

FIGURE 13. Mean increase in plasma TSH after administration of TRH. The response is greater in women than in men and declines in men with increasing age. (From Snyder and Utiger,[193] with permission.)

trast to the negative feedback effects of thyroid hormones on pituitary TSH secretion which require at least 15 minutes to develop *in vitro* and an even longer period *in vivo*. The potency of TRH is indicated by the fact that estimations of the "multiplication factor" of TRH-induced TSH release are of the order of 1 : 100,000; that is, a single molecule of TRH induces release of more than 100,000 molecules of thyroxine through a hormonal cascade mediated by the pituitary TSH response.[135] Averaged TSH responses to TRH in men and women are illustrated in Figure 13.

The prompt action of TRH can be contrasted with the negative feedback effects of thyroid hormone on pituitary TSH secretion, which requires at least 15 minutes to develop *in vitro* and even longer *in vivo*. TRH effects, in contrast to thyroid hormone effects, do not require new protein formation.

Stimulatory effects of TRH are initiated by binding of the TRH molecule to a specific class of receptors on the plasma membrane of the pituitary cell.

Specific receptors for TRH were demonstrated shortly after TRH became available[67,114,115] and have also been extensively studied in a rat tumor line that secretes prolactin and GH.[74,79] Mixed preparations of pituitary cell membranes did not permit differentiation of the receptors of prolactinotropes and thyrotropes, but with homogeneous suspensions of mouse TSH-secreting tumors it has been possible to identify specific TRH receptors on TSH cells.[63] Prolactinotrope and thyrotrope cells probably have different types of receptors and respond differently to steroid hormones.[63] Thyrotropin-releasing hormone action is exerted on the membrane and does not depend on internalization of the peptide. This conclusion is based on the finding that TRH coupled to beads (thus preventing cell entry) is highly effective in stimulating TSH secretion and that the stimulatory effects of TRH are lost as soon as the material is washed from the cell surface. Despite the fact that cell entry is not essential for induction of TSH release, TRH is internalized (probably bound to its receptor) and is presumably inactivated by endocytic phagosomes. Binding is highly hormone specific; neither thyroid hormones nor somatostatin compete for binding on the TRH receptor. Rather, each of these agents can modify, over time, the number of TRH receptors per cell.

TRH action initially was attributed to activation of membrane adenyl-cyclase and formation of cyclic AMP, the classic second messenger demonstrable in most peptide-activated tissues.

Indeed, the effect of TRH in stimulating cyclic AMP production, and the stimulating effect of cyclic AMP on TSH secretion, have been convincingly demonstrated in many studies.[188,219] More recent studies have shown the cyclic AMP accumulation may not occur in some models of TRH-induced TSH release and that certain situations in which intracellular cyclic AMP is increased may not be associated with increased TSH secretion.[64] For these reasons, workers in the field no longer believe that cyclic AMP activation is of primary importance in TRH action; it may be a component of the response when TRH concentrations are sufficiently high.[63]

An alternative mechanism implicates stimulated calcium uptake into cells and mobilization of calcium from intracellular binding sites as essential to TSH release.

TRH treatment is followed almost immediately by an increased inward flux of calcium; the effect of TRH is mimicked by exposure to a calcium ionophore and is abolished or reduced by conducting the experiment in a calcium-free medium or in the presence of a calcium-chelating agent or a calcium-channel blocking agent such as verapamil.[61,62,128]

The most recent work in this area implicates the phosphoinositol system in the response to TRH.[41,107,128,138]

Within seconds of exposure to TRH, the membrane TRH-receptor complex activates membrane-bound phosphodiesterase, which in turn hydrolyses phosphatidylinositol 4,5-biphosphate and phosphatidylinositol 4-phosphate. The activated phospate-containing compounds stimulate protein phosphorylation; this complex presumably becomes the activated second (or third) messenger. Calcium, in this model of TRH action, appears to be essential at least in part because it is required for protein phosphorylation.[41]

This general mechanism appears to hold true for many different tissues, including serotonin release from platelets, lysosomal release from neutrophils, epinephrine secretion from medullary cells, aldosterone secretion from adrenal glomerulosa, insulin release from pancreatic islets, amylase secretion from pancreatic acinar cells, and acetylcholine release from cholinergic nerve endings.[31,54]

THYROTROPIN-RELEASING HORMONE AS A PROLACTIN-RELEASING FACTOR

Thyrotropin-releasing hormone elicits prolactin release both *in vivo* and *in vitro* and follows the same time course and has virtually identical dose/response characteristics. Its role in prolactin-luteotropic hormone regulation is discussed in chapter 7.

THYROTROPIN-RELEASING HORMONE IN BODY FLUIDS

BLOOD

Thyrotropin-releasing hormone was initially detected in hypophysial-portal blood by bioassay.[217] More recently, the peptide has been detectable in portal blood by radioimmunoassay[55] and in the peripheral blood in human beings[130] and in several lower forms including rat, frog, and chicken.[89,91,92]

> Most work has been done with human being and rat, and there are several conflicting estimates of TRH levels in plasma of these species. This is due, in part, to the rapid inactivation of TRH in the blood and also to the low concentrations found. Values have been reported ranging from unmeasurable to as high as 700 pg/ml. Estimates by indirect criteria (production rate and urinary secretion) suggest that normal values in the human being and rat are less than 5 pg/ml. Because of uncertainty about significance of assays, there is controversy about the effects of thyroid status and cold exposure on plasma TRH.

Jackson and collaborators[94] have cautioned that plasma levels should not necessarily be taken as a measure of TRH secretion rate, inasmuch as peripheral turnover shows wide alterations in different thyroid functional states, the turnover being very rapid in hyperthyroidism and low in hypothyroidism. In the newborn rat, blood TSH is relatively high and falls significantly after pancreatectomy.[48]

> In contrast to the situation in mammals in which circulating TRH levels are quite low, high values have been detected in chicken plasma (up to 300 pg/ml); in the leopard frog (but not the bullfrog) the extraordinary level of 150 ng/ml was demonstrated. This material releases TSH from rat pituitary glands *in vivo* and is therefore active. The Mexican axolotl also has exceedingly high plasma TRH levels which appear to have no biologic effects.

URINE

The first report of a TRH-like material in the urine of mammals was that by Shibusawa and associates in 1959. However, subsequent studies by other workers using bioassays failed to confirm these findings.[161] Following the development of the more sensitive radioimmunoassays, TRH was again detected in urine of the human being and rat. The estimation of the precise concentration of TRH in urine has been controversial because of technical problems in the radioimmunoassay.[44,60,99,209] The most comprehensive studies are those of Leppaluoto and colleagues,[122,203,204] who report that urine concentration of TRH in normals is 4.4 ± 1 ng/liter, that it is not altered by states of hyperthyroidism or hypothyroidism but is increased in patients with pancreatitis. These data, together with the results of Engler et al,[48] indicate that the small levels of TRH in urine are derived mainly from the pancreas. Deamido-TRH, a breakdown product of TRH, is also found in urine.[13]

It should be emphasized that because TRH in the blood or urine comes mainly from extrahypothalamic tissues, it is not possible to infer hypothalamic secretion rates from measurements of TRH in blood and urine.

CEREBROSPINAL FLUID

Thyrotropin-releasing hormone has been reported to be present in cerebrospinal fluid, but the precise level is a matter of controversy. Reported concentrations range from 4.9 ± 2.6 pg/ml to 290 pg/ml.[228] We believe that the lower levels are more accurate.

MILK

Immunoreactive TRH has been detected in human and cow's milk. The concentration is higher than in plasma, suggesting that there is a concentrating mechanism or local synthesis. Biologic function as a regulator of the infant's thyroid function has been suggested.[2]

DEVELOPMENTAL ASPECTS

Thyrotropin-releasing hormone is detectable in fetal rat brain as early as the 13th day of gestation. The brain content of TRH increases from 16 pg at 14 days to 388 pg at term (23 days), and over the first 10 days following birth it rises sharply to adult levels. It is also reported that serum TRH rises markedly between the 10th and 35th days of postnatal life. In the human fetus, TRH is detectable as early as 4 1/2 weeks after conception; the highest levels in human fetuses were in the hypothalamus. Significant levels were noted in the cerebellum also in rats. TRH appears in high concentrations in the newborn pancreas and is present for only a few days, gradually declining as hypothalamic levels rise.[48]

EFFECTS OF TRH ON THE BRAIN

In keeping with the view that the extensive neuronal distribution of TRH fibers is physiologically important is the widespread distribution of specific TRH receptors in many parts of the brain. These receptors have been characterized in several regions[28-30,131] and closely resemble the TRH receptors of the anterior pituitary gland.[29,39] The highest concentration in some species is found in the retina and in the nucleus accumbens, an important component of the limbic system. Burt and Taylor[30] point out that there is a wide species difference in receptor concentration in various regions. In some species, receptors in certain regions of the brain are even more numerous than in the anterior pituitary gland.

Also in keeping with the view that TRH is a neurotransmitter is its demonstrated effect on neuronal activity.

> The earliest studies of TRH effects on unit neuronal activity suggested that TRH was an inhibitory neurotransmitter in the cerebral cortex;[43,175,176] other studies indicate that it is an excitatory transmitter on spinal motor neurons.[148,220] In brainstem, TRH produced rhythmic "bursting."[38] Several physiologic effects of TRH (see below) support the idea that TRH is excitatory in most systems. However, because neural responses to TRH appear to show rather early tachyphylaxis, there is some question as to the role of this peptide in regulation of activities over time. Tachyphylaxis has been shown in electrophysiologic studies of neuronal activity[150] and by physiologic studies (see below). For example, the hypertensive response to intrathe-

cal TRH is lost after relatively brief exposure to the peptide.[145] Thyrotropin-releasing hormone receptors in the central nervous system are down-regulated by exposure to a TRH analog.[190]

Among the proposed mechanisms by which TRH acts on the brain is through changes in synthesis and secretion of dopamine.

Evidence supporting this view can be summarized. The rate of release of dopamine from brain slices, the activity of tyrosine hydroxylase (the rate-limiting enzyme of dopamine synthesis),[10] and homovanillic acid (an important degradation product of dopamine[146]) are increased in response to TRH. *In vivo* studies using a push-pull cannula have shown that TRH or a powerful analog, MK-771, increases the release of the dopamine metabolite dihydroxyphenylacetic acid *in vitro*.[147] Not all observations are in agreement with these findings. For example, both increased,[133] and decreased[69] dopamine turnover has been described after TRH administration, and TRH is reported to have no effect on whole brain levels of dopamine or homovanillic acid.

Although the anatomic distribution of TRH and its receptors and several electrophysiologic effects have been well defined, there is a disappointingly large gap between this knowledge and the understanding of TRH physiologic and behavioral effects. This is true for laboratory animals and even more so for the human being.

The best recognized effects of central TRH administration are summarized in and alluded to in several reviews.[157,223] The predominant effects of TRH can be interpreted as being generally excitatory or, as epitomized by Metcalf and Dettman[140] using Hess's term, as ergotropic, that is, central nervous system activating. These ergotropic effects include increased spontaneous motor activity,[221] tremor of the paws,[155,218] arousal from sleep[107] or from hibernation,[199] increased activity of the peripheral sympathetic nervous system (manifested by adrenaline release, tachycardia, hypertension),[22] increased parasympathetic activity leading (in some species) to gastric hypersecretion[209,210] and increased colonic motility,[82,191] increased neuronal activity of the ciliary nerve,[108] tachypnea,[106] antagonism of sedative drugs such as barbiturates and ethanol,[154] potentiation of strychnine-induced seizures,[21] reversal of endorphin effects,[4,206] reversal of neurotensin effects,[151] and reversal of several forms of experimental shock including that of spinal trauma[50-52] and *E. coli* toxemia.[83,84]

Several other neural effects of TRH are less easily categorized. These include inhibition of intake of food[211] and of water,[211] and modification of body temperature.[22] The effects of TRH on body temperature homeostasis are not entirely clearcut because responses are species specific and influenced by ambient temperature. The most consistent effect appears to be that TRH increases core body temperature by increasing sympathetic nervous activity and by shivering (the wet-dog shake seen after intracerebroventricular TRH could be interpreted as being either a shivering response or an antiendorphin effect). However, there must also be an alteration of setpoint, because increase in heat production alone would not significantly alter body temperature. In the rat, TRH reverses the hypothermia induced by intraventricular injection of bombesin.[23] There is an ample anatomic basis for an effect on TRH on body temperature homeostasis inasmuch as

TRH fibers and cell bodies are found in the preoptic area, a region previously recognized as possessing thermoreceptors and being important in the integration of autonomic and endocrine body temperature homeostatic mechanisms (see chapter 11).[159,161]

NEURAL EFFECTS OF TRH IN THE HUMAN BEING

Upon this background of research on neural effects of TRH in animals, we next consider the neural effects of TRH in the human being. The response that has received the most study is its use as a neuroleptic in depression. An extensive literature has accumulated, initially reporting that TRH had antidepressant effects, but later the earlier claims were not confirmed, so most workers now believe that TRH as administered as a single intravenous bolus, or repeatedly as subcutaneous injections, or in massive amounts by mouth is not beneficial.[49,157] An interesting sidelight of these studies is the finding that in approximately one third of patients with classic depression the TSH response to TRH is significantly blunted.[125] Loosen and Prange[125] postulate that blunting is due to excessive endogenous secretion of TRH, and they support this view by citing several reports in which several days of TRH administration led to slight elevation of plasma T_4 and to reduced responsiveness to TRH.[1,196,200] Hypothyroxinemia has been observed in some psychiatrically ill patients.[37,198]

From the perspective of the reports of neural effects of intraventricular injections of TRH in animals, it is important to identify the changes that occur in the human being following central administration. Munsat and collaborators[177] report that intrathecal bolus injections of TRH of 30 μg to 750 μg in 27 patients were followed by a rising sense of warmth reaching the cranium in 30 to 60 minutes in every case. There were shivering in 75 percent, transient hypertension and tachycardia in 50 percent, diaphoresis in 30 percent and nausea in 15 percent. Following 2 to 6 hours of infusions of 3 to 250 μg per hour, wet-dog shakes were observed in 3 of 17 patients. Larger doses of TRH 500 μg twice weekly caused generalized pruritis in 3 of 6 cases. A somewhat similar range of effects followed initiation of chronic infusion, but thereafter the patient became unaware that infusions were continuing (Munsat, personal communication). Several important negative observations were made by this group. In contrast to the response to intravenous TRH, none of the patients described any of the genitourinary symptoms which have been reported. In particular, none of the patients reported previously recognized genitourinary symptoms — a sense of urinary urgency,[16,177] sense of impending orgasm,[68] erotic vaginal feeling.[15] Genitourinary symptoms must therefore arise from peripheral effects of TRH. In contrast to the response in experimental animals, none of the patients complained of diarrhea. Hypertensive responses appear to be more intense and more frequent after central injection than after peripheral injection, thus supporting the view that there is an important central component in this response. The blood pressure response to intravenous TRH is further considered by Laloga and coworkers[115] and Borowski and colleagues.[16]

Thus, in comparison with the effects so far reported in animals, signs of centrally mediated sympathetic activation were the ones most likely to occur in the human being. The finding that these effects wore off over a few days suggest that tachyphylaxis occurs in the human, as has been reported for motor activation measures in the rat.

Any discussion of the neural actions of TRH should consider the possible effects of its metabolic degradation products, deamido TRH (TRH acid), and diketopiperazine (DKP).[9,14,153] Acid TRH has been shown to be inactive in all systems in which TRH is active, except for the induction of "wet-dog shakes."[153] Diketopiperazine is formed as a cyclic dipeptide from the degradation peptide histidyl-proline. The studies of Jackson and colleagues strongly suggest that TRH breakdown is not the principal source of DKP in the brain: TRH and DKP appear at markedly different rates during embryologic development,[116] and destruction of the spinal TRH system by injection of 5–7-dihydroxytryptamine (which destroys the cocontained serotoninergic system) leads to TRH depletion with no change in spinal DKP concentration.[119] Nevertheless, DKP may be an important neuromodulator in its own right. Actions of DKP and TRH have been compared in a number of systems.[153] Diketopiperazine is more potent than TRH in decreasing sleep time and in reversing ethanol narcosis. Like TRH, DKP causes hypothermia in rats, reverses naloxone-induced morphine withdrawal behaviors, inhibits eating, and stimulates motor activity. The possibility thus arises that many, if not all, TRH effects are mediated by its degradation product. However, TRH receptors in brain do not cross-react with DKP, and it has been difficult thus far to demonstrate DKP receptors in neural tissue.[153]

ROLE OF NEUROTRANSMITTERS IN REGULATION OF TSH SECRETION

The principal systems that influence tuberoinfundibular function include the bioamine neurotransmitters (norepinephrine, serotonin, dopamine, histamine, epinephrine), GABA, acetylcholine, and the neuropeptides.[103,109,110,144,168,192,199] Attempts to elucidate the role of specific neurotransmitters in regulation of TSH secretion have often given confusing and contradictory results because neuronal inputs into the hypothalamus are heterogenous and because either stimulatory or inhibitory hypophysiotropic factors may be activated by particular agonists or antagonists. Best established of the neurotransmitter effects is that of norepinephrine. α-Adrenergic agonists injected systemically or into the third ventricle stimulate TSH release in rats, and α-antagonists or catecholamine depletion block TSH secretion in response to cold. Amphetamine, a centrally acting adrenergic agent, elevates plasma thyroxine. In several experiments, norepinephrine has been shown to stimulate TRH release from hypothalamic preparations *in vitro*. However, efforts to show an effect in the human of α-agonists and α-antagonists have been generally inconclusive. Dopamine exerts a direct inhibitory effect on the pituitary gland as shown by the administration of dopamine and analogs, which inhibit responses to TRH. Domperidone (a peripheral-acting dopamine antagonist) stimulates TSH secretion. In addition to this direct pituitary effect, there is an indication that central dopamine inhibits TRH secretion as well. It is likely that dopamine and TRH interact in a negative-feedback loop at one or more levels of the central nervous system. In several studies, dopamine added directly to hypothalamic preparations reportedly releases somatostatin (which would thus inhibit TSH secretion), but not all workers have confirmed this observation.

In the field of neurotransmitter regulation of TSH secretion, the effect of the serotonin system is particularly controversial. Both increased and decreased TSH levels are reported to follow procedures that increase central serotonin activity. Similarly conflicting are the results using serotonin antagonists. Efforts to show serotonergic control of TSH secretion in human beings are inconclusive. Histamine reportedly increases TRH secretion in the rat,[103] but studies in the human being are contradictory.

Morphine and other opiates inhibit TSH secretion in the rat and mouse. For example, the codeine-blocked mouse has low thyroid function and was one of the first effective bioassay preparations used to demonstrate TRH in hypothalamic extracts. Naltrexone, an opiate antagonist, blunts the severity of stress-induced TSH suppression. This documentation of opioid control of TSH secretion in animals notwithstanding, evidence that administration of morphine or of the morphine antagonist, naloxone, influences TSH secretion in human beings is not convincing.[70] A number of other peptides has been reported to influence TSH secretion in the rat. These include neurotensin, vasoactive intestinal polypeptide (VIP), cholecystokinin, bombesin, oxytocin, vasopressin, and substance P. Of these, only bombesin has been adequately studied in human beings and has been shown to have no effect on pituitary-thyroid function. However, adequate studies of the function of the other putative regulatory peptides have not been carried out in human beings, and until suitable specific peptide antagonists become available it will not be possible to determine their physiologic role in pituitary-thyroid regulation.

Because GABA suppresses somatostatin release *in vitro*, it would have been predicted that GABA administration to rats would increase TSH release. In fact, GABA suppresses TSH secretion in the rat. It is likely, therefore, that GABA also suppresses the secretion of TRH. In human volunteers, administration of several benzodiazepines brought about a slight inhibition of basal·TSH secretion.[201] Inasmuch as this class of neuroactive drugs act in part by potentiating GABA at the GABA receptor, it appears likely that in human beings, as in rats, GABA inhibits TRH secretion.

It is disappointing to acknowledge that despite more than two decades of study of neuropharmacologic control of TSH secretion, an unambiguous picture of the neurotransmitter control of its regulator hypophysiotropic neurons has not emerged.

CLINICAL USES

The availability of TRH for clinical studies has resulted in extensive documentation of its use in human beings. Details of testing procedures are given in chapter 15.

Response to TRH: Normals and Thyroid Disease

Intravenous administration of TRH in doses ranging from 10 to 500 μg results in a rapid release of TSH with a peak response at 15 to 30 minutes.[58,72,73,76,182,193] This response is followed by marked increases in T_3 and marginal increases in T_4 2 to 4 hours later. Women tend to have greater responses than men, an effect which appears to be due to estrogen sensitization of the pituitary gland (see Figure 13).[183] Synthetic TRH is also effective when administered orally, but much larger doses are required. Several acute but minor side effects have been noted after rapid intravenous administration which do not occur with administration over a 3- to 5-minute interval. The most common are facial flushing, urinary urgency, and occasionally slight nausea. These are transient effects, and no serious short-term or long-term consequences of TRH administration have been reported. Because about 40 percent of cases develop transient hypertension (up to 40 mm diastolic and systolic), and a much smaller proportion have a slight decline in blood pressure, it is advised that the subject lie supine for 15 minutes after the test dose. The degree of the plasma TSH response to TRH depends upon thyroid state, as might be predicted from the known interaction of TRH and thyroid hormones at the pituitary level.

Primary hypothyroidism results in an exaggerated TSH response in more than 70 percent of cases.[194,210] Subjects with hyperthyroidism, however, show no, or a markedly attenuated, response in more than 95 percent of cases (Fig. 14).[4,58,194] This suppression lasts for several weeks after ade-

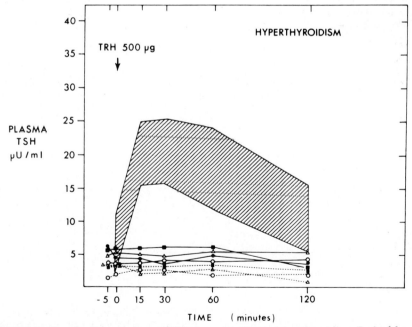

FIGURE 14. Illustrated here is plasma TSH response to TRH in hyperthyroidism. Each of the seven patients failed to release TSH. The shaded area represents the range of responses in a group of normal subjects. (Modified from Gaul, C, et al: *Administration of thyrotropin release hormone (TRH) as a clinical test for pituitary thyrotropin reserve.* Revista de Investagacion Clinica 24:35, 1972.)

quate treatment of the hyperthyroid state. Even minor degrees of hyperthyroidism will block pituitary response.[195] Many patients with "euthyroid" Graves' disease, for example, also fail to respond to exogenous TRH, presumably because their thyroid function is above the upper limit of normal. It is in the evaluation of mild degrees of thyrotoxicosis that TRH testing has achieved its greatest practical utility. It can be assumed confidently that preservation of TSH responsiveness to TRH will exclude thyrotoxicosis in 95 percent of patients. The use of TRH in diagnosis of hypothalamic hypothyroidism is discussed below.

It would be anticipated that patients with TSH deficiency owing to intrinsic pituitary disease would not respond to TRH, whereas patients with TSH deficiency owing to hypothalamic failure would (Figs. 15 and 16). This generalization has proved true in some groups of patients, as in children with idiopathic hypopituitarism, but there is a degree of overlap of responses in hypothalamic-pituitary syndromes, and a few normal individuals may have minimal TSH secretory responses to TRH even in the absence of evident pituitary disease. An appreciable number of normal persons (as much as 15 percent), particularly older men, have TSH responses to TRH of only 2 or 3 mIU/ml, which is in the same range of response as in most patients with intrinsic pituitary disease,[194] but decreased TRH responsiveness in older men has not been observed in all studies.[75] For this reason, preservation of TSH responsiveness in the so-called normal range is not absolute proof that the pituitary gland is normal. Diagnosis of "hypothalamic" hypothyroidism on the basis of retained TRH responsiveness in a TSH-deficient patient alone is insufficient. One must consider the entire clinical picture, including x-ray studies, in making this diagnosis. However, persistent failure of pituitary response in the presence of hypothyroidism is almost certain evidence of intrinsic pituitary failure. As noted in chapter 8, TRH is useful in evaluating patients with acromegaly, and persistence of the paradoxical GH response indicates residual abnormal tissue, even if basal levels of GH are normal. The application of TRH tests for diagnosis of prolactinoma are summarized in chapter 7.

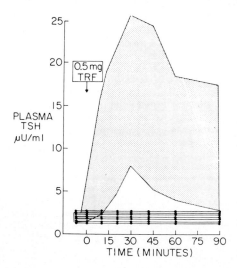

FIGURE 15. Illustrated here is absence of TSH response to TRF in patients with panhypopituitarism secondary to pituitary infarction (Sheehan's syndrome). The shaded area represents the range of responses in a group of normal subjects. (From Fleischer, N, et al,[58] with permission.)

REGULATION OF THE PITUITARY GLAND

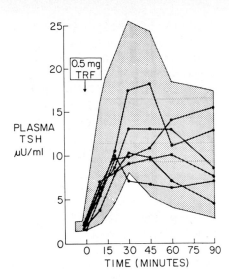

FIGURE 16. Shown here is the normal plasma TSH response to TRF in six patients with idiopathic panhypopituitarism. The finding of TSH release of TRF implicates the hypothalamus as the cause of TSH insufficiency owing to endogenous TRF deficiency. The shaded area represents the range of responses in a group of normal subjects. (From Fleischer, N, et al,[58] with permission.)

Other Factors that Influence TRH Response

A number of other factors that influence the plasma TSH response to TRH are summarized in Table 2.

THERAPEUTIC TRIALS OF TRH IN NEUROLOGIC DISORDER

The use of TRH as a therapeutic agent in human beings was proposed by Sobue and colleagues,[197] who in 1980 reported that intravenous injections of large doses of the peptide produced transient improvement in nystagmus and ataxia in patients with spinocerebellar degeneration. This observation led Engel and colleagues[45] to study the effect of intravenous (IV) TRH in patients with amyotrophic lateral sclerosis (ALS). Transient improvement in several measures of muscle function was reported. Several groups of workers have attempted to repeat this work with some reporting no benefit, and others moderate benefit.[32,46,66,86,142,202] At best, the pace of functional loss has been slowed, but there have been no cures.

One of the rationales underlying the use of TRH in ALS was the finding that cerebrospinal fluid (CSF) TRH levels were reduced in ALS,[45] but subsequent work has shown that CSF levels of TRH in patients with ALS are indistinguishable from normal.[145] Direct TRH assays of spinal cord

TABLE 2. Factors that Influence TRH-induced TSH Release

Factors that Increase	Factors that Decrease
1. Sex—greater response in females (during luteal phase of cycle) 2. Hypothyroidism 3. Estrogen Administration to Men 4. Renal Failure	1. Age—decreased response in elderly 2. Hyperthyroidism 3. Euthyroid Graves' Disease 4. L-dopa 5. Bromocriptine 6. Adrenal Steroids—Cushing's Disease 7. Somatostatin

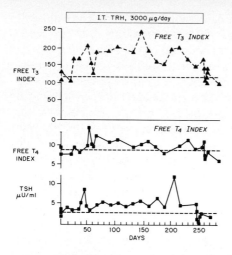

FIGURE 17. Sustained increase in serum T_3, T_4, and TSH follow prolonged infusion of TRH (3000 $\mu g/24$ hr) by intrathecal injection (From Kaplan et al,[105] with permission.)

have given contradictory findings; one group has reported a modest decrease,[141] but others have reported no difference from the cords of patients dying of nonneurologic disease. A potential source of error in this work is the great variability in TRH content from region to region in spinal cord. Increased His-Pro-DKP concentration has been reported,[98] a finding that may implicate abnormalities in TRH depletion (see above).

Owing to the blood-brain barrier, only a small fraction of TRH injected systematically can be expected to reach the brain or CSF. To circumvent this problem, Munsat and colleagues[145] carried out trials of intrathecal therapy with TRH, a procedure that exposes the nervous system to extremely high TRH concentrations. Several patients reportedly showed improvement in some measures of motor function, but the results of double-blind crossover studies have not as yet been reported. A problem that needs to be resolved with either intravenous or intrathecal use of peptides is the defining of the appropriate parameters for administration of peptide, because tachyphylaxis may occur in response to repeated doses. Constant infusion of TRH into the intrathecal space causes a sustained increase in serum TSH, T_3, and T_4 (Fig. 17).

Thyrotropin-releasing hormone is also being tested as an adjunct to treatment of shock in sepsis, and spinal cord shock following spinal cord trauma.[50-52,83,84] Experimental studies have indicated that parenteral administration of the peptide improves the recovery rate of both preparations. Because TRH is distributed to the cells of origin of the sympathetic nervous system (lower-cervical–upper thoracic segments) and is known to elevate blood pressure when given IV or intrathecally, it is reasonable to speculate that the beneficial effect of this peptide in shock is due to central stimulation of the sympathetic nervous system. There is evidence in rats to indicate that TRH raises blood pressure by stimulating vasopressin release.[111]

EVALUATION OF TSH SECRETION

As noted below, it is rare that the physician has to evaluate TSH hypersecretion. However, hypothyroidism is relatively common, and the differen-

REGULATION OF THE PITUITARY GLAND

tial diagnosis between primary thyroid failure (primary hypothyroidism), TSH deficiency due to intrinsic pituitary disease (secondary hypothyroidism), and TSH deficiency caused by hypothalamic TRH deficiency (tertiary hypothyroidism) often must be made. Intrinsic thyroid disease is the most common, and hypothalamic disease, the least common, of the three. Aside from clinical features which may suggest the diagnosis of intrinsic thyroid disease such as goiter, evidence of thyroiditis, and prior thyroidectomy or radioiodine treatment, more than 90 percent of patients with intrinsic thyroid insufficiency have elevated levels of plasma immunoassayable TSH (normal level is 1 to 8 mIU/ml). Clinical and laboratory evidence of hypothyroidism (plasma T_4 levels less than 5 μg/dl, plasma T_3 levels less than 80 ng/ml, in association with normal plasma thyroid hormone-binding proteins), if present in association with low or normal TSH levels, is highly suggestive of TSH failure. Usually, patients with pituitary or hypothalamic disorders that cause hypothyroidism have low TSH levels, and the differential diagnosis is made between these two entities by overall consideration of the clinical picture and by use of the TRH stimulation test (see chapter 15).

Clinical tests of pituitary-thyroid function have generally conformed to the widely accepted theory of control of the pituitary-thyroid axis: TSH levels are high in primary thyroid disease and low in pituitary or hypothalamic disease. The TRH test is of greatest value in the diagnosis of hyperthyroidism, is useful in a minority of cases with primary thyroid failure who do not have elevated plasma TSH levels, and helps differentiate between pituitary and hypothalamic hypothyroidism (see chapter 15 for clinical use of the TRH test).

Several investigators have called attention to the paradoxical finding that a few patients with hypothyroidism caused by pituitary or hypothalamic disease have high normal plasma TSH levels. The most likely explanation is the secretion of a biologically inactive molecule with retained immunoreactivity. These cases also may be caused by a combination of intrinsic thyroid disease and pituitary failure, neither of which alone would have been capable of causing clinical disease. This peculiar syndrome should be borne in mind in the evaluation of hypothyroidism with normal levels of TSH.

HYPOTHALAMIC-PITUITARY-THYROID DISEASE

Modifications in TSH secretion observed in clinical disease of the pituitary gland and thyroid generally conform to predictions based on classic formulations of pituitary-thyroid negative-feedback regulation, with a few paradoxical exceptions.

PRIMARY HYPOTHYROIDISM

Effects on the pituitary gland of long-standing thyroid gland insufficiency were recognized long before the modern concept of pituitary-thyroid feedback or even the understanding of the function of the thyroid gland was developed. In 1847, Niépce reported the autopsy finding of an enlarged pituitary gland in cretins. In more recent times, a number of authors noted enlargement of the pituitary fossa in long-standing hypothyroidism. On superficial study, patients may appear to have a tumor of the pituitary gland with secondary thyroid failure. In cases of this type, elevation of plasma TSH levels in combination with *hypo*thyroidism provides the clue to the underlying pathophysiology. In one series, 10 of 14 cases had evidence of field defects by Goldman isopter perimetry, ranging from early chiasmal compression to bitemporal hemianopsia. Central vision was more commonly affected than was peripheral vision. The sella turcica was enlarged in most cases.[224] Pituitary TSH-secreting tumors rarely may arise in the human being secondary to prolonged hypothyroidism,[88] as is common in the hypothyroid mouse (Furth thyrotropic tumor).

All primary diseases of the thyroid gland with thyroid failure cause an increase in plasma TSH levels. This is true after thyroidectomy, thyroiditis, and treatment with radioactive iodine. Incipient or subclinical thyroid failure, seen, for example, during the evolution of Hashimoto's disease or postradiation thyroiditis, may be followed by an increase in plasma TSH, and it is accentuated when thyroid secretion is reduced further by administration of inorganic iodide in therapeutic doses.[213] Even in normal individuals, the slight lowering of plasma TSH caused by iodide administration may sensitize the pituitary to TRH. In patients with marginal thyroid-secretion defects, plasma TSH levels may be elevated disproportionately in relationship to T_3 hormone levels, suggesting a compensatory stage of thyroid failure in which adequate thyroid function is maintained only by TSH hypersecretion.[117] This phenomenon may account for the disproportionate elevation in TSH levels in thyrotoxic patients after treatment. PRL secretion can also be induced by thyroid insufficiency and, rarely, precocious puberty (see chapters 7 and 9).

Secondary Hypothyroidism

Failure of pituitary TSH secretion causes *secondary* hypothyroidism. As predicted from the concept of negative-feedback control of the pituitary-thyroid axis, most such patients have low or unmeasurable TSH levels in blood and usually do not respond to TRH injection (see Figure 15).[194] A few patients with established pituitary lesions demonstrate an exaggerated response to TRH. It is proposed that in such cases both suprasellar and pituitary involvement has led to a reduction in TRH, as well as to thyrotrope-cell damage, but this has not been proved. Euthyroid acromegalic patients frequently fail to show a normal TSH response to TRH (see above). Paradoxically, a few patients with pituitary lesions and hypothyroidism have been found to have TSH in the blood within the normal or even high range. Faglia and colleagues[53] explain this phenomenon by postulating secretion of an abnormal TSH.

Isolated thyrotropin deficiency with TRH unresponsiveness has been reported, suggesting that, rarely, there may be a true failure of thyrotropes to develop.

HYPOTHALAMIC HYPOTHYROIDISM (TERTIARY HYPOTHYROIDISM)

The introduction of TRH into clinical medicine made it possible to evaluate pituitary secretory reserve in hypothyroid patients with low plasma TSH levels, commonly considered to be due to pituitary insufficiency. A number of patients with secondary hypothyroidism ("thyrotropic failure") now have been shown to have normal or even supranormal responses to exogenous TRH (Fig. 16).[76] Because the pituitary gland can function normally in these individuals, it has been inferred that the defect is due to failure of stimulation by the hypothalamus (discussed above as to limitations in interpretation of the TRH test).

The relative incidence of hypothalamic hypothyroidism as a cause of thyrotropin failure depends upon the population studied. The majority of children suffering from "idiopathic" partial or total hypopituitarism have TRH-responsive pituitary glands.[36] This important observation indicates that idiopathic dwarfism is due in most instances to an intrinsic hypothalamic disorder, a surmise confirmed by use of GHRH (see chapter 8).

In sporadic cases of "hypothalamic hypothyroidism," hypothalamic failure may be due to hypothalamic tumors, inflammation, pituitary stalk section, trauma, in Sheehan's syndrome (rarely, then attributed to hypothalamic damage or stalk infarction), and also occasionally either as a single defect or in association with other pituitary defects. It may be anticipated that a group of such cases will prove to have hypophysiotropic neuron failure and analogous to the atrophy of the supraoptic-hypophysial neurons seen in human cases of idiopathic DI.

Most patients with hypothalamic disease of various types have shown normal or exaggerated TSH responses to administration of TRH, indicating that the primary pathophysiologic mechanism may be a failure to synthesize or to release endogenous TRH. It was proposed at one time that hypothalamic hypothyroid patients characteristically showed a delayed peak response (and thus resemble patients with primary hypothyroidism), but in the series reported by Snyder and Utiger,[193,196] several patients with presumed intrinsic pituitary disease showed a delayed response to TRH. Furthermore, the state of GH secretion was considered by Cobb and colleagues[35] to be the major determinant of TSH response in hypothalamic-pituitary disease. High and prolonged responses occurred in those with low GH.

Criteria for the diagnosis of hypothalamic hypothyroidism are (1) low thyroid function, (2) inappropriately low or undectable plasma TSH levels, (3) a normal or exaggerated response to exogenous TRH, and (4) anatomic evidence of hypothalamic or pituitary stalk disease. A few patients with intrinsic pituitary disease may show TSH responses in the low normal range, and for this reason, the criteria listed above cannot be taken as absolutely diagnostic. The full clinical picture must be considered.

An apparent exception to the rule that TSH secretion is dependent upon an intact hypothalamus is the finding of normal pituitary-thyroid function in anencephalic infants. The minimal brain tissue found in such infants synthesizes TRH when grown in tissue culture, a finding that suggests that some TRH has been available to the developing pituitary gland.

Hyperthyroidism

Although the overwhelming proportion of patients with thyrotoxicosis suffer from primary thyroid disease (Graves' disease, toxic nodular goiter, thyroiditis), there have been at least 46 published cases of primary TSH-secreting tumors of the pituitary gland, and there are a similar number of patients with TSH hypersecretion due to a defect in thyroid hormone feedback control of the pituitary gland.[176] Cases of these types, though exceedingly rare, are detected by documenting inappropriate elevation of TSH in the blood in relation to the level of thyroid hormones. In primary hyperthyroidism, TSH levels would uniformly be below 0.5 mIU/ml, whereas in either of the TSH hypersecretory syndromes the values would be much higher, that is, more than 1.6 mIU/ml and usually much higher. It should be recognized that the routine TSH assays available in most laboratories are not reliable below the level of 2.5 mIU/ml, so a few reported cases of TSH-secreting adenomas might be missed if TSH screening is carried out routinely. One third of reported cases of TSH-secreting adenomas had TSH values below 10 mIU/ml.

TSH-secreting Adenomas. In the 46 reported cases reviewed by Ridgway,[176] all but 3 had thyrotoxicosis, and none had the typical features of infiltrative exopthalmopathy (save for one case who had proptosis owing to tumor involvement of the orbit). Nor did any case have positive Graves' immunoglobulins. About one third of cases had associated acromegaly or hyperprolactinemia. The tumors tended to be quite large at the time of discovery. They occurred in the range 17 to 64 years of age and were approximately equally divided between men and women. None of the patients studied was shown to suppress TSH by exogenous thyroid hormone (although we have seen one case studied by Biedleman, unpublished, who did suppress), and none of the reported cases has shown a TSH response to TRH injection. One of the interesting clues to the diagnosis of TSH-secreting tumors is the inappropriately elevated alpha chain which is usually higher than the TSH β-subunit level.

Although unresponsive to the suppressive effects of thyroid hormone, the majority of TSH-secreting tumors are inhibited by glucocorticoids but not by treatment with bromocriptine (a dopamine agonist).

TSH Hypersecretion due to Pituitary Resistance to Thyroid Hormones. A small number of cases have been described who display thyroid hormone resistance,[176,225] more commonly of all tissues, and less commonly isolated to the pituitary gland. When thyroid hormone resistance is restricted to the pituitary gland, the thyroid gland is stimulated, thyroid-stimulating hormone levels are inappropriately elevated, and the clinical syndrome of thyrotoxicosis ensues. These patients do not display the infiltrative eye signs of Graves' disease, often are found in familial groupings linked as an autosomal dominant trait, and may be quite resistant to antithyroid therapy. They can be differentiated from the primary tumor syndrome by the lack of pituitary tumor (as noted on computerized axial tomography scan), by normal ratios of the α- and β-subunit of TSH, and by their suppression with bromocriptine. Although both syndromes of primary TSH hypersecretion are rare, it is the routine in our clinic to measure TSH levels at least once in every patient being treated for thyrotoxicosis who does not manifest the classical eye signs of Graves' disease and who does not have a nodular goiter.

TRH Hypersecretion. It also has been postulated that TRH hypersecretion might be responsible for TSH hypersecretion, but in the absence of specific measurements of TRH, this hypothesis is only conjectural. That prolonged TRH exposure can cause hyperthyroidism is suggested by the work of Kaplan and colleagues.[105] Three patients suffering from ALS who were given TRH by chronic intrathecal infusion at the rate of 3000 μg per day developed mild persisting elevations of T_4, T_3, and TSH above their baseline, but values remained in the "normal" range.

REFERENCES

1. AHUJA, S, BAUMGARTEN, S, OEFF, K: *Repetitive intravenous TRH-stimulations at short intervals in euthyroid and hypothyroid subjects.* Acta Endocrinol 93:20–24, 1980.
2. AMARANT, TM, FRIDKIN, M, KOCH, Y: *Luteinizing hormone-releasing hormone and thyrotropin-releasing hormone in human and bovine milk.* Eur J Biochem 127:647–650, 1982.
3. AMIR, S, HAREL, M, SCHACHAR, S: *Thyrotropin-releasing hormone (TRH) improves survival in anaphylactic shock: A central effect mediated by the sympatho-adrenomedullary β-adrenoceptive system.* Brain Res 298:219–224, 1984.
4. ANDERSON, MS, BOWERS, CY, KASTIN, AJ, ET AL: *Synthetic thyrotropin releasing hormone.* N Engl J Med 285:1279–1283, 1971.
5. ANDERSSON, B: *Hypothalamic temperature and thyroid activity.* In *Brain-Thyroid Relationships.* Little, Brown & Co, Boston, 1964, pp 35–50.
6. ARANCIBIA, S, TAPIA-ARANCIBIA, L, ASSENMACHER, I, ET AL: *Direct evidence of short-term cold-induced TRH release in the median eminence.* Neuroendocrinology 37:225–228, 1983.
7. ARIMURA, A, GORDIN, A, SCHALLY, AV: *Increases in basal and thyrotropin-releasing hormone-stimulated secretion of thyrotropin and the effects of triiodothyronine in rats passively immunized with antiserum to somatostatin.* Fed Proc 35:782A, 1976.
8. ARIMURA, A, AND SCHALLY, AV: *Increases in basal and thyrotropin-releasing hormone (TRH)-stimulated secretion of thyrotropin (TSH) by passive immunization with antiserum to somatostatin in rats.* Endocrinology 98:1069–1072, 1976.
9. BAUER, K: *Biochemical properties of TRH inactivating enzymes.* In GRIFFITHS, EC, AND BENNETT, GW (EDS): *Thyrotropin-Releasing Hormone.* Raven Press, New York, 1983, pp 103–108.
10. BENNETT, GW, SHARP, T, BRAZELL, M, MARSDEN, GA: *TRH and catecholamine neurotransmitter release in the central nervous system.* In GRIFFITHS, EC, AND BENNETT, GW (EDS): *Thyrotropin-Releasing Hormone.* Raven Press, New York, 1983, pp 253–269.
11. BERG, GR, UTIGER, RD, SCHALCH, DS, REICHLIN, S: *Effect of central cooling in man on pituitary-thyroid function and growth hormone secretion.* J Appl Physiol 21:1791–1794, 1966.
12. BERELOWITZ, M, MAEDA, K, HARRIS, S, FROHMAN, LA: *The effect of alterations in the pituitary-thyroid axis on hypothalamic content and in vitro release of somatostatin-like immunoreactivity.* Endocrinology 107:24–29, 1980.
13. BHANDRAU, L, AND EMERSON, CH: *Evidence for the presence of the putative TRH metabolite, deamido-TRH in urine.* J Clin Endocrinol Metab 5:410–412, 1980.
14. BIGGINS, JA, DAS, S, DODD, PR, EDWARDSON, JA, ET AL: *Studies on the release, degradation and presynaptic actions of thyrotropin-releasing hormone.* In GRIFFITHS, EC, AND BENNETT, GW (EDS): *Thyrotropin-Releasing Hormone.* Raven Press, New York, 1983, pp 241–251.
15. BLUM, M, AND PULINI, M: *Vaginal sensations after injection of thyrotropin-releasing hormone.* Lancet 2:43, 1980.

16. Borowski, GD, Garofano, DC, Rose, LI, Levy, RA: *Blood pressure response to thyrotropin-releasing hormone in euthyroid subjects.* J Clin Endocrinol Metab 58:197–200, 1984.

17. Borst, GC, Osburne, RC, Obrian, JT, et al: *Fasting decreases thyrotropin responsiveness to thyrotropin-releasing hormones: a potential cause of misinterpretation of thyroid function tests in the critically ill.* J Clin Endocrinol Metab 57:380–383, 1983.

18. Boschi, G, Launay, N, Rips, R: *Induction of wet-dog shakes by intracerebral 'acid' TRH in rats.* Neurosci Lett 16:209–212, 1980.

19. Bowers, CY, Schally, AV, Enzemann, F, et al: *Porcine thyrotropin releasing hormone is (pyroglu-his-pro(NH₂).* Endocrinology 86:1143–1153, 1970.

20. Brammer, GL, Morley, JE, Geller, E, et al: *Hypothalamus-pituitary-thyroid axis interactions with pineal gland in the rat.* Am J Physiol 231:E416–E420, 1979.

21. Brown, M, and Vale, W: *Central nervous system effects of hypothalamic peptides.* Endocrinology 96:1333–1336, 1975.

22. Brown, M, and Taché, Y: *Hypothalamic peptides: Central nervous system control of visceral functions.* Fed Proc 40:2565–2569, 1981.

23. Brown, M, River, J, Vale, W: *Actions of bombesin, thyrotropin releasing factor, prostaglandin E₂ and naloxone on thermoregulation in the rat.* Life Sci 20:1681–1687, 1977.

24. Brownstein, JM, Palkovits, H, Saavedra, JM, Bassiri, RM, Utiger, RD: *Thyrotropin-releasing hormone in specific nuclei of rat brain.* Science 185:267–269, 1974.

25. Burger, HG, and Patel, YC: *TSH and TRH: Their physiological regulation and the clinical applications of TRH.* In Martin, L, and Besser, GM (eds): *Clinical Neuroendocrinology.* Academic Press, New York, 1977, pp 67–132.

26. Burgus, R, Dunn, TF, Desiderio, D, Guillemin, R: *Structure moléculaire da facteur hypothalamique hypophysiotrope TRF d'origine ovine: Mise en évidence par spectrométrie de masse de la séquence PCA-XI His-Pro-NH₂.* Compt Rend 269:226–228, 1969.

27. Burgus, R, and Guillemin, R: *Chemistry of thyrotropin-releasing factor (TRF).* In Meites, J (ed): *Hypophysiotropic Hormones of the Hypothalamus.* Williams & Wilkins, Baltimore, 1970, pp 227–241.

28. Burt, DR: *Thyrotropin releasing hormones: Apparent receptor binding in the retina.* Exp Eye Res 29:252, 1979.

29. Burt, DR, and Taylor, RL: *Binding sites for thyrotropin-releasing hormone in sheep nucleus accumbens resemble pituitary receptors.* Endocrinology 106:1416–1423, 1980.

30. Burt, DR, and Taylor, RL: *TRH receptor binding in retina and pituitary: Major species variation.* Exp Eye Res 25:173–182, 1982.

31. Cannico, PL, and MacLeod, RM: *The role of phospholipids in hormone secretory mechanisms.* In Müller, EE, and MacLeod, RM (eds): *Neuroendocrine Perspectives,* vol 2. Elsevier, Amsterdam, 1983, pp 123–172.

32. Caroscio, JT, Cohen, JA, Zawodnisk, J: *A double-blind, placebo-controlled trial of TRH in amyotropic lateral sclerosis.* Neurology 35:106A, 1985.

33. Cheifetz, PN: *Effect of lesions in the globus pallidus upon thyroid function.* J Endocrinol 43:36–37, 1969.

34. Chin, WW: *Biosynthesis of the glycoprotein hormones.* In Black, P McL, Zervas, NT, Ridgway, EC, Martin, JB (eds): *Secretory Tumors of the Pituitary Gland. Progress in Endocrine Research and Therapy,* vol 1. Raven Press, New York, 1984, pp 327–342.

35. Cobb, WE, Reichlin, S, Jackson, IMD: *Growth hormone secretory status is a determinant of the thyrotropin response to thyrotropin-releasing hormone in euthyroid patients with hypothalamic pituitary disease.* J Clin Endocrinol Metab 52:324–329, 1981.

36. Costom, BH, Grumbach, MM, Kaplan, SL: *Effect of thyrotropin-releasing factor on serum thyroid stimulating hormone: An approach to distinguishing hypothalamic from pituitary forms of idiopathic hypopituitary dwarfism.* J Clin Invest 50:2219–2225, 1971.

37. Cowdry, RW, Wehr, T, Zis, AP, Goodwin, FK: *Thyroid abnormalities associated with rapid-cycling bipolar illness.* Arch Gen Psych 40:414–420, 1983.

38. Dekin, MS, Richerson, MS, Getting, PA: *Thyrotropin-releasing hormone induces rhythmic bursting in newborns of the nucleus tractus solitarius.* Science 229:67–69, 1985.

39. Detimar, TW, Lynn, AG, Metcalf, G, Morgan, BA: *Brain TRH receptors are the same as pituitary TRH receptors.* J Pharm Pharmacol 25:389–400, 1983.

40. Dewhurst, KE, el-Kabir, DJ, Harris, GW, Mandelbrote, DM: *A review of the effect of stress on the activity of the central nervous-pituitary-thyroid axis in animals and man.* Confin Neurol 30:161–196, 1968.

41. Drust, DS, and Martin, TF: *Thyrotropin-releasing hormone rapidly activates protein phosphorylation in GH₃ pituitary cells by a lipid-linked, protein kinase c-mediated pathway.* J Biol Chem 259:14520–14530, 1984.

42. Dupont, A, Bastarache, E, Endröczi, E, Fortier, C: *Effect of hippocampal stimulation on the plasma thyrotropin (TSH) and corticosterone responses to acute cold exposure in the rat.* Can J Physiol Pharmacol 50:364–367, 1972.

43. Dyer, RG, and Dyball, REJ: *Evidence for a direct effect of LRF and TRF on single unit activity in nostral hypothalamus.* Nature 252:233–255, 1974.

44. Emerson, CH, Frohman, LA, Szabo, M, Thakkar, I: *TRH immunoreactivity in human urine: Evidence for dissociation from TRH.* J Clin Endocrinol Metab 45:392–399, 1977.

45. Engel, WK, Siddique, T, Nicoloff, JT: *Effect on weakness and spasticity in amyotrophic lateral sclerosis of thyrotropin-releasing hormone.* Lancet ii:73–75, 1983.

46. Engel, WK, Van den Bergh, P, Askanas, V: *Subcutaneous thyrotropin-releasing hormone seems ready for wider trials in treating lower motor neuron produced weakness spasiticity.* Ann Neurol 16:109–110, 1984.

47. Engler, D, and Burger, AG: *The deiodination of the iodothyronines and of their derivatives in man.* Endocrine Rev 5:151–184, 1984.

48. Engler, DM, Scanlon, MF, Jackson, IMD: *Thyrotropin-releasing hormone in the systemic circulation of the neonatal rat is derived from the pancreas and other extraneural tissues.* J Clin Invest 67:800–808, 1981.

49. Evans, LEJ, Hunter, P, Hall, R, Johnston, M, Roy, VM: *A double-blind trial of intravenous thyrotropin-releasing hormone in the treatment of reactive depression.* Br J Psych 127:227–230, 1975.

50. Faden, AI, Jacobs, TP, Holaday, JW: *Thyrotropin-releasing hormone improves neurologic recovery after spinal trauma in cats.* N Engl J Med 305:1063–1068, 1981.

51. Faden, AI, Jacobs, TP, Smith, MT, Holiday, JW: *Comparison of thyrotropin-releasing hormone (TRH) Naloxone and dexamethasone.* Neurology 33:673–678, 1983.

52. Faden, AI, Jacobs, TP, Smith, MT: *Thyrotropin-releasing hormone in experimental spinal injury: Dose response and late treatment.* Neurology 34:1280–1284, 1984.

53. Faglia, G, Beck-Peccoz, P, Ferrari, C, Ambrosi, B, Spada, A, Travaglini, P, Paracchi, S: *Plasma thyrotropin response to thyrotropin-releasing hormone in patients with pituitary and hypothalamic disorders.* J Clin Endocrinol Metab 37:595–601, 1973.

54. Farese, RV: *Phosphoinositide metabolism and hormone action.* Endo Rev 4:78–95, 1984.

55. Fink, G, Koch, Y, Aroya, NB: *Release of thyrotropin releasing hormone into hypophysial portal blood is high relative to other neuropeptides and may be related to prolactin secretion.* Brain Res 243:186–189, 1982.

56. Fisher, DA, and Odell, WD: *Effect of cold on TSH secretion in man.* J Clin Endocrinol Metab 33:859–862, 1971.

57. Fisher, DA, Dussalt, JM, Sack, J, Chopra, IJ: *Ontogenesis of hypothalamic-pituitary-thyroid function and metabolism in man, sheep and rat.* Recent Progr Horm Res 33:59–116, 1977.

58. Fleischer, N, Lorente, M, Kirkland, J, Kirkland, R, Clayton, G, Calderon, M: *Synthetic thyrotropin releasing factor as a test of pituitary thyrotropin reserve.* J Clin Endocrinol Metab 34:617–624, 1972.

59. Flohé, L, Bauer, K, Friderichs, E, Gunzler, WA, Hennies, HH, Herrling, S, Lagler, F, Otting, F, Schwertner, E: *Biological effects of degradation-stabilized TRH analogues.* In Griffiths, EC, and Bennett, GW (eds): *Thyrotropin-Releasing Hormone.* Raven Press, New York, 1983, pp 327–340.

60. Gagel, RE, Jackson, IMD, Deprez, DP, et al: *The significance of urinary thyrotropin releasing hormone (TRH) excretion in man.* In Robinson, J, and Braverman LE (eds): *Thyroid Research.* Amsterdam Excerpta Medica, 8–10, 1976.

61. Geras, EJ, and Gershengorn, MC: *Evidence that TRH stimulates secretion of TSH by two calcium-mediated mechanisms.* Am J Physiol 242(Endocrinol Metab 5):E109–E114, 1982.

62. Gershengorn, MC: *Thyrotropin releasing hormone: A review of the mechanisms of acute stimulation of pituitary hormone release.* Mol Cell Biochem 45:163–179, 1982.

63. Gershengorn, MC: *Thyroid hormone regulation of thyrotropin production and interaction with thyrotropin releasing hormone in thyrotropic cells in culture.* In Oppenheimer, JH, and Samuels, HH (eds): *Molecular Basis of Thyroid Hormone Action.* Academic Press, New York, 1982, pp 387–412.

64. Gershengorn, MC, Rebecchi, MJ, Geras, E, Arevalo, CO: *Thyrotropin-releasing hormone (TRH) action in mouse thyrotropic monophosphate as a mediator of TRH-stimulated thyrotropin release.* Endocrinology 107:665–670, 1980.

65. Gordin, A, Arimura, A, Schally, AV: *Effect of thyroid hormone excess and deficiency on serum thyrotropin in rats immunized passively with antiserum to somatostatin.* Proc Exp Biol Med 153:319–323, 1976.

66. Gracco, VJ, Caliguiri, M, Abbs, JH: *Placebo controlled computerized dynometric measurements on bulbar and somatic muscle strength increase in patients with amyotrophic lateral sclerosis following intravenous infusion of 10 mg/kg thyrotropin-releasing hormone.* Ann Neurol 16:110(A), 1984.

67. Grant, G, Vale, W, Guillemin, R: *Interaction of thyrotropin-releasing factor with membrane receptors of pituitary cells.* Biochem Biophys Res Commun 46:28–34, 1972.

68. Green, PJ: *Sensations after injection of TRH* (letter). Lancet 2:199, 1980.

69. GREEN, AR, HEAL, DJ, GRAHAME-SMITH, DG, KELLY, PH: *The contrasting actions of TRH and cycloheximide in altering the effects of centrally acting drugs: Evidence of the non-involvement of dopamine sensitive adenylate cyclase.* Neuropharmacology 15, 591–599, 1976.

70. GROSSMAN, A, CLEMENT-JONES, V, BESSER, GM: *Clinical implications of endogenous opioid peptides.* Neuroendocrine Perspectives 4:243–294, 1985.

71. HALÁSZ, B, SLUSHER, MA, GORSKI, RA: *Thyrotropic hormone secretion in rats after partial or total interruption of neural afferents to the median basal hypothalamus.* Endocrinology 80:1075–1082, 1967.

72. HALL, R, AMOS, J, GARRY, R, BUXTON, RL: *Thyroid-stimulating hormone response to synthetic thyrotrophin releasing hormone in man.* Br Med J 2:274–277, 1970.

73. HALL, RJ, ORMSTON, BJ, BESSER, GM, ET AL: *The thyrotropin-releasing hormone test in diseases of the pituitary and hypothalamus.* Lancet 1:759–763, 1972.

74. HALPERN, J, AND HINKLE, PM: *Direct visualization of receptors for thyrotropin-releasing hormone with a fluorescin-labeled analog.* Proc Natl Acad Sci USA 78:587–591, 1981.

75. HERMANN, J, HEINEN, E, KROLL, HJ, ET AL: *Thyroid function and thyroid hormone metabolism in elderly men. Low T_3-syndrome in old age?* Klin Wochenschr 59:315–323, 1981.

76. HERSHMAN, JM: *Use of thyrotropin-releasing hormone in clinical medicine.* Med Clin No America 62:313–325, 1978.

77. HERSHMAN, JM, AND PITTMAN, JA, JR: *Control of thyrotropin secretion in man.* N Engl J Med 285:997–1006, 1971.

78. HERSHMAN, JM: *Use of thyrotropin-releasing hormone in clinical medicine.* Med Clin No America 62, 313–326, 1978.

79. HINKLE, PM, AND GOH, KBC: *Regulation of thyrotropin-releasing hormone receptors and responses by L-triiodothyronine in dispersed rat pituitary cell cultures.* Endocrinology 110:1725–1731, 1982.

80. HIROOKA, Y, HOLLANDER, CS, SUZUKI, S, FERDINAND, P, JUAN, S-I: *Somatostatin inhibits release of thyrotropin releasing factor from organ cultures of rat hypothalamus.* Proc Natl Acad Sci 75:4509–4513, 1978.

81. HÖKFELT, T, FUXE, K, JOHANSSON, O, JEFFCOATE, SL, WHITE, N: *Distribution of thyrotropin-releasing hormone (TRH) in the central nervous system as revealed with immunochemistry.* Eur J Pharmacol 34:389–392, 1975.

82. HORITA, A, AND CARINO, MA: *Centrally administered thyrotropin-releasing hormone (TRH) stimulates colonic transit and diarrhea production by a vagally mediated serotonergic mechanism in the rabbit.* J Pharmacol Exp Ther 222:367–371, 1982.

83. HOLADAY, JW: *Neuropeptides in shock and traumatic injury: Sites and mechanisms of action.* In MÜLLER, EE, MACLEOD, RM (EDS): *Neuroendocrine Perspectives,* vol 3. Elsevier, Amsterdam, 1984, 161–199.

84. HOLADAY, JW, AND D'AMATO, RJ: *Thyrotropin-releasing hormone improves cardiovascular function in experimental endotoxic and hemorrhagic shock.* Science 213:216–218, 1981.

85. HOSKINS, RG: *The thyroid-pituitary apparatus as a servo (feedback) mechanism.* J Clin Endocrinol 9:1429–1431, 1949.

86. IMOTO, K, SAIDA, K, IWAMURA, K: *Amyotrophic lateral sclerosis: Blind cross-over trial of thyrotropin-releasing hormone.* J Neurosurg Psychiat 47:1332–1334, 1984.

87. INGBAR, SH: *The Thyroid Gland.* In WILSON, J (ED): *Williams Textbook of Endocrinology,* ed 7. WB Saunders, Philadelphia, 1985, pp 582–815.

88. JACKSON, IMD: *Thyrotropin- and gonadotropin-secreting pituitary adenomas.* In POST, KD, JACKSON, IMD, REICHLIN, S (EDS): *The Pituitary Adenoma.* Plenum, New York, 1980, 141–150.

89. JACKSON, IMD, PAPAPETROU, D, REICHLIN, S: *Metabolic clearance of thyrotropin-releasing hormone in the rat in hypothyroid and hyperthyroid states: Comparison with serum degradation in vitro.* Endocrinology 104:1292–1298, 1979.

90. JACKSON, IMD: *Thyrotropin-releasing hormone.* N Engl J Med 306:145–156, 1982.

91. JACKSON, IMD: *Thyrotropin-releasing hormone (TRH): Distribution in mammalian species and its functional significance.* In GRIFFITH, EC, AND BENNETT, GW (EDS): *Thyrotropin-Releasing Hormone.* Raven Press, New York, 1983, pp 3–18.

92. JACKSON, IMD, AND BOLAFFI, J: *Phylogenetic distribution of TRH: Significance and function.* In GRIFFITHS, EC, AND BENNETT, GW (EDS): *Thyrotropin Releasing Hormone.* Raven Press, New York, 1983, pp 191–202.

93. JACKSON, IMD, AND LECHAN, RM: *Thyrotropin releasing hormone.* In KRIEGER, DT, BROWNSTEIN, MJ, MARTIN, JB (EDS): *Brain Peptides.* John Wiley & Sons, New York, 1983, pp 661–686.

94. JACKSON, IMD, PAPAPETROU, PD, REICHLIN, S: *Metabolic clearance of TRH in the rat in hypothyroid and hyperthyroid states: Comparison with serum degradation in vitro.* Endocrinology 104:1292–1298, 1979.

95. JACKSON, IMD, AND REICHLIN, S: *Thyrotropin-releasing hormone (TRH): Distribution in hypothalamic and extrahypothalamic brain tissues of mammalian and submammalian chordates.* Endocrinology 95:854–862, 1974.

REGULATION OF THE PITUITARY GLAND

96. JACKSON, IMD, AND REICHLIN, S: *Brain-thyrotropin-releasing hormone is independent of the hypothalamus.* Nature 267:853–854, 1977.

97. JACKSON, IMD, AND REICHLIN, S: *Distribution and biosynthesis of TRH in the nervous system.* In COLLU, R, BARBEAU, A, DUCHARME, JR, ROCHEFORT, J-G (EDS): *Central Nervous System Effects of Hypothalamic Hormones and on Other Peptides.* Raven Press, New York, 1978, pp 3–54.

98. JACKSON, IMD, WU, P, LECHAN, RM: *Immunohistochemical localization in the rat brain of the precursor for thyrotropin-releasing hormone.* Science 229:1097–1099, 1985.

99. JEFFCOATE, SL, AND WHITE, N: *Clearance and identification of thyrotrophin releasing hormone in human urine after intravenous injections.* Clin Endocrinol 4:421–426, 1975.

100. JOHANSSON, O, AND HÖKFELT T: *Thyrotropin releasing hormone, somatostatin and enkephalin distribution studies assay immunohistochemical techniques.* J Histochem Cytochem 28:364–366, 1980.

101. JOHANSSON, O, HÖKFELT, T, JEFFCOATE, SL: *Ultrastructural localization of TRH-like immunoreactivity.* Exp Br Res 38:1–10, 1980.

102. JOHANSSON, O, HÖKFELT, T, JEFFCOATE, SL, WHITE, N, STEINBUSCH, HWM, VERNOFSTAD, AAJ, EMSON, PC, SPINDEL, E: *Immunohistochemical support for three putative transmitters in one neuron: Coexistence of 5-hydroxytryptamine substance P- and thyrotropin releasing hormone-like immunoreactivity in medullary neurons projecting to the spinal cord.* Neuroscience 6:1857–1881, 1981.

103. JOSEPH-BRAVO, P, CHARLI, JL, PALACIDS, JM, KORDON, C: *Effect of neurotransmitters on the in vitro release of immunoreactive thyrotropin-releasing hormone from rat mediobasal hypothalamus.* Endocrinology 104:801–806, 1979.

104. KAPLAN, MM: *The role of thyroid hormone deiodination in the regulation of hypothalamo-pituitary function.* Neuroendocrinology 38:254–260, 1984.

105. KAPLAN, MM, MUNSAT, TL, TAFT, J, REICHLIN, S: *Sustained rises of serum thyrotropin, thyroxine, and triiodothyronine during long-term, continuous thyrotropin-releasing hormone treatment in patients with amyotrophic lateral sclerosis.* J Clin Endocrinol Metab 63:808–814, 1986.

106. KOIVUSALA, F, PAAKKARI, I, LEPPALUOTO, J, KARPPANEN, H: *The effect of centrally administered TRH on blood pressure, heart rate and ventilation in the rat.* Acta Physiol Scand 106:83–86, 1979.

107. KOLESNICK, RN, MUSACCHIO, T, THAW, C, GERSHENGORN, MC: *Thyrotropin (TSH)-releasing hormone decreases phosphatidylinositol and increased unesterified arachidonic acid in thyrotropic cells. Possible early events in stimulation of TSH secretion.* Endocrinology 114:671–676, 1984.

108. KOSS, MC: *Stimulant action of thyrotropin-releasing hormones on ciliary nerve activity.* Eur J Pharmacol 65:105–108, 1980.

109. KRULICH, L: *Central neurotransmitters and the secretion of prolactin, GH, LH and TSH.* Ann Rev Physiol 41:603–615, 1979.

110. KRULICH, L: *Neurotransmitter control of thyrotropin secretion.* Neuroendocrinology 35:139–147, 1982.

111. KUNOS, G, NEWMAN, F, FARSANG, C, UNGAR, W: *Thyrotropin releasing hormone and naloxone attenuate the antihypertensive action of central alpha 2-adrenoceptor stimulation through different mechanisms.* Endocrinology 115:2481–2483, 1984.

112. LABRIE, F, DROUIN, J, FERLAND, L, ET AL: *Mechanism of action of hypothalamic hormones in the anterior pituitary gland and specific modulation of their activity by sex steroids and thyroid hormones.* Rec Prog Horm Res 34:25–93, 1978.

113. LABRIE, F, BARDEN, N, POIRIER, G, DeLEAR, A: *Binding of thyrotropin-releasing hormone to plasma membranes of bovine anterior pituitary gland.* Proc Natl Acad Sci USA 69:283–287, 1972.

114. LaHANN, TR, HORITA, A: *Thyrotropin releasing hormones: Centrally mediated effects on gastrointestinal motor activity.* J Pharm Exp Therap 222:66–70, 1982.

115. LALOGA, GP, CNARNOW, B, ZAJCHUK, R, ET AL: *Diagnostic doses of protyrelin (TRH) elevate BP by noncatecholaminergic mechanisms.* Arch Int Med 144:1149–1152, 1984.

116. LAMBERTON, PM, LECHAN, RM, JACKSON, IMD: *Ontogeny of thyrotropin-releasing hormone and histidyl proline diketopiperazine in the rat central nervous system and pancreas.* Endocrinology 115:2400–2405, 1984.

117. LARSEN, PR: *Thyroid-pituitary interactions.* N Engl J Med 306:23–32, 1982.

118. LECHAN, RM, JACKSON, IMD: *Immunohistochemical localization of thyrotropin-releasing hormone in the rat hypothalamus and pituitary.* Endocrinology 111:55–65, 1982.

119. LECHAN, RM, JACKSON, IMD: *Thyrotropin releasing hormone but not histidyl-proline diketopiperazine is depleted from rat spinal cord following 5,7-dihydroxytryptamine treatment.* Brain Res 326:152–55, 1985.

120. LECHAN, RM, SNAPPER, SB, JACOBSON, S, JACKSON, IMD: *Distribution of thyrotropin releasing hormone (TRH) in the Rhesus monkey spinal cord.* Peptides 5:185–194, 1984.

121. LECHAN, RM, WU, P, JACKSON, IMD, WOLFE, H, COOPERMAN, S, MANDELL, G, GOODMAN, RM:

Thyrotropin-releasing hormone precursor: Characterization in rat brain. Science, 231:159–161, 1986.

122. LEPPALUOTO, J, AND SUHONEN, AS: *High pressure liquid chromatography purification of human urinary samples for thyrotropin-releasing hormone radioimmunoassay.* J Clin Endocrinol Metab 54:914–918, 1982.

123. LIPPE, OM, VAN HERLE, AJ, LEFRANCHI, SH, ET AL: *Reversible hypothyroidism in growth hormone-deficient children treated with human growth hormone.* J Clin Endocrinol Metab 40:612–618, 1975.

124. LOOSEN, PT: *The TRH-induced TSH response in psychiatric patients: A possible neuroendocrine marker.* Psychoneuroendocrinology 10:237–260, 1985.

125. LOOSEN, PT, PRANGE, AJ, JR: *Serum thyrotropin response to thyrotropin-releasing hormone in psychiatric patients: A review.* Am J Psych 139:405–416, 1982.

126. LUCKE, C, HOFFKEN, B, MÜHLEN, A: *The effect of somatostatin on TSH levels in patients with primary hypothyroidism.* J Clin Endocrinol Metab 41:1082–1084, 1975.

127. LUPULESCU, A, NICOLESCU, A, GHEORGHIESCU, B, ET AL: *Neural control of the thyroid gland: Studies of the role of extrapyramidal and rhinencephalon areas in the development of goiter.* Endocrinology 70:517–524, 1962.

128. MACPHEE, CH, DRUMMOND, AH: *Throtropin-releasing hormone stimulates rapid breakdown of phosphatidylinositol 4,5-biphosphate and phosphatidyl inositol 4-phosphate in GH3 pituitary tumor cells.* Mol Pharmacol 25:193–200, 1984.

129. MAEDA, K, AND FROHMAN, LA: *Release of somatostatin and thyrotropin-releasing hormones from rat hypothalamic fragments in vitro.* Endocrinology 106:1837–1842, 1980.

130. MALLIK, TK, WILBER, JF, PEGUES, J: *Measurements of thyrotropin-releasing hormone-like material in human peripheral blood by affinity chromatography and radioimmunoassay.* J Clin Endocrinol Metab 54:1194–1198, 1982.

131. MANAKER, S, WINOKUR, A, RHODES, CH, RAINBOW, TC: *Autoradiographic localization of thyrotropin-releasing hormone (TRH) receptors in human spinal cord.* Neurology 35:328–332, 1985.

132. MANAKER, S, WINOKUR, A, ROSTENE, WH, RAINBOW, TC: *Autoradiographic localization of thyrotropin-releasing hormone receptors in the rats central nervous system.* J Neurosci 5:167–174, 1985.

133. MAREK, K, AND HAUBRICH, DR: *Thyrotropin-releasing hormone-increased catabolism of catecholamines in brains of thyroidectomized rats.* Biochem Pharmacol 26:1817–1818, 1977.

134. MARTIN, JB: *Regulation of the pituitary-thyroid axis.* In MCCANN, SM (ED): *Endocrine Physiology: M.T.P. International Review of Science Physiology,* ser 1, vol 5. Butterworth, London, 1974, p 67.

135. MARTIN, JB, AND REICHLIN, S: *Neural regulation of the pituitary-thyroid axis.* In KENNY, AD, AND ANDERSON, RR (EDS): *Proceedings of the Sixth Midwest Conference on the Thyroid.* University of Missouri Press, Columbia, MO, 1970, p 1.

136. MARTIN, JB, BOSHANS, R, REICHLIN, S: *Feedback regulation of TSH secretion in rats with hypothalamic lesions.* Endocrinology 87:1032–1040, 1970.

137. MARTIN, JB, AND REICHLIN, S: *Plasma thyrotropin (TSH) response to hypothalamic electrical stimulation and to injection of synthetic thyrotropin-releasing hormone (TRH).* Endocrinology 90:1079–1086, 1972.

138. MARTIN, TFJ: *Thyrotropin-releasing factor rapidly activates the phosphodiester hydrolysis of polyphosphoinositides in GH$_3$ pituitary cells.* J Biol Chem 258:14816–14822, 1983.

139. METCALF, G: *The neuropharmacology of TRH analogues.* In GRIFFITHS, EC, AND BENNETT, GW (EDS): *Thyrotropin-Releasing Hormone.* Raven Press, New York, 1983, pp 315–326.

140. METCALF, G, AND DETTMAR, PW: *Is thyrotropin-releasing hormone an endogenous substance in the brain?* Lancet 1:586–589, 1981.

141. MITSUMA, T, NOGIMORI, T, ADACHI, K, ET AL: *Concentrations of immunoreactive thyrotropin-releasing hormone in spinal cord of patients with amyotrophic lateral sclerosis.* Am J Med Sci 287:34–6, 1984.

142. MITSUMOTO, H, SALGADO, ED, NEGROSKI, D, ET AL: *Double-blind crossover trials with acute intravenous thyrotropin-releasing hormone infusion in patients with amyotrophic lateral sclerosis: Negative studies.* Ann Neurol 16:109, 1984 (abstract).

143. MORLEY, JE: *Extrahypothalamic thyrotropin releasing hormone (TRH) — Its distribution and its functions.* Life Sci 25:1539–1550, 1979.

144. MORLEY, JE: *Neuroendocrine control of thyrotropin secretion.* Endo Rev 2:396–419, 1981.

145. MUNSAT, TL, MORA, JS, ROBINTON, JE, JACKSON, I, LECHAN, R, HEDLUND, W, TAFT, J, REICHLIN, S, SCHEIFE, R: *Intrathecal TH in amyotrophic lateral sclerosis: Preliminary observations.* Neurology 34:239, 1984 (abstract).

146. NARUMI, S, AND NAGAWA, Y: *Modification of dopaminergic transmission by thyrotropin-releasing hormone.* In SEGAWA, T, YAMAURA, HI, KURIYAMA, K (EDS): *Advances in Biochemical Psychology Pharmacology,* vol 36. Raven Press, New York 1983, pp 185–197.

147. NIELSEN, JA, MOORE, KE: *Thyrotropin-releasing hormone and its analog. MK-771 increase the*

cerebroventricular perfusate content of dehydroxyphenylactic acid. J Neurochem 43:593–596, 1984.

148. NICOLL, RA: *The action of thyrotropin releasing hormones, substance P and related peptides in frog spinal motorneurons.* J Pharmacol Exp Ther 207:817–824, 1978.

149. NIEPCE, B: *Traite de Goitre et du Crétinisme.* Balliere, Paris, 1851.

150. OKA, J-I, AND FUKUDA, H: *Properties of the depolarization induced by TRH in the frog spinal cord.* Neurosci Lett 46:167–72, 1984.

151. OSBAHR, AJ, NEMEROFF, CB, LUTTINGER, D, MASON, GA, PRANGE, AJ, JR: *Neurotensin-induced antinociception in mice: Antagonism by thyrotropin-releasing hormone.* J Pharmacol Exp Ther 217:645–651, 1981.

152. PAWLOWSKI, L, RUCZYNSKA, J, PRZEGALINSKI, E: *The effect of thyroliberin and some effects of its analogues on the hind limb flexor reflex in the spinal rat.* Pol J Pharmacol Pharm 32:539–550, 1980.

153. PETERKOFSKY, A, BATAINI, F, KOCH, Y, TAKAHARA, Y, DANNIES, P: *Histidylproline diketopiperazine: Its biological role as a regulatory peptide.* Mol Cell Biochem 42:45–63, 1982.

154. PORTER, CC, LOTTI, VJ, deFELICE, MJ: *The effect of TRH and related tripeptide L-N-(2-oropiperidin-6-yl carbonyl). Histidyl L-thiazolidine- 4-carboxyamide (MK-771, OHT) on the depressant action of barbiturates and alcohol in mice and rats.* Life Sci 21:811–820, 1977.

155. PORTER, BA, REFETOFF, S, ROSENFIELD, RL, DeGROOT, LJ, LANG, VS, STARK, V: *Abnormal thyroxine metabolism in hyposomatotrophic dwarfism and inhibition of responsiveness to TRH during GH therapy.* Pediatrics 51:668–674, 1973.

156. POTTS, J: Discussion of paper by Burgus R and Guillemin R: *Chemistry of thyrotropin-releasing factor (TRF).* In MEITES, J (ED): *Hypophysiotropic Hormones of the Hypothalamus: Assay and Chemistry.* Williams & Wilkins, Baltimore 1970, p. 238.

157. PRANGE, AJ, JR, NEMEROFF, CB, LOOSEN, PT, ET AL: *Behavioral effects of thyrotropin-releasing hormones in animals and man: A review.* In COLLU, R, BARBEAU, A, DUCHARME, JR, ROCHEFORT, J-G (EDS): *Central Nervous System Effects of Hypothalamic Hormones and Other Peptides.* Raven Press, New York, 1979, p 75.

158. RABELLO, MM, SNYDER, PJ, UTIGER, RD: *Effects on the pituitary-thyroid axis and prolactin secretion of single and repetitive oral doses of thyrotropin-releasing hormone (TRH).* J Clin Endocrinol Metab 39:571–578, 1974.

159. REICHLIN, S: *Thyroid function, body temperature regulation and growth in rats with hypothalamic lesions.* Endocrinology 66:340–354, 1960.

160. REICHLIN, S: *Function of the hypothalamus in regulation of pituitary-thyroid activity.* In *Brain-Thyroid Relationships.* Little, Brown & Co, Boston, 1984, pp 17–32.

161. REICHLIN, S: *Control of thyrotropic hormone secretion.* In MARTINI, L, AND GANONG, E (EDS): *Neuroendocrinology,* vol 1. Academic Press, New York, 445–536, 1966.

162. REICHLIN, S: *Biosynthesis and degradation of hypothalamic hypophysiotrophic factors.* In NAFTOLIN, F, RYAN, KJ, DAVIES, J (EDS): *Subcellular Mechanisms in Reproductive Neuroendocrinology.* Elsevier, Amsterdam, 1976, pp 109–127.

163. REICHLIN, S: *Regulation of thyrotropin and gonadotropin secretion.* In BLACK, P, RIDGEWAY, EC, MARTIN, JB, ET AL (EDS): *Pituitary Adenoma.* Plenum, New York, 1984, pp 309–326.

164. REICHLIN, S: *Neuroendocrinology.* In WILSON, G, AND FOSTER, D (EDS): *Williams Textbook of Endocrinology,* ed 7. WB Saunders, Philadelphia, 1985, pp. 492–567.

165. REICHLIN, S: *Neural function of TRH.* Acta Endocrinologica, (in press).

166. REICHLIN, S: *Neuroendocrine control of TSH secretion.* In INGBAR, S, AND BRAVERMAN, L. (EDS): *The Thyroid,* ed 5. JB Lippincott, Philadelphia, 1986, pp 241–266.

167. REICHLIN, S, BOLLINGER, J, NEJAD, I, SULLIVAN, P: *Tissue thyroid hormone concentration of rat and man determined by radioimmunoassay.* Mt Sinai J Med 40:502–510, 1973.

168. REICHLIN, S, MARTIN, JB, JACKSON, IMD: *Regulation of thyroid-stimulating hormone (TSH) secretion.* In JEFFCOATE, SL, AND HUTCHINSON, JSM (EDS): *The Endocrine Hypothalamus.* Academic Press, New York, 1978, pp. 230–270.

169. REICHLIN, S, MARTIN, JB, MITNICK, MA, BOSHANS, RL, GRIMM, Y, BOLLINGER, J, GORDON, J, MALACARA, J: *Function of the hypothalamus in regulation of pituitary-thyroid activity.* Recent Prog Horm Res 28:229–277, 1972.

170. REICHLIN, S, AND UTIGER, RD: *Regulation of the pituitary-thyroid axis in man: Relationship of TSH concentration to concentration of free and total thyroxine in plasma.* J Clin Endocrinol Metab 27:251–255, 1967.

171. RELKIN, R: *Pineal hormonal interactions.* In RELKIN, R (ED): *The Pineal Gland.* Elsevier, Amsterdam, 1983, pp 225–246.

172. RENAUD, LP, BLUME, HW, PITTMAN, QJ, LAMOUR, Y, TAN, AT: *Thyrotropin-releasing hormone selectively depresses glutamic excitation of cerebral cortical neurons.* Science 205:1275–1277, 1979a.

173. RENAUD, LP, PITTMAN, QJ, BLUME, HW, LAMOUR, Y, ARNAULD, E: *Effects of peptides on central neural excitability.* In COLLU, R, BARBEAU, A, DUCHARME, JR, ROCHEFORTE, J-G (EDS): Raven Press, New York, 1979b, 147–161.

174. RICHTER, K, KAWASHIMA, E, EGGER, R, KREILL, G: *Biosynthesis of thyrotropin releasing hormone in the skin of Xenopus laevis: Partial sequences of the precursor deduced from cloned cDNA.* EMBO J 3:617–621, 1984.

175. RICHMAND, DA, MOLITCH, ME, O'DONNELL, TF: *Altered thyroid hormones levels in bacterial sepsis: The role of nutritional adequacy.* Metabolism 29:936–942, 1980.

176. RIDGWAY, EC: *Glycoprotein hormone production by pituitary tumors.* In BLACK, P, ZERVAS, ZT, RIDGWAY, EC, MARTIN, JB (EDS): *Secretory Tumors of the Pituitary Gland (Progress in Endocrine Research and Therapy,* vol 1). Raven Press, New York, 1984, pp 343–363.

177. ROBINSON, J, BENEDICT, C, TAFT, J, ET AL: *TRH toxicity in humans.* Neurology (Suppl 1), Abstract 135, 1985.

178. ROOT, AW, SNYDER, PJ, REZVANI, I, DIGEORGE, AM, UTIGER, RD: *Inhibition of thyrotropin-releasing hormone-mediated secretion of thyrotropin by human growth hormone.* J Clin Endocrinol Metab 36:103–107, 1973

179. ROWE, JW, ET AL: *Relation of the pineal gland and environmental lighting to thyroid function in the rat.* Neuroendocrinology 6:247–254, 1970.

180. RUPNOW, JH, HINKLE, P, DIXON, JE: *A macromolecule which gives rise to thyrotropin releasing-hormone.* Biochem Biophys Res Commun 89:721–728, 1979.

181. SAFFRAN, M: *Chemistry of hypothalamic hypophysiotropic factors.* In *Handbook of Physiology,* Sect. 7, *Endocrinology* vol. 4, part 2. American Physiological Society, Washington, DC, 1974, pp. 563–586.

182. SAWIN, CT, AND HERSHMAN, JM: *Clinical use of thyrotropin-releasing hormone (TRH).* In BRAY, GA, AND HERSHMAN JM (EDS): *The Thyroid. Physiology and Treatment of Disease.* Pergamon Press, New York, 1979, 597–619.

183. SAWIN, CGF, HERSHMAN, JM, BOYD, AE, III, LONGCOPE, C, BACHARACH, P: *The relationship of changes in serum estradiol and progesterone during the menstrual cycle to the thyrotropin and prolactin responses to thyrotropin-releasing hormone.* J Clin Endocrinol Metab 47:1296–1302, 1978.

184. SCANLON, MF, LEWIS, M, WEIGHTMAN, DR, ET AL: *The neuroregulation of human thyrotropin secretion.* In MARTINI, L, AND GANONG, WF (EDS): *Frontiers in Neuroendocrinology,* vol 6. Raven Press, New York, 1980, pp 333–380.

185. SCHALCH, DS, AND REICHLIN, S: *Stress and growth hormone release.* In PECILE, A, AND MULLER, EE (EDS): *Growth Hormone.* Excerpta Medica, Amsterdam, 1968, pp 211–225.

186. SCHMIDT-ACHERT, KM, ASKANAS, V, ENGEL, WKL: *Thyrotropin-releasing hormone enhances choline acetyltransferase and creatine kinase in cultured spinal ventral horn neurons.* J Neurochem 43:586–589, 1984.

187. SCHONBRUNN, A, AND TASHJIAN, AH: *Modulation of somatostatin receptors by thyrotropin-releasing hormone in a clonal pituitary cell strain.* J Biol Chem 255:190–198, 1980.

188. SCHREY, MP, BROWN, BL, EKINS, RP: *Studies on the role of calcium and cyclic nucleotides in the control of TSH secretion.* Mol Cell Endocrinol 11:249–264, 1978.

189. SILER, T, YEN, S, VALE, W, GUILLEMIN, RJ: *Inhibition by somatostatin of the release of TSH induced in man by thyrotropin-releasing factor.* J Clin Endocrinol Metab 38:742–745, 1974.

190. SIMASKO, SM, AND HORITA, A: *Treatment of rats with TRH analog MK-771. Down-regulation of TRH receptors and behavioral tolerance.* Neuropharmacology 24:157–65, 1985.

191. SMITH, JR, LA HANN, TR, CHESNUT, RM: *Thyrotropin-releasing hormone: Stimulation of colonic activity following intracerebroventricular administration.* Science 196:660–662, 1976.

192. SMYTHE, GA, BRADSHAW, KE, CAI, WY, SYMONS, RG: *Hypothalamic serotonergic stimulation of thyrotropin secretion and related brain-hormone and drug interactions in the rat.* Endocrinology 111:1181–1191, 1982.

193. SNYDER, PJ, AND UTIGER, RD: *Response to thyrotropin releasing hormone (TRH) in normal man.* J Clin Endocrinol Metab 34:380–385, 1972.

194. SNYDER, PJ, JACOBS, LS, RABELLO, MM, ET AL: *Diagnostic value of thyrotropin-releasing hormone in pituitary and hypothalamic disease.* Ann Intern Med 81:751–757, 1974.

195. SNYDER, PJ, AND UTIGER, RD: *Inhibition of thyrotropin response to thyrotropin-releasing hormone by small quantities of thyroid hormones.* J Clin Invest 51:2077–2089, 1972.

196. SNYDER, PJ, AND UTIGER, RD: *Repetitive administration of thyrotropin-releasing hormone results in small elevations of serum thyroid hormones and in marked inhibitions of thyrotropin response.* J Clin Invest 52:2305–2312, 1973.

197. SOBUE, I, YAMAMOTO, H, KONAGAYA, M, IIDA, M, TAKAYANAGI, T: *Effect of thyrotropin-releasing hormone on ataxia of spinocerebellar degeneration.* Lancet 1:418–419, 1980.

198. SPRATT, DI, PONT, A, MILLER, MB, McDOUGALL, IR, BAYER, MF, McLAUGHLIN, WT: *Hyperthyroxinemia in patients with acute psychiatric disorders.* Am J Med 73:41–48, 1982.

199. STANTON, TL, WINOKUR, A, BECKMAN, AL: *Reversal of natural CNS depression by TRH action in the hypocampus.* Brain Res 181:470–475, 1980.

200. STAUB, JJ, GIRARD, J, MUELLER-BAND, J: *Blunting of TSH response after repeated oral administration of TRH in normal and hypothyroid subjects.* J Endocrinol Metab 46:260–265, 1978.

201. STRYKER, T, GREENBLATT, D, REICHLIN, S: *Somatostatin suppression as a possible cause of GH and*

TSH secretory response to benzodiazepines (abstract 2331). Proceedings of the Seventh International Congress of Endocrinology, July 1–7, Quebec City, Canada, 1984.

202. SUFIT, R, BEAULIEU, D, SANGUA, M, ET AL: *Placebo controlled quantitative measurements of neuromuscular function following intravenous infusion of 10 mg/kg thyrotropin-releasing hormones in 16 male patients with ALS.* Ann Neurol 16:110–111, 1984.

203. SUHONEN, AS, LEPPALUOTO, J, SAIMI, J: *Urine TRH immunoreactivity in hypothyroid and hyperthyroid patients.* Acta Endocrinol (Copenh) 105:482–486, 1984.

204. SUHONENMALM, AS, LEPPALUOTO, J, KIVINIEMI, H, LARMI, T: *Increased urinary levels of thyrotropin-releasing hormone immunoreactivity in acute pancreatitis.* Scand J Gastroenterol 20:559–562, 1985.

205. SZENTAGOTHAI, J, FLERKO, B, MESS, B, HALÁSZ, B: *Hypothalamic Control of the Anterior Pituitary.* Akadémiai Kiado, Budapest, 1968.

206. TACHÉ, Y, LIS, M, COLLU, R: *Effects of thyrotropin-releasing hormones on behavioral and hormonal changes induced by β-endorphin.* Life Sci 21:841–846, 1977.

207. TACHÉ, Y, LESEIGE, D, VALE, W, COLLU, R: *Gastric hypersecretion by intracisternal TRH: Dissociation from hypophysiotropic activity and role of central catecholamines.* Eur J Pharmacol 107:149–155, 1985.

208. URMAN, S, AND CRITCHLOW, V: *Long-term elevations in plasma thyrotropin, but not growth hormone concentrations associated with lesion-induced depletion of median eminence somatostatin.* Endocrinology 112:659–664, 1983.

209. VAGENAKIS, AG, ROTI, E, MANNIX, J, BRAVERMAN, LE: *Problems in the measurement of urinary TRH.* J Clin Endocrinol Metab 41(4):801–804, 1975.

210. VAGENAKIS, AG, RAPOPORT, B, AZIZI, F, ET AL: *Hyper-response to thyrotropin releasing hormone accompanying small decreases in serum thyroid hormone concentrations.* J Clin Invest 54:913–918, 1974.

211. VIJAYAN, E, AND McCANN, SM: *Suppression of feeding and drinking activity in rats following intraventricular injections of thyrotropin-releasing hormone (TRH).* Endocrinology 100:1727–1730, 1977.

212. WADE, N: *The Nobel Duel.* Anchor Press/Doubleday, Garden City, New York, 1981.

213. WARTOFSKY, L, AND BURMAN, KD: *Alterations in thyroid function in patients with systemic illness: The "euthyroid sick syndrome."* Endocrine Rev 3:164–217, 1982.

214. WEEKE, J, HANSEN, A, LUNDBAEK, K: *The inhibition by somatostatin of the thyrotropin response to thyrotropin-releasing hormone in normal subjects.* Scand J Clin Lab Invest 33:101–103, 1974.

215. WEHMAN, RE, GREGERMAN, RI, BURNS, WH, SARAL, R, SANTOS, GW: *Suppression of thyrotropin in the low-thyroxine state of severe nonthyroidal illness.* N Engl J Med 213:546–552, 1985.

216. WEI, ET: *Pharmacological aspects of shaking behavior produced by TRH, AG-3-5, and morphine withdrawal.* Fed Proc 40:1491–1496, 1981.

217. WILBER, JF, AND PORTER, JC: *Thyrotropin and growth hormone releasing activity in hypophysial portal blood.* Endocrinology 27:807–811, 1970.

218. WILBER, JF: *Thyrotropin releasing hormone. Secretion and actions.* Annu Rev Med 24:353–364, 1973.

219. WILBER, JF, AND UTIGER, RD: *In vitro studies on mechanism of action of thyrotropin releasing factor.* Proc Soc Exp Biol Med 127:488–490, 1968.

220. WINOKUR, A, BECKMAN, AL: *Effects of thyrotropin-releasing hormone, norepinephrine and acetylcholine on the activity of neurons in the hypothalamus, septum and cerebral cortex of the rat.* Brain Res 150:205–209, 1978.

221. YAMADA, K, MATUSUKI, J, USHIJIMA, I, INOUE, T, FURUKAWA, T: *Behavioral studies of shaking behavior induced by thyrotropin-releasing hormone and morphine withdrawal in rats.* Arch Int Pharmacodyn Ther 262:24–33, 1983.

222. YAMAMOTO, K, SAITO, K, TAKAI, T, NAITO, M, YOSHIDA, S: *Visual field defects and pituitary enlargement in primary hypothyroidism.* J Clin Endocrinol Metab 57:283–287, 1983.

223. YARBROUGH, GG: *On the neuropharmacology of thyrotropin-releasing hormone (TRH).* Prog Neurobiol 12:291–312, 1979.

224. YOUNG, JB, SAVILLE, E, ROTHWELL, NJ, STOCK, MJ, LANDSBERG, L: *Effect of diet and cold exposure on norepinephrine turnover in brown adipose tissue of the rat.* J Clin Invest 69:1061–1071, 1982.

225. DeGROOT, LJ, LARSEN, PR, REFETOFF, S, STANBURY, JB: *The Thyroid and Its Diseases,* ed 5. John Wiley & Sons, New York, 1984.

226. McKELVY, JF: *Thyrotropin-releasing-hormone biosynthesis.* In GRIFFITHS, EC, AND BENNETT, GW (EDS): *Thyrotropin-Releasing Hormone.* Raven Press, New York, 1983, pp 51–60.

227. MITNICK, MA, AND REICHLIN, S: *Enzymatic synthesis of thyrotropin-releasing hormones (TRH) by hypothalamic "TRH" synthetic.* Endocrinology 91:1145–1153, 1972.

228. JACKSON, IMD: *Neuropeptides in the cerebrospinal fluid.* In MÜLLER, EE, AND MacLEOD, RM (EDS): *Neuroendocrine Perspectives,* vol 3, Elsevier, Amsterdam, 1984, pp 121–160.

Chapter 6

REGULATION OF ADRENOCORTICOTROPIC HORMONE (ACTH) SECRETION AND ITS DISORDERS

During the search for the cause of what was then called pernicious anemia, Thomas Addison discovered at autopsy that the adrenal glands in several patients had been destroyed.[5] Addison's first publication, in 1855, prompted Brown-Sèquard to study the effects of adrenalectomy in laboratory animals. A year later, he reported that adrenalectomy led to death within a few days and proposed that these structures were essential for life.[10] The consequences of adrenal hypersecretion and its relationship to the pituitary gland were not well recognized until the work of Cushing in the 1920s, and the concepts that the adrenal cortex was under the control of the central nervous system and was responsive to stress did not emerge until the late 1930s with the work of Selye[147] and subsequently by several others.[23,34,35,96] The existence of a corticotropin-releasing factor (CRF)* as the mediator of the hypothalamic control of adrenocorticotropic hormone (ACTH) secretion was proposed in 1955 by Saffran and Schally[137] and by Guillemin and Rosenberg,[52] and the chemical isolation and identification of this compound finally established by Vale and colleagues[171] 126 years after Thomas Addison's first report.

The function of the hypothalamic-pituitary-adrenal axis can be regarded as a model system illustrating the way that the central nervous system and the glandular secretory system interact to maintain vital homeostatic functions, the response to stress, and the regulation of circadian rhythms (Fig. 1). This system also has received much attention as a model of stress disorder in man. In fact, many regard the hypothalamic-pituitary-adrenal axis as the quintessential neuroendocrine system.

---

*The terms corticotropin-releasing factor (CRF) and corticotropin-releasing hormone (CRH) are used interchangeably in this chapter.

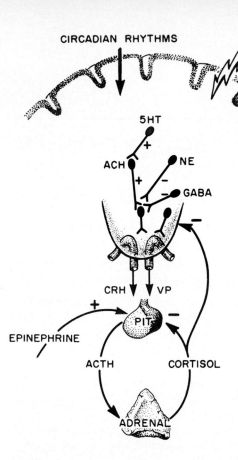

FIGURE 1. Elements of the hypothalamic-pituitary-adrenal cortical system for regulation of cortisol secretion are illustrated here. Secretion of adrenocorticotropic hormone (ACTH) is stimulated by corticotropin releasing factor whose secretion is regulated by a complex set of neurotransmitter neurons that includes two stimulatory components (cholinergic and serotonergic) and an adrenergic inhibitory pathway. These pathways mediate stress-induced and circadian ACTH secretory changes. Feedback effects of cortisol may be exerted on the nervous system as well as on the pituitary gland. This model is based on studies in rats and dogs. In human beings there appears to be an α-adrenergic stimulating pathway. Abbreviations: NE, norepinephrine; ACH, acetylcholine.

HORMONES INVOLVED IN PITUITARY-ADRENAL REGULATION

ADRENOCORTICOTROPIC HORMONE

Adrenocorticotropic hormone (adrenocorticotropin, corticotropin, ACTH) is the principal regulator of glucocorticoid and sex-hormone secretion by the adrenal cortex and a modulator of secretion of salt-retaining hormone.

Human ACTH is a basic 39-amino-acid-containing peptide (Fig. 2). The N-terminal sequence of ACTH (1-19) has nearly full steroidogenic activity, but smaller peptide fragments require concentrations several orders of magnitude greater. Synthetic ACTH 1-24, widely available for clinical testing, is highly active. Alpha-melanotropin (α-melanocyte-stimulating hormone, α-MSH) is a peptide consisting of 13 amino acids which is identical to the 1-13 sequence of ACTH. A peptide that appears to be ACTH 18-39 has been isolated from an MSH-producing human tumor as well as from other species.

Biosynthesis of ACTH

One of the most important recent advances in our understanding of pituitary hormone synthesis and regulation was the discovery that ACTH and

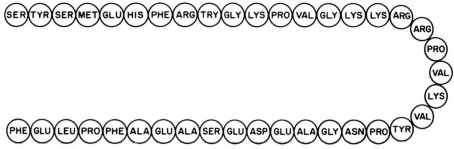

FIGURE 2. The structure of ACTH is illustrated here. ACTH is a linear peptide, 39 amino acids in length. Counting from the free amino end (SER), biologic activity requires a chain 19 amino acids long, and full biologic activity is reached with 20 amino acids. Synthetic ACTH 1-24 is available for clinical use. Segments 1 to 13 of ACTH bear close resemblance to the peptide hormones α-MSH and β-MSH.

several other hormones synthesized in the anterior lobe, intermediate lobe, and brain were all derived from a common prohormone designated pro-opiomelanocortin (POMC) (Fig. 3).[27,81,82,108,109,125,131] The gene coding this peptide is identical in all three regions, and the differences in hormonal product formed are due to different modes of processing of the prohormone by the different cell types. The gene coding for human POMC has been sequenced; it is localized to chromosome 2.

> In the anterior lobe, the principal hormones found are ACTH and β-lipotropin. The β-lipotropin molecule includes sequences corresponding to the endorphins including β-endorphin and metenkephalin (see below). α-MSH, which corresponds to the initial 13 amino acid sequence of ACTH, is not secreted as such; its presence in anterior lobe extract, causing it to be described early as a separate hormone, is now attributed to degradation of the prohormone during the extraction process.
>
> The precursor POMC is itself inactive. The components of POMC that are secreted as such into the blood of man are ACTH, β-LPH, β-endorphin, and a fragment of POMC designated 16 K. Any physiologic factor that changes the secretion of ACTH (such as stress, CRF, or glucocorticoids) correspondingly changes the secretion of its cosecreted peptides.[53] The function of the other secreted POMC

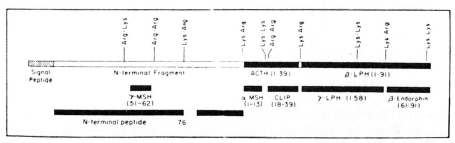

FIGURE 3. This is a schematic representation of the bovine proopiomelanocortin precursor (POMC) molecule. (Note that human β-LPH consists of 89 amino acids.) Note that this molecule codes for ACTH (1-39), β-LPH (1-91), and γ-MSH. Within the ACTH sequence are coded α-MSH (ACTH 1-13), corticotropin like-intermediate lobe peptide (CLIP, ACTH 18-39). Within the β-LPH sequence are coded γ-LPH (1-58), and β-endorphin (61-91). The secretory products found in any tissue containing POMC are determined by patterns of posttranslational processing. Thus in the rat intermediate lobe, ACTH is further degraded to α-MSH and CLIP, but in the human being, this pathway is apparently present only during early fetal life, and possibly during pregnancy. (From Krieger, DT: *The multiple faces of proopiomelanocortin: A prototype precursor molecule.* Clin Res 31:342-353, 1983; with permission.)

REGULATION OF ADRENOCORTICOTROPIC HORMONE   161

peptides is still somewhat controversial. It has been claimed that the release of β-endorphin in stress or after prolonged running is responsible respectively for loss of pain sensation and the "runner's high,"[22,40] but there is still controversy as to whether sufficient β-endorphin can reach the central nervous system from peripheral blood to influence brain function.

In those vertebrate species in which an intermediate pituitary lobe is present, such as frog and rat (but not human being), the POMC prohormone in this lobe is further processed to form α-MSH and a fragment of ACTH which has been called CLIP (corticotropin-like intermediate lobe protein) corresponding to ACTH 18-39 (see Fig. 3).

In the central nervous system defined sets of neurons have been shown to contain and to secrete ACTH (corticotropinergic neurons) and β-endorphin (endorphinergic neurons) and α-MSH.[44,54,65] Their distribution and function are described in chapter 18. The metenkephalin found in brain tissue, which has a much more extensive distribution than β-endorphin arises from two other prohormones (proenkephalin A and B, see below).

The POMC gene is widely distributed. It is found in a population of neurohypophysial neurons, in other regions of the brain, in the adrenal medulla, in well-defined cells in the gastrointestinal tract, and in a variety of neoplasms including pheochromocytoma, medullary thyroid carcinoma, bronchogenic carcinoma, and carcinoid. Its expression in neoplastic tissue accounts for the appearance of Cushing's syndrome as a paraendocrine disorder.

The rate of synthesis of POMC mRNA is regulated by processes specific to the cell type. Thus, in the anterior pituitary gland where ACTH-producing cells are located, glucocorticoids inhibit,[126] and CRF stimulates, mRNA synthesis.[11] In the intermediate lobe, on the other hand, glucocorticoids and CRF have little or no effect and dopamine, the principal inhibitory regulator of these cells, inhibits POMC mRNA formation. In POMC cells in the brain, neither CRF nor glucocorticoids regulate mRNA synthesis.[126]

Adrenocorticotropic hormone acts on the adrenal cortex through specific receptors on cell membranes.[134] As is the case for most peptide hormones, occupancy of the receptor leads to activation of cell membrane enzymes that initiate the formation of active "second messengers," cAMP and the phosphatidylinositol pathway.[30]

ADRENAL HORMONES

Based on their biologic effects, the principal hormones of the adrenal cortex fall into three classes: glucocorticoids, mineralocorticoids, and androcorticoids (Figs. 4 and 5).[8] These are synthesized by an array of enzymes localized in mitochondria and cytoplasm in functional synthesizing units.[91] The principal natural glucocorticoid in human beings is cortisol (hydrocortisone). Cortisol is largely responsible for the clinical manifestations of Cushing's syndrome, and its actions include effects on metabolism of carbohydrate, fat, and protein. Cortisol also has weak mineralocorticoid activity (defined as promoting potassium excretion and sodium retention) and weak androgen activity (defined as causing masculinizing effects). The

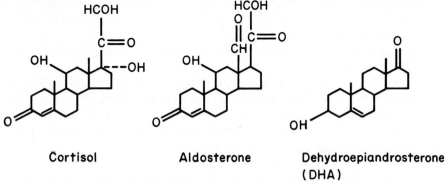

Cortisol   Aldosterone   Dehydroepiandrosterone
(DHA)

FIGURE 4. Structures of major adrenal steroid hormones are shown here. The three principal classes of adrenal steroids are the glucocorticoids, of which cortisol is the most important; mineralocorticoids, of which aldosterone is the most important; and androgenic hormones, of which dehydroepiandrosterone (DHA) is the most important. Small amounts of dehydroepiandrosterone sulfate (DHA-S) δ^4-androstenedione and testosterone are also secreted. Trace amounts of 17 β-estradiol are also synthesized. In pathologic states, the various androgenic and estrogenic hormones may be secreted in excess.

principal mineralocorticoid in humans is aldosterone, more than two hundred times as active as cortisol in promoting sodium retention, and the principal androgen dehydroepiandrosterone (DHA) (see Fig. 4). Adrenal androgens possess little intrinsic androgenic activity but are converted in peripheral tissues to testosterone, the active circulating androgen.

The secretion of cortisol, androsterone, and androstenedione is under

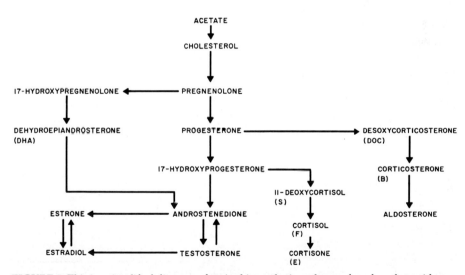

FIGURE 5. This is a simplified diagram of major biosynthetic pathways for adrenal steroidogenesis. These pathways are mediated by specific enzymes localized either to the cytosol or the mitochrondria. Congenital deficiency of specific enzymes leads to underproduction of certain steroids and may give rise to deficiency of aldosterone or cortisol. Loss of cortisol synthesis leads to overproduction of other steroids owing to activation of ACTH production by the negative-feedback loop. Drugs also can interfere with biosynthesis of adrenal hormones. Metyrapone, used for the diagnosis of pituitary-adrenal insufficiency, blocks the formation of cortisol from 11-deoxycortisol, leading to an increase in the secretion of this compound.

REGULATION OF ADRENOCORTICOTROPIC HORMONE   163

moment-to-moment control by ACTH. However, although aldosterone release may be triggered by ACTH administration and continued aldosterone secretion requires a certain level of ACTH stimulation, the principal regulating factor for aldosterone secretion is the renin-angiotensin system (see chapter 4).[43]

Cortisol release following an intravenous pulse of ACTH begins rapidly and can be detected in peripheral blood within 3 minutes. The blood level peaks at about 10 minutes and then declines over a further 10 minutes if the dose is small. With larger intramuscular (IM) doses, the peak response is prolonged, and the decline more gradual (Fig. 6). The half-life of cortisol in blood is about 60 to 90 minutes.

Glucocorticoids circulate in blood in both bound and free forms.

> Under physiologic conditions, about 75 percent of cortisol is bound to transcortin (cortisol-binding globulin), about 15 percent to albumin, and only about 10 percent is free. It is principally the free fraction that is available to cells. Transcortin levels are elevated in pregnancy and during treatment with estrogen, giving rise to increased total plasma cortisol levels; the concentration of free hormone remains constant. Contrariwise, transcortin levels may be low in liver disease, but free-hormone concentrations remain normal. Urinary free cortisol reflects secretion of the unbound fraction.[8]

Glucocorticoids exert two kinds of effects: (1) on the cell membrane, and (2) on genes to stimulate formation of mRNAs coding for specific cellular regulatory proteins.[21] Direct cell membrane effects have a very short latency and are dissipated quickly. Cell regulatory proteins under

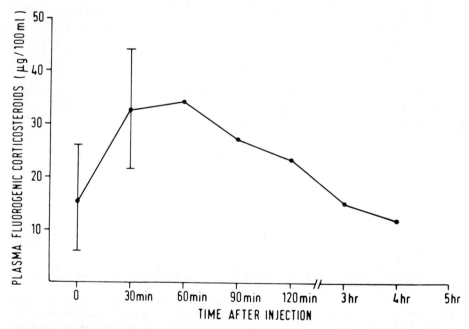

FIGURE 6. Demonstrated here is the effect of an intramuscular injection of synthetic ACTH 1-24 on plasma cortisol levels in the human being. Results shown are means and range in 45 patients and 5 normal subjects. (From Irvine, WJ, and Barnes, EW: *Adrenocortical insufficiency.* In Mason, AS (ed): *Clinics in Endocrinology and Metabolism,* vol 1. WB Saunders, London, 1972, p 562, with permission.)

gene control are mainly enzymes that regulate fat, carbohydrate, and protein metabolism and in some cells stimulate differentiation. Glucocorticoids enter cells by solution through the lipoprotein membrane and bind to a specific intracellular protein to form a protein-steroid complex. Cortisol acts on chromosomes by combining with a specific gene sequence at a "regulatory site." Cortisol receptors are found only in cells that are responsive to this hormone. The synthetic glucocorticoids, such as dexamethasone, widely used in treatment as antiinflammatory steroids, bind to the cellular cortisol receptors, but most do not bind to cortisol-binding globulin (CBG). Recently, antagonists of cortisol that block peripheral effects of the physiologic compound have been developed.[56]

CORTICOTROPIN-RELEASING FACTOR (CRF)/HORMONE (CRH)

The first evidence for CRF was published in 1955 by Guillemin and Rosenberg,[52] who showed that coincubation of hypothalamic tissue and anterior pituitary fragments stimulated the secretion of ACTH, and by Saffran and Schally,[137] who found an active ACTH-releasing substance in extracts of the posterior pituitary gland. Saffran and Schally coined the term CRF, thereby introducing the terminology for what was to be an entirely new class of physiologically important hormones. These observations were followed by intense (but frustrating) efforts in many laboratories to isolate and to identify CRF, a goal achieved finally in 1981 by Vale and colleagues,[168-170] who used extracts of hypothalamic fragments obtained from 500,000 sheep. In retrospect, it is now possible to clarify the numerous factors that made it so difficult to isolate this compound. Early bioassays were insensitive and nonspecific. For example, CRF is present in minute amounts; a rat hypothalamus contains only 1 to 2 ng; hypothalamic extracts contain several biologically active compounds that can release ACTH (such as vasopressin and epinephrine), and these are synergistic with CRF. Finally, the elucidation of the structure of CRF required the development of powerful peptide separation methods, such as high-pressure liquid chromatography and sophisticated microsequencing methods, that were not available 25 years ago.

Ovine CRF shows close homologies with several known peptides: sauvagine, urotensin, calmodulin, and angiotensinogen (Fig. 7).[168]

> Sauvagine was first isolated from frog skin by Erspamer and colleagues[29] and had already been shown to have CRF activity when CRF was discovered. Over 50 percent of the residues in sauvagine are identical to ovine CRF, and the remaining residues often are conservative substitutions, meaning that only minor changes in the base sequences of the triplet code are required to produce the amino acid changes that have occurred (see chapter 18). Urotensin I is a peptide isolated from the fish caudal neurosecretory organ (urophysis). Angiotensinogen is a peptide secreted by the liver that is converted to angiotensin I by renin, an enzyme formed in the kidney, and thence coverted to angiotensin II.

Because angiotensin II regulates the zona glomerulosa of the adrenal cortex, and CRF regulates ACTH secretion — which in turn stimulates the zona reticularis of the adrenal cortex — many regard the homologies between CRF and angiotensinogen as a reflection of a common ancestral molecule whose function is the regulation of the adrenal gland.

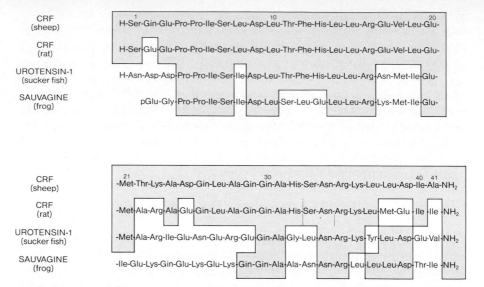

FIGURE 7. This schematic drawing shows areas of homology shaded among the various related peptides, sheep CRF, rat CRF (which is identical with that in human beings), urotensin 1, and sauvagine. Urotensin is a secretion of the caudal gland in fish, and sauvagine is found in the skin of a species of frog. (From Vale and Greer,[168] with permission.)

The structure of CRF has been identified in the human being[149] and rat;[130] it is identical in the two species and different by only six amino acids from the ovine hormone.[152] Synthetic CRF is a potent stimulator of ACTH secretion in the human being (Fig. 8) and in all other species in which it has been used. Unlike most of the other hypothalamic hormones, CRF is cleared relatively slowly from blood after injection. The plasma half-life is 11.6 ± 1.5 min for the initial fast component, and 73 ± 8 min for the slow component of disappearance.[145,146] This explains the rather prolonged effects; ACTH and cortisol remain elevated after intravenous (IV) bolus injections for 2 to 3 hours.[24,105,117] It also stimulates the secretion of β-endorphin, a peptide formed from the ACTH prohormone (see above for discussion of proopiomelanocortin peptides). The search for the structure of porcine CRF also has recently culminated. After more than 25 years of effort, Schally and colleagues have demonstrated that in this species CRF is a 41-residue polypeptide sharing a common amino acid sequence 1-39 with the rat and the human CRF and differs from these only in positions 40 and 41. The sequence of porcine CRF shows 83 percent homology with ovine CRF.[118]

> Structure-activity studies indicate the importance of the C-terminal amide; its deletion reduces biologic activity by a factor of 1000. At the N-terminal, the first three residues can be removed without loss of activity, but removal of the first six results in loss of 75 percent of activity.[169] The double leucine residues at positions 14 to 15 and 37 to 38 are critical for biologic activity. As a pituitary stimulator, CRF is quite specific for ACTH release but has been reported to stimulate GH release in two of six patients with acromegaly[122] and in some patients with affective disorders (Gold, et al[48,49]). Corticotropin-releasing factor infusion in man led to an increase in circulating pancreatic polypeptide but no changes in a number of other gut and pancreatic peptides.[94]

Physiologic Studies of CRF

Corticotropin-releasing factor can be detected in the pituitary portal blood of anesthetized rats. Concentrations of about 100 pmol/ml are detected, sufficient to stimulate ACTH secretion as determined by *in vitro* studies.[45]

Passive immunization studies using antisera to CRF result in a dramatic reduction in ACTH levels in the blood.[129] Stress-induced ACTH secretion is totally blocked by large quantities of anti-CRF antibodies (Fig. 9). CRF is present in human cerebrospinal fluid (normal level 8.6 ± 1.7 fmol/ml). The central POMC system gives rise to POMC peptides in cerebrospinal fluid (CSF).[100,158,165]

Interactions of CRF with Vasopressin and α-Adrenergic Agents

Vasopressin has been known for many years to be an effective stimulator of ACTH secretion; in recent years a debate emerged over its physiologic importance and even over whether it might be CRF itself.[16] The characterization of ovine CRF has now permitted direct comparison with the biologic

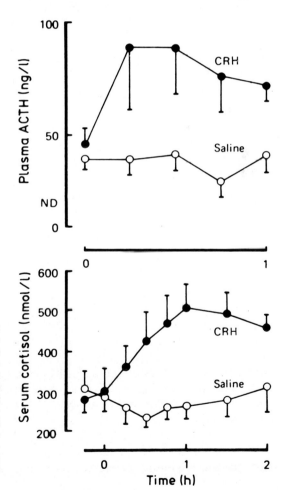

FIGURE 8. Shown here are changes in blood ACTH and cortisol following intravenous injection of either saline (open circles) or corticotropin-releasing hormone (CRH) in a group of six normal men. Initial prompt response of ACTH is followed by a somewhat delayed rise in cortisol (From Grossman, A, Kruseman, ACN, Perry, L, et al: *New hypothalamic hormone, corticotropin-releasing factor, specifically stimulates the release of adrenocorticotropic hormone and cortisol in man.* Lancet 1:921–922, 1982, with permission.)

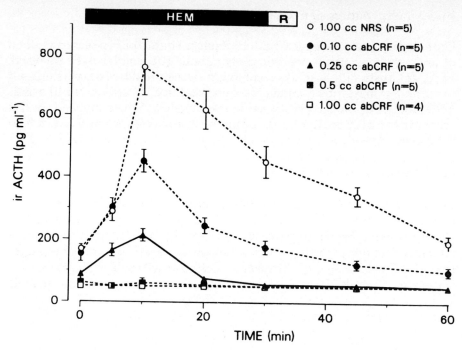

FIGURE 9. To demonstrate the role of CRH (CRF) release in mediating stress-induced ACTH secretion, this experiment utilized the injection of anti-CRH antiserum during the ACTH response to hemorrhage (HEM) in rats. Note that the largest dose of antiserum (1 ml) completely blocked the response. (From Plotsky, PM: *Hypophyseotropic regulation of adenohypophyseal adrenocorticotropin secretion.* Fed Proc 44:207-213, 1984, with permission.)

potencies of vasopressin and a study of their interactions in ACTH regulation. Vasopressin is about 1000-fold less potent than CRF, but its effects are synergistic when given with CRF. At low concentrations of CRF, the synergistic effect of addition of vasopressin is quite dramatic.[46,85] Norepinephrine and epinephrine also are synergistic with CRF in enhancing ACTH/β-endorphin secretion (Fig. 10).[127,163]

Interaction of CRF with Feedback Regulation by Glucocorticoids

On the basis of numerous physiologic studies, glucocorticoids have been postulated to regulate ACTH secretion by effects mediated on both the hypothalamus and the anterior pituitary gland.[31,68,73] Evidence obtained with the use of pure CRF supports this hypothesis: Hypothalamic CRF levels rise after adrenalectomy and fall after glucocorticoid administration, suggesting a feedback effect on the hypothalamus. Glucocorticoid receptor distribution in the brain has been demonstrated using antisera directed against liver glucocorticoid receptor.[38] In addition to a distribution in several telencephalic regions, there is an extensive overlapping distribution with the CRF neurons in the paraventricular nucleus. Exposure to glucocorticoids blunts pituitary response to CRF. The synergistic action of CRF and vasopressin is emphasized by the demonstration that both peptides are colocalized in hypothalamic neurons.[76,142] Oxytocin is also secreted by CRF neurons.[139] However, even very high doses of dexamethasone do not totally abolish the ability of CRF to stimulate some ACTH secretion. This observation may be important in understanding "breakthrough" secretion of ACTH in stress in animals receiving suppressive doses of corticoids. In the pituitary gland, glucocorticoids lower both ACTH and the synthesis of mRNA coding for the ACTH prohormone (POMC, see above); several other aspects of corticotropic activation, such as cAMP production, are also inhibited.

Mechanism of Action of CRF

Corticotropin-releasing factor action is initiated by binding to pituitary membrane receptors.[87,176] The secretion of ACTH stimulated by CRF is accompanied by a rapid increase in 3'5'-cyclic AMP,[84] an effect that is prevented by prior treatment with glucocorticoids. CRF stimulated secretion of ACTH is calcium dependent. Corticotropin-releasing factor also stimulates phospholipid methylation.[61] Corticotropin-releasing factor is highly hormone specific in its actions in the pituitary, but does release GH in some patients with acromegaly, and in others with depression.[48,122]

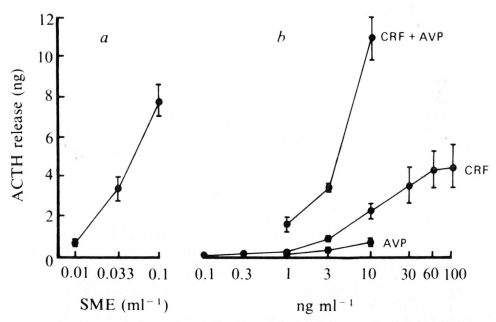

FIGURE 10. Illustrated here is the potentiating effect of vasopressin (AVP) on pituitary ACTH release induced by corticotropin-releasing factor (CRF) compared with the response to extracts of rat stalk median eminence. In this experiment, carried out on isolated rat pituitary cells, AVP was shown to have only a slight releasing effect while it markedly synergized with CRF effects. The dose response to SME resembles that to the combined CRF and AVP, suggesting that the effects of stalk median eminence are mediated by the combined action of the two peptides. (From Gillies, et al,[46] with permission.)

FACTORS REGULATING ACTH SECRETION

PITUITARY-ADRENAL RHYTHMS AND THE SLEEP-WAKE CYCLE

Glucocorticoids in blood vary diurnally; the highest levels occur at about 6 AM in an individual who sleeps from 11 PM to 7:30 AM and the lowest levels in late evening (Fig. 11).[39,79,135,136] There is also evidence of non-ACTH mechanisms in the regulation of circadian rhythms.[32]

Adrenocorticotropic hormone and cortisol secretory bursts occur predominantly during the latter half of the sleep cycle when alternating REM (rapid-eye-movement) and stage II sleep is occurring. Individual secretory bursts of cortisol secretion are not correleated with REM episodes. Adrenocorticortropic hormone and cortisol rise in the early morning occurs even when subjects are deprived of sleep; established secretory patterns persist with little change for several days when the sleep-wake cycle phases are shifted. Plasma levels of ACTH at rest in the morning are usually between 10 and 100 pg/ml, but evening levels may be as low as one tenth of these values. After stress, ACTH may increase tenfold. Adrenocorticotropic hormone is secreted in bursts throughout the day; an average of 8 to 9 major secretory episodes occur in a 24-hour period (Fig. 12), even in the absence of stressful

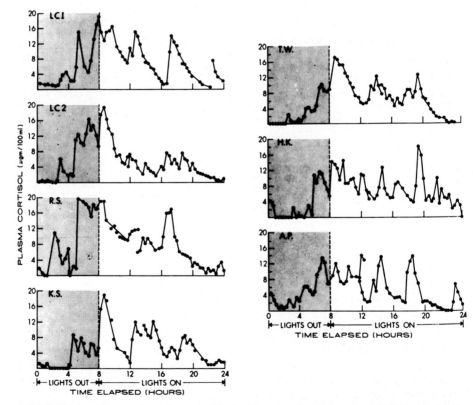

FIGURE 11. Plasma cortisol levels are sampled at intervals in seven unstressed subjects. Levels are highest between 4 and 9 AM, lowest around midnight, and fluctuate during the day without obvious relationship to external events. (From Weitzman, ED, et al: *Twenty-four hour pattern of the episodic secretion of cortisol in normal subjects.* J Clin Endocrinol Metab 33:14, 1971, with permission.)

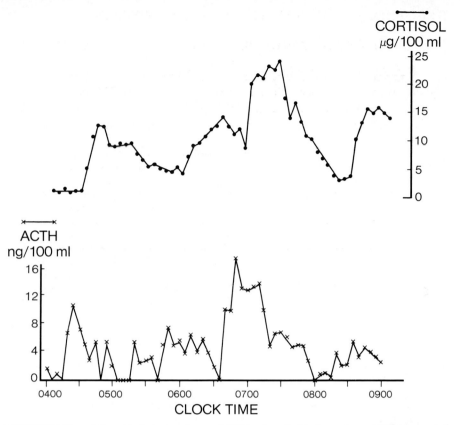

FIGURE 12. The relationship between plasma ACTH and cortisol is shown here. ACTH is secreted in bursts. Each major spurt in cortisol release follows a burst of ACTH secretion. (Adapted from Weitzman, ED et al: *Twenty-four hour pattern of the episodic secretion of cortisol in normal subjects.* J Clin Endocrinol Metab 33:14, 1971.)

stimuli. Most normal persons secrete cortisol only 25 percent of the time. Normal secretion rate of cortisol is about 16 mg per day. The magnitude of an individual ACTH secretory episode bears no relationship to preceding plasma cortisol levels, and ACTH rhythms persist in patients with glucocorticoid deficiency. In such patients, baseline ACTH levels are elevated and fluctuate around this higher level.

Other components of the POMC prohormone including β-endorphin accompany ACTH release in stress such as running.[22,40]

Circadian and episodic release of ACTH are under neural control. The diurnal rhythm is impaired in patients with certain brain disorders, including localized hypothalamic disease, general paresis, Wernicke's encephalopathy, and lesions that result in impaired consciousness.[78] A diurnal rhythm in hypothalamic CRF content has been reported in both normal and adrenalectomized rats, and lesion of the anterior hypothalamus, or treatment with para-chlorophenylalanine, a brain serotonin depletor, abolishes the diurnal changes in plasma cortisol.[60] In the human being, cyproheptadine inhibits nocturnal cortisol secretion. These observations suggest that circadian rhythms are mediated through serotonergic pathways.

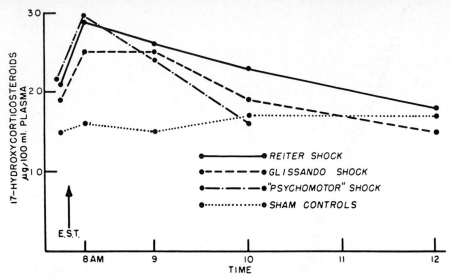

FIGURE 13. The effect of electroconvulsive therapy on level of 17-hydroxycorticosteroids in plasma is shown here. This is an example of stress-induced pituitary-adrenal activation. (From Bliss, EL, et al: *Influence of ECT and insulin coma on levels of adrenocortical steroids in peripheral circulation.* Arch Neurol Psych 72:352, 1954, with permission.)

STRESS

The pituitary-adrenal axis is activated by many different kinds of stressful stimuli, including psychologic stresses, such as apprehension or fear, and physical stresses, such as severe cold exposure, hemorrhage, and electro-shock therapy (Fig. 13). The biologic significance of the stress response is considered in chapter 21.

NEURAL CONTROL OF ACTH SECRETION

TUBEROINFUNDIBULAR SYSTEM

At the level of the pituitary gland, secretion of ACTH is regulated by both CRF and vasopressin, which act synergistically. The *vasopressinergic* system arises in the supraoptic and paraventicular nuclei (see chapter 4). The principal projection of these neurons is to the neural lobe, but some neurons from these nuclei terminate in the median eminence in apposition to the primary plexus of the hypophysial portal capillaries, as is the case for other tuberoinfundibular neurons. In addition, vasopressin secreted from the neural lobe can reach the anterior lobe by retrograde flow. The specific CRF neurons arise mainly in a specific division of the paraventricular nucleus (Fig. 14). This system of neurons cocontains a number of other peptides, including vasopressin, dynorphin, neurotensin, vasoactive intestinal polypeptide (VIP), and peptide histidine isoleucine (PHI). Corticotropin-releasing factor is also cocontained in subsets of oxytocinergic neurons that project to the neural lobe and in some cells in the paraventricular nucleus that project to the brainstem and spinal cord. This descending set of neurons is thought to be involved in autonomic regulation.

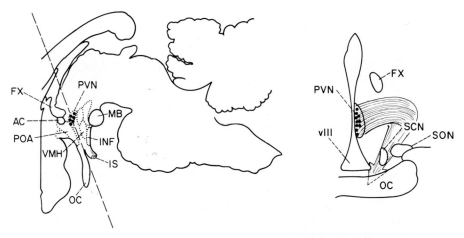

FIGURE 14. This is a schematic depiction of the location of tuberoinfundibular neurons which secrete CRH, based on human and animal studies. Tuberoinfundibular neurons *(solid dots)* are shown in a coronal section through the plane of densest cell bodies and in a sagittal section. The projection pathway of tuberoinfundibular axons toward the median eminence is depicted by the solid lines forming a point. Abbreviations: OC, optic chiasm; IS, infundibular stalk; INF, infundibular nucleus (arcuate nucleus); MB, mammillary body; PVN, paraventricular nucleus; FX, fornix; AC, anterior commissure; POA, preoptic area; VMH, ventromedial hypothalamic nucleus; ME, median eminence; DMH, dorsomedial hypothalmic nucleus; vIII, third ventricle; SON, supraoptic nucleus; SCN, suprachiasmatic nucleus. [From Riskind, PN, and Martin, JB: *Functional anatomy of the hypothalamic-anterior pituitary complex.* In DeGroot, LJ (ed): *Endocrinology,* ed 2. Grune & Stratton, Orlando (in press).]

Corticotropin-releasing hormone neurons, constituting the "final common pathway" for ACTH regulation, are in turn the target for an extensive neural input that brings ACTH secretion under the control of virtually all parts of the nervous system.[70,141]

> The principal afferents to the paraventricular nucleus include (1) nucleus of the tractus solitarius, a structure that receives input by way of vagal and glossopharyngeal afferents from heart, lungs and gastrointestinal tract; (2) three distinct noradrenergic pathways (nucleus of the tractus solitarius, medulla reticular formation, and locus coeruleus); (3) almost all nuclear cell groups in the hypothalamus; (4) nucleus of the subfornical region; and (5) many parts of the limbic system by direct or indirect pathways. These afferents convey impulses generated by stress, volume contraction, and pain. The histologic analysis of CRF afferents corresponds well to earlier classical studies of central "stress" pathways.[15,33,41,42,95,97,172-174]

Certain severely stressful stimuli used experimentally act via systemic mechanisms and appear to bypass the hypothalamus. These include *E. coli* endotoxin, hemorrhage, and laparotomy. These effects may be due to release of CRF from the gut and extrahypothalamic brain.

In addition to its role as a tuberoinfundibular pituitary-regulating hormone, CRF is widely but selectively distributed throughout the brain. Corticotropin-releasing factor-containing neurons are present throughout forebrain, brainstem, spinal cord, and in the limbic system (see also chapter 18) and outside the brain. Immunoreactive CRF has been identified in the adrenal medulla, lung, liver, stomach, duodenum, and pancreas. Its possible role in pancreatic function is suggested by the finding that CRF increases secretion of pancreatic polypeptide.[94]

ACTIONS OF CRF ON BRAIN

Intracerebroventricular administration of CRF to rats or dogs results in a remarkable activation of the sympathetic nervous system.[9,151,179] Adrenal medullary secretion of epinephrine and norepinephrine is increased, and plasma levels of glucagon and glucose rise. Blood pressure and heart rate are elevated. Behavioral changes observed include increased locomotor activity, arousal, and increased emotionality.[160] It has been postulated that CRF may have a general function in the mediation of the animal's response to stress; at the pituitary level it initiates appropriate stimulation of ACTH secretion; within the brain it may serve to activate alerting mechanisms appropriate for a "fight or flight" response.

FEEDBACK REGULATION

The nonepisodic secretion of ACTH is controlled by the negative-feedback effects of cortisol (see Figure 1). Adrenalectomy or spontaneous disease of the adrenal glands leads to a marked increase in plasma ACTH concentration; the administration of cortisol depresses ACTH secretion (Fig. 15).[58,73,74] Glucocorticoids act both in the pituitary gland and on CRF secretion. Glucocorticoids suppress ACTH production by suppressing mRNA coding for POMC (see above) and by reducing CRF receptors. In the brain, adrenal deficiency is followed by increased concentrations of hypothalamic CRF; glucocorticoid excess reduces concentration of brain CRF.[168-170] Adrenal deficiency also leads to increased secretion of vasopressin[76] and the response to CRF.

 The mechanism of glucocorticoid feedback has been analyzed in great detail.[73]

 Three time domains of feedback are described. Fast feedback can be demonstrated by stress in an animal within 30 minutes after intravenous injection of high doses of a glucocorticoid. The time course of glucocorticoid inhibition is too short to be explained by actions at the gene level and are considered to be membrane directed. Intermediate time inhibition, seen between 1 and 6 hours, requires activation of the genome and can be blocked by administering inhibitors of protein synthesis; presumably, steroids induce the synthesis of an inhibitory protein. Long-term

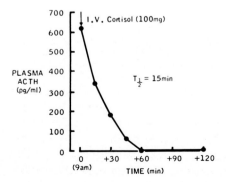

FIGURE 15. Shown here is the response of plasma ACTH to the intravenous injection of cortisol in a patient with adrenocortical insufficiency. The initially elevated levels fall rapidly, illustrating the negative-feedback regulation and the short half-life of ACTH in plasma. (From Irvine, WJ, and Barnes, EW: *Adrenal insufficiency.* In Mason, AS (ed): *Clinics in Endocrinology and Metabolism,* vol 1. WB Saunders Co., Ltd., London, 1972, p. 549, with permission.)

inhibition (12 hours or longer) is accompanied by suppression of mRNA coding for ACTH and decreased ACTH synthesis.

Different kinds of stress (even though they provoke equivalent degrees of adrenal response) are differently inhibited by glucocorticoids. For example, laparotomy combined with intestinal root traction induces ACTH release, which cannot be suppressed by even high glucocorticoid doses. Other stresses, however, such as that provoked by ether exposure, are readily inhibited by glucocorticoids. These differences suggest that feedback effects are predominantly directed at the level of the brain and that there are different neural pathways for different kinds of stress.

Glucocorticoid receptors are present in the pituitary, hypothalamus, and extrahypothalamic brain, but it is not known with certainty which of these serve as the principal target for feedback control.[38,99,155] Because the hippocampus has the largest population of neurons with glucocorticoid receptors and is known to be inhibitory to ACTH secretion, it has been proposed that this region terminates the adrenocortical stress response, a view supported by physiologic studies in aged rats, whose hippocampi are deficient in glucocorticoid receptors.[138]

"Short-loop" feedback of ACTH secretion has also been described.[130]

Increased blood levels of ACTH decrease the release of ACTH from the pituitary, an effect that can be demonstrated in adrenalectomized animals maintained on a constant replacement dose of glucocorticoids. The finding that β-endorphin suppresses ACTH and cortisol levels in man is additional support for a short loop feedback,[162] but studies using a synthetic ACTH do not support the idea of feedback regulation.[177]

ROLE OF NERVOUS STRUCTURES OUTSIDE THE HYPOTHALAMUS

As noted above, a number of extrahypothalamic structures also are involved in ACTH regulation. Isolation of the hypothalamus by cutting fiber connections from the overlying brain results in sustained high plasma corticosterone levels in the rat, providing strong evidence that areas outside the hypothalamus have a tonic inhibitory influence on the hypothalamic secretion of CRF.[34,55] Both activating and inhibitory functions have been described for midbrain structures. Responses to a variety of stressful stimuli depend on the integrity of afferents from the brainstem. This is true for stimuli such as fracture of the leg, surgical trauma, and hemorrhage. Responses to a variety of other stimuli, such as acoustic or photic stimuli and cold stress, also require intact posterior inputs to the hypothalamus.[33]

Several limbic structures are also important in ACTH regulation (Fig. 16).

The amygdala has a predominantly facilitatory effect on ACTH release, as shown by ACTH release following electrical stimulation.[98,123] Studies in which the whole amygdala is lesioned demonstrate in the rat that the amygdaloid complex is essential in ACTH release in response to neurogenic stresses such as fracture of the leg, but not in response to systemic stresses such as tourniquet or ether.[4] Available evidence indicates that this effect is mediated by a direct ventral pathway from the lateral amygdala to the hypothalamus, rather than by the more indirect stria terminalis.

The hippocampus has an inhibitory influence on the pituitary-adrenal axis. Electrical stimulation leads to inhibition and ablation to increased ACTH secretion. Hippocampal glucocorticoid receptors may participate in pituitary-adrenal feedback

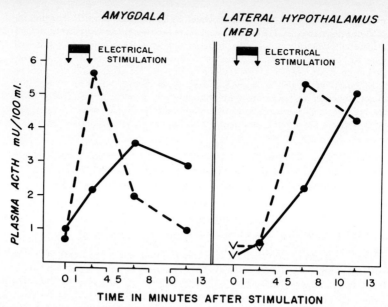

FIGURE 16. Effect of electrical stimulation of the amygdala and lateral hypothalamus (MFB, medial forebrain bundle) on plasma bioassayable ACTH in the cat, showing activation of release. Each line shows a different experiment. Electrical stimulation of the median eminence was without effects. (Plotted from data of Redgate, ES,[123] with permission.)

control (see above). However, Wilson and Critchlow[175] reported that fornix transection or hippocampectomy did not modify rhythms of pituitary-adrenal secretion.

Neurotransmitter Regulation

Adrenocorticotropic hormone secretion is influenced by many different neurotransmitter agonists and antagonists acting through the hypothalamic neuron control network (see Figure 1).[59,68,69] Acetylcholine and serotonin[88] are stimulatory, whereas catecholamines are inhibitory to ACTH release. In the human being, ACTH secretion is enhanced by amphetamines, and the pituitary-adrenal respose to insulin-induced hypoglycemia is augmented by propranolol, a β-adrenergic antagonist, and suppressed by phentolamine, an α-adrenergic blocker, suggesting that there is a stimulating α-adrenergic regulation pathway. Cyproheptadine, a blocker of serotonin, blunts cortisol response to hypoglycemia and the normal cortisol circadian rhythm.[80,82] Fenfluramine, a serotonin-releasing agent, stimulates ACTH in the human being.[88] The relevance of the serotonin stimulatory effect of ACTH regulation in disease is indicated by the inhibitory effects of the serotonin antagonist cyproheptidine on ACTH release in patients with Cushing's disease.[80,82,86] However, this drug also has been shown to act directly on pituitary adenomas,[159] a finding that makes it difficult to be certain about a hypothalamic locus of action.

Adrenocorticotropic hormone secretion is also influenced by neuropeptides, the most important of which are the opioid peptides.

In the human, β-endorphin by systemic infusion lowers circulating ACTH and cortisol levels,[162] as does the injection of met-enkephalin, or the analog DAMME

REGULATION OF THE PITUITARY GLAND

(D-Ala 2.MePhe4, Met (o)-01)-enkephalin).[51]Naloxone, an opiate antagonist, increases cortisol and ACTH. It is likely that these effects are exerted on central CRF neuronal pathways.

NEUROENDOCRINE DISEASE OF THE ADRENAL GLAND

CUSHING'S SYNDROME

Cushing's description in 1932 of the manifestations of excessive secretion of cortisol included virtually all of the features now recognized in florid cases.

> As paraphrased by Ross,[133] Cushing's first case was a 23-year-old woman who had gained 25 pounds in two years and who complained of headaches, nausea, shortness of breath, bruising, baldness, excessive facial hair, and amenorrhea. She had become round-shouldered and had lost four inches in height. On clinical examination, she is described by Cushing as being of most extraordinary appearance: a kyphotic, undersized young woman whose round face was dusky, cyanosed, and abnormally hairy. Her abdomen had the appearance of a full-term pregnancy, her breasts were pendulous, and there were pads of fat over the supraclavicular and posterior cervical regions. Purple striae were present over the abdomen, breasts, shoulders, and hips. Her skin was cyanotic, especially over the trunk and lower extremities, and of marbled appearance, rough and pigmented. The tense and painful adiposity of the trunk contrasted markedly with her thin extremities. The skin bruised easily and often spontaneously, without apparent trauma. Hypertension and glycosuria completed the clinical picture. A definitive description was given by Krieger in 1983.[80,82]

Cushing's syndrome is predominantly a condition of women (women to men ratio 9:1), and when it occurs in men it is much more difficult to detect clinically because most of the symptoms are attenuated. The term *Cushing's syndrome* refers to all patients with excessive amounts of cortisol, whether owing to spontaneous disease of the pituitary or adrenal glands or secondary to steroid therapy. The term *Cushing's disease* is reserved for patients with bilateral adrenal hyperplasia caused by excessive secretion of pituitary ACTH.

The modern clinician, armed with a high index of suspicion and improved laboratory tests for the diagnosis of hypercortisolism, need not wait for the entire array of serious manifestations, and only moderate changes may be noted in patients with clear-cut disease.[154] Today, the most common cause of Cushing's syndrome is the therapeutic use of glucocorticoids in inflammatory and allergic disease. Because of duration of disease, degree of steroid hypersecretion, and the variability of the time at which the disorder comes to the attention of physicians, the relative frequencies of the various manifestations in Cushing's syndrome cannot be given precisely.

The clinical presentation is diagnostic of Cushing's syndrome in only 50 percent of mild or early cases, and frequently the clinician must differentiate between authentic hypercortisolism and the "pseudo-Cushingoid" patient who has primary obesity with hormonal changes secondary to the obesity. Chronic alcoholism also mimics Cushing's disease. These aspects are considered below.

Etiology

The most common pathologic finding in *spontaneous* Cushing's syndrome (approximately 75 percent of cases) is bilateral hyperplasia of the adrenal cortex secondary to excessive ACTH secretion by the pituitary gland. This disease properly fits the designation of Cushing's disease (which Cushing called pituitary basophilism). The other causes, in more or less equal proportions, are adenoma of the adrenal, carcinoma of the adrenal, and the "ectopic" production of ACTH by a malignant neoplasm of an organ such as lung or pancreas. This chapter deals mainly with disorders due to ACTH hypersecretion.

Cushing's Disease/Pituitary Hypersecretion of ACTH

The cases of Cushing's disease with increased pituitary ACTH secretion have the greatest interest to the neuroendocrinologist. Cushing believed that most arose from basophil adenomas of the pituitary gland. Subsequent experience, particularly in patients treated with transsphenoidal surgery, have confirmed the view that a majority of patients (about 85 percent) have demonstrable pituitary adenomas. Approximately 20 percent of cases of Cushing's disease have roentgenographic evidence of sellar abnormality by high resolution computerized axial tomography (CAT) scans, but most patients harbor small adenomas. For example, Boggan and colleagues[7] reported that in the series of 100 patients treated surgically, 82 showed adenomas (60 microadenomas and 22 macroadenomas). Findings in childhood Cushing's disease are similar.[156]

Cushing's original idea that the disease was due to ACTH-producing adenoma appears to be true in most cases. This viewpoint has important implications for ideas of pathogenesis and therapy.

The hypothesis that ACTH hypersecretion could arise from hypothalamic dysfunction was first put forth by Heinbecker,[57] who pointed out that patients dying from Cushing's disease had regressive changes in the paraventricular nucleus.[57] Subsequently, it was found that similar changes could be produced in rat hypothalamus by giving high doses of cortisone[19] (an effect now recognized to be due to suppression of vasopressinergic and CRF-ergic neurons). The idea that central nervous system abnormality was the root cause of Cushing's disease remained strong. In part this was because emotional and physical stress cause ACTH hypersecretion and because, in Cushing's disease, adrenal responses to stress and to suppressive doses of exogenous steroids are qualitatively normal, but quantitatively abnormal, suggesting retention of the normal physiologic regulating mechanisms, but at a new setpoint of control.

In support of a central nervous system etiology it has been pointed out that growth hormone (GH) secretory rhythms are also abnormal in Cushing's disease[47] and that patients with depressive illness have adrenal hypersecretion poorly suppressed by exogenous steroid administration (see chapter 21). Treatment with the drug cyproheptadine, a serotonin-receptor blocker, lowered adrenal cortical function to normal in some cases. Subsequently, more than 100 cases have been treated with the drug, which caused lowering of ACTH in approximately 50 percent.[80,82] However, the demonstration that cyproheptidine can act directly on pituitary adenomas[159] weakens the claim that Cushing's disease is a disorder of the hypothalamus. A few rare cases of Cushing's disease attributable to CRF-secreting hypothalamic gangliocytomas, also have been reported.[5] Most assuredly, these cases have to be considered to be due to hypothalamic disease. A single case has been reported with paroxysmal release of cortisol, responsive to therapy with chlorpromazine (see chapter 11).

Another viewpoint on the pathogenesis of Cushing's disease equally harmonious with clinical observations is that the disorder begins as a pituitary microadenoma that retains normal responsiveness to CRF. This might arise because of the loss or change of feedback receptors for cortisol on a clone of ACTH-producing cells. Numerous cases now have been tested with CRF before and after microadenomectomy. Most show exuberant responses before surgery and flat responses immediately afterward.[20,105,114] This means that the adenoma itself has suppressed normal hypothalamic-pituitary function. The regressive changes in the paraventricular nucleus which can be interpreted as being secondary to hypercortisolism have been cited above. The crucial observation required to establish which of the two hypotheses is correct will require the measurement of CRF concentration in portal-vessel blood. Corticotropin-releasing factor in CSF of patients with Cushing's disease was less than normal (3.7 ± 2.9 (SD) f mol eq/ml versus 8.6 ± 1.7 f mol eq/ml), which can be interpreted to mean that glucocorticoids suppress CRF secretion.[165] However, CRF in CSF probably comes from the entire neuraxis; alterations may therefore reflect altered extrahypothalamic secretion as well as hypothalamic CRF.

Analyses of pituitary-adrenal function in depression give further support to the idea that Cushing's disease is *not* due to a primary hypothalamic disorder. Many patients with psychotic depression have abnormal cortisol circadian rhythms[135] and are resistant to dexamethasone suppression (see chapter 21), an abnormality that reverses with recovery. It has been assumed, therefore, that depressed individuals secrete excessive CRF. Their pituitary-adrenal responses to CRF are blunted.[48] This finding is best explained as being due to the inhibitory effects of the elevated cortisol levels on the pituitary gland. In contrast, the majority of patients with Cushing's disease are hyperresponsive to CRF,[20] a finding best explained by a loss of normal feedback inhibition. In our view it is likely that most cases of Cushing's disease will be found to be due to intrinsic pituitary disease, but that rarely excess CRF secretion may lead to the disorder.

It also should be noted that some corticotropic adenomas are silent, that is, unaccompanied by clinical evidence of Cushing's disease.[62]

ECTOPIC ACTH SECRETION

Hypercortisolism as a paraneoplastic syndrome now is being recognized with some frequency. Oat-cell carcinoma of the lung was the first tumor to be described as associated with Cushing's syndrome, but the etiologic relationship was not appreciated at the time. Reported by Brown in 1928, the case was that of a 45-year-old woman who developed the clinical picture of Cushing's syndrome and died within 5 months of onset of her illness.[37] At postmortem examination she was found to have oat-cell carcinoma of the lung and bilateral adrenal hyperplasia. A number of such cases, associated with a variety of neoplasms, were reported sporadically in the literature[17,18] but only in the early 1960s did three groups of investigators (Liddle, Christy and Holub and their respective collaborators) recognize that the plasma or tumors of such patients contained an ACTH-like material indistinguishable by usual tests from pituitary ACTH.[90,124] It was therefore proposed that ACTH was secreted by the tumor.[17] Detailed studies of the chemical properties of the ACTH secreted by tumors have been carried out. Like ACTH in pituitary glands, large and small forms are recognizable by anti-ACTH antibodies, but only the small form is biologically active. Tumors generally contain and secrete a larger proportion of the large (inactive) form than of the small form of ACTH and other components of the POMC complex such as α-endorphin.[80-82] Virtually all bronchogenic carcinomas contain ACTH prohormone, which in most cases produces no clinical manifestations because it is biologically inactive.

Less common carcinomas causing Cushing's syndrome are thymus, pancreas (including islet-cell tumors), carcinoid, neoplasms of neural-crest tissues (pheochromocytomas, neuroblastoma, paraganglioma, ganglioma, medullary carcinoma of the thyroid), and isolated cases of tumor of the ovary, prostate, breast, thyroid, kidney, salivary glands, testis, stomach, colon, gallbladder, esophagus, appendix, and acute myelogenous leukemia.[120] Adrenocorticotropic-hormone secreting tumors commonly produce more than one peptide, or biogenic amine. Thus, ACTH hypersecretion may be accompanied by secretion of vasopressin, or of serotonin, gastrin, norepinephrine, calcitonin, and glucagon.[112]

The presentation of Cushing's syndrome owing to ectopic ACTH production usually occurs atypically. Marked hypercortisolism may develop almost explosively, either at the beginning of or late in the course of tumor growth, so that many of the usual features (such as obesity and striae) do not have time to develop.[90] Instead, electrolyte abnormalities (notably severe hypokalemic alkalosis), hypertension, and diabetes mellitus may dominate the picture. The electrolyte abnormalties are due to excessive secretion of the mineralocorticoids, desoxycorticosterone (DOC), and 18-hydroxy-DOC. Usually other manifestations of tumor are evident, but in a few cases the differentiation from Cushing's disease is not readily apparent because the primary tumor is occult. Such cases are not easy to distinguish from Cushing's disease; fortunately, they are not common. A striking feature of the ectopic ACTH syndrome is marked pigmentation;[90,143] the producton of cortisol is usually much higher than in Cushing's disease. Plasma cortisol levels over 50 μg/100 ml are virtually pathognomonic of the ectopic disorder.

Corticotropin-releasing factor-secreting tumors also have been reported.[157] These include bronchogenic carcinoma and pheochromocytoma; they cause the disease by stimulating pituitary ACTH secretion. A hypothalamic gangliocytoma secreting CRF has been reported.[5]

Several types of tumors producing ACTH are of particular interest from a neuroendocrine point of view. These are tumors arising from neural-crest cells, and they include medullary carcinoma of the thyroid, islet-cell tumors, gangliomas, and pheochromocytomas. These can secrete an extraordinary range of peptides and neurotransmitters. According to

Pearse,[119] ACTH-producing cells of the pituitary belong to the APUD series (Amine Precursor Uptake Decarboxylase cells), as do the other cells of neural-crest origin, and it is not surprising, therefore, that these other cells might share the primitive capacity to form ACTH. However, other tumors not having similar embryologic origin may form ACTH, suggesting a still more primitive differentiation of protein synthesis and secretion.

DIFFERENTIAL DIAGNOSIS

Details of the metabolic aspects of Cushing's disease are dealt with in standard endocrinology texts, and the important psychologic aspects of this condition are reviewed in chapter 21. This section summarizes the physiologic basis of neuroendocrine tests for the differential diagnosis of cortisol hypersecretion.

From a clinical point of view it is first essential to exclude iatrogenic hypercortisolism. A history of ingestion of glucocorticoids such as prednisone and cortisone may be readily disclosed, but less obvious would be the long-term use of topical steroids (cortisol analogs) which in patients with severe skin disease may be absorbed in amounts sufficient to cause systemic toxicity. Such patients present with evidence of hypercortisolism with suppressed adrenal cortical function, as indicated by the low excretion of cortisol and its metabolites and low plasma ACTH. Factitious hypercortisolism also should be considered and will present the same biochemical findings.

The ectopic ACTH syndrome is associated (as is Cushing's disease) with evidence of atypically high cortisol secretion and high ACTH levels in the blood (over 200 pg/ml and usually greater than 500 pg/ml). Most ectopic-tumor cases have evident systemic disease; more than half show lung tumor, but, rarely, other occult tumors may cause the syndrome. Extremely high cortisol excretion and severe electrolyte abnormality, particularly if it appears abruptly, strongly favor the existence of a tumor. Hypokalemic alkalosis is uncommon in Cushing's disease.

Plasma ACTH measurements permit differentiation of the main forms of Cushing's syndrome into two main groups, the hypersecretors and hyposecretors of ACTH. Adrenocorticotropic hormone measurements now are available in commercial laboratories and are useful in differential diagnosis when the diagnosis is not clearly apparent by the older tests. Computerized axial tomography scans should be taken routinely; these are abnormal in about 20 percent of Cushing's disease cases.

Normal diurnal secretion patterns show maximum values up to 25 μg/dl occurring between 4:00 AM and 8:00 AM and minimum values, usually not exceeding 8 μg, in late afternoon and evening. In psychically and physically stressed patients, particularly during the first day or two of hospitalization, it is not uncommon to see even higher values (up to 40 μg/dl) and loss of normal diurnal variation. Marked and invariable elevation of plasma cortisol throughout the day (15 μg/dl late afternoon, 35 μg/dl in the morning) is strong evidence for hypersecretion. Increased cortisol secretion is reflected in increased urinary excretion of cortisol and its metabolites.[13,26,66,154] Normal values for adult glucocorticoid excretion (17-hydroxycorticoids) are 4 to 12 mg per 24 hours and are a function of muscle mass. Marked elevation of urinary glucocorticoid excretion is seen in well-established Cushing's disease, but there is an overlap with the normal levels; a few very obese patients who have a form of secondary hypercortisolism and a number of patients with Cushing's syndrome may have total corticoid secretion that falls within the normal range. Streeten and coworkers[153,154] have defined carefully the criteria for laboratory diagnosis of Cushing's disease.

Given clinical evidence of hypercortisolism and laboratory evidence of increased cortisol secretion—such as high plasma cortisol, loss of diurnal rhythm, increased glucocorticoid excretion, or increased free cortisol excretion in urine—adrenal suppression tests provide the best confirmatory evidence of adrenal abnormality and give great assistance in classifying the nature of the defect (see below).

ADRENAL CORTICAL INSUFFICIENCY: ADDISON'S DISEASE

Acute or chronic adrenal insufficiency poses a severe threat to the life of the patient. Insufficiency may be primary (adrenal failure) or secondary to pituitary hypofunction. The disease described by Addison and which bears his name is a chronic, primary disease of adrenal glands of diverse causes. In Addison's disease, hypothalamic-pituitary regulation of the adrenal gland is qualitatively normal. Adrenocorticotropic hormone levels are elevated in response to the low plasma glucocorticoids. Negative feedback of plasma glucocorticoids is intact, with normal or slightly diminished sensitivity as assessed by the response to exogenously administered glucocorticoids. Circadian periodicity of plasma ACTH is retained despite the overall elevation in circulating levels.

In Addison's time the most common cause of adrenal failure was tuberculosis. With the decline in the incidence of tuberculosis, the greater number of cases appear to be due to "idiopathic" adrenal atrophy. Most cases probably have autoimmune disorder.[8,64] The majority have adrenal autoantibodies, and the illness is often associated with polyglandular failure, the most common association being with thyroiditis of the Hashimoto type and diabetes mellitus.[28] Schmidt's syndrome is the name given to combined adrenal and thyroid failure. The thyroid usually fails first and the adrenal gland some time later. Rarely does the reverse order occur. Addison's disease is managed by administration of a glucocorticoid (cortisone 25 to 37.5 mg per day; prednisone 5 to 7.5 mg per day), a mineralocorticoid such as Florinef 0.05 to 0.2 mg per day, and in women (to restore libido) testosterone (long-acting preparation such as testosterone enanthate), the equivalent of 1 to 2 mg per day (30 to 50 mg per month IM). The dose should be lowered if excessive hair growth is detected. In all cases of adrenal failure, regardless of cause, the replacement dose must be increased twofold to threefold during stress, and the patient must be instructed to wear a MedicAlert identification to ensure adequate care if found unconscious.

Adrenal insufficiency secondary to pituitary disease may occur with pituitary tumors, infarction, granulomas, or other pituitary lesions. Defects in pituitary function are usually multiple and lead to panhypopituitarism. In the absence of ACTH, cortisol secretion is markedly reduced, but aldosterone secretion is much less affected. In chronic hypopituitarism the adrenal medulla is spared and the response to ACTH may be delayed, owing to secondary atrophy of the adrenal cortex. The clinical presentation of glucocorticoid deficiency in secondary adrenal failure is less severe than in Addison's disease. The clinical findings and management of patients with panhypopituitarism are discussed in chapter 16.

HYPOTHALAMIC HYPOADRENALISM

Disturbance of adrenal function secondary to hypothalamic or other brain lesions occurs less frequently than alteration of gonadotropin, GH, or prolactin secretion. Disturbances of diurnal rhythms of pituitary-adrenal secretion are common with intracranial disease and provide an early, sensitive index to disturbance of neuroendocrine control.[78] Structural lesions of the hypothalamus (tumors, inflammation, hydrocephalus) rarely result in serious adrenal insufficiency. The reason for this is not clear; a relatively large reserve of CRF neurons may be present. Anencephalic infants without any hypothalamic tissue secrete measurable concentrations of cortisol into the blood, and in a few cases respond to insulin hypoglycemia or ADH with further cortisol release. Isolated ACTH deficiency is rare but has been reported in a few cases.[2,63] One may speculate that congenital absence of CRF can occur in a situation analogous to hypothalamic hypothyroidism and hypogonadism.

ADRENOLEUKODYSTROPHY

The association of adrenal insufficiency with demyelination of the brain has been extensively investigated by Schaumberg and collaborators[144] and by Moser and coworkers.[102] This condition, called adrenoleukodystrophy, is sex-linked, occurring almost exclusively in male subjects. It is recognized now that many cases of so-called Schilder's disease fit into this group. The onset is usually in childhood, between the ages of 4 and 16 years. Personality change, dementia, vomiting, unsteady gait and ataxia, increasing pigmentation of extensor surfaces and oral mucosa, cortical blindness, and quadriplegia lead to death in 5 to 10 years in most cases. A rarer form of the disease called *adrenomyeloneuropathy* also may occur, affecting girls and boys and producing a combination of central nervous system and peripheral nerve symptoms.[6,102] The adrenal glands become atrophic and show specific cytoplasmic inclusions. Extensive demyelination occurs in the cerebrum and results in hemianopia, blindness, and dementia. Adrenal failure and central demyelination are believed to be due to an enzymatic defect in myelin metabolism, but the precise abnormality has not been identified. Abnormal accumulation of $C_{24}-C_{26}$ long-chain fatty acids has been documented in the adrenal glands and in the myelin of the central nervous system. Increased secretion of these fatty acids in the urine provides a diagnostic test. There is no treatment for the disorder.

LABORATORY DIAGNOSIS OF ACTH ABNORMALITIES

Because ACTH deficiency and excess have serious consequences for health, their accurate diagnosis is extremely important. Most testing proce-

secretion which stimulates increased steroid biosynthesis. The increased secretion of total 17-hydroxycorticosteroids indicates an adequate ACTH reserve. Either hypothalamic or pituitary disease can cause abnormal responses. Normal responses to decreased plasma cortisol levels (the basis of the metyrapone test) require a certain number of functioning ACTH cells in the pituitary gland and a certain amount of CRF secretion. Loss of either of these components of ACTH regulation may result in failure of the response, and for this reason the test does not discriminate adequately between hypothalamic and pituitary abnormalities.

The standard test is performed by administering metyrapone, 750 mg every 4 hours for six doses. Pituitary, hypothalamic, or adrenal failure can cause impaired responses. A normal response consists of a two-fold or greater increase in urinary 17-hydroxycorticosteroids on the day of administration or the day following, compared with preadministration values. The enzyme-blocking effectiveness is demonstrated by measuring compound S. In Cushing's disease, the response is supranormal.[154] Streeten and colleagues have standardized a one-day metyrapone test.[154]

Stress-induced ACTH Responses

The administration of insulin, pyrogens, and vasopressin all have been used to stimulate ACTH secretion. The most readily available clinical test, the insulin hypoglycemia test, is useful in evaluating simultaneously GH and PRL reserves as well.

All stress tests are at best unpleasant, and at worst dangerous. Both hypoglycemia and vasopressin can induce coronary insufficiency and are contraindicated in older patients or those with known heart disease. Neither pyrogen nor vasopressin evokes stimulatory responses in 10 percent of normal persons, and for this reason failure to respond is not an absolute indicator of hypothalamic-pituitary failure. In practice, it is sometimes useful to evaluate ACTH, GH, and prolactin secretory reserves by measuring plasma hormone levels after the patient has completed a stressful diagnostic procedure. A patient with suspected ACTH deficiency never should be exposed to severe stress without adequate pretreatment with corticoids. This applies particularly to angiography and surgical procedures.

An abnormal stress test does not differentiate between hypothalamic and pituitary causes of insufficiency.

CRH Test in Hypoadrenalism

The CRH test has not as yet been made available for general use, but enough information has been gained to give a relatively clear idea as to its potential value in the differential diagnosis of pituitary-adrenal disease. In normal individuals, CRH has a relatively prolonged action. Indeed, the hormonal response has the longest duration of action of any of the releasing factors owing to the relatively long half-life of CRH in the circulation (half-life of fast component, 11.6 minutes, and of the slow component, 73 minutes); plasma levels of ACTH and cortisol remain elevated for 2 to 3 hours after a single injection.[145,146] The doses that have been used widely for diagnostic purposes have been 100 μg and 1 μg/kg (see above). The National Institutes of Health (NIH) group[49] carries out tests in the evening because baseline levels of ACTH and cortisol are lowest at that time and responses were found to be greater than in the morning,[48,49] but Tsukada and associates[166] reported that despite the differences in baseline levels, increments of both ACTH and cortisol are the same in the morning as in the evening.

Patients with normal pituitary-adrenal reserve have normal responses to CRH, although the CRH-induced responses are not as intense as those to insulin hypoglycemia,[93] possibly reflecting the fact that the stress response includes vasopressin and epinephrine components. Patients who fail to respond to insulin-induced hypoglycemia may respond to CRH (Fig. 18). As far as can be told from the limited number of cases reported,[93,146,167] those who respond have hypothalamic disease, thus suggesting that the CRF tests can differentiate between hypothalamic and

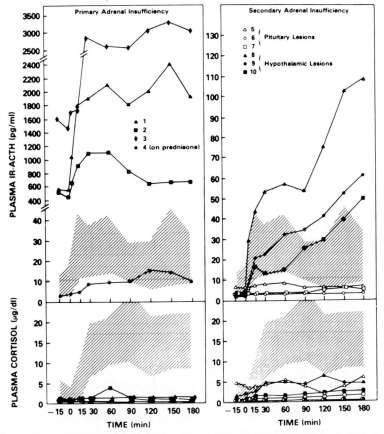

FIGURE 18. Effects of CRH on patients with hypoadrenalism, are plotted here. (*Left*) Patients with primary adrenal cortical disease, (*right*), patients with either hypothalamic or pituitary disease causing ACTH deficiency. Four out of five of the patients with adrenal insufficiency had supra-normal responses, and one had a response within the low range of normal. In patients with secondary adrenal insufficiency, all six of the cases caused by hypothalamic disease had either a normal or increased ACTH response, and the responses of the three cases with pituitary disease were below normal. (From Schulte, HM[146] with permission.)

pituitary failures. It will take more experience to determine whether this generalization holds true for all cases.

DIAGNOSIS OF GLUCOCORTICOID EXCESS

The diagnosis of ACTH hypersecretion is considered in the differential diagnosis of Cushing's syndrome, which can be caused by primary hypersecretion of ACTH by a pituitary adenoma (Cushing's disease), by primary disease of the adrenal gland (adenoma, carcinoma, multinodular hyperplasia), or by the ectopic secretion of ACTH by a cancer such as carcinoma of lung, carcinoid, or medullary thyroid carcinoma. Cushing's syndrome rarely has been caused by CRH-secreting gangliocytoma of the hypothalamus. Depression is associated in some cases with elevated cortisol secretion.

The diagnosis of adrenal hyperfunction is made first, and further tests are carried out for differential diagnosis. Hypersecretion is suggested by demonstrating (1) loss of diurnal variations; (2) serum cortisol levels consistently above 25 μg/ml, urinary-free cortisol levels in excess of 200 μg per 24 hours, or urinary 17-hydroxycorticosteroid levels in excess of 18 mg per 24 hours (corrected for body weight).[154]

Dexamethasone Suppression Test

As a screening test, 1 mg of dexamethasone is administered at 10 to 11 PM. Morning cortisol levels in normal individuals fall to 5 μg/dl or less. If suppression does not occur, more additional sophisticated suppression testing is carried out.

The standard test for Cushing's syndrome was originally developed by Liddle and colleagues[89] (Fig. 19). This test is carried out by first administering dexamethasone at a low dose (0.5 mg every 6 hours for 2 days) and then at a high dose (2 mg every 6 hours for 2 days). Suppression at high doses but not low doses points to pituitary-dependent Cushing's disease. Excess cortisol secretion owing to adrenal tumors or ectopic ACTH secretion is refractory to inhibition at both doses. Almost without exception, the high-dose dexamethasone suppression test will reduce plasma cortisol in Cushing's disease but not affect levels in patients with adrenal disease or ectopic ACTH secretion, although some exceptions have been reported. The greatest problem is in the differentiation of ectopic production of ACTH by occult carcinoids. Pituitary-dependent adrenal nodular hyperplasia may not be suppressed by even high-dose dexamethasone. A few cases of dexamethasone suppression-resistant Cushing's disease have been reported, one of which was suppressed by cortisol, suggesting an abnormality in the dexamethasone receptor.[14]

In most (but not all) patients with Cushing's syndrome of whatever cause, dexamethasone, 2 mg per day, will not inhibit endogenous corticoid secretion, a finding that indicates an elevation of setpoint control (see Figure 19). The main exceptions to this generalization are some patients with obesity who may suppress only after a longer period of administration (up to 4 days), and a few patients with Cushing's disease secondary to hypothalamic tumor or to ectopic ACTH production. Patients with depres-

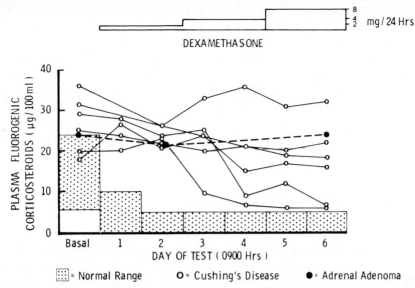

FIGURE 19. Effects of dexamethasone treatment on the secretion of the adrenal cortex in patients with Cushing's disease and adrenal hyperfunction caused by adrenal adenoma are illustrated. In five of the six patients with Cushing's disease (open circles), plasma cortisol gradually decreased, but the dose required for suppression was much greater than that required in normal individuals. In the patient with adenoma, there were no changes in plasma cortisol. Responses in the patient with Cushing's disease indicate an "elevated setpoint" for feedback control of ACTH secretion, whereas the response in the patient with adenoma indicates completely autonomous function. (From Besser, GM, and Edwards, CRW: *Cushing's syndrome.* In Mason, AS (ed): *Clinics in Endocrinology and Metabolism,* vol. 1. WB Saunders, Philadelphia, 1972, p 451, with permission.)

sion may also fail to suppress with low-dose dexamethasone. In rare patients with Cushing's disease who suppress glucocorticoid secretion with the low dose of dexamethasone, associated defects in dexamethasone metabolism lead to abnormally high (and suppressive) levels of this steroid.[75,101] Atypical suppression tests occur in patients with pituitary-dependent nodular hyperplasia of the adrenal cortex. In the patient who fails to suppress corticoid secretion with the 2 mg per day dexamethasone dose, it is recommended that 8 mg per day be administered. In most (but not all) cases of Cushing's disease, this dose will suppress corticoid excretion but will not in patients with adenomas, carcinomas of the adrenal gland or the ectopic-ACTH syndrome. Although this conclusion is generally correct, several rare instances have been reported in which this differentiation was not valid. These cases included patients with adrenal carcinoma and adrenal adenoma. Paradoxic response (that is increased cortisol excretion after dexamethasone) has been observed in one patient who otherwise showed typical Cushing's disease.[36]

The exceptions to the rule, though uncommon, reemphasize the importance of the clinical evaluation and the recognition that no one test is infallible for proper diagnosis of Cushing's disease.[154]

Patients with adrenal tumors usually do not show adrenal response to the administration of ACTH, but patients with Cushing's disease are hyperresponsive. A few patients with adrenal carcinoma, however, are ACTH-responsive.

Obesity with secondary hypercortisolism is a special problem, particularly important because many very obese women develop purple striae, hirsutism, and amenorrhea. The classic, central type of obesity occurs in only half of patients with Cushing's disease. Most obese patients will show suppression of plasma cortisol to less than 5 μg/dl after the administration of a single dose of 1.0 mg dexamethasone at bedtime (screening suppression test), but a few require 2 mg per day for more than 4 days. Urinary free cortisol is rarely elevated in obesity.

Chronic alcoholism or administration of certain drugs, notably phenytoin and estrogens, may give rise to findings suggestive of Cushing's disease. Careful study indicates that these can be distinguished on the basis of reversibility (after withdrawal of alcohol or drugs).

CRH in Adrenal Cortical Hypersecretion

Patients with classical Cushing's disease almost uniformly show either normal or an exuberant response to CRH, whereas patients with primary adrenal hypersecretion owing to adenoma or ectopic ACTH almost always show suppressed responses.[20,113,121,176] Similarly, the administration of glucocorticoids blunts or suppresses responses to CRH. The CRH test thus far appears to be excellent in differentiating between classical Cushing's disease and primary adrenal cortical hypersecretion. The test does not differentiate between adrenal tumor and ectopic ACTH secretion. There have not been any cases reported as yet in which the ectopic ACTH secretion was enhanced by CRH. Hermus and collaborators[180] compared CRH and high-dose dexamethasone suppression for efficacy in distinguishing Cushing's disease from other causes of Cushing's syndrome. A false-negative response to CRH was present in 9 percent (2 of 22) patients with Cushing's disease. A false-negative dexamethasone suppression test occurred in 11 percent (2 of 18). Three patients with Cushing's syndrome owing to adrenal adenoma were unresponsive to both CRH and dexamethasone. One patient with ectopic ACTH secretion showed no response to either CRH or dexamethasone.

One of the fairly frequent problems in differential diagnosis that arises is that between Cushing's disease and depression. In the studies of Gold and colleagues,[48,49] patients with chronic depressive disease showed a blunted response to CRH (in contrast to Cushing's disease).

PHYSICAL METHODS FOR DIAGNOSIS OF ADRENAL DISEASE

Computerized axial tomography (CAT) scanning has become the most useful physical technique for diagnosing adrenal disease.[111,150,164] Adrenal tumors are readily diagnosed because they have become large by the time clinical manifestations of hypersecretion are apparent. Bilateral hyperplasia can be detected in a large proportion of cases, a finding confirmatory of ACTH hypersecretion. Computerized axial tomography scanning is also mandatory for the differential diagnosis of pituitary microadenomas, although, in symptomatic Cushing's disease, only 20 to 30 percent will show diagnostic abnormalities (see chapter 14).

In difficult diagnostic cases of adrenal disease, it may be necessary to carry out angiography or local venous catheterization with measurement of cortisol levels.[111] Large adrenal tumors also can be detected by abdominal echo scans. At one time, intravenous pyelography (IVP) was commonly done to demonstrate distortion of regional anatomy by adrenal tumors, but this approach has been superseded by the methods described above.

Because fewer than 30 percent of patients with Cushing's disease have adenomas detected on CAT scans, and only 80 percent have tumors demonstrable at the time of transsphenoidal adenomectomy, other techniques to localize the tumor have been developed. The most promising is bilateral simultaneous petrosal sinus catheterization.[110] Measurement of ACTH in blood drawn from these vessels provides evidence of a local "step-up" in concentration, permitting appropriate hemihypophysectomy, even when no tumor has been visualized by direct examination.

It is possible that magnetic resonance imaging (MRI) will prove to be especially useful in diagnosis of pituitary adenomas (see chapter 14).

TREATMENT

CUSHING'S SYNDROME

If Cushing's syndrome is due to tumor of the adrenal gland, excision is the treatment of choice. In ectopic ACTH production, the culprit tumor is removed if possible or treated by chemotherapy or roentgenotherapy. If the condition is due to an operable lesion (which is rare), cure may result. The excess cortisol secretion can be controlled by drugs that act on the adrenal cortex to suppress steroid formation.[8] These drugs include metyrapone, aminoglutethemide, and the adrenocortolytic drug o,p'-DDD (Mitotane). Metyrapone blocks the formation of cortisol by blocking the 11β-hydroxylase step. Aminoglutethemide, a drug that is selectively concentrated in the adrenal cortex and interferes with corticoid biosynthesis with damage to the cell is a better choice, and effects are evident within a few days. It is so effective that replacement cortisol therapy is usually required. o,p'-DDD, another adrenal cortical toxin, is widely used for treatment of inoperable and metastatic adrenal carcinoma.

CUSHING'S DISEASE

The use of the antiserotonergic drug cyproheptadine has been advocated by Krieger as a treatment of choice in some patients.[80,81] The rationale for use of the drug developed from experimental observations of the facilitatory function of central nervous system serotonin in the release of ACTH. Cyproheptadine, which is a serotonin receptor blocker (it also has antihistaminic and antidopaminergic actions), has been shown in some patients with Cushing's disease to reduce ACTH levels to normal and to restore circadian rhythmicity and dexamethasone suppressibility. Remission of clinical symptoms occurs simultaneously with the return of biochemical parameters to normal. Administration of 24 to 32 mg daily in divided doses is required. Significant side effects of hyperphagia and somnolence occur in most patients. In over 100 patients treated to date, the response rate is less than 50 percent. Relapses occur in some patients despite continued medication and in most on cessation of drug treatment, although permanent remission has been reported in a few cases. Responses also have been observed in a few patients with Nelson's syndrome. It is our opinion that the drug may be useful as an adjunct to radiation or in preparation of patients with fulminant symptoms of the disease for surgery but that its use as a primary form of therapy is unwarranted. Cyproheptadine has been used successfully to manage Cushing's disease in pregnancy.[50]

Unlike the situation in tumor-induced Cushing's syndrome, whether of adrenal or extraadrenal origin, in which the course of therapy is usually straightforward, the treatment of Cushing's disease has passed through many fashions and is still subject to continuing revisions. Before synthetic corticoids were developed, these patients were treated by adrenalectomy on one side and subtotal adrenalectomy on the other, the idea being that sufficient adrenal tissue would be left to maintain health. However, in most cases, this procedure led either to adrenal insufficiency or to relapse, and so it is no longer used. Instead, bilateral total adrenalectomy became widely practiced, the patient then being maintained on regular replacement therapy with the equivalent of 25 to 37.5 mg of cortisone per day and 9-α-fluorohydrocortisone, a mineralocorticoid, at a dose of 0.1 to 0.2 mg per day. However, such patients almost invariably show increasing pigmentation, increasing high ACTH levels in blood (over 500 to 750 pg/ml), and in 10 to 15 percent, evidence of pituitary tumor. This occurrence, called Nelson's syndrome, requires radiotherapy and/or neurosurgical removal, because this type of tumor is especially likely to behave like a carcinoma by invading the base of the skull and to cause optic and cranial nerve damage.

Because bilateral adrenalectomy is followed by the lifetime requirement for adrenal cortical replacement, and by development of Nelson's syndrome in about 15 percent, there has been continuing study of effective ways of directing therapy at the pituitary gland. In many centers, conventional roentgenotherapy (5000 rads) is used and will cause a remission in about 50 percent of cases and virtually completely prevent the late occurrence of Nelson's syndrome.[116,148] Success rate is higher in children.[67] Because the response is quite slow, this approach is not advised in severe cases unless there is direct therapy of the adrenal glands with drugs such as aminoglutethemide or metyrapone. Proton-beam irradiation[77] is said to ameliorate Cushing's disease in a much higher proportion of cases — 85 percent or more — and in 80 percent in Nelson's syndrome, but this procedure is limited to only a few centers. Its full therapeutic effectiveness remains to be determined. Pituitary microsurgery is recommended as the treatment of choice in cases with evident adenomas. Microsurgery in cases with normal CAT scans reveals tumors in 80 to 85 percent of cases; 70 percent or more are cured. Newer procedures to improve the success of surgery include preoperative venous catheterization of the sinus to detect asymmetrical ACTH secretion[110] and the use of central "wedge" resection if tumors are not found. Despite the apparent success of unilateral hypophysectomy, it should be pointed out that in approximately two thirds of cases with adenomas the tumor is located in the central region of the pituitary gland.[55,171] Wedge secretion would be expected to cure two thirds of cases. Total hypophysectomy may be necessary. In such cases, the choice is between hypophysectomy and bilateral adrenalectomy. Most clinical endocrinologists opt for adrenalectomy when this decision must be made.

The true recurrence rate after apparently successful adenomectomy is not known with accuracy and varies from center to center (range from 4 to 50 percent).[12] The problem of maintaining normal pituitary function after either microsurgery or proton-beam irradiation must be considered. Only a small proportion (about 10 percent) are reported to develop hypopituitarism, but this possibility is a consideration, especially in patients who want to have children. A small number of cases have successfully been treated with bromocriptine.[72]

In our opinion, in the future, all patients with Cushing's disease will be treated first by pituitary microsurgery unless some contraindication exists. This is true for children as well.[156] If the hypercortisolism is severe, medical measures directed against adrenal steroidogenesis are available until the pituitary disorder can be attacked directly. Proper choice of treatment now depends on access to treatment resources, such as radiation therapy and skilled neurosurgeons.

REFERENCES

1. ABRAMS, HL, SIEGELMAN, SS, ADAMS, DF, SANDERS, R, FINBERG, HJ, HESSEL, SJ, McNEIL, BJ: *Computed tomography versus ultrasound of the adrenal gland: A prospective study.* Radiology 143:121–129, 1982.
2. ABRAMSON, EA, AND ARKY, RA: *Coexistent diabetes mellitus and isolated ACTH deficiency: Report of a case.* Metabolism 17:492–495, 1968.
3. ADDISON, T: *On the constitutional and local effects of disease of the supra-renal capsules.* Samuel Highley, London, 1855.
4. ALLEN, JP, AND ALLEN CF: *Role of the amygdaloid complexes in the stress-induced release of ACTH in the rat.* Neuroendocrinology 15:220–230, 1974.
5. ASA, SL, KOVACS, K, TINDALL, GT, BARROW, DL, GHORVATH, E, VECSEI, P: *Cushing's disease associated with an intrasellar gangliocytoma producing cortico-trophin-releasing factor.* Ann Int Med 101:789–793, 1984.
6. BERKOVIC, SF, ZAJAC, JD, WARBURTON, DJ, MERORY, JR, FELLENBERG, AJ, POULOS, A, POLLARD, AC: *Adrenomyeloneuropathy—clinical and biochemical diagnosis.* NZ J Med 13:594–600, 1983.
7. BOGGAN, JE, TYRELL, JB, WILSON, CB: *Transsphenoidal microsurgical management of Cushing's disease.* J Neurosurg 59:195–200, 1983.
8. BONDY, PK: *Disorders of the adrenal cortex.* In WILSON, JD, AND FOSTER, DW (EDS): *Willliams Textbook of Endocrinology,* ed 7. WB Saunders, Philadelphia, 1985; pp 816–890.
9. BROWN, MR, AND FISHER, LA: *Corticotropin-releasing factor: Effects on the autonomic nervous system and visceral systems.* Fed Proc 44:243–248, 1985.
10. BROWN-SEQUARD, CE: (1856; cited by Medvei, VC) *A History of Endocrinology.* MTP Press Limited, Lancaster, 1982, pp 230–231.
11. BRUHN, TO, SUTTON, RE, RIVIER, CL, VALE, WW: *Corticotropin-releasing factor regulates proopiomelanocortin messenger ribonucleic acid levels in vivo.* Neuroendocrinology 39:170–175,1984.
12. BURCH, W: *A survey of results with transsphenoidal surgery in Cushing's disease.* (Letter) N Engl J Med 308:103–104, 1983.
13. BURKE, CW, AND BEARDWELL, CG: *Cushing's syndrome and internal hydrocephalus producd by a cerebellar tumor.* Q J Med 42:175–184, 1973.
14. CAREY, RM: *Suppression of ACTH by cortisol in dexamethasone-suppressible Cushing's disease.* N Engl J Med 302:275–279, 1980.
15. CARLSON, DE, DORNHORST, A, GANN, DS: *Organization of the lateral hypothalamus for control of adrenocorticotropin release in the cat.* Endocrinology 107:961–969, 1980.
16. CARLSON, DE, DORNHORST, A, SEIF, SM, ET AL: *Vasopressin-dependent and independent control of the release of adrenocorticotropin.* Endocrinology 110:680–682, 1982.
17. *Case records, Cushing's disease (pancreatic tumor).* N Engl J Med 304:591–599, 1981
18. *Case records, Cushing's disease (lung tumor).* N Engl J Med 305:1637, 1981.

19. CASTOR, CW, BAKER, BL, INGLE, DJ, LI, CH: *Effects of treatment with ACTH or cortisone on anatomy of the brain.* Proc Soc Exp Biol 76:353–357, 1951.

20. CHROUSOS, GP, SCHULTE, HM, OLDFIELD, EH, GOLD, PW, CUTLER, PW, CUTLER, GBJR, LORIAUX, JL: *The corticotropin-releasing factor stimulation test: An aid in the evaluation of patients with Cushing's syndrome.* N Engl J Med 310:622–626, 1984.

21. CLARK, JH, SCHRADER, WT, O'MALLEY, BW: *Mechanism of steroid hormone action.* In WILSON, JD, FOSTER, DW, (EDS): *Williams Textbook of Endocrinology,* ed 7. WB Saunders, Philadelphia, 1985, pp 33-75.

22. COLT, EW, WARDLAW, SL, FRANTZ, AG: *The effect of running on plasma betaendorphin.* Life Sci 28:1637–1640, 1981.

23. DEGROOT, J, AND HARRIS, GW. *Hypothalamic control of the anterior pituitary gland and blood lymphocytes.* J Physiol (London) 111:335–346, 1950.

24. DEBOLD, CR, DECHERNEY, GS, JACKSON, RV, SHELDON, WR, ALEXANDER, N, ISLAND, DP, RIVIER, J, VALE, W, ORTH, DN: *Effect of synthetic ovine corticotropin-releasing factor: Prolonged duration of action and biphasic response of plasma adrenocorticotropin and cortisol.* J Clin Endocrinol Metab 57:294–298, 1983.

25. DREYFUSS, F, BURLET, A, TONON, MC, VAUDRY, H: *Comparative immunoelectron microscopic localization of corticotropin-releasing factor (CRF-41) and oxytocin in the rat median eminence.* Neuroendocrinology 39:284–287, 1984.

26. EDDY, RL, JONES, AC, GILLILAND, PF, ET AL: *Cushing's syndrome. A prospective study of diagnostic methods.* Am J Med 55:621–630, 1973.

27. EIPPER, BA, MAINS, RE: *Structure and biosynthesis of proadrenocorticotropin/endorphin and related peptides.* Endocrine Rev 1:1-27, 1980.

28. EISENBARTH, GS: *The immunoendocrinopathy syndromes.* In WILSON, JD, AND FOSTER, DW (EDS): *Williams Textbook of Endocrinology,* ed 7. WB Saunders, Philadelphia, 1985, pp 1290–1300.

29. ERSPAMER, V, MELCHIORRI, P: *Actions of amphibian skin peptides on the central nervous system and the anterior pituitary.* In MÜLLER, EE, MACLEOD, RM (EDS): *Neuroendocrine Perspectives,* vol 2. Elsevier, Amsterdam, 1983, pp 37–106.

30. FARESE, RV: *Phosphoinositide metabolism and hormone action.* Endocrine Rev 3:78–95, 1983.

31. FEEK, CM, MARANTE, DJ, EDWARDS, CRW: *The hypothalamic-pituitary adrenal axis.* In SCANLON, MR (ED): *Clinics in Endocrinology and Metabolism.* WB Saunders, Philadelphia, 1983, pp 597–618.

32. FEHM, HL, KLEIN, E, HOLL, R, VOIGHT, KH: *Evidence of extrapituitary mechanisms mediating the morning peak of plasma cortisol in man.* J Clin Endocrinol Metab 58:410–414, 1984.

33. FELDMAN, S: *Neural pathways mediating adrenocortical responses.* In VALE, W, AND GREER, M (EDS): *Corticotropin-releasing Factor,* Fed Proc 44:169–176, 1985.

34. FORTIER, C: *Nervous control of ACTH secretion.* In HARRIS, GW, AND DONOVAN, BT (EDS): *The Pituitary Gland.* Butterworth, London, 1966, vol 2, pp 195–234.

35. FORTIER, C, AND SELYE, H: *Adrenocorticotrophic effect of stress after severance of the hypothalamo-hypophyseal pathways.* Am J Physiol 159:433–439, 1949.

36. FRENCH, FS, MACFIE, JA, BAGGETT, B, WILLIAM, TF, VAN-WYK, JJ: *Cushing's syndrome with a paradoxical response to dexamethasone.* Am J Med 47:619–624, 1969.

37. FRIEDMAN, M, MARSHALL-JONES, P, ROSS, EJ: *Cushing's syndrome: Adrenocortical hyperactivity secondary to neoplasm arising outside the pituitary-adrenal system.* Q J Med 34:193–214, 1966.

38. FUXE, K, WIKSTROL, AC, OKRET, S, AGNATI, LF, HARFSTRAND, A, YU, ZY, GRANHOLD, LL, ZOLI, M, VALE, W, GUSTAFSSON, JA: *Mapping of glucocorticoid receptor immunoreactive neurons in the rat tel- and diencephalon using a monoclonal antibody against rat liver glucocorticoid receptor.* Endocrinology 117:1803–1812, 1985.

39. GALLAGHER, TF, YOSHIDA, K, ROFFWARG, HD, FUKUSHIMA, DK, WEITZMAN, ED, HELLMAN, L: *ACTH and cortisol secretory patterns in man.* J Clin Endocrinol Metab 36:1058–1073, 1973.

40. GAMBERT, SR, GARTHWAITE, TL, PONTZER, CH, COOK, EE, TRISTIANI, FE, DUTHIE, EH, MARTINSON, DR, HAGEN, TC, MCCARTY, DJ: *Running elevates plasma beta-endorphin immunoreactivity and ACTH in untrained human subjects.* Proc Soc Exp Biol Med 168:1–4, 1981.

41. GANN, DS, ALLEN-ROWLANDS, CF, BEREITER, DA, PLOTSKY, PM: *Pituitary adrenal regulation in relation to affective disorder.* In BROWN, GM, KOSLOW, SH, REICHLIN, S (EDS): *Neuroendocrinology and Psychiatric Disorder.* Raven Press, New York, 1984, pp 229–239.

42. GANN, DS, BEREITER, DA, CARLSON, DE, THRIVIKAMEN, KV: *Neural interaction in control of adrenocorticotropin.* Fed Proc 44:161–168, 1985.

43. GANONG, WF, BARBIERI, C: *Neuroendocrine components in the regulation of renin secretion.* In GANONG, WF, AND MARTINI, L (EDS): *Frontiers in Neuroendocrinology,* vol. 7. Raven Press, New York, 1982, pp 231–262.

44. GEE, CE, CHEN, CL, ROBERTS, JL, THOMPSON, R, WATSON, SJ: *Identification of proopiomelanocortin neurons in rat hypothalamus by in situ cDNA-mRNA hybridization.* Nature 306:374–376, 1983.

45. Gibbs, DM: *Measurement of hypothalamic corticotropin-releasing factors in hypophyseal portal blood.* In Vale, W, and Greer, M (eds): *Corticotropin-releasing Factor.* Fed Proc 44:203–206, 1985.

46. Gillies, GE, Linton, EA, Lowry, PJ: *Corticotropin-releasing activity of the new CRF is potentiated several times by vasopressin.* Nature 299:355–357, 1982.

47. Gold, PW, and Chrousos, GP: *Clinical studies with corticotropin releasing factor: Implications for the diagnosis and pathophysiology of depression, Cushing's disease, and adrenal insufficiency.* Psychoneuroendocrinology. 10(4):401–419, 1985.

48. Gold, PW, Kellner, CH, Rubinow, DR, Altemus, M, Post, RM: *Abnormal growth hormone responses to corticotropin releasing factor in patients with primary affective disorder.* Endocrine Society, p. 191, 1983.

49. Gold, PW, Loriaux, DL, Roy, A, Kellner, CH, Post, RM, Picker, D, Galluci, W, Avgerinos, P, Schulte, H, Paul, S, Nieman, L, Oldfield, EH, Cutler, GB, Chrousos, GP: *Responses to corticotropin-releasing hormone in the hypercortisolism of depression and Cushing's disease.* N Engl J Med 314:1329–1335, 1986.

50. Griffith, DN, Ross, EJ: *Pregnancy after cyproheptadine treatment for Cushing's disease* [letter]. N Engl J Med 305:893–894, 1981.

51. Grossman, A, Clement-Jones, V, Besser, GM: *Clinical implications of endogenous opioid peptides.* In Müller, EE, MacLeod, RM, Frohman, LA (eds): *Neuroendocrine Perspectives,* vol 4. Elsevier, Amsterdam, 1985, pp 243–294.

52. Guillemin, R, Rosenberg, B: *Humoral hypothalamic control of anterior pituitary: A study with combined tissue cultures.* Endocrinology 57: 599–607, 1955.

53. Guillemin, R, Vargo T, Rossier, J, Minick, S, Ling, N, Rivier, C, Vale, W, Bloom, F: *Beta-endorphin and adrenocorticotropin are secreted concomitantly by the pituitary gland.* Science 197:1367–1369, 1977.

54. Guy, J, Vaudry, H, Pelletier, G: *Differential projections of two immunoreactive alpha-melanocyte stimulating hormone (alpha-MSH) neuronal systems in the rat brain.* Brain Res 220:199–202, 1981.

55. Hardy, J: *Transsphenoidal microsurgical treatment of pituitary tumors.* In Linfoot, JA (ed): *Recent Advances in the Diagnosis and Treatment of Pituitary Tumors.* Raven Press, New York, 1979, pp 375–388.

56. Healy, DL, Chrousos, GP, Schulte, HM, Gold, PW, Hodgen, GD: *Increased adrenocorticotropin, cortisol, and arginine vasopressin secretion in primates after the antiglucocorticoid steroid RU 496: Dose response relationships.* J Clin Endocrinol Metab 60:1–11, 1985.

57. Heinbecker, P: *The pathogenesis of Cushing's disease.* Medicine 23:225–247, 1944.

58. Hermus, AR, Pieters, GFFM, Smals, AGH, Benraad, TJ, Kloppenborg, PWC: *Plasma adrenocorticotropin, cortisol, and aldosterone responses to corticotropin-releasing factor: Modulatory effect of basal cortisol levels.* J Clin Endocrinol Metab 58:187–191, 1984.

59. Hillhouse, EW, Burden, J, Jones, MT: *The effect of various putative neurotransmitters on the release of corticotropin releasing hormone from the hypothalamus of the rat in vitro.* Neuroendocrinology 17:1–11, 1975.

60. Hiroshige, T, and Abe, K: *Role of brain biogenic amines in the regulation of ACTH secretion.* In Yagi, K, and Yoshida, S (eds): *Neuroendocrine Control.* John Wiley & Sons, New York, 1973, p 205.

61. Hook, VYH, Heisler, S, Axelrod, J: *Corticotropin-releasing factor stimulates phospholipid methylation and corticotropin secretion in mouse pituitary tumor cells.* Proc Natl Acad Sci USA 79:6220–6224, 1982.

62. Horvath, E, Kovacs, K, Killinger, DW, Smyth, HS, Platts, ME, Singer, W: *Silent corticotropic adenomas of the human pituitary gland.* Am J Pathol 98:617–638, 1980.

63. Hung, W, and Migeon, CJ: *Hypoglycemia in a two-year-old boy with adrenocorticotrophic hormone (ACTH) deficiency (probably isolated) and adrenal medullary unresponsiveness to insulin induced hypoglycemia.* J Clin Endocrinol Metab 28:146–152, 1968.

64. Irvine, WJ: *Autoimmune mechanisms in endocrine disease.* Proc Roy Soc Med 67:499–502, 1974.

65. Jacobowitz, DM, and O'Donohue, TL: *Alpha-melanocyte stimulating hormone: Immunohistochemical identification and mapping in neurons of rat brain.* Proc Natl Acad Sci USA 75:6300–6304, 1978.

66. James, VHT, and Landon, J (eds): *The investigation of hypothalamic-pituitary-adrenal function.* Memoirs of the Society for Endocrinology 17. Cambridge University Press, Cambridge, 1968.

67. Jennings, AS, Liddle, GW, Orth, DL: *Results of treating childhood Cushing's disease with pituitary irradiation.* N Engl J Med 297:957–962, 1977.

68. Jones, MT: *Control of corticotropin (ACTH) secretion.* In Jeffcoate, SL, Hutchinson, JSM (eds): *The Endocrine Hypothalamus.* Academic Press, New York, 1978, pp 385–420.

69. Jones, MT, Hillhouse, EW: *Neurotransmitter regulation of corticotropin-releasing factor in vitro.* Ann NY Acad Sci 297:536–560, 1977.

70. JOSEPH, SA AND KNIGGE, KM: *Corticotropin releasing factor: Immunocytochemical localization in rat brain.* Neurosci Lett 35:135–141, 1983.

71. JOSEPH, SA, PILCHER, WH, KNIGGE, KM: *Anatomy of the corticotropin-releasing factor and opiomelanocortin systems of the brain.* Fed Proc 44:100–107, 1985.

72. KAPCALA, LP, AND JACKSON, IMD: *Long term bromocriptine therapy in Cushing's disease.* J Endocrinol Invest 5:117–120, 1982.

73. KELLER-WOOD, ME, AND DALLMAN, MF: *Corticosteroid inhibition of ACTH secretion.* Endocrine Rev 5:1–14, 1984.

74. KENDALL, JW: *Feedback control of adrenocorticotrophic hormone secretion.* In MARTINI, L, AND GANONG, WF (EDS): *Frontiers in Neuroendocrinology,* Oxford University Press, New York, 1971, pp 177–207.

75. KING, LW, POST KD, YUST, JY, REICHLIN, S: *Suppression of cortisol secretion by low-dose dexamethasone testing in Cushing's disease.* J Neurosurg 58:129–132, 1983.

76. KISS, JZ, MEZEY, E, SKIRBOLL, L: *Corticotropin-releasing factor-immunoreactive neurons of the paraventricular nucleus become vasopressin positive after adrenalectomy.* Proc Natl Acad Sci USA 1854–1858, 1984.

77. KJELLBERG, RN, KLIMAN, B, SWISHER, B, BUTLER, W: *Proton beam therapy of Cushing's disease and Nelson's syndrome.* In BLACK, PM, ZERVAS, NT, RIDGWAY, EC, MARTIN, JB (EDS): *Secretory Tumors of the Pituitary Gland.* Raven Press, New York 1984, p. 295–307.

78. KRIEGER, DT: *Pathophysiology of central nervous system regulation of anterior pituitary function.* In *Biology of Brain Dysfunction,* vol II. Plenum Press, New York, 1973, pp 351–408.

79. KRIEGER, DT: *Rhythms in CSF, ACTH, and corticosteroids.* In KRIEGER, DT (ED): *Endocrine Rhythms.* Raven Press, New York, 1979, pp 123–142.

80. KRIEGER, DT: *Physiopathology of Cushing's disease.* Endocrine Rev 4:22–43, 1983.

81. KRIEGER, DT: *Medical management of Cushing's disease.* In BLACK, PM, ZERVAS, NT, RIDGWAY, EC, MARTIN, JB (EDS): *Secretory Tumors of the Pituitary Gland.* Raven Press, 1984, pp 273–285.

82. KRIEGER, DT AND GLICK, SM: *Sleep EEG stages and plasma growth hormone concentration in states of endogenous and exogenous hypercortisolemia or ACTH elevation.* J Clin Endocrin Metab 39:986–1000, 1974.

83. KRIEGER, DT, LIOTTA, AS, BROWNSTEIN, MJ, ET AL: *ACTH, beta-lipotropin, and related peptides in brain, pituitary, and blood.* Recent Prog Horm Res 36:277–344, 1980.

84. LABRIE, F, VEILLUS, R, LEFEVRE, G, COY, DH, SUEIRAS-DIAZ, J, SCHALLY, AV: *Corticotropin-releasing factor stimulates accumulation of adenosine 3',5'-monophosphate in rat pituitary corticotrophs.* Science 216:1007–1008, 1982.

85. LAMBERTS, SWJ, VERLEUN, T, OOSTEROM, R, DEJONG, F, HACKENG, WHL: *Corticotropin-releasing factor (ovine) and vasopressin exert a synergistic effect on adrenocorticotropin release in man.* J Clin Endocrin Metab 58:1087–1089, 1984.

86. LANFORD, HV, ST. GEORGE TUCKER, J, BLACKARD, WG: *A cyproheptadine reversible defect in ACTH control persisting after removal of the pituitary tumor in Cushing's disease.* N Engl J Med 305:1244–1248, 1981.

87. LEROUX, P, PELLETIER, G: *Radioautographic study of binding and internalization of corticotropin-releasing factor by rat anterior pituitary corticotrophs.* Endocrinology 114:14–21, 1984.

88. LEWIS, DA, AND SHERMAN, BM: *Serotonergic stimulation of adrenocorticotropin secretion in man.* J Clin Endocrinol Metab 58:458–462, 1984.

89. LIDDLE, GW, ISLAND, D, MEADOR, CK: *Normal and abnormal regulation of corticotropin secretion in man.* Rec Prog Horm Res 18:125–153, 1962.

90. LIDDLE, GW, GIVENS, JR, NICHOLSON, WE, ISLAND DP: *The ectopic ACTH syndrome.* Cancer Res 25:1057–1061, 1965.

91. LIEBERMAN, S, GREENFIELD, NJ, WOLFSON, A: *A heuristic proposal for understanding steroidogenic processes.* Endocrine Rev 5:128–148, 1984.

92. LIU, JH, MUSE, K, CONTRERAS, P, GIBBS, K, VALE, W, RIVIER, J, YEN, SSC: *Augmentation of ACTH-releasing activity of synthetic corticotropin-releasing factor (CRF) by vasopressin in women.* J Clin Endocrinol Metab 57:1087–1089, 1983.

93. LYTRAS, N, GROSSMAN, A, PERRY, L, TOMLIN, S, WASS, JAH, COY, DH, SCHALLY, AV, REES, LH, BESSER, GM: *Corticotropin releasing factor: Responses in normal subjects and patients with disorders of the hypothalamus and pituitary.* Clin Endocrinol 20:71–84, 1984.

94. LYTRAS, N, GROSSMAN, AS, REES, LH, SCHALLY, AV, BLOOM, SR, BESSER, GM: *Corticotropin releasing factor: Effects on circulating gut and pancreatic peptides in man.* Clin Endocrinol 20:725–729, 1984.

95. MAKARA, GB, STARK, E, RAPPAY, G, KARTESZI, M, PALKOVITS, M: *Changes in corticotropin releasing factor of the stalk median eminence in rats with various cuts around the medial basal hypothalamus.* J Endocrinol 83:165–173, 1979.

96. MANGILI, G, MOTTA, M, MARTINI, L: *Control of adrenocorticotropic hormone secretion.* In MARTINI, L, AND GANONG, WF (EDS): Neuroendocrinology, vol 1, Academic Press, New York, 1966, pp 297–370.

97. Maran, JW, Carlson, DE, Grizzle, WE, Ward, DG, Gann, DS: *Organization of the medial hypothalamus for control of adrenocorticotropin in the cat.* Endocrinology 103:957–970, 1978.

98. Matheson, GK, Branch, BJ, and Taylor, AN: *Effects of amygdaloid stimulation on pituitary-adrenal activity in conscious cats.* Brain Res 32:151–167, 1971.

99. McEwen, BS, Biegon, A, Davis, PG, Krey, LC, Luine, VN, McGinnis, MY, Paden, CM, Parsons, B, Rainbow, TC: *Steroid hormones: Humoral signals which alter brain cell properties and functions.* Rec Progr Horm Res 8:41–92, 1982.

100. McLoughlin, L, Lowry, PJ, Ratter, SJ, Hope, J, Besser, GM, Rees, LH: *Characterization of the pro-opiocortin family of peptides in human cerebrospinal fluid.* Neuroendocrinology 32:209–212, 1981.

101. Meikle AW: *Dexamethasone suppression tests: Usefulness of simultaneous measurement of plasma cortisol and dexamethasone.* Clin Endocrinol 16:401–408, 1982.

102. Moser, HW, Moser, AE, Singh, I, O'Neill, BP: *Adrenoleukodystrophy: Survey of 303 cases: Biochemistry, diagnosis, and therapy.* Ann Neurol 16:628–641, 1984.

103. Motta, M, Fraschini, F, Martini, LH: *"Short" feedback mechanisms in the control of anterior pituitary function.* In Ganong, WF, and Martini, L (eds): *Frontiers in Neuroendocrinology.* Oxford University Press, London, 1969, pp 211–254.

104. Motta, M, Mangili, G, Martini, L: *A "Short" feedback loop in the control of ACTH secretion.* Endocrinology, 77:392–395, 1965.

105. Müller, OA, Stalla, GK, Hartwimmer, J, Schopol, J, von Werder, K: *Corticotropin releasing factor (CRF): Diagnostic implications.* Acta Neurochirurgica 75:49–59, 1985.

106. Müller, OA, Stalls, GK, von Werder, K: *Corticotropin releasing factor: A new tool for the differential diagnosis of Cushing's syndrome.* J Clin Endocrinol Metab 57:227–229, 1983.

107. Nakahjara, M, Shibasaki, T, Shizume, K, Kiyosawa, Y, Odagiri, E, Suda, T, Yamaguchi, H, Tsushima, T, Demura, H, Maeda, T, Wakabayashi, I, Ling, N: *Corticotropin-releasing factor test in normal subjects and patients with hypothalamic-pituitary-adrenal disorders.* J Clin Endocrinol Metab 57:963–968, 1983.

108. Nakanishi, S, Inoue, A, Kita, T, Nakamura, M, Chang, ACY, Cohen, SN, Numa, S: *Nucleotide sequence of cloned cDNA for bovine corticotropin-beta-lipotropin precursor.* Nature 278:423–427, 1979.

109. Nakanishi, S, Inoue, A, Kita, T, et al: *Construction of bacterial plasmids that contain the nucleotide sequence for bovine corticotropin-beta-lipotropin precursor.* Proc Natl Acad Sci USA 75:6021–6025, 1978.

110. Oldfield, EH, Chrousos, GP, Schulte, HM, Schaaf, M, McKeever, PE, Krudy, AG, Cutler, GB, Jr., Loriaux, DL, Doppman, JL: *Preoperative lateralization of ACTH-secreting pituitary microadenomas by bilateral and simultaneous inferior petrosal venous sinus sampling.* N Engl J Med 312:100–103, 1985.

111. Older, RA, Van Moore, A Jr, Glenn, JF, Hidalgo, HJ: *Diagnosis of adrenal disorders.* Radiol Clin North America 22:433–455, 1984.

112. O'Neal, LW, Kipnis, DM, Luse, SA, Lacy, PE, Jarett, L: *Secretion of various endocrine substances by ACTH-secreting tumors-gastrin, melanotropin, norepinephrine, serotonin, parathormone, vasopressin, glucagon.* Cancer 21:1219–1232, 1968.

113. Orth, DN: *The old and the new in Cushing's syndrome* (editorial). N Engl J Med 310:649–651, 1984.

114. Orth, DN, DeBold, CR, DeCherney, G, Jackson, RV, Alexander, AN, Rivier, J, Rivier, C, Speiss, J, Vale, W: *Pituitary microadenomas causing Cushing's disease respond to corticotropin-releasing factor.* J Clin Endocrinol Metab 55:1017–1019, 1982.

115. Orth, DN, DeBold, CR, DeCherney, GS, Jackson, RV, Sheldon, WR, Jr, Nicholson, WE, Uderman, H, Alexander, AN, Island, DP, Rivier, J, Vale, WW. *Clinical studies with synthetic ovine corticotropin-releasing factor.* Fed Proc 44:197–202, 1985.

116. Orth, DN, and Liddle, GW: *Results of treatment in 108 patients with Cushing's syndrome.* N Engl J Med 285:243–247, 1971.

117. Orth, DN, DeBold, CR, DeCherney, GS, Jackson, RV, Sheldon, WR, Nicholson, WE, Uderman, H, Alexander, AN, Island, DP, Rivier, J, Vale, WW: *Clinical studies with synthetic ovine corticotropin-releasing factor.* Fed Proc vol 44, no. 1, pt. 2, 1985, pp 197–202.

118. Patthy, M, Horvath, J, Mason-Garcia, M, Szoke, B, Schlesinger, DH, Schally, AV: *Isolation and amino-acid sequence of corticotropin releasing factor (CRF) from pig hypothalami.* Proc Natl Acad Sci USA 82:8762–8766, 1985.

119. Pearse, AGE: *The diffuse neuroendocrine system and the APUD concept: Related "endocrine" peptides in brain, intestine, pituitary, placenta and anuran cutaneous glands.* Med Biol 55:115–125, 1977.

120. Pfluger, KH, Gramse, M, Gropp, C, Havemann, K: *Ectopic ACTH production with autoantibody formation in a patient with acute myeloblastic leukemia.* N Engl J Med 305:1632–1636, 1981.

121. Pieter, GFFM, Hermus, ARMM, Smals, AGH, Bartelink, AKM, Benraad, TH, Kloppen-

BORG, PWC: *Responsiveness of the hypophyseal-adrenocortical axis to corticotropin-releasing factor in pituitary dependent Cushing's disease.* J Clin Endocrinol Metab 57:513–516, 1983.

122. PIETERS, GFFM, HERMUS, ARMM, SMALS, AGH, KLOPPENBORG, PWC: *Paradoxical responsiveness of growth hormone to corticotropin-releasing factor in acromegaly.* J Clin Endocrinol Metab 58:560–562, 1984.

123. REDGATE, ES: *ACTH release evoked by electrical stimulation of brain stem and limbic system sites in the cat: The absence of ACTH release upon infundibular area stimulation.* Endocrinology 86:806–823, 1970.

124. REES, LH, AND RATCLIFFE, JG: *Ectopic hormone production by nonendocrine tumors.* Clin Endocrinol (Oxf) 3:263–299, 1974.

125. REES, LH: *Human adrenocorticotropin and lipotropin (MSH) in health and disease.* In MARTINI, L, AND BESSER GM (EDS): *Clinical Neuroendocrinology.* Academic Press, New York, 1978, pp 402–442.

126. ROBERTS, JL, CHEN, C-LC, EBERWINE, JH, ET AL: *Glucocorticoid regulation of proopiomelanocortin gene expression in rodent pituitary.* Rec Prog Horm Res 38:227–256, 1982.

127. RIVIER, C, AND VALE, W: *Effects of corticotropin-releasing factor, neurohypophyseal peptides, and catecholamines on pituitary function.* Fed Proc 44, no 1, pt 2, 1985, pp 189–196.

128. RIVIER, C, AND VALE, W: *Modulation of stress-induced ACTH release by corticotropin-releasing factor, catecholamines and vasopressin.* Nature 305:325–327, 1983.

129. RIVIER, C, RIVIER, J, VALE, W: *Inhibition of adrenocorticotropic hormone secretion in the rat by immunoneutralization of corticotropin-releasing factor.* Science 218:377–379, 1982.

130. RIVIER, J, SPEISS, J, VALE, W: *Characterization of rat hypothalamic corticotropin-releasing hormone factor.* Proc Natl Acad Sci USA 80:4851–4855, 1983.

131. ROBERTS, JL, HERBERT, E: *Characterization of a common precursor to corticotropin and beta-lipotropin: Identification of beta-lipotropin peptides and their arrangement relative to corticotropin in the precursors synthesized in a cell-free system.* Proc Natl Acad Sci USA 74:5300–5304, 1977.

132. ROBERTS, JL, CHEN, CL, CHEN, C, EBERWINE, JH. *Glucocorticoid regulation of proopiomelanocortin gene expression in rodent pituitary.* Recent Progr Horm Res 38:227–256, 1982.

133. ROSS, EJ, MARSHALL-JONES, P, FRIEDMAN, M: *Cushing's syndrome: Diagnostic criteria.* Q J Med 35:149–192, 1966.

134. ROTH, J, AND GRUNFELD, C: *Mechanism of action of peptide hormones and catecholamines.* In WILSON, JD, AND FOSTER, DW (EDS): *Williams Textbook of Endocrinology,* ed 7. WB Saunders, Philadelphia, 1985, pp 76–122.

135. RUBIN, RT, AND POLAND, RE: *The chronoendocrinology of endogenous depression.* In MÜLLER, EE, AND MACLEOD, RM (EDS): *Neuroendocrine Perspectives.* Elsevier Biomedical, Amsterdam, 1982, pp 305–338.

136. SACHAR, EJ, HELLMAN, L, ROFFWARG, HP, HALPERN, FS, FUKUSHIMA, DK, GALLAGHER, TF: *Disrupted 24-hour pattern of cortisol secretion in psychotic depression.* Arch Gen Psychiatry 28:19–24, 1973.

137. SAFFRAN, M, AND SCHALLY, AV: *Release of corticotropin by anterior pituitary tissue in vitro.* Can J Biochem 33:408–415, 1955.

138. SAPOLSKY, RM, KREY, KC, MCEWEN, BS: *Glucocorticoid-sensitive hippocampal neurons are involved in terminating the adrenocortical stress response.* Proc Natl Acad Sci USA. 81: 6174–6177, 1984.

139. SAWCHENKO, PE, AND SWANSON, LW: *Localization, colocalization, and plasticity of corticotropin-releasing factor immunoreactivity in rat brain.* Fed Proc 44, no 1, pt 2, 1985, pp 221–228.

140. SAWCHENKO, PE, AND SWANSON, LW: *The organization and biochemical specificity of afferent projections to the paraventricular and supraoptic nuclei.* Prog Brain Res 60:19–29, 1983.

141. SAWCHENKO, PE, SWANSON, LW, VALE, WW: *Corticotropin-releasing factor: Co-expression within distinct subsets of oxytocin-, vasopressin-, and neurotensin-immunoreactive neurons in the hypothalamus of the male rat.* J Neurosci 4:1118–1129, 1984.

142. SAWCHENKO, PE, SWANSON, LW, VALE, WW: *Co-expression of corticotropin-releasing factor and vasopressin immunoreactivity in parvocellular neurosecretory neurons of the adrenalectomized rat.* Proc Natl Acad Sci USA 81:1883–1887, 1984.

143. SAWIN, CT, ABE, K, ORTH, DN: *Hyperpigmentation due solely to increased plasma beta-melanotropin.* Arch Int Med 125:708–710, 1970.

144. SCHAUMBERG, HH, POWERS, JH, ET AL: *Adrenoleukodystrophy: Similar ultrastructural changes in adrenal cortical and Schwann cells.* Arch Neurol 30(5):406–408.

145. SCHULTE, HM, CHROUSOS, GP, BOOTH, JD, OLDFIELD, EH, GOLD, PW, CUTLER, GB, JR, LORIAUX, DL: *Corticotropin-releasing factor: Pharmacokinetics in man.* J Clin Endocrinol Metab 58:192–196, 1984.

146. SCHULTE, HM, CHROUSOS, GP, AVGERINOS, P, OLDFIELD, EH, GOLD, PW, CUTLER, GB, JR, LORIAUX, DL: *The corticotropin-releasing hormone stimulation test: A possible aid in the evaluation of patients with adrenal insufficiency.* Clin Endocrinol Metab 58:1054–1067, 1984.

147. SELYE, H: *The physiology and pathology of exposure to stress.* Acta, Montreal, Canada, 1950.

REGULATION OF THE PITUITARY GLAND

148. SHELINE, GE: *Radiation therapy of pituitary tumors.* In GIVENS, JR (ED): *Hormone-secreting Pituitary Tumors.* Yearbook Medical Publishers, Chicago, 1982, pp 121–143.

149. SHIBIHARA, S, MORIMOTO, Y, FURUTANI, Y, NOTAKI, M, TAKAHASHI, H, SHIMUZU, S, HORIKAWA, S, NUMA, S: *Isolation and sequence analysis of the human corticotropin-releasing factor precursor gene.* Embo J 2:775–779, 1983.

150. SHIRKHODA, A: *Current diagnostic approach to adrenal abnormalities.* J Comput Tomogr 8:277–285, 1985.

151. SIGGINS, GR, GRUOL, D, ALDENHOFF, J, PITTMAN, Q: *Electrophysiological actions of corticotropin-releasing factor in the central nervous system.* Fed Proc 44, no 1, pt 2, 1985, pp 237–242.

152. SPIESS, J, RIVIER, J, RIVIER, C AND VALE, W: *Primary structure of corticotropin-releasing factor from ovine hypothalamus.* Proc Natl Acad Sci USA 78:6517–6521, 1981.

153. STREETEN, DHP, ET AL: *The diagnosis of hypercortisolism. Biochemical criteria differentiating patients from lean and obese normal subjects and from females and oral contraceptives.* J Clin Endocrinol Metab 29:1191–1211, 1969.

154. STREETEN, DHP, ANDERSON, GH, JR, DALAKOS, TG, SEELEY, D, MALLOV, JS, EUSEBIO, R, SUNDERLIN, FS, BADAWY, SZA, KING, RB: *Normal and abnormal function of the hypothalamic-pituitary-adrenocortical system in man.* Enodocrine Rev 5, 1984, pp 371–394.

155. STUMPOF, WE, AND SAR, M: *Anatomical distribution of corticosterone concentrating neurons in rat brain.* In STUMPOF, WE, AND GRANT, LD (EDS): *Anatomical Neuroendocrinology.* S Karger, Basel, 1975, pp 254–261.

156. STYNE, DM, GRUMBACH, MM, KAPLAN, SL, WILSON, CB, CONTE, FA: *Treatment of Cushing's disease in childhood and adolescence by transsphenoidal microadenomectomy.* N Engl J Med 310:889–893, 1984.

157. SUDA, T, TOMORI, N, TOZAWA, F, DEMURA, H, SHIZUME, K, MOURI, T, MIURA, Y, SASANO, N: *Immunoreactive corticotropin and corticotropin-releasing factor in human hypothalamus, adrenal, lung cancer and pheochromocytoma.* J Clin Endocrinol Metab 58:919–924, 1984.

158. SUDA, T, TOZAWA, F, MOURI, T, DEMURA, H, SHIZUME, K: *Presence of immunoreactive corticotropin-releasing factor in human cerebrospinal fluid.* J Clin Endocrinol Metab 57:225–226, 1983.

159. SUDA, T, TOZAWA, F, MOURI, T, SASAKI, A, SHIBASAKI, T, DEMURA, H, SHIUME, K: *Effects of cyproheptadine, reserpine and synthetic corticotropin-releasing factor on pituitary glands from patients with Cushing's disease.* J Clin Endocrinol Metab 56:1094–1099, 1983.

160. SUTTON, RE, KOOB, GF, LEMOAL, M, ET AL: *Corticotropin releasing factor produces behavioral activation in rats.* Nature 297:331–333, 1982.

161. SWANSON, LW, SAWCHENKO, PE, RIVIER, J, VALE, WW: *Organization of ovine corticotropin-releasing factor immunoreactive cells and fibers in the rat brain: An immunohistochemical study.* Neuroendocrinology 36:165–186, 1983.

162. TAYLOR T, DLUHY, RG, WILLIAMS, GH: *Beta-endorphin suppresses adrenocorticotropin and cortisol levels in normal human subjects.* J Clin Endocrinol Metab 57:592–596, 1983.

163. TILDERS, FJH, BERKENBOSCH, F, VERNES, I, LINTON, EA, SMELIK, PG: *Role of epinephrine and vasopressin in the control of the pituitary-adrenal response to stress.* Fed Proc vol 44, no. 1, pt. 2, 1985, pp 155–160.

164. TISNADO, J, CHO, SR, WALSH, JW, BEACHLEY, MC, GOLDSCHMIDT, RA: *Computed tomography versus angiography in the diagnosis of large right adrenal carcinomas.* J Comput Tomogr 8:287–299, 1984.

165. TOMORI, N, SUDA, T, TOZAWA, F, DEMURA, H, SHIZUME, K AND MOURI T: *Immunoreactive corticotropin-releasing factor concentrations in cerebrospinal fluid from patients with hypothalamic-pituitary-adrenal disorders.* J Clin Endocrinol Metab 57:1305–1307, 1983.

166. TSUKADA, T, NAKAI, Y, KOH, T, TSUJII, S, IMURA, H: *Plasma adrenocorticotropin and cortisol responses to intravenous injection of corticotropin-releasing factor in the morning and evening.* J Clin Endocrinol Metab 57:869–871, 1983.

167. TSUKADA, T, NAKAI, Y, KOH, T, TSUJII, S, INADA, M, NISHIKAWA, M, SHINODA, H, KAGAI, I, TAKEZAWA, N, IMURA, H: *Plasma adrenocorticotropin and cortisol responses to ovine corticotropin-releasing factor in patients with adrenocortical insufficiency due to hypothalamic and pituitary disorders.* J Clin Endocrinol Metab 58:758–760, 1984.

168. VALE, W, AND GREER, M: *Corticotropin-releasing factor.* Fed Proc 44:145–146, 1984.

169. VALE, W, RIVIER, C, BROWN, MR, SPEISS, J, KOOB, G, SWANSON, L, BILEZIKJIAN, L, BLOOM, F, RIVIER, J: *Chemical and biological characterization of corticotropin releasing factor.* Rec Prog Horm Res 39:245–270, 1983.

170. VALE, WW, RIVIER, C, SPEISS, J, RIVIER, J: *Corticotropin releasing factor.* In KRIEGER, DT, BROWNSTEIN, MJ, MARTIN, JB (EDS): *Brain Peptides.* John Wiley and Sons, New York, 1983, pp 963–974.

171. VON WERDER, K, EVERSMAN, T, FAHLBUSCH, R, MULLER, OA, RJOSK, HK: *Endocrine-active pituitary adenomas: Long-term results of medical and surgical treatment.* In CAMANNI, F, AND MÜLLER, EE (EDS): *Pituitary Hyperfunction, Physiopathology and Clinical Aspects.* Raven Press, New York, 1984, pp 385–406.

172. WARD, DG, AND GANN, DS: *Inhibition and facilitatory areas of the dorsal medulla mediating ACTH release in the cat.* Endocrinology 99:1213–1219, 1976.

173. WARD, DG, BOLTON, MG, GANN, DS: *Inhibitory and facilitatory areas of the ventral midbrain mediating release of corticotropin in the cat.* Endocrinology 102:1147–1154, 1978.

174. WARD, DG, GRIZZLE, WEE, GANN, DS: *Inhibitory and facilitatory areas of the rostral pons mediating ACTH release in the cat.* Endocrinology 99:1220–1228, 1976.

175. WILSON, M, AND CRITCHLOW, V: *Effect of fornix transection or hippocampectomy on rhythmic pituitary-adrenal function in the rat.* Neuroendocrinology 13:29–40, 1973/74.

176. WYNN, PC, AGUILERA, G, MORELL, J, ET AL: *Properties and regulation of high-affinity pituitary receptors for corticotropin-releasing factor.* Biochem Biophys Res Commun 110:602-608, 1983.

177. CAVAGNINI, F, INVITTI, C, DANESI, L, PASSAMONTI, H, FOSSATI, R: *Evidence against a self-inhibiton of ACTH secretion in man.* Neuroendocrinology 41:518–525, 1985.

178. KRIEGER, DT, AND GLICK, SM: *Growth hormone and cortisol responsiveness in Cushing's syndrome. Relation to a possible central nervous system etiology.* Am J Med 52:25–40, 1972.

179. TACHE, Y, AND GUNION, M: *Corticotropin-releasing factor: Central action to influence gastric secretion.* Fed Proc vol 44, no 1, pt 2, 1985, pp 255-258.

180. HERMUS, AR, PESMAN, GJ, BENRAAD, TJ, ET AL: *The corticotropin-releasing-hormone test versus the high-dose dexamethasone test in the differential diagnosis of Cushing's syndrome.* Lancet II:540–544, 1986.

Chapter 7

REGULATION OF PROLACTIN SECRETION AND ITS DISORDERS

Long recognized as an important hormone in lower vertebrates, it was not until 1970 that prolactin (PRL) was shown to be a distinct hormone in primates, including human beings.[13,36,43,65,66,86–88,98,120,122,139] Prolactin is essential to the stimulation of milk production in mammals. Indeed, prolactin-dependent milk production has been crucial to the evolution of mammals whose offspring require a relatively long period of time after birth to become self-sufficient.

Prolactin secretion is influenced by many different stimuli. In addition to suckling (Fig. 1), PRL is released in response to physical and emotional stress,[24] meals,[16,140] arginine infusion, hypoglycemia, and estrogen administration. Prolactin secretion also is regulated by sleep-related rhythms. In its lability, PRL secretion resembles the secretion of growth hormone (GH) and of adrenocorticotropic hormone (ACTH).

Although many neural stimuli can induce PRL release, secretion is inhibited tonically by the hypothalamus; PRL secretion can be increased by any process that interferes with hypothalamic-pituitary continuity.

PITUITARY PROLACTIN SECRETION

Prolactin is a protein hormone secreted by specific cells of the anterior pituitary gland designated *lactotropes.* These generally stain chromophobic by classical methods because they have relatively small storage pools of hormone, but they are readily differentiated by specific immunohistochemical techniques and have characteristic secretory granules demonstrable by electron microscopy.[28,142] At least two cell subtypes are present in human pituitaries. Prolactin circulates in the blood and is present in the pituitary gland in several molecular forms. Only one gene codes for prolactin, but there are many posttranslational changes.[60] The smallest form has been characterized, and the gene for human PRL sequenced by molecular biologic methods.[128] Prolactin is related chemically to GH and chorionic somatotropin (the placental GH-like hormone); all are thought to have arisen by serial mutations from a common ancestral gene at least 400 million years ago.[77]

Basal PRL levels in resting and nonstressed adult human subjects show a great deal of variability from individual to individual and from time to time. Normal values vary from 5 to 25 ng/ml during the day but can rise

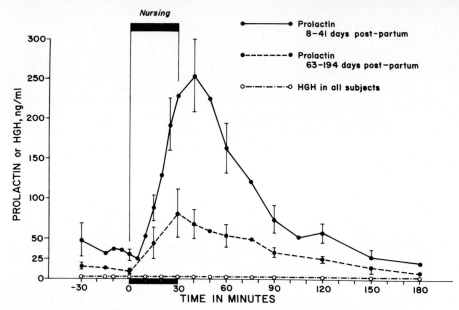

FIGURE 1. Illustrated here are prolactin and growth hormone release during nursing showing effect of time postpartum. Growth hormone is not released during suckling. (From Noel, GL, Suh, HK, Frantz, AG: *Prolactin release during nursing and breast stimulation in postpartum and nonpostpartum subjects.* J Clin Endocrinol Metab 38:413, 1974, with permission.)

to double these values during spontaneous surges that occur at night (see below).[34] Mean 24-hour level in normal women is approximately 13 ng/ml[52] (Fig. 2). Although there is no known function for PRL in men, levels of the hormone are approximately the same as in women. During the last two thirds of pregnancy, PRL levels are quite high (50 to 200 ng/ml),

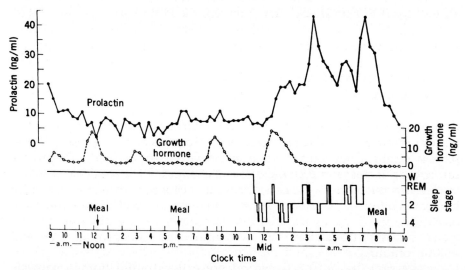

FIGURE 2. Shown here are prolactin and growth hormone secretion during a 24-hour period. Blood samples were taken every 20 minutes. There is an episodic rise in plasma prolactin between 3 and 8 AM, with a fall to low values after awakening. (From Sassin,[104] with permission.)

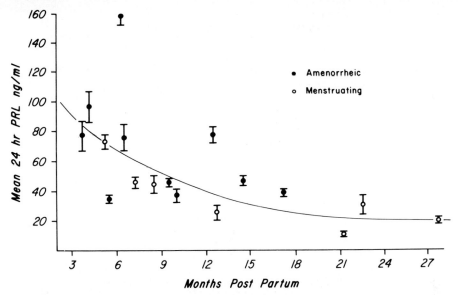

FIGURE 3. Shown here is the decline of mean PRL over time following delivery. This figure shows integrated 24-hour PRL levels in a group of 20 nursing mothers studied at various times after delivery. Note that there is a gradual decline in values, and some variability in the level at which menses resume. (From Stern, et al,[118] with permission.)

and after delivery they may rise still higher during individual nursing episodes. In women who nurse their babies, mean PRL levels gradually decline with the passage of time (Fig. 3), owing in part to the decreasing frequency of nursing bouts.[118]

Serum PRL levels are increased episodically during sleep (see Figure 2), with peak elevations occurring during the latter part (usually 2:00 to 8:00 AM).[104,105] This late nocturnal rise in plasma PRL levels is followed by a decline immediately after awakening.

HYPOTHALAMIC CONTROL OF PROLACTIN SECRETION

Control of basal pituitary PRL secretion by the hypothalamus is predominantly inhibitory; disruption of hypothalamic-pituitary connection by stalk section, pituitary transplantation, or placement of hypothalamic lesions all result in an increase in PRL secretion while secretion of other tropic hormones is reduced (Fig. 4). This effect has been reproduced *in vitro;* the incubated pituitary gland synthesizes and releases large quantities of PRL, while secretion of other hormones steadily declines. The isolated pituitary gland of the rat incubated *in vitro* secretes three times as much PRL per day as the pituitary *in situ,* and human pituitaries behave similarly. These results illustrate the powerful restraint normally imposed by the hypothalamus on PRL secretion and thus prompted the search for PRL inhibitory factors.

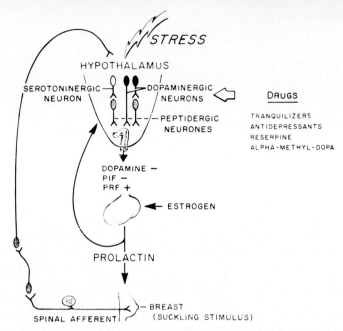

FIGURE 4. Illustrated here is the mechanism of hypothalamic regulation of prolactin secretion. Two hypothalamic factors, prolactin-inhibiting factor (PIF) and prolactin-releasing factor (PRF), regulate pituitary prolactin secretion. Neural inputs such as stress and suckling act upon the hypothalamus. Estrogen from ovary and placenta regulates pituitary sensitivity to hypothalamic factors.

PROLACTIN-INHIBITING AND PROLACTIN-RELEASING FACTORS

Prolactin-inhibiting Factors

Several PRL inhibitory factors have been isolated from hypothalamic extracts. Most important is dopamine, a bioamine secreted into the hypophysial portal vessels by a group of specific tuberoinfundibular cells located in the arcuate nucleus (see chapters 2 and 3). Dopamine is present in portal vessel blood in concentrations sufficient to suppress PRL secretion, and its concentration is shown to vary in response to suckling.[87] Administration of dopamine-agonist drugs like the phenothiazines and metoclopramide stimulate PRL release. These effects are mediated by specific dopamine receptors located on the lactotrope cells.[22]

Although important in determining basal levels, the tonic inhibitory actions of dopamine do not account for all the regulatory effects of the hypothalamus. For example, nipple stimulation, which causes PRL release, leads to inhibition of dopamine release into the portal blood, but the time course and magnitude of the effect does not correspond to the pattern of PRL secretion and hence cannot account entirely for the suckling-induced changes.[87]

A number of different prolactin-inhibiting factors (PIF) are demonstrable in hypothalamic extracts: gamma-aminobutyric acid (GABA), an inhibitory neurotransmitter;[107] His-Pro diketopiperizine, a metabolic breakdown product of thyrotropin-releasing hormone (TRH);[94] and additional factors not well characterized.[29] A potent PIF has been found to be coded within the prohormone for gonadotropin-releasing hormone (GnRH).[90] The term GAP (gonadotropin-releasing factor associated peptide) has been applied to this factor, which is localized to the GnRH neurons (Fig. 5). The physiologic role of each of these substances as PIF's has not been demonstrated.

Prolactin-releasing Factor(s)

Because physiologic studies anticipated the identification of PIF, it came as a surprise when investigators discovered that hypothalamic extracts contain several factors that release PRL.[132] One of the prolactin-releasing factors (PRF) has been shown to be TRH, administration of which brings about a rise in plasma PRL levels in the human being and several other species.[38,49] Prolactin and thyroid-stimulating hormone (TSH) responses to TRH share many similarities (Fig. 6). The threshold dose for the PRL response to TRH is similar to the threshold dose for the TSH response, and like the TSH response, PRL release is inhibited by thyroxine excess and enhanced by thyroxine deficiency. The mechanisms whereby TRH stimulates PRL secretion resembles effects on TSH secretion, because radiolabeled TRH binds to membrane receptors of lactotrope as well as thyrotrope cells (see below). However, the PRL response to TRH is reduced only partially after thyroxine treatment, whereas that for TSH release is completely abolished. Because TRH influences PRL secretion in the same range of doses that control TSH secretion, it is likely that TRH may function as a PRL regulatory factor. Several lines of evidence, however, argue against TRH being the only PRF, or the one involved in reflex PRL release. The acute burst of PRL release caused by suckling or by stress, or the rise associated with certain stages of sleep is not associated with the change in plasma TSH levels which would be anticipated if TRH secretion was activated.[38] Attempts to resolve the role of TRH in PRL regulation by using TRH antisera have given contradictory results.[44,55] Content of TRH in hypophysial portal blood of the rat has been reported to be increased by nipple stimulation.[30]

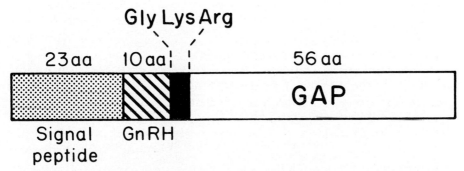

FIGURE 5. This is a diagram of the structure of prepro GnRH isolated by genetic recombinant methods from human placenta. The region coding for GnRH is followed by a sequence coding for a peptide 56 amino acid residues in size. This has been designated gonadotropin-releasing hormone associated peptide. This peptide has potent PRL-inhibiting properties. (Adapted from Nikolics, et al.[90])

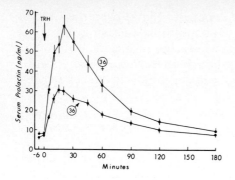

FIGURE 6. TRH-stimulated prolactin release in 36 men and 36 women is shown here. The response is greater and more rapid in women. (From Jacobs, et al,[49] with permission.)

Other candidate PRF's are vasoactive intestinal peptide (VIP),[6] peptide histidine isoleucine-27 (PHI),[50] neurotensin,[5] angiotensin II,[2,23] bombesin,[109,137] substance P,[134] cholecystokinin,[67] GRF 1–40,[40] vasopressin[10,114] and oxytocin.[63] All these substances have been reported in one or more studies to stimulate PRL release, but their physiologic relevance has not been established.[72]

Of these, VIP and PHI are most likely to be "the" physiologic PRF(s).

Vasoactive intestinal peptide is a potent PRF when added to pituitaries *in vitro*,[67] VIP increases PRL mRNA in GH_3 cells,[17] there are VIP receptors on lactotropes,[151] VIP administration raises blood PRL levels in patients with prolactinoma,[61] VIP has been reported to be present in hypophysial-portal blood in physiologically meaningful concentrations,[114] and its concentration is increased by serotonin, a neurotransmitter that stimulates PRL release.[114] Further evidence for a role of VIP as a regulator of PRL secretion is the finding that VIP antisera reduce the PRL response to suckling[1] and inhibit the response to serotonin (in the rat).[92] VIP can be demonstrated in typical paraventricular tuberoinfundibular neurons whose hormone content is markedly elevated in lactating (and adrenalectomized) rats.[45] Finally, destruction of the paraventricular nucleus in the rat abolishes the PRL response to suckling and to stress.[149]

Peptide histidine isoleucine-27 is a 27-amino-acid peptide with relatively weak PRF potency as compared with VIP, but it is present in a particular population of tuberoinfundibular cells located in the parvocellular division of the paraventricular nucleus. These cells cocontain corticotropin-releasing factor (CRF) and hence must be activated during stress.[45] Peptide histidine isoleucine-27 is an analog of VIP. Moreover, there is evidence that both peptides are secreted by the same neurons: Recombinant DNA analysis of pre-pro-VIP from a human VIPoma revealed a sequence coding for a peptide, designated PHM, differing by only two amino acids from PHI.[48] Both VIP and PHI are secreted in hypophysial portal blood.[114] That both VIP and PHI are active as PRF is indicated by the studies of Kaji et al[51] who find that the combined administration of anti-VIP and anti-PHI has a greater inhibitory effect on the PRL response to ether stress than either antiserum alone.

Oxytocin has its advocates as a PRF.

It acts directly on the pituitary gland as a relatively weak releaser of PRL,[63] is secreted with PRL during suckling, and is present in portal blood in relatively high concentrations.[150] In human beings however, detailed studies of the time course of oxytocin and PRL release during suckling reveal striking dissociated responses during the presuckling period when oxytocin, but not prolactin, is released as a conditioned response to the sound of the baby's crying.[73]

It is quite possible that the three peptides, VIP, PHI, (PHM in the human being), and oxytocin are all PRF's and that they may synergize in their effects on PRL release. This hypothesis has not been tested, but if it proved to be true it would be analogous to the multiple factors that release ACTH secretion during stress, including synergistic interactions among CRF, vasopressin, epinephrine, and norepinephrine (see chapter 6).

At the level of the hypothalamus, biogenic amines also regulate PRL secretion by modulating secretion of dopamine and PRF's[20,58,65,86,87]

The morphologic and histochemical evidence of a monoamine neural control system in the basal hypothalamus has been reviewed (see chapter 3). Dopamine agonists inhibit, and serotonin agonists stimulate, PRL secretion. Administration of L-dopa, the precursor of both dopamine and norepinephrine, causes an acute lowering of plasma prolactin levels in human beings. Pretreatment with L-dopa is effective in blocking the PRL response to TRH, suggesting an effect at the pituitary level (see Figure 5). That this effect is mediated by dopaminergic receptors is indicated by the observation that apomorphine, a specific dopamine-receptor-stimulating agent, also causes acute suppression of PRL.[71]

> Further studies are necessary to determine the extent to which dopamine acts through its effects on the hypothalamus. If exerted at the level of the hypothalamus, the effects would not be directed on the tuberoinfundibular neurons because these lack dopamine receptors.[83]

Additional support for the idea that dopamine plays a role in PRL control comes from observations of effects of several drugs such as the phenothiazines, which affect monoamine transmission in brain. This class of drugs, which block dopaminergic receptor sites, cause an acute increase in plasma PRL levels in the human being and in other species.[53] The administration of α-methyldopa or reserpine (agents that interfere with central catecholamine synthesis or storage) also can cause increased PRL secretion and may result in the production of abnormal lactation (galactorrhea). Systemic administration of 5-hydroxytryptophan, a serotonin precursor which readily crosses the blood-brain barrier, also causes PRL release.

These observations indicate that PRL, like GH, is under a complex double regulatory system that involves both specific hypothalamic regulatory factors (releasing and inhibiting) and a dual monoaminergic control system. Most evidence suggests that serotonergic fibers are excitatory, and dopaminergic nerve fibers, inhibitory.

Central opioid pathways are also involved in PRL regulation.[18,42]

> Both humans and laboratory species of animals show increased blood PRL levels after administration of either morphine or opioid peptides, an effect associated with and possibly owing to decreased hypothalamic dopamine secretion. That endogenous opioids are involved in physiologic control of PRL is indicated by the demonstration that naloxone, an opiate antagonist, stimulates PRL in normal women but only late in the follicular and in the mid luteal phases of the menstrual cycle.[18] This is a highly selective effect, inasmuch as, with the possible exception of severe exercise-induced PRL release,[84] naloxone does not block other physiologically induced rises in plasma PRL.[18]

NEURAL PATHWAYS IN REGULATION
OF PROLACTIN RELEASE

Three different types of environmental stimuli are recognized to bring about release of prolactin in rats. These are the suckling stimulus (a reflex abolished by nipple denervation); mechanical stimulation of the uterine cervix, which brings about the hyperprolactinemic state of pseudopregnancy (in rodents);[43] and physical and emotional stress. The suckling stimulus can be duplicated by direct stimulation of the mammary nerves.[87] In addition, in the female rat, but not the male rat, administration of estrogen brings about the acute release of PRL.[86] Inasmuch as systemic estrogen administration[86] or direct intrahypothalamic estrogen implants[97] can induce PRL release, it is possible that the PRF pathway is also estrogen sensitive, as is the pituitary gland itself. Although estrogens increase basal levels of plasma PRL in both sexes, only in the female sex does estrogen cause acute PRL release. This sexually dimorphic response depends upon the early steroid milieu in the perinatal period (see chapters 9 and 20). The emotion- and suckling-reflex-induced release of PRL is also readily demonstrated in other species.

> Attempts to trace the neural pathways mediating these responses have utilized electric stimulation experiments,[54,69,123] circumscribed electrolytic lesions,[19,86] and deafferentation of the hypothalamus by the Halasz technique.[135] All forms of stimuli known to elicit PRL release appear to converge upon the hypothalamus via an anterior route because most responses can be abolished by lesions in the preoptic region. The importance of this region is further demonstrated by electric stimulation, which also brings about increased PRL release. The VIP pathway involving a population of paraventricular neurons would probably receive the same inputs as the CRF neurons. In addition to the acute release pathway, a prolactin-inhibitory pathway can be demonstrated by sectioning the pituitary stalk[86] or by electrolytic lesions[19] of the median eminence or the arcuate nucleus.

The course of the prolactin-release pathway has been traced in goats, guinea pigs, and rabbits. Tindal and collaborators report that the pathways for milk ejection and prolactin release are similar.[122-124]

> In the midbrain, the afferent path of the reflex is compact, lying in the lateral tegmentum of each side and passing forward to lie medioventral to the medial geniculate body. On entering the diencephalon, the pathway on each side bifurcates: a dorsal pathway passing forward in association with the extreme rostral central gray and periventricular regions, and a ventral path ascending through the subthalamus.[124]
>
> The prolactin-release pathway follows the course of the dorsal pathway for oxytocin release and then, like the dorsal pathway, swings into the far-lateral hypothalamus to ascend in the medial forebrain bundle. However, whereas the oxytocin-release path moves dorsally and then medially by means of medial forebrain bundle collaterals at the level of the paraventricular nucleus, the prolactin-release pathway continues forward in the medial forebrain bundle and then spreads out in the preoptic region.[123]

FEEDBACK REGULATION OF PROLACTIN SECRETION
SHORT-LOOP FEEDBACK

Prolactin, unlike other anterior pituitary hormones, does not have a specific target gland with which it interacts in a negative-feedback loop. Instead,

PRL secretion appears to be self-regulated by a short-loop mechanism. Implants of PRL in the hypothalamus of the rat cause a decrease in pituitary PRL concentration and a fall in plasma PRL levels. In suckling rats, intra-hypothalamic PRL inhibits lactation. This effect is probably mediated through the effects of PRL on hypothalamic dopaminergic neurons, because rapid and significant increase in dopamine turnover in the hypothalamus follows PRL administration. In hypophysectomized animals, elevation of circulating levels of PRL (by introduction of multiple pituitary implants), also leads to increased dopamine levels in the hypothalamus. Feedback effects of PRL on the hypothalamus probably inhibit GnRH secretion as well. This view is supported by the finding that removal of PRL-secreting microadenomas, or treatment with bromocriptine in women with galactorrhea-amenorrhea syndromes, generally restores normal menses without changing the responsiveness of the pituitary glands of such patients to test doses of GnRH.[2,6,35,46,127,133] The effect of PRL on PRF secretion has not been evaluated.

EFFECTS OF SEX STEROIDS

Estrogenic hormones have striking effects on lactotrope cells. In rodents and monkeys, estrogen administration increases the number of lactotropes and the rate of PRL synthesis.[64] In the rat, this striking stimulation commonly induces tumor formation. The hyperplasia of the pituitary gland seen in pregnant women mainly is due to increased numbers and size of lactotrope cells formed under the influence of placental estrogens. This stimulating effect explains the vulnerability of the pituitary gland of the pregnant woman to infarction and the tendency of chromophobe PRL-secreting adenomas to grow during pregnancy.[31,33] The effects of progesterone have not been as thoroughly explored. In rats, progesterone inhibits the estrogen-induced increase in PRL secretion, but its effects in humans are not known. Also unknown is the effect of androgenic hormones on PRL secretion in humans.[116]

FACTORS THAT INFLUENCE PRL SECRETION IN THE HUMAN BEING

A number of stimuli that cause acute changes in PRL secretion, such as stress and sleep-associated release, are probably mediated by extra-hypothalamic inputs to the medial basal hypothalamus.[91] The precise areas involved have not been determined, but involvement of the limbic system would seem almost a certainty. Factors that influence PRL secretion are listed in Table 1.

STRESS-ASSOCIATED RELEASE

A variety of stresses cause significant elevation of plasma PRL levels. Prolactin is released during anesthesia and surgical procedures. In one study, mean plasma PRL levels increased from 38.8 ng/ml to 173.8 ng/ml in 19 women undergoing surgical explorations under general anesthesia.[91] The increase in PRL was maintained during the entire operation and re-

TABLE 1. Factors that Influence Serum Prolactin Levels in Human Beings

Physiologic	Pathologic	Pharmacologic
Increase in Serum Prolactin		
1. Pregnancy	1. Prolactin-secreting	1. TRH
2. Postpartum	pituitary tumors	2. Psychotropic drugs
a. Nonnursing mothers	2. Hypothalamic-pituitary	a. Phenothiazines
(days 1–7)	disorders:	b. Reserpine
b. Nursing mothers after	a. ("functional"?)	3. Oral contraceptives
suckling	b. Tumors (craniopharyn-	4. Estrogen therapy
3. Nipple stimulation (males	gioma), metastases	5. Methyldopa
and females)	c. Histiocytosis X	
4. Coitus (some subjects)	d. Inflammation-	
5. Stress	sarcoidosis	
6. Exercise	3. Pituitary stalk section	
7. Neonatal period (2–3	4. Hypothyroidism	
months)	5. Renal failure	
8. Sleep	6. Ectopic production by	
	malignant tumors	
Decrease in Serum Prolactin		
1. Water loading	1. Isolated pituitary prolactin	1. Levodopa
	deficiency	2. Apomorphine
		3. Bromocriptine

mained elevated for 20 minutes after completion of surgery. Prolactin levels had returned to preoperative levels the following day. Slightly less marked increases were observed in men. The rise in plasma GH was considerably less. Less stressful procedures such as gastroscopy and proctoscopy also cause a rise in PRL, without significant rise in GH. Acute myocardial infarction also causes PRL release. The effects of psychologic stress on PRL release have been systematically tested. In a few studies one of the most surprising (and negative) studies utilized as a stimulus exposure to a phobic object. Despite induction of severe anxiety the experimental subjects showed no change in blood PRL levels. This finding underlines the specificity of emotional factors inducing PRL release. Prolactin levels and prolactin responses to phenothiazines are normal in schizophrenic patients.[75]

A teleologically satisfactory rationale for stress-induced PRL release in the human being is not readily apparent. General metabolic effects of PRL have not been described except for possible electrolyte and water-retaining effects (see below). In fact, patients with PRL-secreting pituitary tumors may have plasma levels as high as 5,000 to 10,000 ng/ml without manifesting any apparent metabolic change that could be interpreted as being helpful in stress.[127]

SEIZURE-ASSOCIATED RELEASE

Several studies have documented a close association of temporal lobe seizures and PRL release. It appears that seizure activity in deep limbic structures (hippocampus and amygdala) and not the motor component of the seizure is responsible for the PRL response. Determination of serum PRL levels 30 to 90 minutes after seizures is now advocated as a potential discriminator between true seizures and pseudoseizures. In the latter case, even vigorous motor activity is not accompanied by elevation of PRL in blood.

SLEEP-ASSOCIATED RELEASE

Sleep-related rise in plasma PRL levels now has been demonstrated consistently. The increase in PRL occurs as a series of episodic bursts of secretion, the first of which occurs within 60 to 90 minutes after sleep.[93,105] Subsequent pulses carry the plasma level to a peak at approximately 4:00 to 6:00 AM (see Figure 2). Values reached occasionally exceed 40 ng/ml. The rise in PRL is not related to a specific phase of the sleep. Soon after morning awakening, plasma PRL levels begin to fall, and the lowest levels of the 24-hour period are reached 1 to 3 hours later. Nocturnal rise in PRL is not simply a circadian rhythm but is related to sleep itself; delay in sleep onset or sleep reversal results in concurrent delay in the response, which is consistently entrained to the episode of sleep.[105] In this respect, sleep-associated PRL release resembles GH release and differs from ACTH release, which, although also occurring in an episodic pulsatile manner during the night, is only loosely entrained to sleep. The teleologic function or significance of sleep-associated PRL release (which occurs in both sexes) is unknown.

The pineal gland may be involved in the regulation of the diurnal variations in PRL secretion. Melatonin, which is synthesized in the pineal gland, has been shown to enhance PRL secretion in the rat, perhaps by stimulation of hypothalamic-serotonergic neurons.[62] Because activity of the pineal is increased during darkness in this species, it was hypothesized that the pineal gland affected PRL secretion and that this effect might be related to the light-dark cycles. In confirmation of this hypothesis, plasma PRL levels in the rat were found to be significantly increased at 6:00 AM compared with levels obtained at 6:30 PM. This rise was completely abolished by pinealectomy.[62]

EPISODIC RELEASE

In addition to the overall nocturnal rise, PRL, like other pituitary hormones, is secreted in a pulsatile manner throughout the day and night (see Figure 2).[29,105] It is probable that episodic neural drive is responsible for these patterned responses. Whether such secretory bursts have physiologic importance remains to be demonstrated.

LACTATION

The sequence of hormonal events responsible for growth of the breast and for lactation are complex (see also chapter 9). As shown in rat experiments, duct growth requires the combined action of glucocorticoids, GH, and estrogen; growth of the alveolar lobules requires progesterone and PRL in addition. During human pregnancy, placental lactogen (human placental lactogen [HPL] also called chorionic mammosomatotropin [CMS]) and pituitary PRL are secreted in increased amounts. Delivery of the child initiates lactation mainly because placental estrogen and progesterone are suddenly withdrawn. Experimental work in rats indicates that secretions of PRL, insulin, and glucocorticoids are required for sustained milk production. Once lactation has developed, its maintenance depends on PRL released after mechanical stimulation of the nipples by suckling. Reflex discharge of PRL from the pituitary gland is abolished by denervation of the nipples or by lesions in the spinal cord and brainstem. Impulses carried over these pathways ultimately impinge upon the hypothalamus, where they bring about the release of PRL. Release of PRL is due to two factors: disinhibition of dopamine secretion, and increased release of PRF(s) (see above).

Suckling brings about two additional neurogenic responses: milk let-down and gonadotropic inhibition. Milk let-down refers to the appearance of milk in the nipple ducts a few seconds after nipple stimulation begins (see chapter 4). As noted above, this component of the suckling response is frequently triggered in anticipation of suckling. Contraction of the myoepithelial cells of the parenchymal acini is responsible for the appearance of milk in the larger ducts, a response caused by the direct effects of oxytocin, in turn released by neural stimuli reaching the hypothalamus. This reflex can be blocked by stress or by epinephrine administration.

The effect of suckling in blocking ovulation is biologically important because it is the most important mechanism by which pregnancies are spaced in societies that do not practice birth control. Pregnancy is delayed by approximately six months in suckling women, but ovulation may begin earlier than this time, so that the contraceptive effect is only partial. The gradual return of ovulation is mainly due to decrease in the frequency of nursing episodes. Introduction of solid food into the infant's diet is a major factor in the decrease in suckling frequency, and with that, the return of periods and restoration of ovulation.[115] Suckling inhibits the luteinizing hormone (LH) ovulatory surge through two mechanisms, indirectly by reflex release of prolactin, which has an inhibitory effect on GnRH secretion, and directly by inhibition of LRF secretion.[106] Prolactin also appears to interfere with the action of gonadotropins on the ovaries.[25]

In addition to stimulation of milk production, in certain species PRL has an important supporting role in initiating and maintaining the corpus luteum of the ovary. For this reason it is also termed luteotropic hormone (LTH).

ACTIONS OF PROLACTIN OTHER THAN ON MAMMALIAN BREAST

As is so often the case, the given name of a hormone tends to blind one to its overall functions. This is particularly true for prolactin, which in addition to its milk-stimulating action in mammals has a diversity of actions unmatched by any other hormone. In Nicoll's comprehensive review[88] more than 85 different functions are described in creatures throughout the animal kingdom (see Table 2A, B, C for summary). In virtually all species PRL has distinct effects on reproduction. In many mammals, PRL induces nest building and "fostering" behavior. In many species of birds PRL induces broodiness (egg sitting), and in pigeons, PRL induces the formation of *pigeon milk:* the secretion of specialized sacs of gut epithelia with which the young are fed. In many species of fish, PRL promotes nest building, the guarding of young, and in some species, increased secretion of skin mucus which serves as a food source for fry. In certain amphibia (like the salamander), PRL promotes migratory behavior.

The effects of PRL in promoting migratory behavior in amphibia is echoed through eons of evolution by the effects of PRL in stimulating migratory behavior in certain species of birds. In response to the changing season (probably signalled by change in day length relative to night), PRL secretion is enhanced, the birds increase their food intake (teleologically adaptive because the excess calories stored as body fat will be utilized in the long migratory flight), and display preovulatory restlessness, "zugenruhe."[74]

PRL effects in broodiness and concern for their offspring's welfare may have analogs in the human. The nursing experience is described by many women as "tranquilizing" (whether due to hormonal effects or the associated psychologic interaction with the offspring), and both women and men with elevated PRL levels describe a loss of libido which is reversed only partially, if at all, by therapy with sex steroids.[120] Prolactin inhibits the turnover of catecholamines in the median eminence after binding to specific receptors.[82]

In lower forms, PRL is an important hormone for regulation of serum osmolarity. This homeostatic regulation is both behavioral — it determines migration of fish to fresh water — and visceral — it regulates renal function. Prolactin receptors have been demonstrated in the kidneys of most animal species, including the mammal, although there is no convincing evidence that PRL influences salt water balance in higher forms.

Prolactin is also a regulator of metamorphosis, especially in frogs in which it is inhibitory to the effects of thyroid hormones.

When one considers the wealth of data documenting behavioral effects of PRL in lower animals, the striking evidence indicating that PRL-related functions are identifiable over vast stretches of evolutionary time, and the reduced libido associated with high PRL in human beings, it is likely that PRL will prove to have a number of psychologic effects in the human being. However, these have not been adequately defined as yet because of the lack of sufficient amounts of PRL for studies.

CLINICAL ABNORMALITIES OF PRL SECRETION

Before sensitive immunoassays for PRL became available, the only indication of disordered PRL secretion apparent to the clinician was the appearance of inappropriate milk secretion. Although this manifestation remains in many cases the clinical hallmark of abnormal PRL secretion, it now is known that PRL secretion may be increased in both men and women without recognizable clinical symptoms. In fact, only one in six patients with elevated PRL levels has galactorrhea, and in long-standing galactorrhea, PRL levels may fall into the normal range.[127,140]

NONPUERPERAL GALACTORRHEA

Abnormal lactation occurs in a number of clinical disorders, usually attributable to excessive secretion of PRL (Fig. 7).[80,108,120] There is considerable

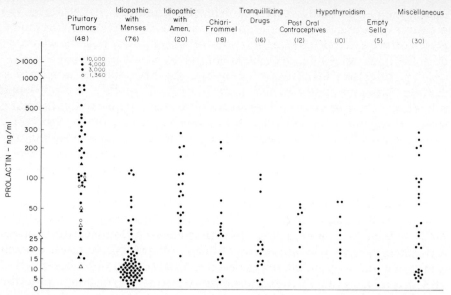

FIGURE 7. Shown here are serum prolactin concentrations in 235 patients with galactorrhea owing to various causes. The usual upper limit of normal for serum prolactin is 20 to 25 ng/ml. (From Kleinberg, DL, Noel, GL, Frantz, AG: *Galactorrhea: A study of 235 patients.* N Engl J Med 296:589–600, 1977, with permission.)

variability in the expression of this condition, inasmuch as only a small proportion of individuals with hyperprolactinemia show lactation. In order for galactorrhea to develop in the presence of high PRL, the breast parenchyma must have been properly primed by normal amounts of insulin, GH, glucocorticoids, estrogens, and progesterone, and estrogen secretion must be low or relatively low. In the normal sequence of development of lactation at the time of delivery, the crucial initiating signal is the sudden decline in placental estrogen secretion which, though necessary for breast growth and development, inhibits milk secretion. It is not known with certainty whether a similar sequence of ovarian steroid withdrawal is needed for the development of nonpuerperal galactorrhea, but most patients with severe galactorrhea have amenorrhea and variable degrees of estrogen deficiency. In a few cases, treatment with estrogens will inhibit the lactational effects of PRL on the breast. In one of the galactorrhea syndromes, so-called postpill amenorrhea, lactation begins when contraceptive therapy is stopped. Lactation may occur in patients with Cushing's disease and acromegaly.[138] In some cases of acromegaly both GH and PRL are secreted in excess. Most such cases probably are due to simultaneous hypersecretion of PRL by mixed tumors.

Understanding the nature of hyperprolactinemic states has unfolded gradually with the description of a number of clinical syndromes which bear eponymic descriptions of historic interest.[31] It is now possible to classify these conditions according to pathophysiologic principles.

The first category of nonpuerperal galactorrhea to be recognized, the Chiari-Frommel syndrome, is recognized as the persistence of postpartum lactation accompanied by amenorrhea and ovarian deficiency.[20,37] A somewhat similar illness, but independent of pregnancy, was later described as

REGULATION OF THE PITUITARY GLAND

the Argonz del Castillo syndrome.[4] Forbes, Henneman, Griswald, and Albright recognized that approximately one half of their patients with galactorrhea had "chromophobe" tumors of the pituitary and suggested that occult tumors might be the cause of the disease in the others.[32] Subsequently, pituitary stalk section in women was found to cause lactation, indicating that the syndrome could also occur as a hypothalamic deficiency disorder.[23a] These findings, together with the observation that certain neuroleptic drugs, such as reserpine and chlorpromazine, could induce lactation, provide the clinical bases for basic neuroendocrine insights into the mechanism of regulation of PRL secretion and for a classification of lactational disorders. The older terminology is no longer used. Rather, the general designations are galactorrhea or galactorrhea-amenorrhea syndrome, further characterized by etiology.

Galactorrhea (and PRL hypersecretion) occurs either as primary hypersecretion of a pituitary adenoma or as a disorder secondary to hypothalamic dysfunction thought to be a deficiency of PIF secretion. A few cases of unknown etiology are believed to be due to occult pituitary tumor or of psychosomatic origin. The major causes of hyperprolactinemia are listed in Table 2.

TABLE 2. Etiologies of Hyperprolactinemia

Pituitary disease
   Prolactinomas (microadenomas, macroadenomas)
   Acromegaly
   "Empty sella syndrome"
   Pituitary stalk section
Hypothalamic disease
   Craniopharyngiomas
   Sarcoidosis
   Neuraxis irradiation
Neurogenic
   Chest wall lesions
   Spinal cord lesions
   Breast stimulation
Pregnancy
Hypothyroidism
Chronic renal failure
Laennec's cirrhosis
Stress
   Physical
   Psychologic
   Pseudocyesis
Medications
   Neuroleptics (phenothiazines, thioxanthenes, butyrophenones)
   Sulpiride
   Metoclopramide
   Opiates
   Monoamine oxidase inhibitors
   Amoxepin
   Clomipramine
   Reserpine
   Cimetidine (intravenous)
   Alpha-methyldopa
   Estrogens
   Licorice
   Verapamil
Idiopathic

PROLACTIN-SECRETION ADENOMAS

The most common pituitary tumors are chromophobe adenomas. For many years these were believed to be nonfunctional, but radioimmunoassay methods now show that approximately one third or more such tumors secrete PRL into the blood and that the removed tumors contain PRL.[80,108] Acidophilic staining in these tumors is difficult to demonstrate because of their relatively small hormone storage pool, but characteristic secretory granules are demonstrable by electron microscopy, and explants grown in organ culture synthesize PRL.[56] Specific immunohistochemical stains prove the presence of PRL. Mixed PRL and GH tumors are reasonably common; most are made up of mixed cell types, but a few are secreted by the same cell (see chapters 8 and 12).

> A single case of mixed prolactinoma and somatotropinoma associated with intrasellar ganglioneuroma has been reported.[15] Inasmuch as acromegaly with GRH-secreting ganglioneuroma has been recognized, it is possible that the prolactin adenoma was due to excess secretion of a PRF. A combination of hyperplasia of both somatotrope and lactotrope cells has been identified as the cause of hyperprolactin-emia in patients with polyostotic fibrous dysplasia.[57,102]

With increasing experience it has become apparent that galactorrheic patients with PRL levels above 150 to 200 ng/ml almost always have PRL-secreting microadenomas (over 90 percent in the series of Tolis[126]), even when radiologic findings are normal. Several patients desirous of becoming pregnant who failed to respond to treatment with bromocriptine or had marked elevation of PRL have been explored by the transsphenoidal route and have been cured by removal of microadenoma. This kind of clinical experience raises the important suggestion that a substantial proportion of the "idiopathic" cases may have occult tumors. Clinical techniques for identifying these tumors depend most on roentgenographic study (chapter 14). Details of testing methods and management are discussed below.

PITUITARY ISOLATION

Galactorrhea or hyperprolactinemia also may occur after damage to the ventral hypothalamus or to the pituitary stalk–pituitary isolation syndrome. This syndrome has been reported in patients with craniopharyngioma, granulomas (including sarcoidosis), histiocytosis X, empty sella, and large nonfunctioning tumors with suprasellar extension.[81]

External head trauma and pituitary stalk section rarely may cause galactorrhea. In the series reported by Turkington and colleagues,[129] plasma PRL levels (by bioassay) were elevated in 9 of the 11 patients, but galactorrhea was not observed in any of the cases. Gynecomastia is sometimes a manifestation of PRL excess in men, and galactorrhea does rarely occur.

ABNORMALITIES IN PERIPHERAL RECEPTOR CONTROL

Prolonged irritative lesions of the anterior chest wall, notably after thoracotomy or herpes zoster, may cause galactorrhea.[80] Even prolonged mechanical stimulation of the nipples as by suckling has been known to initiate lactation in nonpregnant or even virgin women. A foster mother may thus be enabled to suckle her adopted child.

Galactorrhea with hyperprolactinemia has been observed in women with neurologic lesions of the thoracic spinal cord.[11] The mechanism by which a lesion of ascending pathways could cause PRL hypersecretion is not known. Presumably this is a stimulatory effect.

NEUROLEPTIC DRUGS

Large doses of drugs that interfere with central catecholamine metabolism may induce excessive PRL secretion, presumably by disrupting hypothalamic dopaminergic mechanisms that normally inhibit PIF secretion. Drugs commonly implicated are the phenothiazines, reserpine, and α-methyl-dopa (see Table 2).[80] Amenorrhea may occur also. This is a practical problem in the long-term management of chronic schizophrenia.

Hyperprolactinemia, occasionally with galactorrhea, is common in advanced renal insufficiency.[24] The underlying mechanism is unknown. Although delayed clearance of PRL may be a factor, it is also possible that there is a disturbance in central catecholamine metabolism or a form of metabolic encephalopathy.

HYPOTHYROIDISM

Somewhat less than half of severely hypothyroid patients have elevated plasma PRL levels, and in this group, a small proportion have galactorrhea, usually with amenorrhea.[143] The pathogenesis of this syndrome is a matter of controversy (see chapter 5). One theory is that TRH secretion is increased in hypothyroidism, thereby leading to increased release of both TSH and PRL. It also has been postulated that PRL hypersecretion comes about through TRH stimulation of PRL secretion from the pituitary gland, which is known to be more sensitive to TRH in the hypothyroid state. Also, the hypothyroid state may cause a deficit of PIF biosynthesis, with resultant PRL hypersecretion. Precocious puberty as well as lactation may result from hypothyroidism in young girls (see chapter 9). Hypothyroidism must be ruled out in any patient with the galactorrhea-amenorrhea syndrome.

POSTPILL AMENORRHEA-GALACTORRHEA

A small but significant proportion of women (less than 0.2 percent) fail to resume normal menses after taking contraceptive pills and show hyperprolactinemia. Although early work suggested that these women had an abnormally high incidence of menstrual disturbance prior to use of the contraceptive agents, more recent studies indicate that this is not true.[46,49] Nor is the duration of therapy. The disturbance is often transient but may become permanent. The underlying pathophysiology is not known; nor is it known whether the progesterone or the estrogen component of the pill is more important. The syndrome increasingly is recognized to be associated with PRL-secreting microadenomas. However, as shown by case control studies, prior use of contraceptive pills does not account for the incidence of hyperprolactinemia.[49,113]

Idiopathic Hyperprolactinemia

Although some cases undoubtedly harbor microadenomas not revealed by computerized axial tomography (CAT) scanning, extended observation has shown that the majority of patients without evident prolactinomas continue to show normal pituitary CAT scans even after prolonged periods.[68] Furthermore, a few patients show marked fluctuations of PRL over time, and others have spontaneous, permanent remissions. The pathogenesis of this disorder is unknown. A few may be due to psychogenic factors (see below), but this has been difficult to prove. The majority of patients with established adenomas also remain stable over many years.[70]

Psychogenic Hyperprolactinemia

Cases that would have been classified as having pseudocyesis may be examples of stress-induced hyperprolactinemia (see chapter 9). The authors have seen a patient whose transient hyperprolactinemia and lactation were coincident with a severe emotional episode.

Prolactin Deficiency

Prolactin deficiency occurs mainly in panhypopituitarism and only rarely as an isolated defect that first comes to light due to failure to lactate following pregnancy. In normal individuals, prolactin secretion is uniformly increased by the administration of TRH, but if patients with initially low PRL fail to respond to TRH, it can be concluded that the disorder is intrinsic to the pituitary gland. Normal individuals uniformly show an increase in serum PRL levels following insulin-induced hypoglycemia — failure to respond is indicative of PRL failure but does not distinguish between a hypothalamic and a pituitary cause. The use of dopamine antagonists as tests of secretory reserve is discussed below.

DIAGNOSIS OF PROLACTIN DISORDERS

Determination of plasma PRL levels is essential in the workup of all patients with suspected hypothalamic and pituitary disease, even in patients without galactorrhea.[35,80] Normally, PRL levels in men are 1 to 20 ng/ml, in nonpregnant women, 1 to 25 ng/ml. In a large series reported by Frantz,[34] men had a mean serum prolactin level of 4.7, and women, 8.0 ng/ml (see Figure 7). Normal children have values in the same range, but neonatal infants (during the first 4 weeks) have slightly elevated levels during the early morning hours. Most patients with galactorrhea-amenorrhea have elevated serum PRL levels. However, galactorrhea is observed in only 1 of 6 women with hyperprolactinemia.[80] Galactorrhea alone in the absence of gonadotropin inhibition usually is not due to hyperprolactinemia. In patients with chromophobe adenomas, 30 to 50 percent have elevated prolactin levels, indicating that the tumor is hypersecretory, or, in a few cases with suprasellar extension, that compression of the hypothalamus or stalk has led to PIF deficiency. Lesions of the hypothalamus and the empty sella syndrome also may cause an elevation. In such cases, even minimal amounts of residual pituitary may be capable of maintaining normal levels of PRL, presumably owing to loss of PIF activity.

The most difficult problem in differential diagnosis of the etiology of hyperprolactinemic states is the detection of microadenoma before distinctive roentgenographic changes have occurred. Even in cases that appear to be "functional" and unrelated to any obvious etiology, an occult adenoma may be present. A number of workers have tried to develop dynamic secretory tests based on physiologic principles, but none are entirely satisfactory. This field has been studied extensively and reviewed in several publications.[35,81] The principal tests used have been administration of TRH; dopamine antagonists, such as chlorpromazine (which acts on both central and peripheral dopamine receptors); domperidone and metoclopramide, which are relatively specific peripheral dopamine antagonists; insulin-induced hypoglycemia, which mobilizes central control mechanisms; L-dopa (which acts on both central and peripheral dopamine receptors); and the combination of L-dopa and the peripheral dopa decarboxylase inhibitor, carbidopa, which has been postulated to exert its dopamine agonist action at the central control levels. Most workers now believe that none of the functional tests adequately discriminate among the various causes of hyperprolactinemia. In part, this unsatisfactory conclusion may come about because persistent hyperprolactinemia from whatever cause probably changes central PRL regulatory mechanisms. Furthermore, most states of hyperprolactinemia probably are associated with a small PRL pool that is turning over rapidly. This is true for most prolactinomas as judged by histologic findings.[56,89,117,119] No pharmacologic test was able to distinguish between pituitary isolation syndrome and microadenoma.[80,81]

The best hormonal guide to differential diagnosis is the basal level of PRL, repeated a few times to exclude spontaneous or stress-induced elevations. In the series of Tolis and coworkers,[127] PRL levels in excess of 200 ng/ml were associated with adenomas in over 90 percent of cases. Prolonged followup may be needed for diagnosis. In one case, an adenoma was removed from a patient whose sella was completely normal roentgenographically; a number of "negative" explorations also have been reported. Thus the diagnosis is made by consideration of the known causes (see above), repeated measurements of basal levels, and careful radiologic study (see chapter 14).

MANAGEMENT OF HYPERPROLACTINEMIA

The means chosen for treatment of prolactin excess depends upon the specific etiology (Table 2), the age and sex of the patient, and in the case of women, the desired reproductive state.[8,9,78-80,120,148] When the cause can be corrected, for example, as in hypothyroidism, the therapy is obvious. Substitution of one class of drugs for another (for example, hydralazine instead of methyldopa for treatment of hypertension) may ameliorate the problem. More difficult is the patient who has phenothiazine-induced hyperprolactinemia. Agents that reverse the hyperprolactinemia, such as bromocriptine, are contraindicated on theoretic grounds in schizophrenia, because such drugs have a tendency to exacerbate symptoms. Tricyclic antidepressants have not been implicated as causes of hyperprolactinemia.

MICROPROLACTINOMA

No Active Intervention

A number of alternatives are open for treatment of PRL-secreting microadenoma. One option is to carry out no active treatment at all and simply to keep the patient under surveillance. Accumulating evidence indicates that the adenoma in most women will remain stable. For example, March and colleagues[70] followed 43 women with hyperprolactinemia and tomographic evidence of a microadenoma (admittedly not a highly specific radiologic method) without treatment for 3 to 20 years. Of this group, tomograms and CAT scans did not change in 41 women, and in 13 women PRL levels fell to normal, galactorrhea resolved, and normal menses resumed spontaneously. In two patients, PRL levels did not change, but CAT scans showed growth of the tumor; microadenomas were found at surgery. One of the patients had become pregnant while taking bromocriptine, and tumor growth became apparent only following delivery. In short, 95 percent of the women in this study were essentially unchanged for prolonged periods. Are there any problems with this approach, which involves monitoring serum PRL at reasonable intervals, that is, every 6 months with CAT scans repeated only if PRL levels showed persistent increases? First, a few women may wish to menstruate or may suffer loss of libido and dyspareunia due to the hypogonadal (estrogen-deficient) state. Bone loss also occurs, presumed to be the equivalent of a premature menopause.[146] It is not known whether the use of calcium supplements, 1 to 1.5 gm per day, prevents bone loss in this group of patients as it may do in postmenopausal osteoporosis. Estrogen administration probably would reverse this bone loss, but endocrinologists generally have considered the presence of an adenoma as a contraindication to estrogen use because of the hormone's well-known lactotrope-stimulating properties.

The single largest problem with the no treatment option is that the patient remains infertile; if pregnancy is desired, more aggressive therapeutic intervention is warranted.

The natural history of microadenoma in men has not been elucidated.

Selective Transsphenoidal Adenomectomy

This procedure is now widely available in most large medical centers and is an attractive therapeutic option. Initial cure rates approximate 85 percent for microadenomas and 40 to 50 percent for moderate-size macroadenomas (excluding large lesions with local invasion)[8,27,80,101,110] (see chapter 16). The incidence of significant complications is relatively low but is not negligible.

In a series of cases from a multicenter collaborative report by neurosurgeons, Zervas[141] reported that in 2104 microadenomas operated on for all causes (acromegaly, prolactinoma, Cushing's disease) there were 7 deaths (meningitis, vascular injury, cardiac, hemorrhage, and anesthetic) and 48 complications (including meningitis, diabetes insipidus, pulmonary embolus, ocular palsy, transient hemiparesis, visual loss). The largest single complication was cerebrospinal fluid rhinorrhea in 33 cases. This overall mortality is 0.3 percent, the morbidity rate, 2.3 percent. These figures would undoubtedly be somewhat lower for prolactinoma alone, inasmuch as patients with Cushing's disease and acromegaly made up about half of the cases reported upon, and, by and large, these individuals are older and have a higher incidence of general medical problems.

Enthusiasm for adenomectomy for treatment of microadenomas has waned recently as results of long-term followup studies have begun to appear. The incidence of late recurrences is summarized in several series. In the series of Rodman and colleagues[101] approximately 17 percent of initially "cured" patients relapsed within 5 years; other centers have reported similar, or even higher, relapse figures—up to 50 percent in the series reported from Serri's group.[110] Thus, taking the most conservative estimates, approximately 15 percent of patients with microadenoma are initially not cured and an additional 15 percent relapse within 5 years, for a total failure rate of 30 percent or more. This relatively high failure rate has made most endocrinologists rather cautious in recommending surgery over medical treatment (see below) in a disease that does not represent a major threat to health.

Bromocriptine Therapy

The treatment of galactorrhea-amenorrhea syndromes has been revolutionized by the introduction of the dopamine agonist drug bromocriptine (2-bromo-alpha-ergocryptine mesylate) (Fig. 8), which was developed by Fluckiger and colleagues at Sandoz in the 1960s for the purpose of inhibiting PRL secretion without the uterotonic or vasospasm properties of other ergots.[9,80,120,148] The drug is now available throughout the world and is in wide use. A number of other analogs, including pergolide and lisuride, also have been evaluated but are not approved for use in the United States except as research drugs.

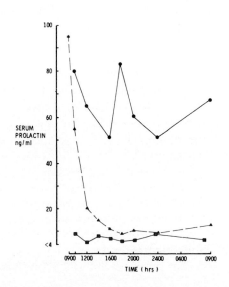

FIGURE 8. Changes in circulating serum prolactin concentration in a woman with idiopathic amenorrhea and galactorrhea after the first 5mg dose of bromocriptine and when maintained on 7.5 mg daily. (● = Control day; ▲ = 5.0 mg at 0900 hours, 2.5 mg at 1800 hours; ■ = 2.5 mg three times a day for 2 months.) (From Besser, GM, and Thorner, MO: *Bromocriptine in the treatment of the hyperprolactinaemia-hypogonadism syndromes.* Postgrad Med J 52(Suppl 1):64–70, 1976, with permission.)

Administered by mouth, bromocriptine produces a rapid fall in PRL in most hyperprolactinemic cases, regardless of etiology, that persists for more than 12 hours (Fig. 8). The long action of this agent is in part due to its relatively slow rate of absorption (peak at 3 hours after ingestion) and relatively long half-life in the blood of 3½ to 4½ hours. In 80 to 90 percent of cases, the manifestations of hyperprolactinemia, that is, galactorrhea, anovulation, short luteal phase, and amenorrhea — are reversed, permitting normal pregnancy to occur. Approximately 40 percent of patients with idiopathic hyperprolactinemia showed a return of menses by 1 month, and more than 80 percent at the end of 2 months. Patients with adenomas show a somewhat slower rate of response (60 percent at 3 months); by 10 months nearly 85 percent of patients with idiopathic disease have a restitution of normal periods, and 70 percent of the tumor cases.

The main side effects encountered in 10 to 15 percent of cases have been nausea and anorexia, hypotension, peripheral vasospasm, headaches, nasal stuffiness, and depression.[8,9,148] Psychotic reactions have been recognized to occur in 1 to 2 percent of patients with parkinsonism treated with high doses of bromocriptine (50 to 100 mg per day) and in patients with a prior history of psychiatric disease, but they have generally not been a problem with the usual low doses required in management of prolactinomas which seldom exceed 7.5 mg per day. However, Turner and colleagues[130] described the occurrence of serious psychotic reactions in 8 of 600 cases treated for functioning tumors with either bromocriptine or lisuride who had no prior history of psychiatric disease. Symptoms that came on as late as 52 months after initiation of therapy (onset as early as 4 months) included auditory hallucinations, delusional ideas, and mood changes necessitating discontinuation of the drug. The illness was schizophreniform for the most part.

To circumvent the gastrointestinal and hypotensive effects, the drug should be taken after meals, and the dose should be increased gradually. The occurrence of postural hypotension should be evaluated carefully. The lowest effective dose should be used. Several regimens have been advocated by experienced physicians.[7,126,148] In our clinics we usually initiate therapy with 1.25 mg per day, increased stepwise in 1.25 mg doses at one-week intervals. Prolactin levels are tested when a dose of 2.5 mg twice daily is reached and further increased until PRL is normalized.

When the drug is used to promote fertility, several important cautions must be emphasized. Patients must be told to use mechanical contraceptives until normal menstrual cycling has been established by the therapy. This precaution is taken so that the patient will be able to tell as soon as possible that she may be pregnant. Although the use of this drug has not been associated with any definite increased incidence of congenital malformations,[78,80,120] it is widely recommended that it be discontinued as soon as possible after diagnosis of pregnancy. *In the United States bromocriptine has been approved by the FDA for the induction of pregnancy in women with idiopathic, that is nontumorous, hyperprolactinemia but not for pregnancy induction in women with established tumors.* However, in practice this drug is being widely used in the United States and throughout the world even in patients with tumor.

No pituitary complications have been reported during pregnancy in patients with idiopathic hyperprolactinemia. In those with microadenomas reviewed by Gemzell and Wang,[39] of 91 pregnancies in 85 patients with untreated microadenomas, headaches occurred in 3, headache and visual disturbance in 1, and diabetes insipidus in 7.[78] In the series reviewed by Molitch,[78,79] only 1.6 percent showed significant pituitary enlargement. Pregnancy in patients with microadenoma is relatively safe, but the patients should remain under surveillance and undergo monthly visual field tests during pregnancy. In contrast, patients with macroadenomas encounter a very significant incidence of pituitary tumor growth. In the series of Gemzell and Wang,[39] in 56 pregnancies in 46 women with untreated macroadenomas, headache and visual disturbances occurred in 14 pregnancies requiring pituitary surgery in 5 and radioactive yttrium pellet implantation in 1. Thus the complication rate is on the order of 25 to 35 percent.[78] Visual complications during pregnancy have been treated successfully with bromocriptine so that surgical intervention is not necessarily indicated.

Because of the unquestioned risk for significant aggravation of the pituitary tumor during pregnancy in patients with macroadenoma, Besser and colleagues[8,9] have advocated prophylactic treatment with conventional x-irradiation therapy prior to pregnancy in such patients. A typical course of therapy would be a total dose of 4500 rads in 26 fractions given over a 5-week period. With this regimen these workers claim to have seen no incidence of tumor growth. In most centers, surgical decompression by transsphenoidal adenomectomy (preceded by a brief course of bromocriptine) is used as prophylactic management of patients who have macroadenomas and are desirous of becoming pregnant.

Although not generally advocated for therapy of pregnant patients with tumor, sufficient information is now available to suggest that there is no increase in minor or major congenital malformations in babies born of bromocriptine-treated mothers.

One of the most important aspects of bromocriptine is its ability to cause tumor regression. This antineoplastic effect in the human being was first described by Thorner and colleagues,[121] and Cornblum and colleagues[21] and has been widely confirmed.[148] In a large multicenter study,[79] 50 percent of cases showed a dramatic reduction in tumor size; 25 percent, a significant decrease; and in the remainder, no regression but no increase in size. The beneficial effects may begin within a week or two, as manifested by improvement in visual acuity and visual fields and decreased density and size of the tumor demonstrable by serial CAT scans.

Bromocriptine and other dopamine agonists have been used for treatment of acromegaly (see chapter 8), for hypersecretion of TSH in both idiopathic and adenoma cases (see chapter 5), and for therapy in Cushing's disease (see chapter 6). Responses are somewhat variable, and probably about one third of cases of acromegaly benefit from treatment. However, in a few cases bromocriptine may be the only alternative and merits a trial. In acromegaly, a small percentage of cases show complete remission while patients are on the medication.

Many endocrinologists have taken the position that they will initiate therapy for microadenomas with bromocriptine, and then at a later time when it is more convenient or if the patient tires of the medication they will recommend adenomectomy. This seemingly reasonable approach has been brought into question by the recent studies of Landholt and co-workers,[59] who reported that the cure rate of microadenomas in patients who had been on bromocriptine for 1 year or more was markedly reduced when compared with that of patients who had never taken the agent. Presumably this is because the tumor regression leads to difficulties for the surgeon in determining boundaries of the tumor. In contrast, the cure rate of macroadenomas is not appreciably different. Not every group has made the same observations (see Faglia and coworkers[26]). The difference may lie in the interval between surgery and the discontinuation of therapy. In the study by Landholt and associates, the medication was continued almost up to the time of surgery, but in the studies of Faglia and colleagues, intervals ranged from 2 to 24 months (mean 8.4 months). This issue remains to be resolved. Until it is settled by specific studies, the physician must keep this in mind when embarking on a treatment plan. The practical consideration has to be that if surgery is part of the treatment plan, it should be carried out earlier rather than later. If bromocriptine is used, a decision for surgery should be made within a year. Alternatively, the drug should be discontinued for some period of time before surgery. We do not as yet have guidelines to determine this interval. It is our recommendation now that surgery should be postponed after discontinuation of the drug until the microadenoma is clearly defined on CAT scan if it has shrunk during bromocriptine therapy. But it must be emphasized that there is no scientifically grounded basis for this recommendation.

Macroadenomas

Management of these cases is also controversial. Most endocrinologists now recommend that the tumor be treated initially with bromocriptine. In tumors that are too large to be cured by surgery, the use of this agent in most cases can shrink the tumor and in a surprisingly high percentage reverse the local compressive changes (including visual loss).

In the large series summarized by Molitch,[78] PRL levels returned to normal in 18 of 27 cases. In 46 percent, tumor size was reduced by more than 50 percent; in 18 percent, by about 50 percent; and in 36 percent, by approximately 10 to 25 percent. In more than half of the cases reduction in tumor size was evident by 6 weeks, but in the remainder, reduction was not noted until 6 months. Tumor regrowth occurred in 3 of 4 cases after 1 year of discontinuation of the medication. Visual fields improved in 9 of the 10 patients who initially had abnormal findings. A number of neurosurgeons believe that a course of bromocriptine can make a subsequent "debulking" procedure more effective. Others believe that if what appears to be an inoperable tumor is effectively controlled by bromocriptine (or other dopamine agonists), long-term medical management is indicated and that surgery is not needed. This issue has become a source of continuing controversy at pituitary disease meetings round the world (see, for example, the debate between Besser and Tindall[7]). In part the choice of medical therapy versus surgery depends upon the availability of skilled neurosurgeons.

The majority neurosurgic view is to attempt a surgical cure, followed by radiation if unsuccessful. Although perhaps no more than 40 percent of cases will benefit from surgery, the benefit/risk ratio may be acceptable to many patients. In our view the patient is best served by a frank discussion of the options of treatment. There cannot be any single best way to manage these cases at this time.[100]

Radiation Therapy

Radiation therapy by conventional means is indicated in any patient whose prolactinoma is not adequately controlled with surgery and dopamine agonist therapy unless specific contraindications are present. The doses required are the same as those needed for therapy of nonfunctioning and GH-secreting tumors.

Results of x-ray therapy of prolactinoma has been reviewed by Sheline and others.[111,112,148]

The early experience with "chromophobe" adenomas is relevant because more than half were probably prolactinomas not recognized as such at the time. In this group, 93 percent recurrence free rate at 5 years declined to 71 percent at 10 years, and this figure is probably still true at 15 years.

In Antunes and others'[3] series of prolactinomas, none of 6 normalized, though all responded. In Gomez and others'[41] series, only 1 of 8 normalized, although 4 menstruated.

In the St. Bartholomew's Hospitals series, 36 women with microadenomas were treated with 4500 rads over 5 weeks.[112] Bromocriptine was used as interval treatment, and the drug was stopped periodically to determine baseline levels. Progressive fall in PRL was noted in 25 of 28 women studied thus far. Eight showed values less than 18 ng/ml (2 to 10 years), and fertility was achieved in 24 of 33 patients (attributable to concomitant bromocriptine). No cases have shown growth of tumor during pregnancy. In the St. Bartholomew experience, no patient developed ACTH deficiency, 2 patients became gonadotropin deficient, and 21 became GH deficient, but the clinical significance of GH deficiency in the adult is not known. In the series studied by von Werder and colleagues,[148] 12 patients with failed surgical removal were treated with x-ray therapy with 5000 rads. Mean levels gradually fell from 100 to 25 ng/ml at 20 to 30 months. The potential side effects include GH failure, possible ACTH and TSH failure (though these are rare), and local complications. In patients receiving only the recommended dose of x-ray therapy, a total of seven sarcomas of the brain have been reported, and two cases of brain necrosis.[111,112] As pointed out by Sheline and coworkers, these must be looked upon as rare occurrences.

REFERENCES

1. ABE, H, ENGLER, D, MOLITCH, ME, BOLLINGER-GRUBER, J. REICHLIN, S: *Vasoactive intestinal peptide is a physiological mediator of prolactin release in the rat.* Endocrinology 111:1383–1390, 1985.
2. AGUILERA, G, HYDE, CL, CATT, KJ: *Angiotensin II receptors and prolactin release in pituitary lactotrophs.* Endocrinology 111:1045–50, 1982.
3. ANTUNES, JL, HOUSEPIAN, EM, FRANTZ, AG, HOLUB, DA, HUL, RM, CARMEL, PW, QUEST, DO: *Prolactin-secreting tumors.* Ann Neurol 2:148–153, 1977.
4. ARGONZ, J, AND DEL CASTILLO, EB: *A syndrome characterized by estrogen insufficiency and decreased gonadotropin.* J Clin Endocrinol Metab 13:79–87, 1953.

5. ASKEW, RD, RAMSDEN, DB, SHEPPARD, MC: *The affect of neurotensin on pituitary secretion of thyrotrophin and prolactin in vitro.* Acta Endocrinol (Copenh) 105:156–60, 1984.

6. BESSER, GM, PARKE, L, EDWARDS, CRW, FORSYTH, IA, MCNEILLY, AS: *Galactorrhoea: Successful treatment with reduction of plasma prolactin levels by bromergocryptine.* Br Med J 3:669–672, 1972.

7. BESSER, GM, AND TINDALL, GT: *The great debate: Medical vs surgical treatment of prolactinomas.* In GIVENS, JR, (ED): *Hormone-secreting Pituitary Tumors.* Year Book Medical Publishers, Chicago, 1982, pp 299–312.

8. BESSER, GM, WASS, JAH, GROSSMAN, A, ROSS, R, DONIACH, I, JONES, AE, REES, LH: *Clinical and therapeutic aspects of hyperprolactinemia.* In MACLEOD, RM, AND THORNER, MO (EDS): *Prolactin, Basic and Clinical Correlates.* Scapagnini U, Fidia Research Series vol 1, Liviana Press, Padua, 1985, 833–847.

9. BESSER, GM: *Medical management of prolactinomas.* In GIVENS, JR, (ED): *Hormone-Secreting Pituitary Tumors.* Year Book Medical Publishers, Chicago, 1982, 255–298.

10. BLASK, DE, VAUGHAN, MK, CHAMPNEY, TH, JOHNSON, LY, VAUGHN, GM, BECKER, RA, REITER, RJ: *Opioid and dopamine involvement in prolactin release induced by arginine vasotocin and vasopressin in the male rate.* Neuroendocrinology 38:56–61, 1984.

11. BOYD, AE, III, SPARE, S, BOWER, B, ET AL: *Neurogenic galactorrhea-amenorrhea.* J Clin Endocrinol Metab 47:1374–1377, 1978.

12. BOYD, AE, III, SANCHEZ-FRANCO, F, SPENCER, E, PATEL, YC, JACKSON, IMD, REICHLIN, S: *Characterization of hypophysiotropic hormones in porcine hypothalamic extracts.* Endocrinology 103:1075–1083, 1978.

13. BOYD, AE, AND REICHLIN, S: *Neural control of prolactin secretion in man.* Psychoneuroendocrinology 3:113–130, 1978.

14. BOYD, AE, III, SPENSER, E, JACKSON, IMD, REICHLIN, S: *Prolactin releasing factor (PRF) in porcine hypothalamic extract distinct from TRH.* Endocrinology 99:861–871, 1976.

15. BURCHIELD, KJ, SHAW, CM, KELLY, WA: *A mixed functional microadenoma and ganglioneuroma of the pituitary fossa.* J Neurosurg 58:416–420, 1983.

16. CARLSON, HE, WASSER, HL, LEVIN, SR, WILKINS, JN: *Prolactin stimulation by meals is related to protein content.* J Clin Endocrinol Met 57:334–338, 1983.

17. CARRILLO, AJ, POOL, TB, SHARP, ZD: *Vasoactive intestinal peptide increases prolactin messenger ribonucleic acid content in GH$_3$ cells.* Endocrinology 116:202–206, 1985.

18. CETEL, NS, QUIGLEY, ME, YEN, SSC: *Naloxone-induced prolactin secretion in women: Evidence against a direct prolactin stimulatory effect of endogenous opioids.* J Clin Endocrinol Metab 60:191–196, 1985.

19. CHEN, CL, AMENOMORI, Y, LUK, H, VOOGT, JL, MEITES, J: *Serum prolactin levels in rats with pituitary transplants or hypothalamic lesions.* Neuroendocrinology 6:220–227, 1970.

20. CHIARI, JBVL, BRAUM, C, SPAETH, J: *Klinik der Geburtschilfe und Gynaekologie.* Erlangen, 1855, pp 371–372, quoted by BRYNER, JR, AND GREENBLATT, R. In ALLEN, MB, JR, AND MAHESH, VB (EDS): *The Pituitary—A Current Review.* Academic Press, New York, 121–138, 1977.

21. CORNBLUM, B, WEBSTER, BR, MORTIMER, CB, EZRIN, C: *Possible anti-tumor effects of 2-bromoergocryptine (CB-154, Sandoz) in 2 patients with large prolactin-secreting pituitary adenomas.* Clin Res 23:614A, 1975.

22. CRONIN, MJ: *The role and direct measurement of the dopamine receptor(s) in the anterior pituitary.* In MÜLLER, EE, AND MACLEOD, RM (EDS): *Neuroendocrine Perspective, vol 1.* Elsevier Biomedical Press, Amsterdam, 1982, pp 169–210.

23. DUFY-BARBE, L, RODRIQUEZ, F, ARSAUT, J, VERRIER, D, VINCENT, JD: *Angiotensin II stimulates prolactin release in the rhesus monkey.* Neuroendocrinology 35:242–247, 1982.

24. EMMANOUELL, DS, LINDHEIMER, MD, KATZ, A: *Pathogenesis of endocrine abnormalities in uremia.* Endocrine Rev 1:28–44, 1980.

25. EVANS, WS, CRONIN, MJ, THORNER, JO: *Hypogonadism in hyperprolactinemia: Proposed mechanisms.* GANONG, WF, MARTINI, L (EDS): *Frontiers in Neuroendocrinology.* Raven Press, New York, 1982, pp 77–122.

26. FAGLIA, G, MORIONDO, P, TRAVAGLINI, P, GIOVANELLI, MA: *Influence of previous bromocriptine therapy on surgery for microprolactinoma (letter).* Lancet 1:133–134, 1983.

27. FAHLBUSCH, R, AND SCHRELL, U: *Surgical therapy of lesions within the hypothalamic area.* Acta Neurochirurgica 75:125–135, 1985.

28. FARQUHAR, MG: *Multiple pathways of exocytosis, endocytosis, & membrane recycling: Validation of a Golgi route.* Fed Proc 42:2407–2413, 1983.

29. FINK, G: *Has the prolactin inhibiting peptide at last been found?* Lancet 316:487–488, 1985.

30. FINK, G, KOCH, Y, BEN AROYA, N, ET AL: *Release of thyrotropin releasing hormone into hypophysial portal blood is high relative to other neuropeptides and may be related to prolactin secretion.* Brain Res 243:186–189, 1982.

31. FORBES, AP: *The amenorrhea-galactorrhea syndrome: Clinical features.* In GIVENS, JR (ED): *Hormone-Secreting Pituitary Tumors.* Year Book Medical Publishers, 1982, pp 237–254.

32. FORBES, AP, HENNEMAN, PH, GRISWOLD, GC, ALBRIGHT, F: *Syndrome characterized by galac-*

torrhea, amenorrhea, and low urinary FSH: Comparison with acromegaly and normal lactation. J Clin Endocrinol 14:265–271, 1954.

33. FRANKS, S, JACOBS, HS, HULL, MGR: *The oral contraceptive and hyperprolactinemic amenorrhea.* In CAMANNI, F, AND MÜLLER, EE (EDS): *Pituitary Hyperfunction: Physiopathology and Clinical Aspects.* Raven Press, New York, 1984, pp 175–178.

34. FRANTZ, AG: *The regulation of prolactin secretion in humans.* In GANONG, WF, AND MARTINI, L (EDS): *Frontiers in Neuroendocrinology.* Oxford University Press, New York, 1973, pp 337–374.

35. FRANTZ, AG: *Endocrine diagnosis of prolactin-secreting pituitary tumors.* In BLACK, PM, ZERVAS, NT, RIDGWAY, EC, MARTIN, JB (EDS): *Secretory Pituitary Tumors.* Raven Press, New York, 1984, pp 45–52.

36. FRIESEN, H, AND HWANG, P: *Human prolactin.* Annu Rev Med 24:251–270, 1973.

37. FROMMEL, R: *Uber puerperale Atrophie des Uterus.* Z Geburtshilfe Gynaekol 7:305–314, 1882.

38. GAUTVIK, KM, TASHJIAN, AH, JR, KOURIDES, IA, WEINTRAUB, BD, GRAEBER, CT, MALOOF, F, SUZUKI, K, ZUCKERMAN, JE: *Thyrotropin-releasing hormone is not the sole physiologic mediator of prolactin release during suckling.* N Engl J Med 290:1162–1165, 1974.

39. GEMZELL, C, AND WANG, CF: *Outcome of pregnancy in women with pituitary adenoma.* Fertil Steril 31:363–72, 1979.

40. GOLDMAN, JA, MOLITZH, ME, THORNER, MO, RIVIER, J, VALE, W, REICHLIN, SR: *Growth Hormone Releasing Hormone 1-40-OH (GHRA) is a Prolactin (PRL)-releasing factor.* Endo Soc. 1984, p 606.

41. GOMEZ, F, REYES, FI, FAIMAN, C: *Nonpuerperal galactorrhea and hyperprolactinemia. Clinical findings, endocrine features and therapeutic responses in 56 cases.* Am J Med 62:648–660, 1977.

42. GROSSMAN, A, CLEMENT-JONES, V, BESSER, GM: *Clinical implications of endogenous opioid peptides.* In MÜLLER, EE, MACLEOD, RM, FROHMAN, LA (EDS): *Neuroendocrine Perspectives,* vol 4. 1985, pp 243–294.

43. GUNNETT, JW, AND FREEMAN, ME: *The mating-induced release of prolactin: A unique neuroendocrine response.* Endocrine Rev 4:44–61, 1983.

44. HARRIS, AC, CHRISTIANSON, D, SMITH, MS, ET AL: *The physiological role of thyrotropin-releasing hormone on the regulation of thyroid-stimulating hormone and prolactin secretion in the rat.* J Clin Invest 61:441–448, 1978.

45. HÖKFELT, T, FAHRENKRUG, J, TATEMOTO, K, MUTT, V, WERNER, S, HULTING, AL, TERENIUS, L, CHANG, KJ: *The PHI (PHI-27)/corticotropin-releasing factor/enkephalin immunoreactive hypothalamic neuron: Possible morphological basis for integrated control of prolactin, corticotropin, and growth hormone secretion.* Proc Natl Acad Sci USA 80:895–898, 1983.

46. HULL, MGR, BROMHAM, DR, SAVAGE, PE, BARLOW, TM, HUGHES, AO, JACOBS, HS: *Post-pill amenorrhea: A causal study.* Fertil Steril 36:472–476, 1981.

47. ISHIZUKA, B, QUIGLEY, ME, YEN, SSC: *Pituitary hormone release in response to food ingestion: Evidence for neuroendocrine signals from gut to brain.* J Clin Endocrinol Metab 57:1111–1116, 1983.

48. ITOH, N, OBATA, K, YANAIHARA, N, OKAMOTO, H: *Human preprovasoactive intestinal polypeptide contains a novel PHI-27-like peptide, PHM-27.* Nature 304:547–549, 1983.

49. JACOBS, LS, SNYDER, PJ, UTIGER, RD, DAUGHADAY, WH: *Prolactin response to thyrotropin-releasing hormone in normal subjects.* J Clin Endocrinol Metab 36:1069–1087, 1973.

50. KAJI, H, CHIHARA, K, ABE, H, MINAMITANI, N, KODAMA, H, KITA, T, FUJITA, T, TATEMOTO, K: *Stimulatory effect of peptide histidine isoleucine amide 1-27 on prolactin release in the rat.* Life Sci 35:641-7, 1984.

51. KAJI, H, CHIHARA, K, KITA, T, KASHIO, Y, OKIMURA, Y, FUJITA, T: *Administration of antisera to vasoactive intestinal polypeptide and peptide histidine isoleucine attenuates ether-induced prolactin secretion in rats.* Neuroendocrinology 41:529–531, 1985.

52. KAPCALA, L, MOLITCH, M, ARNO, J, KING, L, REICHLIN, S, WOLPERT, S: *Twenty-four-hour prolactin secretory patterns in women with galactorrhea, normal menses, normal random prolactin levels and abnormal sellar tomograms.* J Endocrinol Invest 7:455–465, 1984.

53. KLEINBERG, DL, NOEL, GL, FRANTZ, AG: *Chlorpromazine stimulation and L-dopa suppression of plasma prolactin in man.* J Clin Endocrinol Metab 33:873–876, 1971.

54. KNAGGS, GS, MCNEILLY, AS, TINDAL, JS: *The afferent pathway of the milk-ejection reflex in the mid-brain of the goat.* J Endocrinol 52:333–341, 1972.

55. KOCH, Y, GOLDHABER, G, FIREMAN, I, ZOR, U, SHANI, J, TAL, E: *Suppression of prolactin and thyrotropin secretion in the rat by antiserum to thyrotropin-releasing hormone.* Endocrinology 100:1476–1478, 1977.

56. KOVACS, K., AND HORVATH, E: *Pathology of pituitary adenomas.* In GIVENS, JR (ED): *Hormone Secreting Pituitary Tumors.* Year Book Medical Publishers, Chicago, 1982, pp 97–119.

57. KOVACS, K, HORVATH, E, THORNER, MO, ROGOL, AD: *Mammosomatotroph hyperplasia asso-*

ciated with acromegaly and hypeprolactinemia in a patient with McCune-Albright syndrome. Virchows Archiv A 403:77–86, 1985.

58. KRULICH, L: *Central neurotransmitters and the secretion of prolactin, GH, LH and TSH.* Ann Rev Physiol 41:603–15, 1979.

59. LANDHOLT, AM, KELLER, PJ, FROESCH, ER, MUELLER, J: *Bromocriptine: Does it jeopardize the result of later surgery for prolactinomas?* (letter) Lancet 2:657–658, 1982.

60. LEWIS, UJ, SINHA, YN, MARKOFF, E, VANDER LAAN, WP: *Multiple forms of prolactin: Properties and measurement.* In MÜLLER, EE, MACLEOD, RM, FROHMAN, LA (EDS): *Neuroendocrine Perspectives,* vol 4. Elsevier, Amsterdam, 1985, pp 43–58.

61. LIGHTMAN, SL, UNWIN, RJ, GRAHAM, K, DIMALINE, R, McGARRICK, G: *Vasoactive intestinal polypeptide stimulation of prolactin release and renin activity in normal man and patients with hyperprolactinaemia: Effects of pretreatment with bromocriptine and dexamethazone.* Eur J Clin Invest 14:444–448, 1984.

62. LU, KH, AND MEITES, J: *Effects of serotonin precursors and melatonin on serum prolactin release in rats.* Endocrinology 93:152–155, 1973.

63. LUMPKIN, MD, SAMSON, WK, McCANN, SM: *Hypothalamic and pituitary sites of action of oxytocin to alter prolactin secretion in the rat.* Endocrinology 112:1711–1717, 1983.

64. MACLEOD, RM: *Regulation of prolactin secretion.* In MARTIN, L, AND GANONG, WF (EDS): *Frontiers in Neuroendocrinology,* vol 4. Raven Press, New York, 1975, pp 169–194.

65. MACLEOD, RM, AND LEHMEYER, JE: *Studies on the mechanism of the dopamine-mediated inhibition of prolactin secretion.* Endocrinology 94:1077–1085, 1974.

66. MACLEOD, RM, AND SCAPAGNINI, U, THORNER, MO: *Prolactin: Basic and Clinical Correlates.* Liviana Press, Padova, 1985.

67. MALARKEY, WB, O'DORISIO, TM, KENNEDY, M, CATALAND, S: *The influence of vasoactive intestinal polypeptide and cholecystokinin on prolactin release in rat and human monolayer cultures.* Life Sci 28:2489–2495, 1981.

68. MALARKEY, WB, MARTIN, TL, KIM, M: *Patients with idiopathic hyperprolactinemia infrequently develop pituitary tumors.* In Prolactin. MACLEOD, RM, THORNER, MO, SCAPAGNINI, A (EDS): Liviana Press, Padova, 1985, pp 705–708.

69. MALVEN, PV: *Prolactin release induced by electrical stimulation of the hypothalamic preoptic area in unanesthetized sheep.* Neuroendocrinology 18:65–71, 1975.

70. MARCH, CM, KLETZKY, OA, DAVAJAN, V, TEAL, J, WEISS, M, APUZZO, MLJ, MARRS, RP, MISHELL, DR: *Longitudinal evaluation of patients with untreated prolactin-secreting pituitary adenomas.* Am J Obstet Gynecol 139:835–844, 1981.

71. MARTIN, JB, LAI, S, TOLIS, G, FRIESEN, HG: *Inhibition by apomorphine of prolactin secretion in patients with elevated serum prolactin.* J Clin Endocrinol Metab 39:180–182, 1974.

72. McCANN, SM: *The role of brain peptides in the control of anterior pituitary hormone secretion.* In MÜLLER, EE, AND MACLEOD, RM (EDS) *Neuroendocrine Perspectives,* vol 1. Elsevier Biomedical Press, Amsterdam, 1982, 1–22.

73. McNEILL, AS, ROBINSON, ICAF, HOUSTON, MJ, HOWIE, PW: *Release of oxytocin and prolactin in response to suckling.* BMJ 286:257–259, 1983.

74. MEIER, AH, FARNER, DS, KING, JR: *A possible endocrine basis for migratory behaviour in the white-crowned sparrow.* Zonotrichia leucophrys gambelli. Animal behaviour 13:453–465, 1965.

75. MELTZER, HY: *Neuroendocrine abnormalities in schizophrenia: Prolactin, growth hormone, and gonadotrophins.* In BROWN, GM, KOSLOW, SH, REICHLIN, S (EDS): *Neuroendocrinology and Psychiatric Disorders.* Raven Press, New York, 1984, pp 1–28.

76. MEZEY, E, AND KISS, JZ: *Vasoactive intestinal peptide-containing neurons in the paraventricular nucleus may participate in regulating prolactin secretion.* Proc Natl Acad Sci USA Jan 82(1) 1985, pp 245–247.

77. MILLER, WL AND EBERHARDT, NL: *Structure and evolution of the growth hormone gene family.* Endocrine Rev 4:97–130, 1983.

78. MOLITCH, ME: *Pregnancy and the hyperprolactinemic woman.* N Engl J Med 312:1364–1370, 1985.

79. MOLITCH, ME, ELTON, RL, BLACKWELL, RE, ET AL: *Bromocriptine as primary therapy for prolactin secreting macroadenomas: Results of a prospective multicenter study.* J Clin Endocrinol Metab 60:698–705, 1985.

80. MOLITCH, MM, AND REICHLIN, S: *Hyperprolactinemic disorders.* DM 28:1–58, 1982.

81. MOLITCH, ME, AND REICHLIN, S: *Hypothalamic hyperprolactinemia: Neuroendocrine regulation of prolactin secretion in patients with lesions of the hypothalamus and pituitary stalk.* In MACLEOD, RM, THORNER, MO, SCAPAGNINI, U (EDS): *Prolactin.* Liviana Press, Padua, 1985, pp 709–720.

82. MOORE, KE, AND DEMAREST, KT: *Tuberoinfundibular and tuberohypophyseal dopaminergic neurons.* In *Frontiers in Neuroendocrinology,* vol 7. GANONG, WF, MARTINI, L (EDS): Raven Press, New York, 1982, pp 161–190.

83. MOORE, KE, AND DEMAREST, KT: *Prolactin secretion and dopaminergic neurons: An evaluation of*

neuropharmacologic strategies. In *Neuroendocrinology and Psychiatric Disorder.* BROWN, GM, KOSLOW, SH, REICHLIN S (EDS): Raven Press, New York, 1984, pp 75–84.

84. MORETTI, C, FABBRI, A, GNESSI, L, CAPPA, M, CALZOLARI, A, FRAIOLI, F, GROSSMAN, A, BESSER, GM: *Naloxone inhibits exercise-induced release of PRL and GH in athletes.* Clinical Endocrinology 18:135–138, 1983.

85. MÜLLER, EE, LOCATELLI, V, PENALVA, A, CAVAGNINI, F, NOVELLI, A, MIYOSHI, H, COCCHI, D: *Neuropharmacologic control of pituitary function in neuroendocrine disorders.* In CAMANNI, F, MÜLLER, EE (EDS): *Pituitary Hyperfunction: Physiopathology and Clinical Aspects.* Raven Press, New York, 1984, 179–191.

86. NEILL, JD: *Prolactin: Its secretion and control.* In GREEP, RO, ET AL (EDS): *Handbook of Physiology, Section 7: The Pituitary Gland and Its Neuroendocrine Control,* vol 4, part 2. American Physiological Society. Williams & Wilkins, Baltimore, 1974, pp 469–488.

87. NEILL, JD: *Neuroendocrine regulation of prolactin secretion.* In MARTINI, L, AND GANONG, WF (EDS): *Frontiers in Neuroendocrinology,* vol 6. Raven Press, New York, 1980, pp 129–155.

88. NICOLL, CS: *Physiological actions of prolactin.* In KNOBIL, E, AND SAWYER, WH (EDS): *Handbook of Physiology, Section 7: Endocrinology. The Pituitary Gland and Its Neuroendocrine Control,* vol 4, part 2. Am Physiol Society, Washington, DC, 1974, pp 253–292.

89. NICOLL, CS, SWEARINGEN, KC: *Preliminary observations on prolactin and growth hormone turnover in rat adenohypophyses in vivo.* In MARTINI, L, MOTTA, M, FRASCHINI F (EDS): *The Hypothalamus.* Academic Press, New York, 1970, pp 449–462.

90. NIKOLICS, K, MASON, AJ, SZONYI, E, RAMACHANDRAN, J, SEEBURG, PH: *A prolactin-inhibiting factor within the precursor for human gonadotropin-releasing hormone.* Nature 316:511–517, 1985.

91. NOEL, GL, SUH, HK, STONE, JG, FRANTZ, AG: *Human prolactin and growth hormone release during surgery and other conditions of stress.* J Clin Endocrinol Metab 35:840–851, 1972.

92. OHTA, H, KATO, Y, SHIMATSU, A, TOJO, K, KABAYAMA, Y, INOUE, T, YANAIHARA, N, IMURA, H: *Inhibition by antiserum to vasoactive intestinal polypeptide (VIP) of prolactin secretion induced by serotonin in the rat.* Eur J Pharmacol 109:409–12, 1985.

93. PARKER, DC, ROSSMAN, LG, VANDER LAAN, EF: *Sleep-related, nyctohemeral and briefly episodic variation in human plasma prolactin concentrations.* J Clin Endocrinol Metab 36:1119–1124, 1973.

94. PETERKOFSKY, A, BATTAINI, F, KOCH, Y, TAKAHARA, Y, DANNIES, P: *Histidyl-proline diketopiperazine: Its biologican role as a regulatory peptide.* Mol Cell Biochem 42: 45–63, 1982.

95. PHILLIPS, HS, NIKOLICS, K, BRANTON, D, SEEBURG, PH: *Immunocytochemical localization in rat brain of prolactin release-inhibiting sequence of gonadotropin-releasing hormone.* Nature 316:542–545, 1985.

96. PITUITARY ADENOMA STUDY GROUP: *Pituitary adenomas and oral contraceptives: A multicenter case-control study.* Fertil Steril 39:753–760, 1983.

97. RAMIREZ, VD, AND MCCANN, SM: *Induction of prolactin secretion by implants of estrogen into the hypothalamo-hypophysial region of female rats.* Endocrinology 75:206–214, 1964.

98. REICHLIN, S: *Etiology of pituitary adenomas.* In POST, KD, JACKSON, IMD, REICHLIN, S (EDS): *The Pituitary Adenoma.* Plenum, New York, 1980, pp 29–46.

99. REICHLIN, S, AND MOLITCH, M: *Neuroendocrine aspects of pituitary adenoma.* In CAMANNI, F, MÜLLER, EE (EDS): *Pituitary Hyperfunction.* Raven Press, New York, 1984, pp 47–70.

100. ROBINSON, A: *Prolactinomas in women: Current therapies.* Ann Int Med 99:115–118, 1982.

101. RODMAN, EF, MOLITCH, ME, POST, KD, BILLER, BJ, REICHLIN, S: *Long-term follow-up of transsphenoidal selective adenomectomy for prolactinoma.* JAMA 252:921–4, 1984.

102. RODMAN, EF, ADELMAN, L, DAYAL, Y, ET AL: *Acromegaly and hyperprolactinemia in polyostotic fibrous dysplasia* (in preparation).

103. SAMSON, WK, LUMPKIN, MD, MCDONALD, JK, MCCANN, SM: *Prolactin-releasing activity of porcine intestinal peptide (PHI-27).* Peptides (Fayetteville) 4:817–819, 1983.

104. SASSIN, JF, FRANTZ, AG, WEITZMAN, ED, KAPEN, S: *Human prolactin: 24-hour pattern with increased release during sleep.* Science 177:1205–1207, 1972.

105. SASSIN, JF, FRANTZ, GF, KAPEN, S, WEITZMAN, ED: *The nocturnal rise of human prolactin is dependent on sleep.* J Clin Endocrinol Metab 37:436–440, 1973.

106. SCHALLENBERGER, E, RICHARDSON, DW, KNOBIL, E: *Role of prolactin in the lactational amenorrhea of the rhesus monkey (Macaca mulatta).* Biol Reprod 25:370–374, 1981.

107. SCHALLY, AV, REDDING, TW, ARIMURA, A, DUPONT, A, LINTHICUM, GL: *Isolation of gamma-amino butyric acid from pig hypothalami and demonstration of its prolactin release-inhibiting (PIF) activity in vivo and in vitro.* Endocrinology 100:681–691, 1977.

108. SCHLECHTE, J, SHERMAN, B, HALMI, N, VAN GILDER, J, CHAPLER, F, DOLAN, K, GRANNER, D, DUELLO, T, HARRIS, C: *Prolactin-secreting pituitary tumors in amenorrheic women: A comprehensive study.* Endocrine Rev 1:294–308, 1980.

109. SCHRAMME C, DENEF C: *Stimulation of spontaneous and dopamine-inhibited prolactin release from anterior pituitary reaggregate cell cultures by angiotensin peptides.* Life Sci 34:1651–8, 1984.

110. SERRI O, RASIO E, BEAUREGARD H, HARDY J, SOMMA M: *Recurrence of hyperprolactinemia after selective transsphenoidal adenomectomy in women with prolactinoma.* N Engl J Med 309:280–283, 1983.

111. SHELINE GE: *Radiation therapy of pituitary tumors.* In GIVENS, JR (ED): *Hormone-Secreting Pituitary Tumors.* Year Book Medical Publishers Inc, Chicago, 121–144, 1982.

112. SHELINE, GE, GROSSMAN, A, JONES, AE, BESSER, GM: *Radiation therapy for prolactinomas.* In BLACK, PMcL, ZERVAS, NT, RIDGWAY, EC, MARTIN JB (EDS): *Secretory Tumors of the Pituitary Gland.* Raven Press, New York, 1984, pp 93–108.

113. SHERMAN, BM, WALLACE, RB, CHAPLER, FK, LUCIANO, AA, BEAN, JA: *Prolactin-secreting pituitary tumors: An epidemiologic approach.* In CAMANNI, F, AND MÜLLER, EE (EDS): *Pituitary Hyperfunction: Physiopathology and Clinical Aspects.* Raven Press, New York, 1984, pp 167–174.

114. SHIMATSU, A, KATO, Y, OHTA, H, TOJO, K, KABAYAMA, Y, INOUE, T, YANAIHARA, N, IMURA, H: *Involvement of hypothalamic vasoactive intestinal polypepide (VIP) in prolactin secretion induced by serotonin in rats.* Proc Soc Exp Biol Med 175:414–416, 1984.

115. SHIN, SH: *Vasopressin has a direct effect on prolactin release in male rats.* Neuroendocrinology 34:55–58, 1982.

116. SHORT, RV: *Breast feeding.* Sci Am 250:35–41, 1984.

117. STACHURA, ME: *Sequestration of an early-release pool of growth hormone and prolactin in GH_3 rat pituitary tumor cells.* Endocrinology 111:1769–1777, 1982.

118. STERN, JM, KONNER, M, HERMAN, TN, REICHLIN, S: *Nursing behavior, prolactin and postpartum.* Clin Endocrinology (in press).

119. SWEARINGEN, KC, AND NICOLL, C: *Prolactin turnover in rat adenohypophyses in vivo: Its evaluation as a method for estimating secretion rates.* J Endocrinol 53:1–15, 1972.

120. THORNER, MO: *Prolactin: Clinical physiology and the significance and management of hyperprolactinemia.* In MARTINI, L, AND BESSER, GM (EDS): *Clinical Neuroendocrinology.* Academic Press, New York, 1978, 320–361.

121. THORNER, MO, BESSER, GM, JONES, A, DACIE, J, JONES, AE: *Bromocriptine treatment of female infertility: Report of 13 pregnancies.* Br Med J 4:694–697, 1975.

122. TINDAL, JS: *Control of prolactin secretion.* In JEFFCOATE, SL, AND HUTCHINSON, JSM (EDS): *The Endocrine Hypothalamus.* Academic Press, New York, 1978, 333–361.

123. TINDAL, JS, AND KNAGGS, GS: *Pathways in the forebrain of the rabbit concerned with the release of prolactin.* J Endocrinol 52:253–262, 1972.

124. TINDAL, JS, KNAGGS, GS, TURVEY, A: *The afferent path of the milk-ejection reflex in the brain of the rabbit.* J Endocrinol 43:663–671, 1969.

125. TINDAL, JS, AND KNAGGS, GS: *Pathways in the forebrain of the rat concerned with the release of prolactin.* J Brain Res 119:211–221, 1977.

126. TOLIS, G, GOLDSTEIN, M, FRIESEN, HG: *Functional evaluation of prolactin secretion in patients with hypothalamic-pituitary disorders.* J Clin Invest 52:783–788, 1973.

127. TOLIS, G, SOUMA, M, VAN CAMPENHOUT, J, FRIESEN, H: *Prolactin secretion in sixty-five patients with galactorrhea.* Am J Obstet Gynecol 118:91–101, 1974.

128. TRUONG, AT, DUEZ, C, BELAYEW, A, RENARD, A, PICTED, R, BELL, G, MARTIAL, JA: *Isolation and characterization of the human prolactin gene.* The EMBO Journal 3:429–437, 1984.

129. TURKINGTON, RW, UNDERWOOD, LE, VAN WYK, JJ: *Elevated serum prolactin levels after pituitary-stalk section in man.* N Engl J Med 285:707–710, 1971.

130. TURNER, TH, COOKSON, JC, WASS, JAH, DRURY, PL, PRICE, PA, BESSER, GM: *Psychotic reactions during treatment of pituitary tumors with dopamine agonists.* Br Med J 289:1101–1103, 1984.

131. VALE, W, RIVIER, C, BROWN, M, CHAN, L, LING, N, RIVIER, J: *Applications of adenohypophyseal cell cultures to neuroendocrine studies.* Curr Top Mol Endocrinol 3:397–429, 1976.

132. VALVERDE, C, CHIEFFO, V, REICHLIN, S: *Prolactin releasing factor in porcine and rat hypothalamic tissue.* Endocrinology 91:982–993, 1972.

133. VARGA, L, WENNER, R, DEL POZO, E: *Treatment of galactorrhea-amenorrhea syndrome with Bromergocryptine (CB-154): Restoration of ovulatory function and fertility.* Am J Obstet Gynecol 117:75–79, 1973.

134. VIJAYAN, E, AND McCANN, SM: *In vivo and in vitro effects of substance P and neurotensin on gonadotropin and prolactin release.* Endocrinology 105:64–68, 1979.

135. WEINER, RI, BLAKE, CA, SAWYER, CH: *Integrated levels of plasma LH and prolactin following hypothalamic deafferentation in the rat.* Neuroendocrinology 10:349–357, 1972.

136. WERNER, S, HULTING, AL, HOKFELT, T, ENEROTH, P, TATEMOTO, K, MUTT, V, MARODER, L, WUNSCH, E: *Effect of the peptide PHI-27 on prolactin release in vitro.* Neuroendocrinology 37:476–478, 1983.

137. WESTENDORF, JM, AND SCHONBRUNN, A: *Characterization of bombesin receptors in a rat pituitary cell line.* J Biol Chem 258:7527–35, 1983.

138. YAMAJI, T, ISHIBASHI, M, TERAMOTO, A, FUKUSHIMA, T: *Hyperprolactinemia in Cushing's disease and Nelson's syndrome.* J Clin Endocrinol Metab 58:790–795, 1984.

139. YEN, SSC: *Physiology of human prolactin.* In YEN, SSC, AND JAFFE, RB (EDS): *Reproductive*

Endocrinology: Physiology, Pathophysiology and Clinical Management. WB Saunders, Philadelphia, 1978, 152–170.

140. YUEN, BH, KEYE, WR, JR, JAFFE, RB: *Human prolactin: Secretion, regulation and pathophysiology.* Obstet Gynecol Surg 28:527, 1973.

141. ZERVAS, NT: *Surgical results for pituitary adenomas: Results of an international survey.* In BLACK, P McL, ZERVAS, NT, RIDGWAY, EC, MARTIN, JB (EDS): *Secretory Tumors of the Pituitary Gland.* Raven Press, New York, 1984, pp 377–385.

142. ZIMMERMAN, EA, DEFENDINI, R, FRANTZ, AG: *Prolactin and growth hormone in patients with pituitary adenomas: A correlative study of hormone in tumor and plasma by immunoperoxidase technique and radioimmunossay.* J Clin Endocrinol Metab 38:577–585, 1974.

143. HONBO, KS, VAN HERLE, AJ, KELLETT, KA: *Serum prolactin levels in untreated primary hypothyroidism.* Am J Med 64:782–787, 1978.

144. CLEMENS, JA, SAR, M, MEITES, J: *Termination of pregnancy in rats by a prolactin implant in median eminence.* Proc Soc Exptl Biol Med 130:628–630, 1969.

145. EHNI, G, ECKLES, NE: *Interruption of the pituitary stalk on the patient with mammary cancer.* J Neurosurg 16:628–652, 1959.

146. KLIBANSKI, A, NEER, RM, BEITENS, IZ, RIDGWAY, EC, ZERVAS, NT, McARTHUR, JW: *Decreased bone density in hyperprolactinemic women.* N Engl J Med 303:1511–1514, 1980.

147. MINAMITANI, N, LECHAN, RM, REICHLIN, S: *Paraventricular nucleus (PVN) mediates prolactin (PRL) secretory responses to restraint stress, ether stress and 5-hydroxy tryptophan (5-HTP) injection in the rat.* Abstract, 1986 Endocrine Society Meeting.

148. VON WERDER, K, EVERSMAN, T, FAHLBUSCH, R, MÜLLER, OA, RJOSK, HK: *Endocrine-active pituitary adenomas: Long-term results of medical and surgical treatment.* In CAMANNI, F, AND MÜLLER, EE: *Pituitary Hyperfunction: Physiopathology and Clinical Aspects.* Raven Press, New York, 1984, pp 385–406.

149. KISS, JZ, KAMJICSKA, B, NAGY, GY: *The hypothalamic paraventricular nucleus has a pivotal role in regulation of prolactin release in lactating rats.* Endocrinology 119:870–873, 1986.

150. SAMSON, WK, LUMPKIN, MD, McCANN, SM: *Evidence for a physiological role for oxytocin in the control of prolactin secretion.* Endocrinology 119:554–560, 1986.

151. ROSSELIN, G.: *The receptors of the VIP family peptides. Specifications and identity.* Peptides, 7(suppl. 1):89–100, 1986.

Chapter 8

REGULATION OF GROWTH HORMONE SECRETION AND ITS DISORDERS

Neural control of growth hormone (GH) secretion is mediated by GH-releasing hormone (GRH or GHRH) and somatostatin (GH-release inhibiting hormone, SRIF), both secreted into the hypophysial-portal circulation from specialized groups of tuberoinfundibular neurons. In turn, these GH-regulating tuberoinfundibular neurons are influenced by a complex array of monoaminergic and peptidergic neurons and by feedback hormonal effects. The pituitary response to neural factors is modulated by hormonal influences that include thyroid hormone, cortisol, estrogens, and somatomedin C, a circulating peptide whose secretion is regulated by GH (Fig. 1). A comprehensive review of GH has recently been published.[271]

PITUITARY GROWTH HORMONE

Human growth hormone (hGH) occurs in two forms, most of it as a single-chained polypeptide of 21,500 dalton molecular weight (Fig. 2).

The molecule contains 191 amino acid residues and two intramolecular disulfide bonds and has a molecular weight of 21,500 daltons.[142,170] Approximately 15 percent of total pituitary hGH consists of a slightly smaller molecule with a 15 amino acid deletion between residues 32 and 46. This variant (GH variant) possesses growth-promoting activity but lacks the insulin-like activity characteristic of the larger GH form. Growth hormone from other primates resembles hGH in many physical properties and cross-reacts with it in radioimmunoassay systems. Growth hormone accounts for 4 to 10 percent of the wet weight of the anterior pituitary gland in the adult human (5 to 15 mg/gland). Content of GH in the pituitary gland is not related to age, although secretion rate is (see below).

Growth hormone is secreted by specific anterior pituitary cells, the somatotropes.[55] Histochemical and immunofluorescence methods have shown that these cells are distinct from those which synthesize other pituitary tropic hormones, including prolactin. Morphologically distinct, round, secretory granules 300 to 400 nm in diameter and containing GH can be demonstrated in these cells and serve as an identifying characteristic of the somatotrope and its secretory product. By classical staining methods GH granules are acidophilic (stain with acidic dyes like eosin), but many GH-

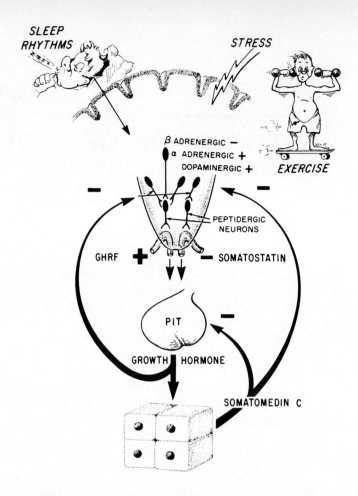

SLEEP RHYTHMS

STRESS

β ADRENERGIC —
α ADRENERGIC +
DOPAMINERGIC +

EXERCISE

PEPTIDERGIC NEURONS

GHRF **+**

— SOMATOSTATIN

PIT

GROWTH HORMONE

SOMATOMEDIN C

HYPOTHALAMIC – GROWTH HORMONE – SOMATOMEDIN AXIS

FIGURE 1. Regulation of GH secretion. GH secretion by the pituitary gland is stimulated by GHRH and inhibited by somatostatin. Negative feedback control of the pituitary is exerted at the pituitary level by somatomedin C. Somatomedin also acts on the hypothalamus to stimulate secretion of somatostatin. Based on indirect pharmacologic data, it appears that release of GHRH is stimulated by acetylcholine, α-adrenergic stimuli, and dopaminergic stimuli and is inhibited by β-adrenergic stimuli. Secretion of somatostatin, studied by direct assay *in vitro,* is stimulated by acetylcholine and VIP and inhibited by GABA. Secretion of GH is modified by endogenous sleep rhythms, by stress, and by exercise.

containing cells do not stain with eosin and would be classified by old-fashioned methods as "chromophobes."

In common with other secretory cells, the hormone is synthesized within the endoplasmic reticulum. From the endoplasmic reticulum, the nascent hormone, in the process of being formed, is packaged into secretory granules within the Golgi apparatus of the cell. In humans, the gene directing GH synthesis is located on chromosome 17.[170] The genetic sequence coding for hGH has been determined, and genetic recombinant techniques have been used to synthesize hGH in colonies of *E. coli.* This biosynthetic GH can be used to treat pituitary dwarfism.

Release of GH from pituitary cells, as is true for the release process of other peptide hormones, occurs by exocytosis, that is, the expulsion of

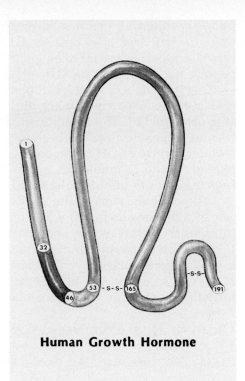

Human Growth Hormone

FIGURE 2. Structure of hGH. The protein contains 191 amino acids and two intramolecular disulfide bonds. About 15 percent of pituitary GH is synthesized as a 20 kd protein with the deletion from residue 32 to 46 as shown.

membrane-bound storage granules. This process is brought about by the translocation of the granule from its site of packaging within the Golgi complex to the plasma membrane where fusion of the granule and plasma membranes occurs. Movement of granules within the cell is mediated by an energy-requiring process that involves contractile elements of the intracellular microtubular cytoskeleton.

Growth hormone circulates unbound in plasma. Its half-life of disappearance is between 17 and 45 minutes, and its estimated secretion rate in normal adults is approximately 400 μg/day.[4] Men and women secrete approximately the same amount of hormone. Growth hormone acts at many sites and in this respect is similar to insulin and thyroid hormone and different from other pituitary hormones such as TSH, ACTH, and the gonadotropins, which have specific target organs.

The actions of GH are numerous and include stimulation of skeletal and muscle growth, regulation of lipolysis, and promotion of cellular uptake of amino acids. Growth hormone has insulin-like effects and is also diabetogenic, with anti-insulin effects. These apparently contradictory effects are partly due to different actions of portions of the hGH molecule that are cleaved from the parent hormone[142] and to the stimulating effect of GH on somatomedin synthesis.[55]

Most of the effects of GH on growth are mediated indirectly through a basic peptide, somatomedin C, which is formed in the liver and perhaps the kidney.[55,188] Somatomedin C, which is called insulin-like growth factor I (IGF I), is one of a family of circulating substances that stimulates proliferation of cartilage and synthesis of cartilage matrix chondroitin sulfate. The other somatomedin that has been identified is IGF II, a neutral peptide. Other factors have been described, including somatomedin A, which is now considered to be a fragment(s) of IGF I or IGF II and somatomedin B, a peptide not dependent on GH. In addition to their ability to stimulate cartilage growth, IgG I and IgG II possess intrinsic insulin-like activity and are closely homologous to proinsulin in structure. Both IGF I and IGF II are stimulated by GH. This is important from a GH-regulatory point of view because somatomedin C has been shown to be part of a negative feedback loop for control of GH secretion. This somatomedin acts directly on the pituitary gland to inhibit the action of GHRH[97,262] and directly on the hypothalamus to stimulate the release of somatostatin[1,240] (see Figure 1).

Although the work of the last two decades has firmly established the role of somatomedin in GH action on bone, GH can act directly on chondrocytes,[146] presumably by stimulating local production of somatomedin C[272] as it can on hypothalamic secretion of somatostatin.[240] Somatomedin C levels are measurable by radioimmunoassay and serve as a useful index of the GH-secretory state of patients with abnormalities of GH secretion, including acromegaly and hypopituitarism.[50]

GROWTH HORMONE SECRETORY PATTERNS

Factors that stimulate GH secretion are presented in Table 1.

Spontaneous Fluctuations

Basal (resting or nonstressed) levels of immunoassayable hGH in plasma taken at random in the adult man or woman are usually less than 5 ng/ml and are often below the lower limit of most radioimmunoassays (less than 2 ng/ml). However, if one samples blood frequently throughout the day and night, striking variations in plasma GH concentration are observed in both human beings and experimental animals.[63,89] Growth hormone levels in the human being may surge as high as 20 to 40 ng/ml, the largest bursts often occurring during the first part of sleep.[72]

Magnitude and the number of the spontaneous bursts of GH secretion in the human being are age-dependent.[72,169] Transition from early puberty to adolescence is associated with an increased number of GH surges, occurring as frequently as 8 times per 24-hour period (Fig. 3).[72] Those occurring during the first few hours of night sleep are the highest. Age and total 24-hour GH secretory rates are closely correlated. In the study of Finkelstein and coworkers[72] prepubertal children had a mean 24-hour secretory rate of 91 μg; adolescents, 690 μg; and young adults, 385 μg. Because spontaneous bursts of GH secretion can occur, studies of provocative agents must be controlled with placebo periods.

Growth hormone also follows a developmental pattern.

Growth hormone secretion occurs as early as 70 days of gestation; average plasma levels were 14.5 ng/ml at this time. Growth hormone levels peaked at 20 to 24 weeks (mean GH 119.3 ng/ml). Plasma levels fall to a mean of 33.5 ng/ml at birth and then decline over the next 2 to 3 months to reach the low basal levels characteristic of the prepubertal child.[118] The age-related changes in aging men appear to be due in part to loss of pituitary sensitivity to GHRH as shown by

TABLE 1. Factors that Stimulate Growth Hormone Secretion in Primates

Physiologic	Pharmacologic	Pathologic
1. Episodic, spontaneous	1. Insulin hypoglycemia	1. Acromegaly
2. Exercise	a. 2-Deoxyglucose	a. TRH
3. Stress	2. Amino acid infusions	b. LHRH
a. Physical	a. Arginine	c. Glucose
b. Psychological	b. Leucine	d. Arginine
4. Sleep	c. Lysine, etc.	2. Pyrogens
5. Postprandial glucose decline	3. Small peptides	3. Protein depletion
	a. GHRH	4. Fasting and starvation
	b. ADH	5. Anorexia nervosa
	c. α-MSH	
	d. ACTH (1-24)	
	e. Glucagon	
	4. Monoaminergic stimuli	
	a. Epinephrine, α-receptor stimulation	
	b. Levodopa	
	c. Apomorphine	
	d. Bromocriptine	
	e. Clonidine	
	f. 5-Hydroxytryptophan	
	g. Fusaric acid (dopa-β-hydroxylase inhibitor)	
	h. Propranolol	
	i. Melatonin	
	5. Nonpeptide hormones	
	a. Estrogens	
	b. Diethylstilbestrol	
	6. Potassium infusion	
	7. Dibutyryl-cAMP	

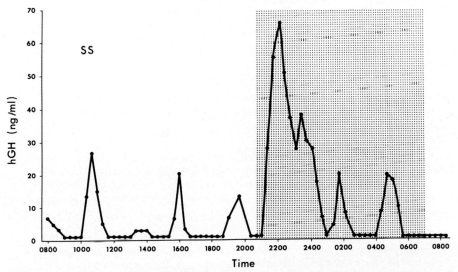

FIGURE 3. Episodic secretion of GH in a normal adolescent male subject. Eight distinct secretory episodes are evident with a large surge of secretion shortly after onset of sleep *(shaded area)*. (Adapted from Finkelstein, JW et al.[72])

progressive loss of responsiveness with successive decades.[220] Women at the time of menopause show a decline in spontaneous GH secretion, response to exercise, and response to GHRH apparently related to loss of estrogens.[57]

The lower GH levels of older individuals have been regarded as a form of acquired hyposomatotropinism thought by some to be responsible for certain aspects of the aging process.

Secretory pulses of GH often show a strikingly abrupt onset, with rapid rise in plasma GH followed by a decline consistent with the known half-life of disappearance of the hormone from the blood, suggesting that GH secretion is totally turned off at the completion of the burst. In this respect, GH secretory patterns resemble the episodic secretion of ACTH, prolactin, and the gonadotropins.

Metabolic Regulation of GH Secretion

All three of the major classes of metabolic substrate (carbohydrate, protein, and fat) affect GH secretion. The first to be recognized was the effect of altered glucose concentration. In 1963, soon after they had developed their immunoassay method, Roth and his associates observed that hypoglycemia produced by insulin administration in the human being triggered GH secretion and that glucose administration lowered basal levels of GH.[208] They also found that GH levels rose during the falling phase of the standard glucose tolerance test and that 2-deoxyglucose, an analog of glucose that causes intracellular glucose deficiency, also triggered GH release. These responses were not observed in a patient with section of the pituitary stalk. On this basis they proposed that glucoreceptors within the nervous system sensed plasma glucose levels and modulated homeostatic GH regulatory responses. This hypothesis appeared reasonable in view of the fact that GH has antiinsulin effects and is a potent lipolytic substance. Further studies of this control system (reviewed in detail by Reichlin,[198,199]) indicate a far greater degree of complexity than was initially conceived. It is now recognized that GH secretion is not regulated in relation to an absolute blood glucose level but, rather, is responsive to change in glucose levels, rising levels suppressing and falling levels exciting GH release. The GH response to hypoglycemia is not truly homeostatic, inasmuch as normal blood sugar levels are restored before the GH response has affected carbohydrate metabolism; also, GH secretion is not related to an absolute level of glucose. In part, response to hypoglycemia can be viewed as a stress response. However, there is a glucoreceptor mechanism unrelated to the stress response, inasmuch as glucose administration inhibits GH secretion in the basal state or after exercise.

> Although these observations indicate that glucose affects GH secretion, review of the available data provides "relatively weak evidence to support the thesis that reflex alterations in GH secretion are important in glucose homeostasis except possibly as an emergency mechanism, as in immature organisms. Even if it could be shown that minor degrees of hypoglycemia induced greater GH responses, the effects of exercise, sleep, psychological stress, random GH bursts, and postprandial glucose decline, are so much more important in determining the secretion rate of GH that these factors, and not the demands of glucose homeostasis, dominate the controlling mechanisms of GH secretion."[199]

Growth hormone secretion is also linked to protein metabolism. Ingestion of a high-protein meal or the intravenous injection of a number of amino acids leads to release of GH, a response that may be blunted by hyperglycemia. Because amino acids are ineffective in releasing GH in patients with hypothalamic disease, it has been assumed that this amino acid acts on a neural site in the hypothalamus. There are specific amino acid receptors in the brain and these may be responsible for the increase in GH secretion. A plasma volume-sensitive mechanism may exist that regulates GH secretion.[199]

Fasting in men of normal weight leads to a rise in GH levels usually within two days, commonly with increased number and amplitude of GH secretory peaks. Severe protein-calorie malnutrition and anorexia nervosa also are associated with an elevation of GH levels. This effect is postulated to be due to the loss of the normal feedback inhibitory effects of somatomedin C, in turn related to starvation-induced deficiency of somatomedin C precursors. Because GH stimulates lipolysis, with release of fatty acids, starvation-induced GH release may play a role in the homeostatic response to fasting. However, the bulk of reported work indicates that the major hormonal regulator of lipolysis is insulin and that starvation leads to suppression of insulin secretion. Under well-defined conditions elevated fatty acids suppress GH secretion in response to certain provocative stimuli including arginine, hypoglycemia, and sleep.[111]

Obese subjects show striking disturbance in GH regulation. Responses to provocative stimuli such as hypoglycemia, stress, and L-dopa are blunted. The introduction of GHRH as a test of intrinsic pituitary responsiveness has shown that the abnormality is mediated at the level of the pituitary gland.[265] Remarkably small degrees of obesity can modify responsiveness. Growth hormone response to exercise was blunted in women whose body weight was 115 percent above ideal,[57] and the response in men to benzodiazepine injection (a stimulator of GH release) also was blocked in individuals whose weight was similarly elevated.[234]

Effects of Activity

Growth hormone levels are usually unmeasurable in normal subjects on bed rest after an overnight fast.[199] Exercise causes GH release in both men and women. Even minor activity such as getting out of bed in the morning (particularly in women or in estrogen-treated men) causes an elevation in plasma GH levels. Walking at the rate of 1 mile per hour for an hour increases GH secretion by approximately 50 percent in older women.[57]

This lability can be utilized in provocative screening for GH deficiency in children. Vigorous stair climbing will raise GH plasma levels to above 7 ng/ml in about 70 percent of normal children.

Responses to Stress

Stimulation. Most stressful stimuli in the human being stimulate GH secretion in a manner analogous to the release of ACTH and of catecholamines under similar circumstances.[38] Surgical operations cause a rise in GH, as does electroshock therapy, even when carried out with neuromuscular blockade. Growth hormone levels are also increased following pyrogen administration, acute trauma, and arterial puncture. A stress effect may explain the GH response to insulin hypoglycemia, but there appear to be central glucoreceptors that control GH secretion.[106]

> Recent studies in patients with complex partial seizures (temporal lobe epilepsy), show that GH fails to rise after an acute seizure, whereas prolactin nearly always increases. This difference can be useful clinically in distinguishing true from pseudoseizures (see chapters 7 and 11).[194]

In contrast to the situation with regard to physical stimuli, little is known of the psychophysiologic regulation of GH secretion. In one study, a systematic investigation was undertaken of the psychologic factors involved in the release of both GH and cortisol.[38] Patients undergoing diagnostic cardiac catheterization were rated psychologically by two independent observers. Cortisol elevations were seen in all patients who showed overt manifestations of anxiety. In contrast, only those anxious patients who did not engage in conversation showed GH elevation. In the same study, low GH levels were observed in "depressed" patients who appeared uninvolved and withdrawn. Sadness induced by viewing a documentary film was found in one study to be associated with an elevation in plasma GH levels.

Further evidence that depression can cause abnormalities in GH secretion is the finding that in many such cases the usual stimulating effects of hypoglycemia, amphetamines, clonidine, and L-dopa[211] on GH secretion are blunted. This finding has been interpreted to indicate an abnormality in α-adrenergic receptors, reflected in simultaneous disturbances in affect and hormonal regulation (see chapter 21). Growth hormone secretion in the nonhuman primate is also markedly stress responsive, with dramatic elevation occurring following a variety of stressful stimuli including noise, pain, pinching of the abdomen, aversive conditioning, capture from the cage, and ether anesthesia.[38] In marked contrast with the human being, GH release in the rat is inhibited by stress.[244] Growth hormone studies in stress and psychiatric disorders are also discussed in chapter 21.

Functional Inhibition (Psychosocial Dwarfism, Maternal Deprivation).
Clinicians have long recognized that gross emotional deprivation may be associated with growth failure (maternal deprivation syndrome, psychosocial deprivation syndrome)[193] and that growth rate may accelerate dramatically when the psychosocial environment has been improved. Many of these children have impaired GH response to hypoglycemia and also may show deficiency of ACTH secretion and delayed sexual development, all of which are reversed by a suitable environment. Children of this type have been reported to have abnormal sleep patterns, leading to the view that GH deficiency is caused by reduction in sleep-related GH release.

> James Barrie, the English playwright and novelist who wrote *Peter Pan*, may be a case in point. The seventh of eight children, he was subjected to severe maternal deprivation when his mother, after the accidental death of James's elder brother, "got into bed and stayed there for over a year." The emotionally deprived James never grew up, remaining less than 5 feet tall and sexually underdeveloped. Like

REGULATION OF THE PITUITARY GLAND

Peter Pan, he may have "chosen" not to grow up. Oskar, the protagonist of Gunter Glass's novel, *The Tin Drum,* is another literary character who also refused to grow because of emotional stress. In the rat, stress lowers and "gentling" (systematic fondling) raises GH levels.

Sleep-associated Release

One of the most characteristic features of GH regulation in the human being is the rise in plasma levels that occurs within an hour or two of onset of sleep.[72,182,235] Evidence that the nocturnal rise is related to sleep onset and not simply to diurnal variations can be summarized thus: (1) The major burst of GH secretion occurs within 2 hours of sleep (Fig. 4);[235] (2) if onset of sleep is postponed, the onset of GH secretion is postponed; (3) if awakened and permitted to fall asleep again, subjects show a second GH secretory peak within 2 hours of sleep; and (4) daytime naps may be associated with GH secretory peaks. The release of GH during early sleep has been used as a test of physiologic secretion in children. About 70 to 80 percent of children tested 90 minutes after nocturnal sleep onset show elevated GH levels.

Sleep-related GH secretion may be correlated with characteristic EEG changes of slow-wave sleep (SWS, stages III and IV).

Earlier investigators believed that the two phenomena were correlated, but later studies indicate that the association may be only fortuitous. Evidence for correlation of SWS with nocturnal GH secretion came initially from the experiments of Takahashi and coworkers,[235] who found that many, but not all, GH surges were correlated

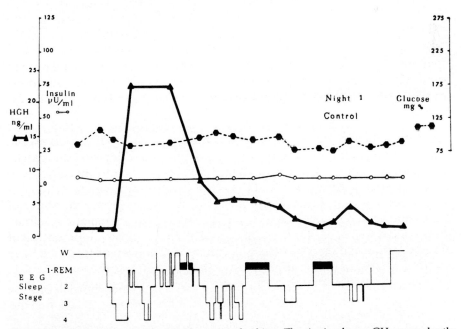

FIGURE 4. GH secretion during sleep in a normal subject. The rise in plasma GH occurs shortly after sleep onset and is not associated with any change in glucose or insulin levels. (From Lucke, C, and Glick, SM: *Experimental modification of the sleep-induced peak of growth hormone secretion.* J Clin Endocrinol Metab 32:729, 1971, with permission.)

with SWS. Subsequently it was found that blind persons, who have less SWS, have less sleep-associated GH release, that ontogenetic development of nocturnal GH secretory patterns correlates somewhat with the appearance of SWS, and that narcoleptic patients (who frequently enter directly into rapid-eye-movement (REM) sleep without an intervening period of SWS) may fail to secrete GH early in sleep.[152]

On the other hand, a number of observations indicate that the two phenomena are associated but not directly interdependent. If there were a common neural mechanism that simultaneously triggers SWS and release of GH, the two events would coincide uniformly, in some constant temporal relationship. Several reports of nocturnal GH secretion have been published which permit a test of this hypothesis. In one experiment, seven subjects were studied for two nights. In two episodes, GH was released before sleep onset. In 10 episodes, the first occurrence of SWS preceded GH secretion by 0 to 60 minutes, but in four of these, GH release appeared to precede the onset of SWS on four occasions. Therefore, there appears to be a frequent but not consistent temporal relationship between SWS and GH release. A number of investigators also have pointed out the lack of concurrence of these two phenomena in some normal persons and in the blind. Dissociation between SWS and GH secretion also has been described in a number of disease states in which both abnormal SWS and abnormal GH secretion occur. These include Cushing's disease (both active and in the early stages of recovery), Nelson's syndrome, hypothalamic tumors, Addison's disease, cerebral lupus erythematosus (on steroids), and in patients with the maternal deprivation syndrome. In addition, several pharmacologic agents can cause dissociation of SWS and GH secretion: imipramine, chlorpromazine, phenobarbital, flurazepam, medroxyprogesterone, acute high-dose glucose infusion, Zn-tetracosactrin (ACTH), and free fatty acids. Thyrotropin-releasing hormone inhibits sleep induced GH release *(vide infra)*.

Our interpretation of the significance of nocturnal GH release is that it is sleep-related as a circadian event but not directly caused by the neural mechanisms that generate SWS. The electroencephalogram characteristics of SWS reflect cortical electrical activity and probably do not accurately reflect changes in the subcortical mechanisms involved in neuroendocrine control of the pituitary. Thus the two phenomenon (SWS and GH release) can be dissociated by factors acting at a number of levels in the central nervous system.

Episode (Pulsatile) Secretion of GH

The spontaneous surges of GH secretion documented by frequent sampling in the human being have been studied in several animal species. Episodic GH secretion has been documented in experimental animals including monkeys, baboons, dogs, rabbits, and rats.[157,158,241,242,266] The episodic secretion in the rat has been studied most extensively, especially to elucidate neuroendocrine control mechanisms. Regular sampling in this species has demonstrated striking variations in plasma GH which are characterized by prominent, high-amplitude bursts that may reach levels of 300 to 1000 ng/ml (Fig. 5). The pulses of GH secretion in this species show a regular 3- to 4-hour pattern that are entrained to the light-dark cycle. Bursts of GH secretion are independent of fluctuations in corticosterone, prolactin, or TSH and are not related to stress. As in man, episodic secretion in the rat is not regulated primarily by glucose or other substrates inasmuch as it is not affected by fasting, feeding, or glucose administration. Studies of the neurotransmitter and neuroanatomic basis of this response are discussed below.

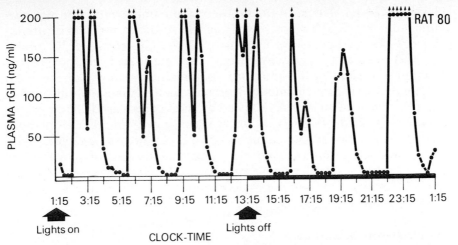

FIGURE 5. Twenty-four-hour secretory pattern of GH release in the rat. (From Tannenbaum and Martin,[238] with permission.)

NEURAL MECHANISMS CONTROLLING GROWTH HORMONE SECRETION

Disturbance in body growth as a result of lesions of the hypothalamus was recognized by clinicians early in this century, but the pathogenesis of this abnormality was not understood until the development of methods for measurement of GH made it possible to differentiate among the various mechanisms by which the hypothalamus can influence growth.[152,196] In addition to GH deficiency, hypothalamic lesions can cause impaired growth by reducing food intake and by causing deficiencies of ADH, ACTH, TSH, and the gonadotropins.[196] The history of development of our knowledge of neural control of GH secretion is summarized in several reviews.[154,197–199]

HYPOTHALAMIC REGULATION

Prior to the elucidation by immunohistochemical techniques of GHRH- and somatostatin-containing neurons, regions of the hypothalamus involved in GH regulation were demonstrated by lesion and electrical stimulation studies. Lesion studies implicated the ventromedial and arcuate nuclei (VMN-ARC) together with the median eminence as the final common pathway of control of GH release.[198,199] Destruction of the VMN-ARC area blocks pulsatile GH release and impairs growth, without interfering with the vascular supply to the pituitary gland. In the squirrel monkey, lesions of the anterior lip of the median eminence blocked stress-induced GH release.[39] The neural component for GH regulation is readily damaged. Growth hormone failure is one of the earliest signs of hypothalamic damage in human beings and laboratory animals. In the work of Brown and colleagues,[39] stress-induced GH release in squirrel monkeys was blocked by only a small lesion in the upper stalk median eminence region which left intact more than 70 percent of the tissue. The arcuate nucleus (ARC) also is related to GH regulation. In the rat, neonatal administration of monosodium glutamate, which destroys this nucleus, results in permanent attenuation of GH secretion; lesions of this region block GH release.[7,28,168] Inhibitory GH regulatory pathways were also elucidated by physiologic techniques. Lesions of the anterior hypothalamus, removal of the brain anterior to the septum, or anterior (coronal) deafferentation at the level of the optic chiasm in rats are all followed by signs of increased GH secretion, including elevated GH levels and more rapid growth. In the squirrel monkey and rat, anterior hypothalamic lesions were found to be associated with exaggerated GH secretory responses (suggesting the loss of an inhibitory component). In the human being, paradoxic GH release has been reported to follow lesions of the anterior hypothalamus, as, for example, in association with optic nerve glioma.

Hypothalamic Stimulation

Electric stimulation of the hypothalamus gave even more convincing evidence of the presence of specific regions controlling secretion of GH than did the study of effects of hypothalamic lesions. Plasma GH levels rise after electric stimulation of the basal hypothalamus in the monkey, and of the VMN and the adjacent ARC nucleus in the rat (Fig. 6).[77,151,154] Electric stimulation of the medial basal hypothalamus in the rat elicits GH secretion within 5 to 15 minutes after the onset of pulsed square waves. The effective stimulation sites are strictly confined to the VMN-ARC complex. Stimula-

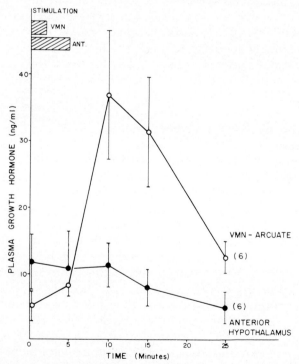

FIGURE 6. GH response to electrical stimulation of the VMN-arcuate region in the rat. Stimulation of other hypothalamic sites is ineffective. (From Martin, JB,[151] with permission.)

REGULATION OF THE PITUITARY GLAND

tion of the preoptic area caused a significant inhibition of GH, a finding that was initially interpreted to mean that inhibitory pathways also exist, a prediction now well substantiated by the discovery of the anterior hypothalamic somatostatinergic system.

Anatomy of GHRH and Somatostatin Peptidergic Pathways

Immunohistochemical studies of the anatomic location of the GHRH and somatostatin pathways have confirmed fully the presumptions based on lesion and electric stimulation studies. Antisera developed against GHRH was shown by Block and collaborators[26,27] to stain hypothalamic neurons in the posterior part of the ARC nucleus and in the premammillary area. Fibers were noted in several hypothalamic regions, including the external zones of the median eminence (Fig. 7)[37,119,223] Antibodies to GHRH stain neuronal perikarya in the VMN and ARC nuclei and nerve fibers ending in the median eminence (Fig. 7)[143,150,165] (see chapter 2).

The somatostatinergic system has been much more extensively studied (Fig. 8)[5,42,53,54,60] (see chapter 2). The principal anterior pituitary regulating pathways arise in the anterior region of the periventricular nuclei, project laterally through the substance of the hypothalamus, and enter the median eminence from its anterior aspect. Other somatostatinergic fibers arise from a well-defined parvocellular (small-cell) subdivision of the paraventricular nucleus.

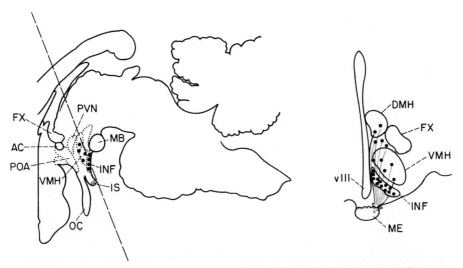

FIGURE 7. This is a schematic depiction of the location of tuberoinfundibular neurons that secrete GRH, based on human and animal studies. Tuberoinfundibular neurons *(solid dots)* are shown in a coronal section through the plane of densest cell bodies, and in a sagittal section. The projection pathway of GRH axons toward the median eminence is depicted by the solid lines forming a point. Abbreviations: OC, optic chiasm; IS, infundibular stalk; INF, infundibular nucleus; (arcuate nucleus); MB, mammillary body; PVN, paraventricular nucleus; FX, fornix; AC, anterior commissure; POA, preoptic area; VMH, ventromedial hypothalamic nucleus; ME, median eminence; DMH, dorsomedial hypothalamic nucleus; vIII, third ventricle; SON, supraoptic nucleus; SCN, suprachiasmatic nucleus. (From Riskind, P, and Martin, JB: Functional anatomy of the hypothalamic-anterior pituitary complex. In DeGroot, LJ (ed): *Endocrinology*, ed 2. Grune & Stratton, Orlando [in press], with permission.)

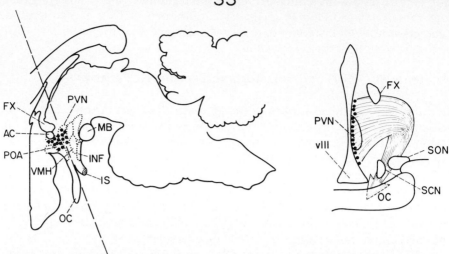

FIGURE 8. This is a schematic depiction of the location of tuberoinfundibular neurons that secrete somatostatin (SS). Abbreviations: OC, optic chiasm; IS, infundibular stalk; INF, infundibular nucleus (arcuate nucleus); MB, mammillary body; PVN, paraventricular nucleus; FX, fornix; AC, anterior commissure; POA, preoptic area; VMH, ventromedial hypothalamic nucleus; ME, median eminence; DMH, dorsomedial hypothalamic nucleus; vIII, third ventricle; SON, supraoptic nucleus; SCN, suprachiasmatic nucleus. (From Riskind, P, and Martin, JB: *Functional anatomy of the hypothalamic-anterior pituitary complex.* In DeGroot, LJ (ed): *Endocrinology,* ed 2. Grune & Stratton, Orlando [in press], with permission.)

Extrahypothalamic Regulation

Physiologic studies demonstrating the effects of stress and sleep on GH secretion point to a probable role of extrahypothalamic structures in GH control. The isolated hypothalamus appears capable of maintaining nearly normal basal secretion of GH, including pulsatile release, but selective hypothalamic cuts indicate that disconnection of specific inputs to the medial basal hypothalamus can have differential excitatory or inhibitory effects on GH secretion, at least in the rat.[157]

Electric stimulation of the hippocampal formation causes GH release, whereas stimulation of the amygdala can elicit either a rise or a fall in plasma GH, depending upon the precise site stimulated.[151,154] Thus, stimulation of the basolateral amygdala causes prompt GH release, which appears to be entrained to the stimulus, plasma levels increasing within 5 minutes of the onset of stimulation and declining immediately after its termination (Fig. 9). This response is blocked by placement of bilateral hypothalamic VMN lesions, indicating that the GH release effects are mediated through the medial basal hypothalamus. Stimulation of the corticomedial amygdala, on the other hand, causes a fall in plasma GH levels comparable with that observed with preoptic stimulation. Because an important component of the efferent system of the corticomedial amygdala travels in the stria terminalis to end in the septum and preoptic area, it remains to be shown whether the corticomedial inhibitory response is mediated via connections in these areas. It is significant that coronal cuts through the anterior hypothalamus cause an increase in growth in the rat and an elevation in plasma GH levels. Such cuts would interrupt the stria terminalis, but they might also disconnect inhibitory effects of the preoptic area.

Complete medial basal hypothalamic deafferentation, in which the VMN and ARC are isolated from the overlying brain, is reported to result in an increased growth rate and elevated plasma GH levels. Preoptic lesions block stress-induced

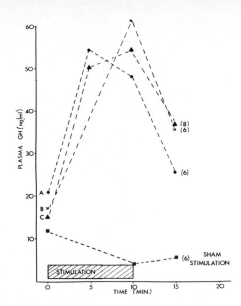

FIGURE 9. Plasma GH responses to stimulation of the basolateral amygdala in three separate groups of animals. Sham stimulation had no effect on GH. Number of animals in each group is shown in parentheses. (From Martin, JB,[153] with permission.)

inhibition of GH secretion in the rat; such lesions permit emergence of a stress GH-release mechanism in this species. These observations suggest that extrahypothalamic inhibitory inputs to the medial basal hypothalamus are important in maintaining a degree of tonic inhibition of GH for mediation of stress-induced GH suppression. Histochemical demonstration of the anterior somatostatinergic pathway supports this hypothesis.

Stimulation of other brain regions also can cause a rise in plasma GH. One effective site is the ventral tegmental area of Tsai surrounding the interpeduncular nucleus, a region giving rise to dopaminergic inputs to higher brain regions. Electric stimulation of the raphe nucleus, the site of serotonergic neurons in the brainstem and of the locus coeruleus, results in GH release.[154] Further investigation of these brain areas will be required to elucidate their role, now a potential one, in GH regulation. The results of locus coeruleus and raphe nucleus stimulation are of interest because both norepinephrine (NE) and serotonin have been implicated in the regulation of GH secretion (see below).

Because emotional state is believed to be based on limbic function, and because GH release is stress modulated, it is reasonable to speculate that these limbic structures influence physiologic GH secretion. The hippocampus, part of the limbic system, is involved in several aspects of behavior—such as the alerting response—and in the recording of new information—as in learning and memory storage. The amygdala is important in establishing emotionality and in the mediation of aggressive behavior. The amygdala is also important in regulation of feeding and drinking. The locus coeruleus is the origin of the ascending noradrenergic fiber system, lesions of which have been implicated in the "sham rage" associated with the "VMH syndrome." The raphe nuclei have been shown to have a role in induction of sleep. Lesions of the raphe nuclei lead to insomnia, as does inhibition of serotonin synthesis by p-chlorophenylalanine.

The anatomic pathways connecting these parts of the limbic system to the medial basal hypothalamus, in general, and the VMN-ARC complex, in particular, have been most clearly defined in the rat (Fig. 10) and are summarized below.

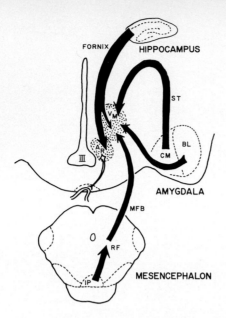

FIGURE 10. Diagram of major afferent pathways to the ventromedial (VM) and arcuate (AR) nuclei in the rat. A large direct hippocampal-arcuate pathway has been described. Amygdaloid inputs arise by two separate pathways. Interpeduncular (IP) inputs to the hypothalamus ascend in the medial forebrain bundle (MFB) after relay in the reticular formation (RF). Abbreviations: BL, basolateral amygdala; CM, corticomedial amygdala; ST, stria terminalis; III, third ventricle. (From Martin, JB: *Plasma growth hormone (GH) response to hypothalamic or extrahypothalamic electrical stimulation.* Endocrinology 91:107, 1972, with permission.)

Direct monosynaptic inputs from a portion of the hippocampus reach the arcuate nucleus via the medial corticohypothalamic tract. The amygdala has a large monosynaptic connection from its corticomedial subdivision which reaches the VMN via the stria terminalis. The connection(s) of the basolateral amygdala to the medial basal hypothalamus has not been as clearly defined. Electrophysiologic studies in the cat have indicated an inhibitory pathway from the corticomedial amygdala via the stria terminalis to the VMN and a complementary excitatory pathway from the basolateral amygdaloid complex to the hypothalamic VMN. It is postulated that this latter pathway is carried in the ventral amygdalohypothalamic tract.[154]

PINEAL INFLUENCES

Relatively little data is available linking the pineal gland and GH regulation. Significant depression of body weight, tibial length, and pituitary GH content are caused in rats by combined blinding and olfactory-lobe removal. These effects are partially reversed by pinealectomy, an indication that the pineal gland exerts tonic inhibitory effects on GH secretion in this species. The mechanism by which this effect is exerted has not been established.

NEUROPHARMACOLOGIC REGULATION OF GH

Monamines

Each of four biogenic amines, NE, dopamine (DA), serotonin, and epinephrine (Epi) has a distinct and separate stimulatory role in GH regulation in the primate.[44,156,157] Oral administration of L-dopa, the precursor of Epi, NE, and DA, readily crosses the blood-brain barrier and causes release of GH in the human being[34] (Fig. 11). Evidence that the L-dopa effect is mediated at least in part through its conversion to either NE or Epi is

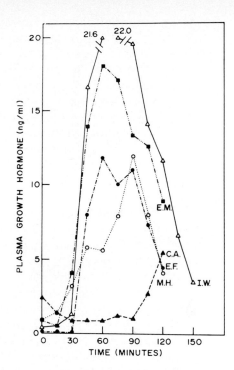

FIGURE 11. Plasma GH response to L-dopa administered orally. The peak of the response occurs 60 to 90 minutes after L-dopa administration. (From Boyd, A,[34] with permission.)

derived from experiments showing that L-dopa-induced GH release is blocked by phentolamine, an α-adrenergic receptor blocking agent.[105] However, subemetic doses of apomorphine, a centrally active, dopamine-receptor-stimulating agent, also release GH;[127] evidently there may be an additional dopaminergic control mechanism independent of conversion to NE.

A role of α-adrenergic receptors in GH control is supported further by the reports that clonidine, a central α_2-adrenergic agonist stimulated GH release in the human being.[128,131,132] Intrahypothalamic infusion of NE is effective in releasing GH in the baboon. Moreover, cerebral intraventricular or hypothalamic injections of systemically ineffective doses of phentolamine, an α-blocker, prevent hypoglycemia-induced GH release in this species. Clonidine is reported to stimulate growth in some growth-retarded children.[190]

Epinephrine may also be important as a GH regulator. Pretreatment of rats with SKF 64139, a drug that inhibits synthesis of Epi, was shown by Terry and colleagues[245] to prevent the characteristic episodic surges of GH in this species. Because the effects of the Epi synthesis inhibitor were reversed by administration of antisomatostatin antiserum, it was concluded that E acted by inhibiting somatostatin release.

Growth hormone release induced by L-dopa and apomorphine is attenuated by prior glucose administration, the glucoreceptor stimulation partially overriding catecholaminergic stimuli for GH release. Dopamine may also act at the pituitary somatotrope level to inhibit GH secretion. This observation, made in short-term cultures of human pituitary glands, may help explain the effectiveness of dopamine agonists in suppression of GH secretion in acromegaly.

Most stimuli that cause GH release appear to act via central α-adrenergic receptors.[64] In the human being, GH release induced by insulin hypoglycemia, arginine, exercise, ADH, L-dopa, and certain stresses are all prevented by phentolamine[152] (Fig. 12). Propranolol, a β-adrenergic blocker, enhances GH release induced by glucagon, ADH, and L-dopa. The β-agonist isoproterenol is reported to inhibit GH release. These studies indicate that GH secretion is facilitated by both dopaminergic and noradrenergic α-receptor stimulation, and it is inhibited by noradrenergic β-receptor stimulation. Pharmacologic blockade of GH release by drugs like chlorpromazine, pimozide, and haloperidol is thought to occur at a hypothalamic level, probably by competitive blockade of dopaminergic receptor sites.

Serotonin also may be involved in GH release in primates. Oral administration of L-tryptophan or 5-hydroxytryptophan (5-HTP) in human beings causes GH release, although the response is not great.[110] The release of GH in response to hypoglycemia is blocked by the serotonin antagonists methysergide and cyproheptadine.[22]

Melatonin is reported both to facilitate GH release and to block release in response to insulin hypoglycemia; these apparently conflicting effects were explained by differences in the time course of melatonin action.[154]

Physiologic GH release, as in sleep, may be regulated by yet another mechanism. Neither α-adrenergic nor β-adrenergic receptor blockade nor dopaminergic blockade affects nocturnal sleep-associated GH release.[158] Blockade of serotonin receptors with methysergide has resulted in an increase in GH release during sleep. Cholinergic mechanisms may be involved in sleep-related GH release.[157]

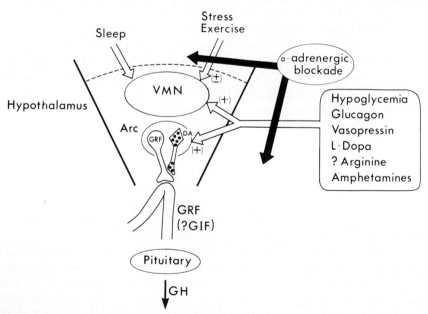

FIGURE 12. Diagram of hypothalamic mechanisms for regulation of GH secretion. α-adrenergic blockade (with phentolamine) partially or completely blocks GH release to the stimuli shown. Sleep-release of GH is not affected. (Modified from Martin, JB.[152])

Acetylcholine

Cholinergic elements also play an important role in GH regulation, especially in humans. Atropine and other muscarinic receptor antagonists inhibit pharmacologically stimulated GH secretion[273] and the response to GHRH.[274] Because ACh does not appear to act directly on the pituitary, it can be postulated that somatostatin secretion is tonically inhibited by hypothalamic cholinergic fibers. Indeed, it has been reported that acetylcholine inhibits somatostatin secretion by rat hypothalamic fragments,[275] although in dispersed fetal cells ACh is stimulatory.[276,277]

> Species seem to differ with respect to GH responses to pharmacologic stimuli. In the rhesus monkey, intravenous clonidine and 5-hydroxytryptophan are potent stimulants for GH release, whereas apomorphine is ineffective except at doses that induce vomiting (and therefore may act as a nonspecific stress effect).[44] In studies by Chambers and Brown,[44] the administration of dihydroxyphenylserine, a precursor of norepinephrine and epinephrine but not dopamine, also was effective in releasing GH. Similarly, in the dog, systemic administration of L-dopa and clonidine released GH, but apomorphine had no effect. These findings suggest that there may be no animal model available that precisely duplicates GH control in man. In the rat, blockade of α-adrenergic receptors is the most effective way to abolish spontaneous, pulsatile GH secretion totally. Inhibitors of dopamine-β-hydroxylase and of serotonin biosynthesis or serotonin receptors are also partially effective. Blockade of dopamine receptors has only a minor effect in the rat.

Experimental studies in the rat have indicated that catecholamines also are involved in the relay of GH release induced by stimulation of extrahypothalamic structures.

> Depletion of central catecholamines by administration of α-methyl-p-tyrosine, an inhibitor of catecholamine synthesis, has no effect on GH release induced by hypothalamic stimulation but prevents GH release after stimulation of the hippocampus or basolateral amygdala.[159] Depletion of serotonin with p-chlorophenylalanine also prevented GH release after amygdaloid stimulation, but did not affect GH release induced by hypothalamic stimulation.[159]
> Electric stimulation studies in the rat described above suggest that dopaminergic, noradrenergic, and serotonergic neurons all are effective in releasing GH.[159] These observations are consistent with a role of both catecholamines and serotonin acting as neurotransmitters in the relay of responses from extrahypothalamic brain regions to tuberoinfundibular neurons.

Amino Acids and Small Peptides

Several amino acids—including arginine, histidine, leucine, phenylalanine, and lysine—bring about the release of GH when injected intravenously or after absorption into the systemic circulation following a large protein-containing meal.

A number of peptides other than the GHRH stimulate GH release under certain well-defined circumstances. Whether any of them is involved in physiologic regulation of GH is not known. The most important are described below.

Thyrotropin-releasing Hormone. Thyrotropin-releasing hormone will release GH from pituitary glands incubated *in vitro*,[67] but it will not stimulate GH in normal individuals.[46] However, TRH stimulates GH release in approximately two thirds of patients with acromegaly.[70] This reaction, considered to be one of the "paradoxic" GH regulatory responses that acromegalic patients manifest, is a useful indicator of the presence of abnormally functioning pituitary tissue.[139] Persistence of TRH-induced GH release postoperatively indicates that adenoma tissue has been left behind. Almost every worker who has described this phenomenon has speculated that TRH responsiveness is due to dedifferentiation of the abnormal somatotrope so that TRH receptors appear on the plasma membrane of the cells. The recent demonstration that acromegaly can occur as the result of excessive ectopic secretion of GHRH has shed new light on this problem. As reported by Thorner and his colleagues,[248] a patient with this syndrome was found to release GH in response to TRH injection; following complete resection of the offending pancreatic tumor and normalization of GH levels, the patient no longer released GH in response to TRH. Several other patients whose acromegaly was due to ectopic GHRH secretion also manifested paradoxical GH responses to TRH. These observations mean that TRH responsiveness can result directly or indirectly from excessive stimulation by GHRH, a response that has been duplicated *in vitro*. However, it has not been shown that TRH responsiveness means that GHRH is being secreted in excess.

Several other pathologic conditions are associated with paradoxical TRH-induced GH release. These include chronic renal failure, anorexia nervosa, and depression. The physiologic basis of the abnormality in these disorders is unknown; the abnormal responsiveness reverts to normal following reversal of the underlying disease.

In several circumstances the administration of TRH is followed by *inhibition* of GH release. The burst of GH secretion that occurs during the first hours of sleep[46] and that induced by arginine and hypoglycemia[47] is blocked by the administration of TRH. It was postulated that in these situations TRH acts at the level of the hypothalamus to cause inhibition of GH release.

Gonadotropin Hormone Releasing Hormone (GnRH). Approximately one third of acromegalic patients (unlike normal subjects) will release GH in response to the administration of GnRH. As with the paradoxical TRH test in this disorder, response to GnRH is indicative of the presence of abnormally functioning tissue even if the basal GH level is only modestly elevated. The mechanism underlying this response is unknown.

Vasopressin. Vasopressin (antidiuretic hormone, ADH) in "pharmacologic" doses releases GH in human being, monkey, and rat. This response in fact is the basis of a test of GH reserve in the human being that is not widely used because vasopressin can induce coronary artery spasm and because the response is inconsistent. Although vasopressin and neurophysin are present in extremely high concentrations in the pituitary-portal blood of surgically stressed monkeys,[269] it can be argued convincingly that vasopressin is not a physiologic GHRH. Rats with hereditary vasopressin deficiency (Brattleboro rats) have normal blood levels of GH and release GH normally after electric stimulation of the VMN.[158] Stimulation of the supraoptic nuclei, which is effective in releasing neurophysin and vasopressin, has no effect on GH release. In the rhesus monkey, vasopressin-induced GH release is blocked by pentobarbital anesthesia, suggesting that this peptide acts indirectly through the hypothalamus.

α-MSH. Several workers have reported that partial or complete amino acid sequences of ACTH release GH in the human being.[158] α-MSH, which consists of an amino acid sequence identical to the first 13 residues of ACTH (with a terminal amide group), causes a rise in GH 30 to 45 minutes after intravenous administration. The physiologic significance of this observation is unknown.

Corticotropin-releasing Hormone (CRH). CRH does not release GH in normals but has been reported to do so in acromegaly[189] and in depressed individuals.[86]

Glucagon. Glucagon releases GH in most normal individuals and has been advocated as a test of GH reserve, especially when combined with a β-blocker such as propranolol, which sensitizes the response.[158] The site of action of glucagon in bringing about this response is unknown. The structural similarities of glucagon and GHRH are described below.

Other Gut-Brain Peptides. A number of peptides present in the hypothalamus can release GH. As summarized by Martin and coworkers,[158] they include met-enkephalin, β-endorphin, substance P, neurotensin, bombesin, vasoactive intestinal peptide (VIP),[45,67] gastrin, and myelin basic protein. None is the authentic GHRH, but each probably acts indirectly through hypophysiotropic neurons.

Endorphins and GH Regulation. Enkephalin, endorphins, and their analogs, including morphine, bring about increase in plasma GH in a number of species, including human beings. It is reasonable, therefore, to consider that central opioid peptidergic pathways may be involved in stress-related GH release. Efforts to establish this relationship in the human being have been surprisingly unrewarding. Conventional or high doses of naloxone (an inhibitor of most central endorphin activities) have little or no effect on basal GH or sleep-associated GH release, hypoglycemia-stimulated GH release, and only modest effects on exercise-induced GH secretion.[225] Growth hormone release brought about by extremely severe physical exertion (80 percent of maximum achieveable workload for 8 minutes) led to GH release that was almost completely blocked by naloxone administration.[174] It would appear, therefore, that only the GH release associated with extreme stress is mediated by an endogenous opioid pathway.

SHORT LOOP FEEDBACK CONTROL

Growth hormone is capable of inhibiting its own secretion (see Figure 1).[1,2] This has been well established in the rat in a number of ways. In older studies, systemic administration of GH, direct intrahypothalamic placement of GH pellets, or subcutaneous implantation of a GH-secreting tumor all were found to decrease pituitary content of GH. More recently, it has been shown that intrahypothalamic and intracerebroventricular injection of GH inhibits GH secretion and blocks the spontaneous surges of GH that are characteristic of this species. The direct exposure of hypothalamic tissue, incubated *in vitro* to GH, brings about the release of somatostatin, thus providing at least one possible mechanism by which GH inhibition could be brought about.[16]

Inasmuch as GH induces formation of somatomedin C in peripheral tissue, it is relevant to ask whether the feedback might be mediated via this hormone-dependent factor. Direct evidence now has been obtained that indicates that somatomedin C can inhibit GH secretion from the pituitary gland, and, when placed into the cerebral ventricles, it can inhibit GH secretion by stimulating somatostatin secretion.[1,16,240] Intraventricular administration of GH also inhibits GH secretion, presumably by enhancing somatostatin release, an effect that has been observed directly *in vitro*.[16] Laron-type dwarfs, who lack normal peripheral-tissue production of somatomedin, have strikingly elevated levels of GH, consistent with a failure in normal feedback regulation.[130] Similarly, the high GH levels of kwashiorkor are associated with low plasma somatomedin.

Experiments in rats infested with the tapeworm *Spirometra mansonoides* have provided further evidence for a short-loop feedback control of GH, mediated by somatomedin.[188] This tapeworm produces a substance(s) that is not immunoreactive in GH assays but that does compete with GH in radioreceptor assays and is capable of stimulating somatomedin production. Infestation with the worm leads to depletion of radioimmunoassayable GH in the pituitary gland, indicating a feedback effect either via the tapeworm substance or via somatomedin.

Efforts to demonstrate GH feedback in human beings and other primates have not been as convincing as those in the rat. Elevation of serum GH levels by exercise in human beings prevented a further rise in response to arginine, but several alternative explanations can be proposed to explain this finding. Prior administration of GH to human beings and monkeys partially blocked GH release induced by arginine or by hypoglycemia.[2] However, studies by Spiler and Molitch[225] have been unable to demonstrate any effects of prior GH administration on either exercise or hypoglycemia-induced GH release. These results may relate in part to the fact that an acute stimulation of GH secretion, induced by any means, is followed by a refractory period, lasting minutes to hours, when a second stimulus is less effective in eliciting GH secretion.

HYPOPHYSIOTROPIC HORMONES INVOLVED IN GH SECRETION

Growth Hormone-releasing Hormone (GHRH)

Despite compelling evidence derived from studies of the effects of hypothalamic lesions, of hypothalamic electrical stimulation, and of hypothalamic extracts on GH secretion that a GHRH must exist, attempts to isolate and chemically to identify such a factor from the hypothalamus were frustrated for many years.[199] The earliest experiments suffered from the insensitivity and lack of specificity of available bioassays, but even with better assays, research was slowed by the exceedingly small amount of biologically active material that was found in hypothalamic extracts. The early history of efforts to isolate GHRH have been reviewed in several publications.[149,154,197-199,246]

The precise nature of *hypothalamic* GHRH finally was elucidated by studies of a GHRH-like material isolated from human pancreatic tumors that caused acromegaly. This is the first example of the structure of a hypophysiotropic hormone having been suggested by isolation of a peptide responsible for a paraneoplastic syndrome and as such is an elegant example of clinical investigation with a fascinating bit of medical history.

The idea that tumor-derived substances can stimulate excessive GH secretion by the pituitary gland emerged over the past decade with the reports of more than a dozen patients who presented with acromegaly and a carcinoid, or pancreatic adenoma. Frohman and his collaborators[78] partially purified extracts of such tumors, showed that they contained specific GH-releasing activity, and provided evidence that the activity was peptide-like in nature. Subsequently, Thorner and his colleagues[246,248] observed a patient who manifested symptoms and signs of acromegaly who was found to have hyperplasia of the somatotrope cells and clinical findings of pituitary tumor by skull x-ray examination. Ultimately, the patient was shown to have a large pancreatic tumor, removal of which cured the GH hypersecretion after partial hypophysectomy had been ineffective. From the pancreatic tumor Rivier and collaborators[203] isolated an exceedingly potent GH-releasing substance which was sequenced and synthesized by chemical means. Working independently and simultaneously, Guillemin and his collaborators[100,101,144] isolated a GH-releasing peptide from another patient with acromegaly who had two pancreatic tumors and a nontumorous pituitary gland. The structure of the peptide isolated by Rivier and colleagues[203] is that of a 40-amino-acid-containing linear peptide (see Figure 10, chapter 2). The structure of the peptide isolated by Guillemin and colleagues is 44 amino acids long (see Figure 10, chapter 2); the first 40 amino acids are identical with the Rivier peptide. Guillemin also identified smaller amounts of the 40 amino acid material in the tumor extract from his patient and from Thorner's patient. The "Guillemin peptide" possesses a terminal amide group, whereas the "Rivier peptide" does not. Rat GHRH has also been characterized.[224]

The active peptide was given the name human pancreatic growth hormone releasing factor (hpGRF). Guillemin proposed to replace the acronym GRF by the name *somatocrinin,* from the Greek *somato,* abbreviated from somatotropin, a trivial name for GH, and *crinin,* meaning to secrete. Somatocrinin would thus be the terminologic counterpart of somatostatin.[97,100,101]

It remains to be established whether the difference in structure between the two peptides found in pancreatic tumor is the result of degradation of the peptide or reflects a difference in posttranslational processing by the tumor cells. Human hypothalamic hormone is identical with pancreatic GHRH. The molecular sequences of the preprohormone of both human and rat GHRH have been elucidated;[96,162] they differ substantially in amino acid structure but are equally potent in releasing GH.

Tissue extracts of the tumor GHRH reported by Guillemin and others

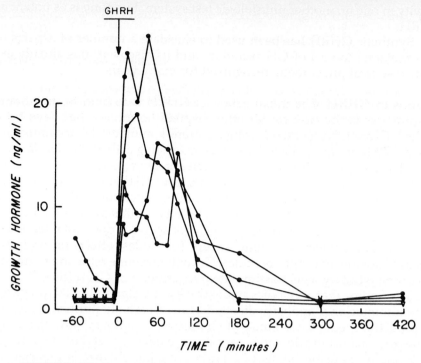

EFFECT OF GHRH ON GH SECRETION IN NORMAL ADULTS

FIGURE 14. Stimulation of GH secretion in six adult men by hpGRF (1-40)-OH. (From Thorner, et al,[246] with permission.)

between excitatory and inhibitory factors. The claims of Krulich and collaborators were not widely accepted when first introduced, largely because there appeared to be no rationale for the existence of a GH inhibitory factor, and because inhibitory effects in the assay system used could be attributed to nonspecific toxic effects. Brazeau and collaborators[35] later rediscovered growth hormone inhibiting factor in ovine hypothalamic tissue, isolated it, identified it chemically, and finally achieved its total chemical synthesis (see Fig. 11, chapter 2). Their work was facilitated by the development of a sensitive bioassay system that utilized pituitary cell cultures and by a highly sophisticated approach to peptide analysis and synthesis that had grown out of earlier work on the isolation of TRH and GnRH. They applied the term *somatostatin* to the new peptide. Since its discovery in 1973, a tremendous amount of investigation has led to new insights into understanding the mechanism of regulation of the pituitary gland and, unexpectedly, into the function of several other secretory systems, including the islets of the pancreas and the gastrin-producing cells of the stomach.

A number of molecular forms of somatostatin are found in tissues.

Subsequent work has considerably expanded the initially simple concept of somatostatin as a tetradecapeptide (14-amino-acid-containing peptide) primarily involved in the regulation of GH secretion. Somatostatin-like peptides are now seen to constitute a family of related molecules, including the originally identified somatostatin (designated somatostatin 14), amino-terminal extended somatostatin (so-

REGULATION OF THE PITUITARY GLAND

matostatin 28), and still larger forms, which range in molecular weight according to location and species from 11.5 to 15.7 K daltons.[15,200,202] In addition, a number of fragments of the prohormone can be found in tissue including a peptide corresponding to the first 12 amino acids of somatostatin 28 (somatostatin 28$_{(1-12)}$) and still others.[15,278] When the larger forms of somatostatin were first recognized, it was reasonable to consider them to be prohormones, but more recent studies have shown that under some circumstances somatostatin 28 and even the larger forms can be secreted as such and possess biologic activity, suggesting that these larger forms can constitute both prohormone and hormone. All mammalian and most submammalian somatostatin-like molecules include a sequence identical to the originally described tetradecapeptide, but in at least one lower animal, the catfish, relatively large differences in sequence have been detected, and recombinant DNA studies show the existence of a number of different genes coding for somatostatin.[91,173] The original name, somatostatin, is therefore somewhat inappropriate, because this compound is distributed widely in cells throughout the nervous system and in many extraneural tissues where it exerts effects on a broad range of structures, including neurons, epithelia, endocrine and exocrine glands.

Important further steps in somatostatin research were the findings that the peptide inhibited TSH release and pancreatic secretion of insulin and glucagon (Fig. 15). When immunohistochemical study established the presence of somatostatin in a subpopulation of pancreatic islet cells (D cells), it became evident that this peptide might exert paracrine secretory control on the pancreas (see below). This paracrine model was then extended to the control of gastrointestinal (GI) secretions when it was established that somatostatin was present in both epithelial and neural elements

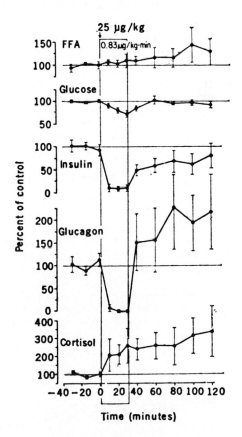

FIGURE 15. Effects of somatostatin on plasma-free fatty acids (FFA), glucose, insulin, glucagon, and cortisol. Somatostatin causes immediate suppression of insulin and glucose, which is followed by a decline in glucose. (From Koerker, DJ, et al: *Somatostatin: Hypothalamic inhibitor of the endocrine pancreas.* Science 184:482, 1974, with permission.)

in the gut and that it suppressed most gut secretions. Finally, the demonstration of the presence of somatostatin in many nerve cells throughout the brain even in areas unrelated to pituitary regulation,[5,68,73,108,180] and the demonstration of its effect on neuronal function have suggested for somatostatin a role in nervous system function of considerable importance. In a word, somatostatin is a quintessential gut-brain peptide. The extra-hypothalamic functions are considered in chapter 18.

Actions of GHRH and Somatostatin on Pituitary GH Release. Somatostatin exerts potent inhibitory actions on GH secretion, both *in vitro* and *in vivo*, in all species of animals in which it has been used, including rat, baboon, dog, sheep, and the human being. It is effective regardless of the stimulus used to induce secretion. For example, in the human being, somatostatin blocks the GH secretory response to insulin-induced hypoglycemia, arginine infusion, L-dopa ingestion, and that associated with sleep. It effectively lowers GH plasma levels in most acromegalic patients.[19] Somatostatin also has been demonstrated to have a role in the suppression of GH that occurs between the physiologic surges of secretion.

The physiologic relevance of somatostatin secretion for GH regulation also has been demonstrated in other ways. Lesions of the somatostatinergic tuberoinfundibular tract lead to depletion of median eminence somatostatin and to increased basal levels of GH (and of TSH).[53,68] Contrariwise, electric stimulation of the anterior periventricular area in the rat corresponding to the cells of origin of the principal hypothalamic-median eminence projection leads to inhibition of GH secretion and, appropriately, to increased release of somatostatin into the hypophysial-portal vessels.[158] That somatostatin is involved in regulation of GH release under normal circumstances is shown in studies in which endogenous somatostatin is neutralized by administration of antisera to the peptide. Acute release of GH[158,244] and reversal in the rat of the characteristic inhibition of GH release caused by physical stress[8] and by starvation[239] are observed.

> Somatostatin secretion also appears to be at least one of the factors mediating short-loop feedback control of GH secretion. GH deficiency (as produced by hypophysectomy) leads to decrease in somatostatin content of the median eminence, a change reversed by GH administration. Exposure of the hypothalamus to GH, either by addition to incubated hypothalamic blocks or via intracerebroventricular injection, brings about somatostatin release, an effect mirrored in the suppression of GH release that follows intraventricular GH injection. Growth hormone may be effective in somatostatin regulation in two different ways, the first as a direct regulator, as outlined above, and the second through somatomedin C, the mediator of GH effects on the musculoskeletal system. Exposure *in vivo* of hypothalamic blocks to somatomedin C (the mediator of GH stimulation) brought about somatostatin release; intraventricular injection of somatomedin C in the rat inhibited GH secretion. Intraventricular injection of somatostatin elevates GH release, an effect possibly explained by the suppression of endogenous somatostatin.

Extensive studies have been carried out in an attempt to elucidate the role of altered hypothalamic somatostatin secretion as the mediator of the effects on GH release of neurotransmitters and neuropeptides. These are summarized by Martin and coworkers and Reichlin.[157,158,201]

Somatostatin Receptors. The action of somatostatin is initiated by binding to a specific cell membrane receptor. Somatostatin-binding receptors have been identified by competitive binding assays in rat pituitary cells, in plasma membranes isolated from bovine pituitaries, in whole brain synaptosome membranes, and in isolated rat islet cells.[201]

> According to Schönbrunn and Tashjian, rat pituitary tumor cells (GH$_4$ C$_1$ strain) have a single class of high affinity binding sites (K$_d$ = 6 × 10^{10} M at 37°C), and a maximum binding capacity of 13,000 receptor sites per cell [see Martin and others[158] for review]. Membranes derived from rat cerebral cortex show two types of somatostatin receptors, one with a single high affinity site and the second of low affinity. Cell function modulation by alteration in somatostatin receptor population is emerging as a possible mode of cell control. Schönbrunn and Tashjian have shown that exposure of rat pituitary tumor cells to TRH acutely increases the number, but not the affinity, of somatostatin receptors. Exposure to cortisol also causes a decrease in somatostatin receptor numbers but by different mechanisms. Glucose concentration was shown by Mehler and colleagues to regulate the number of somatostatin receptors on islet cells. These workers postulated that the change is due to the appearance on the cell membrane of a larger number of secretory vesicles which they have previously shown to have a higher affinity than the membranes themselves.

In detailed analysis of structure–function relationships, Srikant and Patel[227-230] find that pituitary somatostatin receptors as compared with brain receptors behave differently toward several analogs, from which they have inferred that there may be more than one class of somatostatin receptors.

Action of Somatostatin. Efforts to define a general mechanism to explain the action of somatostatin on a wide variety of cell types have only partially been successful (see Gerich[82] and Schönbrunn et al[279] for review).

In pituitary cells somatostatin exerts prompt and striking inhibition of secretion of GH and TSH; in pancreas somatostatin inhibits insulin and glucagon. Although the concentration of 3',5'-cyclic AMP (cAMP) is reduced in both the pituitary gland and pancreas by exposure to somatostatin, the stimulatory effects on hormone secretion of cAMP or of agents which increase intracellular concentration of cAMP also are reduced by somatostatin. It has been concluded, therefore, that somatostatin acts "downstream" from cAMP to inhibit secretion.

> Somatostatin reduces membrane permeability to calcium, and the inhibitory actions of somatostatin on hormone release are partially or completely reversed by exposure to A23187, an ionophore that opens calcium channels in both the external membrane and membranes of intracellular organelles. These findings generally have been interpreted to mean that somatostatin acts to block calcium-mediated intracellular activation.[20]
>
> Pace and Tarvin have provided even more insight into the way that somatostatin may act to inhibit islet cell function (see Reichlin[210] for review). The crucial new finding in their work is that somatostatin, in addition to inhibiting Ca^{++} uptake by islet cells, also increases the permeability of cells to K$^+$ (as inferred from ^{86}rubidium washout). Since chemical agents which interfere with outward K$^+$ flux from islet cells (quinine and tetraethylammonium) block somatostatin effects on both insulin secretory response and the electrophysiological effects of high glucose on islet cells, these workers postulate that SRIF may activate P$_k$ as its primary mode of action, an

event that may be sufficient to reduce the accumulation of intracellular Ca^{++} thereby disrupting glucose-induced stimulus-secretion coupling.

Schönbrunn and colleagues[279] suggest that "the S-14 receptor is coupled to the guanine nucleotide binding protein, N_1, and that a functional N_1 is necessary for S-14 to elicit its biological effects." N_1 can exert effects both through cyclic AMP generation, and by reduction of intracellular calcium by an effect on calcium channels.

Degradation of Somatostatin. Elucidation of the mechanisms of enzyme degradation of somatostatin is relevant to understanding the role of local inactivation in control of activity of the peptide and to the development of longer-acting analogs resistant to proteolysis. This topic has been summarized by Reichlin.[201] Somatostatin is quickly broken down by both soluble and particulate fractions of tissue and by plasma. In plasma an active metabolite is formed.

> Enzymes responsible for this effect are endopeptidases, including cathepsin M and lysosomal cathepsin D. The latter enzyme from brain attacks the -Phe-Phe-bond in position 6-7. Digestion also takes place, but more slowly at the Try-Lys-bond, and this region of vulnerability can be modified by substituting D-Trp in position 8, a change which makes the molecule longer acting and increases its biologic potency. Activity of both cathepsin D and pepsin are blocked by pepstatin. Regulation of hepatic degradation of somatostatin has been studied by Conlon and others (see Reichlin[201]). Somatostatin degradation in blood is reduced by high concentrations of EDTA and aprotinin. That aprotinin is active suggests that plasmin-like activity is responsible for plasma breakdown, but the fact that this agent is not sufficient to block all degradation indicates that other enzymes are involved. Brain-degrading activity is present in both particulate and supernatant fractions of all regions of brain, although the activity is greatest in the supernatant fraction. There is little difference in total activity in various regions of the brain, but that in the cerebellum is the greatest, and that of the hypothalamus is the least of regions studied.

As in the case of other degrading systems found at the site of somatostatin action, little is known about factors regulating its breakdown.

Somatostatin Analogs. Extensive efforts to synthesize analogs that possess clinically advantageous properties have been made. These include peptides that are longer acting, effective by mouth, and relatively selective for one or other of the target tissues, namely, pituitary gland, pancreatic islet cells, and gastrointestinal tract. None so far has met all these critera, but several are already sufficiently useful that they have made their way into clinical trials.

The principles that have been used by pharmacologists in developing analogs have been to define the sites of enzymatic cleavage, to introduce resistant peptide bonds (for example, using D amino acids), and to define the essential conformational requirements for binding and biologic effect. The chemical processes involved in this approach have been described.[178,258,280,281]

Two synthetic peptides so designed have recently been introduced into clinical investigation. Both are smaller than the parent peptide, contain D-tryptophan, and include a ring structure that duplicates the normal β-turn in the peptide. One of these compounds, the octapeptide SMS 201-995 (Fig. 16), given in a dose of 50 μg s.c., lowered serum GH in 6 of 7

H–(D-Phe)–Cys–Phe–(D-Trp)–Lys–Thr–Cys–Throl, acetate

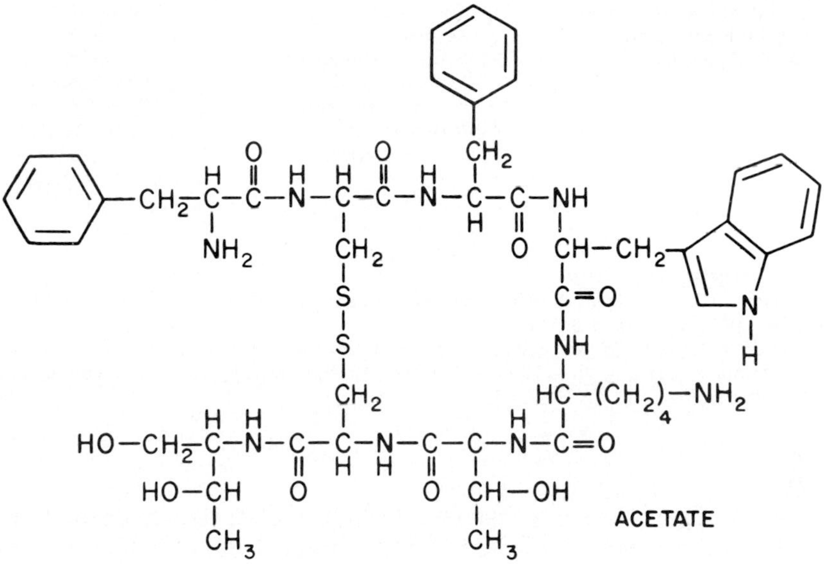

FIGURE 16. Structure of somatostatin analog SMS 201-995.

acromegalics into the normal range with only minimal effects on carbohy-drate-regulating hormones.[192] The same agent has been used to treat a patient with the syndrome of ectopic GHRH secretion owing to metastatic tumor in whom plasma levels of both GHRH and GH were brought into the normal range, indicating an inhibitory effect on both pituitary gland and tumor. Inhibition of diarrhea in pancreatic cholera (VIPoma)[161] and post-ileostomy has also been reported. SMS 201-995 has been used successfully to treat carcinoid flushing.[126] Summarizing progress reports in clinical use of somatostatin and analogs have been published.[29,178,183,195,202,258,281]

DISORDERS OF GROWTH HORMONE SECRETION

GROWTH HORMONE DEFICIENCY

Factors that inhibit GH secretion are presented in Table 2. In childhood, severe GH deficiency leads to dwarfism; lesser degrees of deficiency cause some degree of growth failure. In addition, skeletal maturation is delayed, and loss of the antiinsulin properties of GH may lead to hypoglycemia, especially in the fasting state or if there is an associated deficiency of adrenal cortical function. Decreased basal levels of GH may accompany any hypothalamic-pituitary lesion. Growth hormone secretion is very vul-nerable to hypothalamic-pituitary disease and is one of the earliest pitui-tary functions to be lost in disease of this region. Neuroendocrine reflexes for GH release may be lost in patients with widely differing intracranial

TABLE 2. Factors that Inhibit Growth Hormone Secretion in Primates*

Physiologic	Pharmacologic	Pathologic
1. Postprandial hyperglycemia	1. Somatostatin	1. Acromegaly
2. Elevated free fatty acids	2. Melatonin	a. Levodopa
3. Elevated GH levels	3. Serotonin antagonists	b. Apomorphine
	a. Methysergide	c. Phentolamine
	b. Cyproheptadine	d. Bromocriptine
	4. Phentolamine	2. Hyperthyroidism
	5. Chlorpromazine	3. Hypothyroidism
	6. Morphine	4. Hypothalamic lesions
	7. Cosyntropin	5. Pituitary lesions
	8. Progesterone	
	9. Theophylline	

*In many instances, the inhibition can be demonstrated only as a suppression of GH release induced by a pharmacologic stimulus.

Modified from Martin JB, Brazeau P, Tannenbaum GS, et al. Neuroendocrine organization of growth hormone regulation. In: Reichlin S, Baldessarini RJ, Martin JB, eds. The Hypothalamus. New York: Raven Press, 1978: 329–357.

disorders, and such loss may be an early sign of disturbance of the hypo-thalamic-pituitary axis. For example, following cranial radiation, GH hyposecretion is the first and often the only pituitary deficit.[23,95,206]

Growth failure due to GH deficiency may be apparent as early as 6 months, but it usually is not diagnosed until age 1 to 3 years, when the child is observed to fall behind his or her peers in body size. Growth failure is commonly defined as a growth rate less than 4.5 cm per year. Etiologic causes of GH deficiency are summarized in a comprehensive review.[282]

Organic Lesions of Pituitary or Hypothalamus

Virtually any destructive lesion of the hypothalamus or pituitary gland can bring about GH deficiency (see chapters 11, 13). One characteristic lesion of the hypothalamus that commonly involves GH secretion is the disorder septo-optic dysplasia (de Morsier's syndrome), a disorder in which varying degrees of defects in midline fusion are expressed, including absence of the septum pellucidum, and the iris, and an abnormal third ventricle and lamina terminalis.[232] In one series of six patients, all had GH deficiency, and four of the six had more than one pituitary disturbance, all presumably caused by defects of hypothalamic hypophysiotropic hormones.

Idiopathic Hypopituitarism

Complete hypopituitarism (panhypopituitarism) or partial hypopituitarism may occur in either a sporadic or a familial form. The response to TRH and GnRH in such patients with secondary hypopthyroidism or hypogonadotropism has indicated that the pituitary gland is responsive to these hypothalamic hormones. A subset of such GH-deficient children responds to GHRH. About 50 percent of hypopituitary children with GH deficiency show a response to a single dose of GHRH, but the responses are subnormal.[215] However, the finding of any response to GHRH, when no responses were present after other stimuli (hypoglycemia, arginine infusion, or L-dopa), indicates that endogenous GHRH deficiency probably is the cause of the growth failure in such children. One case has been examined at autopsy (Martin, unpublished). Hypothalamic structures appeared normal, but GHRH cell bodies, although present, when stained by immunocytochemistry were greatly reduced in numbers and less widely distributed in the medial basal hypothalamus. Autopsy studies in cases of pituitary dwarfism have shown biochemical and morphologic evidence for GH within pituitary somatotropes.

These studies provide convincing evidence that the disorder in many patients with idiopathic hypopituitarism is in hypophysiotropic hormone synthesis or release, occurring in either a multiple or monotropic form. Growth hormone deficiency, whether occurring in a sporadic or a familial form, is not usually recognized until early childhood. Rare cases are reported of GH deficiency associated with abnormalities of the structure of GH.[256]

Laron Dwarfism. A form of dwarfism associated with high levels of circulating GH was first described by Laron and colleagues.[130] The GH in the pituitary gland and plasma of such patients is immunologically, biochemically, and biologically indistinguishable from that of normal subjects, and they fail to grow when given exogenous GH.[55,56,87] Somatomedin levels are reduced in the Laron dwarf;[56] hepatic GH receptors may be defective. This interesting pathophysiologic disorder provides indirect evidence for a negative-feedback regulation of GH, involving somatomedin C (see above). Deficiency of somatomedin C leads to excessive GH secretion, which is ineffective in producing normal growth. There is no currently available treatment for these patients. Administration of purified or synthetic somatomedin might provide an effective treatment, but this is not available at this time, although somatomedin production by recombinant DNA techniques is within the realm of possibility.

Dwarfism in Pygmies. Merimee and coworkers[166] showed that IGF I levels are reduced in pygmies, whereas IGF II levels are normal. Defects in the carrier protein or in liver receptors have been postulated.

Maternal Deprivation Syndrome (Psychosocial Deprivation Syndrome). Many reports have documented impairment of GH secretion apparently due to emotional factors.[93,172,193] This disorder, which occurs in children, is characterized by growth failure in the context of severe emotional deprivation. These children have deficient GH release in response to stimuli such as insulin-induced hypoglycemia or arginine infusion and, in a smaller proportion, deficiency in release of ACTH and gonadotropins. This disorder is rapidly reversed by placing a child in a supportive hospital milieu; growth and GH neuroendocrine responses return rapidly. Excessive β-adrenergic inhibitory effects may be one of the causative factors in the syndrome. In one such patient, normal GH secretion could be restored immediately by acute treatment with propranolol. If confirmed, this observation has important implications in the understanding of the physiologic significance of adrenergic systems in the control of GH secretion. It is important in each individual case to exclude malnutrition as a causative or contributory factor to the GH deficiency.

Manifestations of GH Hyposecretion in the Adult. In the adult, a deficiency of GH does not produce readily recognizable clinical symptoms or signs. Whether decreased GH deficiency over many years has deleterious metabolic effects in the aging person is of considerable theoretic interest and is currently undergoing clinical investigation.

HYPERSECRETION OF GH

GIGANTISM AND ACROMEGALY

Hypersecretion of GH occurring *before* closure of the epiphyses results in gigantism, and *after* closure of the epiphyses, acromegaly.[115,116,163,171] Growth hormone levels may be above the normal range, unaccompanied by clinical signs of hypersomatotropism in a number of other conditions, many of which appear in the context of metabolic disturbance.

Pathophysiology

It has long been recognized that excessive GH secretion by a pituitary tumor is the cause of acromegaly and gigantism in the majority of cases.[155,163] In cases with normal pituitary fossae on roentgenography, evidence obtained by careful neuropathologic study of tissue removed at transsphenoidal surgery indicates that almost all harbor an adenoma, in some instances only a few millimeters in size. Although the tinctorial properties of the GH-secreting adenomas classically have been viewed as acidophilic, many are chromophobic by conventional stains.[163] Growth hormone hypersecretion as determined by blood hormone measurements and GH staining in the adenoma are highly correlated regardless of the tumor's conventional tinctorial properties.[163] Only three of eight cases in one series had eosinophilic-staining cells, but all stained with the antibody technique. Cell characteristics of GH-secreting tumors are summarized in chapter 12. The major exception to the rule that hypersomatotropinism is due to adenomas is the syndrome of acromegaly owing to ectopic GHRH production. The tumors reported to cause this syndrome have been reviewed.[283] In 10 cases, 6 were carcinoids (bronchial and intestinal) 2 pancreatic adenomas, 1 small cell carcinoma of the lung, and 1 adrenal adenoma. They emphasize that most of the cases had somatotrope hyperplasia, but several had pituitary tumors. The ectopic GHRH secreting tumors usually express more than 1 neuropeptide. Rarely, acromegaly may be caused by a hypothalamic gangliocytoma, which apparently secretes GHRH.[12] Six such cases now have been reported. Acromegaly also may be due to pituitary hyperplasia in polyostotic fibrous dysplasia[123,204] or rarely to ectopic secretion of GH by a tumor.[164,286]

The diagnosis of acromegaly (or gigantism before epiphyseal closure) is based upon the clinical features of the disease and the documentation of persistent elevation of GH levels above 5 ng/ml, accompanied by failure of GH to suppress normally after administration of glucose. In addition, in about 80 percent of cases of acromegaly, there is a paradoxical inhibition of GH secretion after administration of dopamine receptor agonists such as L-dopa, apomorphine, or bromocriptine. Between 50 and 70 percent of patients also demonstrate paradoxical stimulation of GH secretion after administration of TRH. Most GH-secreting tumors respond to injections of GHRH, but some are unresponsive. Variability in response is sufficient to make the GHRH response a relatively poor tool in differential diagnosis. X-ray therapy may blunt the response to GHRH, even in cases with elevated basal levels.

Early diagnosis of GH hypersecretion is occasionally made in the absence of any radiologic evidence of a pituitary adenoma. On the basis of such cases and the observed paradoxical pharmacologic responses, it has been postulated that acromegaly may be of hypothalamic origin. This is certainly true for cases of gangliocytoma of the hypothalamus, but in a survey of 177 patients with acromegaly, only one had elevated blood levels of GHRH.[247] Most cases thus appear to arise from autonomous pituitary adenomas (for discussion of pathogenesis, see chapter 12).

The paradoxical responses in GH secretion (suppression by dopamine and stimulation by TRH) that occur in acromegaly can be explained by the direct effects of these drugs on cells of the pituitary tumor. Clinical evidence in support of this has been documented in several studies performed before and after pituitary surgery. Growth hormone secretory dynamics return to normal after successful removal of the adenoma.[109] *In vitro* studies of pituitary tumor tissue removed at transsphenoidal surgery indicate that both dopamine and bromocriptine inhibit GH secretion and that TRH is stimulatory.[3] These studies provide convincing evidence that GH-producing adenoma cells respond directly to these agents. Presumably, the effects are mediated via cell surface receptors.

These secretory responses are similar to those that occur in the normal lactotrope. Moreover, approximately 10 to 15 percent of patients with acromegaly have elevated PRL levels, which in many cases is due to concomitant hypersecretion of PRL by the tumor. In the majority of examined cases, it appears that the two hormones are produced in separate cells rather than in the same cell, although a few tumors containing cells secreting both GH and PRL have been reported (see chapter 7). The tendency for these two tumor cell types to occur together in the same adenoma suggests a possible common pathophysiologic process. One possibility is that both PRL- and GH-secreting cells arise from a common precursor stem cell and that adenomas represent a dedifferentiation to a common cell type. In the case of the GH-secreting tumor, changes in membrane receptor characteristics occur as part of the adenomatous dedifferentiation to give rise to cellular responses similar to those in the normal PRL-secreting cell. Furthermore, in experimental pituitary tumors, it has been shown that treatment of the rat with estrogens in high dosage induces GH-secreting tumors that also secrete large amounts of PRL. In these animals, the primary lesion does in fact appear to lie in the pituitary gland, although an effect of estrogens on hypophysiotropic hormone secretion cannot be excluded.

> Experimental studies of cloned rat pituitary tumor cells (GH_3, GH_4) have provided direct evidence for the coproduction of GH and PRL in the same cell. Like normal PRL cells, they bear TRH receptors. They also have somatostatin receptors.

The clinical and experimental findings, taken together with the many similarities in the molecular sequence and biologic effects of PRL and GH, provide strong evidence for a close relationship between prolactinotrope and somatotrope cells.

The delineation of the syndrome of ectopic GHRH as a cause of acromegaly has modified our interpretation of the TRH and L-dopa tests in acromegaly. Acromegaly due to ectopic GHRH shows paradoxical responses to both TRH and L-dopa, and these revert to normal when the offending pancreatic islet cell tumor is removed. This finding means that paradoxical responses can arise secondary to excessive GHRH, and that paradoxical responses *alone* do not prove that in any given case the disease arises in the pituitary gland as a primary disorder.

Specific GHRH radioimmunoassays now have been developed. The incidence of elevated GHRH levels as a cause of acromegaly appears to be very low (0.5 percent).[247] Until such tests are more widely available, we believe that it is reasonable to do computerized axial tomography (CAT) scans of the chest and pancreas to exclude the rare cases of ectopic GHRH syndrome. It must be recognized that *small* islet cell adenomas, such as those causing insulinoma, are identifiable by CAT scanning or ultrasound examination in only half of cases, so conceivably one could not exclude all cases of ectopic GHRH secretion by CAT scanning. Neuroendocrine tumors of carcinoid or pancreatic adenoma display GHRH immunoreactivity in about 18 percent of cases.[11,52,58,59] However, this high incidence is not associated with clinical acromegalic changes.

ELEVATED GROWTH HORMONE LEVELS UNRELATED TO ACROMEGALY

Increased basal GH levels now have been described in several conditions in addition to acromegaly which have in common a disturbance in nutrition. Thus, elevations in GH have been reported in anorexia nervosa, starvation, kwashiorkor, renal failure, mucoviscidosis, and hepatic cirrhosis. The most likely mechanism of this effect is a secondary deficiency of somatomedin C (postulated to be the functional link between GH and feedback control).

Anorexia Nervosa

In a significant percentage of cases of anorexia nervosa, GH levels are markedly elevated.[79] The elevation in GH correlates closely with the degree of malnutrition. Growth hormone elevation is related directly to deficient caloric intake. Refeeding rapidly leads to normalization of plasma GH levels and GH responses. The disturbance in GH is distinct from the alteration in menstrual function. The gonadotropin deficiency is more closely related to reduction in body weight and usually is reversed only after increase in body weight occurs (see chapter 9). The possibility has not been excluded, however, that the disorder in food intake might be due in part to abnormalities in adrenergic control of appetite mechanisms. Concurrent anomalies of adrenergic control of GH might also be present.

Paradoxical Release

In many clinical conditions associated with GH hypersecretion, the responses of GH to provocative stimuli are, on occasion, paradoxical. Thus there is rise, rather than the expected fall, in plasma GH levels after glucose administration, or suppression after administration of dopaminergic agents. Such paradoxical responses occur normally in the neonatal period. It is commonly noted in acromegaly (see above) and occurred in a child with an optic glioma. Paradoxical GH responses to glucose also have been described in renal failure, breast carcinoma, anorexia nervosa, and Turner's syndrome. Paradoxical responses in Huntington's chorea, Wilson's disease, and acute intermittent porphyria suggest that neuroendocrine abnormalities may exist in such cases. The mechanism of these effects is unknown.

Hypersecretion in Diabetes Mellitus

A majority of patients with diabetes show hyperresponsiveness of GH release to stimuli such as exercise, and this response is blocked by phentolamine, an α-adrenergic blocker. Careful clinical control of the diabetic patient reduces this excesive GH responsivity. Further characterization of this anomaly might be important, inasmuch as GH has been implicated (although a role for it is not proven) in the vascular complications arising in diabetes. Hypophysectomy has been carried out in diabetic patients to treat proliferative retinopathy.

Non-GH-related Growth Disturbances

A number of clinical instances have been described in which a normal or exaggerated growth pattern occurs in the absence of elevated radioimmunoassayable GH levels. Intrauterine and early prenatal growth do not require GH. Cerebral gigantism — a condition associated with an increased growth rate in early childhood, mental retardation, and cerebral ventricular dilatation — is not accompanied by measurable elevation in plasma GH levels. Studies to determine whether the total 24-hour secretion of GH may be elevated in such cases have not yet been reported. A similarly perplexing group of disorders are the postoperative hypothalamic or pituitary tumor cases which often show remarkable "catch-up" growth in the absence of measurable GH in plasma. In a group of patients displaying "catch-up" following removal of a craniopharyngioma, Bucher and colleagues[43] showed a close correlation with high insulin levels. They postulate that obesity-induced hyperinsulinism is responsible for increased growth *in the absence* of detectable levels of GH.

Abnormalities of Nocturnal Release

Growth hormone release during the first 90 minutes of nocturnal sleep is sufficiently reproducible in normal subjects to be useful as a physiologic test for pituitary GH reserve. A number of conditions have now been described in which such release is absent or diminished. Elevation of GH levels, either endogenously as in acromegaly or following exogenous GH administration, prevents nocturnal GH release. Cushing's disease (bilateral adrenal hyperplasia) or chronic steroid administration also is reported to block sleep-related GH secretion, whereas acute steroid administration has little effect. The disturbance in Cushing's disease may persist for months following effective treatment of adrenal cortical hypersecretion. The recovery of nocturnal GH responses appears to precede the return of GH release in response to other provocative stimuli. Other metabolic factors that suppress nocturnal GH release include elevated plasma-free fatty acid levels and obesity.

Slow-wave-sleep-related GH release is abnormal in several central nervous system disorders. Blindness, whether congenital or acquired, is associated with lack of nocturnal GH responses in some subjects, a disturbance that was found to correlate with the decrease in percentage of time spent in the third and fourth stages of sleep. Individuals with narcolepsy, who have a sleep disorder typified by direct transition from waking to REM sleep without an intervening period of SWS, have been noted in a single report to lack GH release during sleep (see above).

Pharmacologic blockade of SWS-related GH release has been reported after administration of both imipramine, a tricyclic antidepressant that blocks postsynaptic uptake of both norepinephrine and serotonin, and medroxyprogesterone. The site of action of the latter is unknown.

Effects of Corticosteroids on GH Secretion

Anti-inflammatory doses of glucocorticoids, as used in the treatment of asthma and rheumatoid arthritis, lead to impaired growth in children, owing mainly to direct catabolic effects on bone matrix. However, GH secretion is also moderately or markedly suppressed as well. Inasmuch as GHRH effects on the pituitary release of GH are actually enhanced by glucocorticoids,[260] it is probable that the steroids act on the hypothalamus to suppress GHRH. As a practical matter it is important to know that steroid-induced growth failure occurs even when the associated GH hyposecretion is reversed by GH treatment.

TESTS OF GH SECRETION

Normal patterns of secretion must be considered in diagnosis. Basal serum levels of GH (in the early morning, at rest) rarely exceed 5 ng/ml and are usually less than 1 ng/ml in normal subjects. Spontaneous bursts of GH release may occur at any time and can result in values as high as 20 to 30 ng/ml. Plasma levels of GH are elevated (over 10 ng/ml) in infants during the first few weeks of life, with values as high as 30 to 50 ng/ml. During the early part of nocturnal sleep, especially in adolescents, GH values may rise to 20 to 50 ng/ml.

It is important to determine the status of GH secretion in cases with suspected pituitary deficiency and in cases with suspected GH excess. The strategies of differential diagnosis of these two conditions differ. To determine GH insufficiency, it is necessary to stimulate GH secretion; in the case of hypersecretion one must determine whether glucose, a physiologic inhibitor of GH secretion, can suppress the elevated GH levels. Because random values in normal persons may fall into the "hypopituitary" or the "acromegalic" range, it is necessary to carry out standard provocative and suppression tests.

There are inherent errors in all assays, including radioimmunoassay, and these are greater when assays are performed in different laboratories possibly using different standards.

GROWTH HORMONE SECRETORY RESERVE TESTS IN SUSPECTED GH DEFICIENCY

The choice of tests and their sequences of presentation depend upon the age of the patient, the index of diagnostic suspicion, and factors such as convenience to the patient and doctor. It also must be emphasized that different tests may test different neuroendocrine pathways and that there are some poorly growing children who have "normal" provocative tests, normal patterns of sleep-related GH release, but who may nevertheless benefit from the usual therapeutic doses of GH, thus suggesting that they may have partial GH deficiency.[210,257] This controversial subject and the decision to administer GH in patients without documented GH deficiency has been the subject of much discussion.[226,282,284] A subgroup of patients has been identified who have normal induced GH secretion, reduced 24-hour GH output, and low-somatomedin C levels to which the term *GH neurosecretory dysfunction* has been applied. Reasons to consider that GH deficiency is present is a growth rate below the third percentile at any age, growth rates of less than 4.5 cm a year, or a change in growth rate continuing for more than 6 months in the absence of medical disorders such as infection, malnutrition, or gastrointestinal disease. Measurement of plasma somatomedin C is the most useful indirect index of GH secretion, but it is not entirely definitive because it is affected by nutritional status, varies with age, and has a fairly wide normal range.

If the clinical evaluation suggests that the patient has normal pituitary function (the most common situation in the short child with "constitutional" short stature), most endocrinologists will recommend an exercise provocative test done as an outpatient screening procedure. The details of these tests vary from clinic to clinic, but the procedure used in this clinic is to ask the child to run up and down stairs as quickly as possible for 10 minutes. A single blood sample 5 minutes after completion of the exercise is collected. Approximately 60 percent of normal children will achieve a value of 6 ng/ml or more after this procedure (a somewhat higher figure—90 percent or more—is quoted by Frasier,[75] and others use a level of 8 ng/ml as the normal cutoff level). If the child fails to achieve this level, it is necessary to proceed with more definitive tests.

It is important to recognize that the responsiveness of the GH secretory system is markedly reduced by thyroidal or gonadal deficiency. Hypothyroidism, the prepubertal state, or acquired gonadal deficiency, if evident, should be corrected. The gonadal effect can be reversed by administration of a single priming dose of conjugated estrogens (Premarin), 2.5 mg by mouth, or of diethylstilbestrol, 1.0 mg by mouth 24 hours before the test. Thyroxine replacement should be given for at least 6 weeks.

Adults are not usually tested with exercise, and no standards exist for this procedure, although there is no reason that this would not be feasible inasmuch as adults respond to exercise with elevations of GH level.

If the exercise test is not diagnostic, we usually carry out an insulin-tolerance test as the definitive procedure because it permits the simultaneous testing of ACTH-adrenal and PRL secretory reserve (see chapters 6 and 7). The hypoglycemia tests are not generally done in individuals over the age of 50 because of concern over precipitating cardiac arrhythmias or myocardial infarction.

The best alternative to the hypoglycemia test for GH reserve is the clonidine test, which now is being used widely because of its simplicity and safety. Clonidine, an α-adrenergic agonist, is presumed to act on the GHRH neuronal system to release GHRH and would be abnormal in defects of either hypothalamus or pituitary gland (which is the case for all provocative tests of GH reserve except for the GHRH test). As recommended by Laron and coworkers,[131,132] clonidine can be given either as a screening test (a single dose of 25 μg by mouth with a single blood sample taken 70 to 90 minutes later) or as a more definitive test (single dose of 75 μg/m^2 with bloods drawn through a butterfly catheter at 60 and 120 minutes). In more than 90 percent of children, peak GH levels of 10 ng/ml or more are achieved by this dose.

In children, two other tests are commonly used, the intravenous arginine infusion or the sleep GH test. Unfortunately, arginine for intravenous use is not readily available in many hospitals, and the sleep test requires that a blood sample be drawn about 1 to 1½ hours after the child has fallen asleep. Although the sleep test logically would be the most satisfactory test if a screening study was negative, its inconvenience restricts its use to inpatient workups or research studies.

In adults as an alternative (if hypoglycemia is contraindicated), the L-dopa test can be used. 500 mg of L-dopa is given by mouth. Blood samples are drawn before the test and at intervals thereafter. It should be recalled that treatment with monoamine oxidase inhibitors (i.e., for depression) contraindicates use of L-dopa. Many other provocative tests of GH reserve have been proposed including the use of glucagon, glucagon after propranolol priming, and benzodiazepine. None are widely used at present for routine clinical testing.

Several other factors can alter GH secretory reserve. Older individuals are much less responsive to provocative stimuli; most do not show nocturnal GH release after the age of 50; obesity blunts GH responses to all stimuli, including that to GHRH.[265]

REGULATION OF THE PITUITARY GLAND

GHRH Test in GH Deficiency

Although GHRH has not yet been approved for general use, sufficient clinical experience has been gained with this agent to assess its potential usefulness in the diagnosis of GH deficiency.[31,32,95,205,207,215,219,250] The usual mode of administration is by a single intravenous bolus of 1.0 μg/kg, samples for blood being taken serially. Peak responses to lower doses of GHRH are observed at 15 to 30 minutes in children and as late as 60 minutes in adults with GH deficiency. It will probably be sufficient for routine use to measure serum GH at these intervals. Approximately two thirds of patients with any form of GH deficiency will show a markedly blunted or absent GH response (peak values less than 6 ng/ml).[215,236] Hence the GHRH test has a lower yield than either clonidine or hypoglycemia in documenting the presence of GH deficiency. On the other hand, its main use may be in differentiating intrinsic pituitary disease from hypothalamic disease as the cause of GH deficiency (Fig. 17). Approximately one third of GH-deficient patients show normal responses to GHRH, and in this group, the assumption is that they have GHRH deficiency. On the other hand, failure to show GH responses to a single bolus injection of GHRH does not mean that the patient suffers from intrinsic pituitary disease. Patients have been reported who initially had no detectable re-

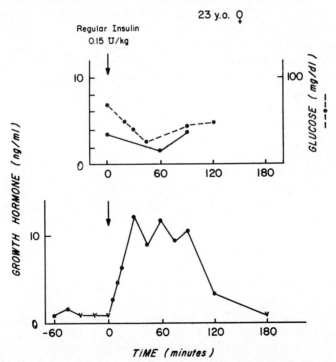

FIGURE 17. GH responses to GHRH in a patient with hypothalamic GH failure owing to eosinophilic granuloma of the hypothalamus, and comparison with response to insulin-induced hypoglycemia. This figure illustrates the failure of GH response to a physiologic stimulus involving the hypothalamus *(top panel)* and the normal response to direct pituitary stimulation *(bottom panel)*. GHRH *(not labeled)* was given as a bolus *(arrow, bottom panel)*. (From Goldman, J, Molitch, ME, Reichlin, S. 1984, unpublished.)

sponse to GHRH but who demonstrated response after repeated injections. Furthermore, several patients with documented hypothalamic disease have blunted GHRH responses. It is reasonable to conclude that prolonged GHRH deficiency can lead to impaired pituitary responsiveness, as in the case of GnRH.

Growth hormone releasing hormone responses in adult normal males are clearly age dependent, decreasing in successive decades.[220] Normal women show a larger response to GHRH than do men. Growth hormone releasing hormone is also effective by intranasal administration.[69]

It is worth emphasizing that in the Laron type of dwarfism, serum GH levels are normal or markedly elevated. This defect is due to abnormality in the generation of somatomedin C with loss of somatomedin C feedback.

GROWTH HORMONE SUPPRESSION TEST AND PARADOXICAL GH RESPONSES

In patients with acromegaly or gigantism, the diagnosis readily can be confirmed simply by demonstrating that random GH levels are consistently above 10 ng/ml. However, GH levels of only 5 ng/ml, or even lower, occasionally can be observed in active acromegaly. Random GH levels in normal adults are usually less than 2 ng/ml. From a diagnostic point of view, the provocative tests are used in ambiguous cases and to serve as a baseline in the monitoring of response to therapy. The provocative tests have been used extensively for research purposes. The most important provocative tests are glucose administration, TRH, and GHRH. Paradoxical GH responses to GnRH and to VIP also are seen in active acromegalics and not in normal subjects.

Glucose Administration

In response to a standard oral glucose tolerance test (75 g glucose by mouth), GH levels in normal individuals are suppressed to less than 3 ng/ml quite consistently, with a small rebound about 2 hours later. About one half of acromegalics show a paradoxical increase in GH levels and the remainder partial suppression, but not to below 5 ng/ml.

Thyrotropin-releasing Hormone

In normal individuals, TRH does not stimulate GH secretion. On the other hand, somewhat more than half of acromegalics will release GH in response to TRH ("paradoxical TRH response").[139] This effect is important in documenting the persistence of abnormally functioning tissue even when baseline values have returned to normal after treatment. Paradoxical responses to TRH are seen in the common forms of acromegaly due to an adenoma, in acromegaly due to the ectopic secretion of GHRH, and in the somatotrope hyperplasia associated with polyostotic fibrous dysplasia.[204] In nonacromegalics, paradoxical GH responses to TRH are seen in some patients with anorexia nervosa, depression, renal failure, and metabolic encephalopathy. The details of the test are described in chapter 15.

Growth Hormone Releasing Hormone

The GHRH test has proven to be of little help in evaluating the clinical state of patients with acromegaly.[81,267] A small proportion show exuberant responses, with values going into the hundreds of ng/ml. Most show responses proportional to their initially high values, and about 20 percent show blunted or no release after GHRH. The test does not indicate the level of disease activity any more clearly than does the basal level and somatomedin C determination. Prior irradiation therapy is one of the causes of blocked responses (indicating damage to the pituitary gland), but even untreated patients may show no responses. Further work with this agent will be needed to define its usefulness as a clinical investigative tool.

Gonadotropin-releasing Hormone

Approximately one fourth of acromegalic patients show a paradoxical release of GH following intravenous injection of 100 μg of GnRH, as is done for the evaluation of gonadotropin secretory reserve.

Miscellaneous

Other provocative stimuli have been used to evaluate acromegalics. Approximately one half show increases after hypoglycemia, but they are blunted as compared with the normal (thus demonstrating persistence of some normal control mechanisms). Responses to vasoactive intestinal peptide (VIP)[45] occur in a subpopulation of patients.

MANAGEMENT OF GH DEFICIENCY

The treatment of documented GH deficiency in children traditionally has used injections of cadaver-derived hGH in doses of approximately 2 mg three times a week.[74,209] On this regimen children grow well but have not reached normal heights.

In mid 1985, the National Institutes of Health (NIH) and private drug companies processing human pituitary glands for GH discontinued distribution because of reports that three patients who had received hGH prepared prior to 1977 had developed Creutzfeldt-Jakob disease,[40,84,122] a uniformly fatal brain infection caused by a slow virus related to Kuru and to the sheep disease Scrapie. It will take several years before the necessary virologic tests are performed to satisfy safety criteria. Indeed, such criteria may never be fulfilled adequately, and it is probable that natural GH may never again be used and that biosynthetic GH, made by recombinant techniques, will be the treatment of choice. This agent is now available for clinical use.

> The first preparation to be released commercially (Somatonorm) differs slightly from hGH in that it contains an additional methionyl group at the amino terminal. This modified GH appears to be slightly more antigenic than pituitary-derived hormone, which also induces antibodies. Several new preparations of terminal methionine-free recombinant GH soon will be available. Nevertheless, it does seem that the appearance of antibodies is correlated with poor responses to GH therapy.

Recent studies of children with impaired growth (less than 4.5 cm per year) have shown a subpopulation who may have normal provocative tests or normal sleep-induced GH but who show increased growth following administration of usual therapeutic doses of GH.[83,210,226,257] In some rare individuals, the GH secreted may be chemically abnormal,[256] but in most the secreted GH is chemically normal. These individuals have generally been classified as having "normal variant short stature."[210] The problem of differentiation from cases with the syndrome of constitutional short stature is a major problem for pediatric endocrinologists.

Faced with a very short child who is growing either slowly or who has "fallen off the growth curve" and who has ambiguous GH reserve tests, the clinical endocrinologist is faced with a difficult decision at this time. It is not known whether therapy of the "normal variant" short-statured child with GH, even if growth is enhanced during treatment, will lead to an *ultimately* greater height than if the child was untreated. Based on observations of children with GH excess, as in gigantism, it is likely that given sufficient amount of hormone, such children will grow, but it is not clear that the large amounts of GH that somatotropic tumors secrete could be duplicated by medical treatment. Unfortunately, the results of several therapeutic trials now underway will not be available to guide the therapy of children who are presently at the crucial phase of their growth curves. It is important to recognize that GH deficiency can be temporary, as judged by serial provocative tests over prolonged periods of time.[92,176,254] The use of GHRH has been reported to stimulate growth;[249] presently underway are trials to determine the optimum regimen of treatment. Clonidine, an α-adrenergic agonist presumed to act by stimulating GHRH secretion, also has been reported to stimulate growth, but insufficient data are available to conclude that this will provide long-term benefits.[191]

Parenthetically, it is important to recognize that even with presently recommended GH regimens, growth achieved in documented hypopituitary dwarfs is suboptimal as compared with the normal population,[76] suggesting that conventional treatment is inadequate, perhaps the consequences of the relatively small amounts of GH that have been available from natural sources. Treatment of hypopituitarism is also discussed in chapter 16.

MANAGEMENT OF ACROMEGALY

Management of acromegaly must take into consideration a number of factors: age, general health, extent of local damage, severity of diabetes and other systemic manifestations of GH hypersecretion, and the importance of preserving residual pituitary function. Ideal therapy of acromegaly requires that morbidity and mortality be less than that of the untreated disease, that GH levels be reduced to less than 5 ng/ml without induction of hypopituitarism, that extrasellar-pressure effects are prevented or cured, and that the reduction in GH levels be relatively rapid. No single mode of treatment presently available fully meets these requirements for all cases.

Therapeutic benefit is demonstrated objectively by a decline in the elevated levels of GH and by the regression of characteristic acromegalic signs and symptoms. When GH levels are reduced, most acromegalic patients show improved carbohydrate tolerance, although the abnormality may not clear completely, and the increased abnormal excess sweating decreases or disappears. Soft-tissue overgrowth, so striking a feature of acromegaly, may show remarkable regression. The hands and feet decrease in volume, the nose becomes less prominent, and the skin becomes much less coarse. These changes, which can occur over a few days or weeks after hypophysectomy, are accompanied by marked excretion of nitrogenous products in the urine. Back pain and other skeletal complaints also may improve dramatically, and blood pressure often falls into the normal range. Regressive changes may continue for several years.

The older literature commonly referred to "burned-out" acromegaly. The development of radioimmunoassays for GH has put this notion largely to rest; virtually all cases of untreated acromegaly have elevated GH levels.[11] Although blood GH levels may be less than 5 ng/ml in an active case, if sustained throughout the 24-hour day, they can be associated with active disease. Acromegaly is a progressive disease, and a decision not to treat must take into consideration the fact that morbidity and mortality in acromegaly are twice that expected in the general population.[268] The progression of the disease and its complications do not correlate with levels of radioimmunoassayable GH in plasma; a definition of "mild" acromegaly is, therefore, difficult to find. Most patients should be treated unless age, general health, or psychosocial factors prevent treatment.

Radiation Therapy

Conventional high-voltage radiation of the pituitary gland has long been a standard therapy for acromegaly;[65] the value of this form of treatment is a subject of controversy.[24,71] Conventional therapy is defined by Sheline[217] as being "megavoltage radiation given in a single fractionated course of about 5 treatments per week to a total dose of approximately 4500 to 5000 rads in 5 to 6 weeks." By clinical criteria (and before immunoassay was developed) it was believed that 50 to 75 percent of treated patients had a remission of their disease, but early studies utilizing radioimmunoassay indicated that most patients (75 percent) did not have a decrease in GH levels below 7.5 ng/ml. As experience has accumulated, a number of workers have pointed out that a large proportion of patients show adequate benefit after conventional treatment but that this response takes a long time to develop fully. For example, in the series of Sheline,[217] 13 of 17 patients studied between 2 and 24 years after therapy had complete return to normal GH levels. Similar findings by Eastman and coworkers[65] indicate that in patients followed for 10 years after treatment with 4000 to 4500 rads, 69 percent had GH levels under 5 ng/ml. Twenty-five to 50 percent of these patients develop partial or complete hypopituitarism. Conventional radiation has the advantage of being available in most communities, being applicable to patients with irregularly shaped tumors with lateral or inferior extension, having a very low incidence of complications such as visual disturbance, and rarely causing pituitary insufficiency (see chapter 16).

The main disadvantage of conventional radiation is the long delay in curing GH hypersecretion and the fact that effects are not usually seen before 6 months. In cases of severe diabetes, skeletal manifestations, progressive disfigurement, and cardiac disease, this long lag may not be tolerable. Other disadvantages are that a significant proportion of patients are not brought under control (as many as 25 percent at 5 years), the treatment requires daily visits to the hospital for 5 to 6 weeks and this may not be feasible for many patients, and transient epilation of the target skin area is very common.

Some clinicians hesitate to give x-irradiation because of their concern that there may be subtle neurologic defects. It has been demonstrated, for example, that the majority of individuals receiving 5000 rads to the hypothalamic-pituitary region for treatment of tumors other than GH-producing lesions will develop impaired GH secretory responses, shown by GHRH tests to be due to hypothalamic damage. A recent study of 1200 patients found evidence of hypothalamic dysfunction in 15.[285] The most common abnormalities were behavioral (14 of 15) and hyperprolactinemia (9 of 15). The possibility of vascular endothelial damage to the lining of the carotid artery by x-irradiation therapy also has been considered on theoretic grounds.

In the rare cases of acromegaly associated with polyostotic fibrous dysplasia in whom x-ray therapy might be considered, it is possibly relevant that the bone lesion in this disorder may become sarcomatous, and that the majority of sarcomas in this syndrome occur in bones that have been treated with x-ray therapy.[222]

The most widely used alternative form of radiation therapy in the United States and Canada is the proton beam. This technique depends on the availability of cyclotron-generated protons delivered to the pituitary region under carefully controlled conditions[120,134] (see chapter 16 for detailed description).

The data reported recently by Kliman and coworkers[120] show that plasma GH levels under 10 ng/ml were achieved in 47.5 percent of patients at 2 years, 65 percent at 4 years, 87.5 percent at 10 years, and 97.5 percent at 20 years after treatment.[120] Using more rigorous criteria for treatment success, that is, GH levels under 5 ng/ml, they quote figures of 75 percent at 10 years and 92.5 percent at 20 years.

Proton beam radiation has the following advantages: It produces maximum effects earlier than conventional radiation therapy, requires only a two- to four-day hospitalization instead of a six-week course of daily treatments, and is usually unaccompanied by epilation. The incidence of side effects, however, is somewhat greater after proton-beam radiation than after conventional radiation. In the compilation of Kliman and colleagues[120] of their 435 cases who have been followed since therapy, the following complications were observed: temporary disturbance in extraocular movements, 6 cases; visual impairment, 8 cases; partial or total hypopituitarism, 9.7 percent; hypothyroid, 9.7 percent; adrenal insufficiency, 9 percent; hypogonadal, 6.7 percent. Other complications, observed in a small number of cases, were temporal-lobe seizures and disturbed mentation, but evidence is lacking that these are direct effects of treatment.

Proton-beam radiation has the disadvantages of requiring high-level technology available in only two centers in the United States, being applicable only when the tumor is confined to the sella, and not being fully effective in an appreciable number of cases.

Because of the high incidence of optic-nerve and cranial-nerve damage and brain necrosis in patients treated with more than 5000 rads by conventional methods or 15,000 rads by proton beam, it is widely recommended that patients not be given a second course of radiation therapy if they have already received one full course. Also, the incidence of sarcoma is increased in patients given more than one course of treatment. Twelve instances of radiation-induced sarcoma were reported up to 1966, all but two of whom had had multiple courses of therapy. However, this rare complication can occur after radiation doses less than 5000 rads.[217]

Alpha particle pituitary irradiation has been carried out by Linfoot and Lawrence and associates[135] in 314 cases, and data are available on 299. By 1 year posttreatment, median fasting GH had fallen to approximately 9.5 from an initial median of 23 ng/ml, and by 4 years to a median of 5 ng/ml. Levels continued to fall over the ensuing 18 years of followup. Growth hormone levels fell to 5 ng/ml in 30 percent of patients within 2 years, 68 percent within 6 years, and 95 percent within 8 years. Relapse was usually the result of some degree of extrasellar extension: suprasellar, intrasphenoidal, or posterior-inferior. In the series treated prior to the use of CAT scans, there is an appreciable incidence of these abnormalities.

Approximately 34 percent of the patients developed ACTH deficiency or TSH deficiency, and 25 percent developed gonadotropic insufficiency (but these values are not certain because gonadotropin deficiency was not tested in older individuals). Neurologic complications included partial field cuts in 29 percent (asymptomatic). Three patients developed unilateral extraocular motor nerve lesions, usually third nerve abnormalities, but the symptoms usually cleared and were relatively asymptomatic. Three developed temporal lobe epilepsy (all in cases treated previously by other modalities). The overall central nervous system complication rate in 298 cases was 4 percent.

Other radiation methods to destroy the pituitary (implantation of particles of radioactive yttrium [^{90}Y] or of radioactive gold [^{198}Au]) have been abandoned mainly in favor of surgical ablation.

MICROSURGERY

This technique, first used by Cushing and later abandoned in favor of the transfrontal approach, was reestablished by Guiot and Thibaut[98,99] in 1958 in France. Subsequently, Hardy and Wigser[103,104] developed a number of technical improvements in Montreal and extended the indications for its use. The results of transsphenoidal treatment in acromegaly have been encouraging. Hardy reports a reduction in GH to normal levels in 80 percent of patients with noninvasive tumors. The morbidity is minimal; patients routinely are up and about on the day after surgery and discharged from the hospital within five to seven days. There are no deaths in his series. Endocrine replacement was required in less than 15 to 20 percent of cases; recurrence was rare in patients who had not received prior radiation and who had normal postoperative GH levels. In a series of 100 cases of acromegaly reported by Williams and coworkers[264] in London, the initial treatment of 68 was surgical (nine underwent transfrontal hypophysectomy and 59 transsphenoidal hypophysectomy). The remainder were not treated because of age, concurrent illness, apparent mildness of the condition, or refusal of treatment. There was no death owing to treatment in the 59 patients operated by the transsphenoidal route; one patient died at home weeks later of a pulmonary embolus, one developed CSF rhinorrhea that stopped spontaneously after two weeks, and three suffered acute frontal sinusitis that responded to antibiotics. A satisfactory response to operation, defined as a fall in plasma GH to less than 5 ng/ml, was achieved in 39 of 59 patients (66 percent). Seven patients required subsequent treatment consisting of either roentgenotherapy (five patients) or implantation of radioactive yttrium (two patients).

Several more recent series now have been published.[241,255] Hardy reports complete biological and clinical follow-up data on 120 of 150 patients. Of the 120, 94 had postoperative GH levels of less than 5 ng/ml (78 percent). Twenty-seven of 33 Grade I patients and 48 of 59 Grade II patients were cured. The success rate declined abruptly with larger tumors; only 1 of 7 patients with a Grade IV tumor had postoperative GH levels less than 5 ng/ml. Of the 120 patients operated in this series, 91 had no postoperative pituitary insufficiency, and 16 showed recovery from postoperative deficits.

A cooperative group of 12 German university clinics reported results of 230 patients with acromegaly.[216] Although treatment modality was not randomized, 152 were treated by transsphenoidal surgery with normalization of GH to less than 5 in 60 percent. It was uncommon for GH normalization to occur in larger (grade III) or more invasive (grade IV) tumors.

Laws and associates have reported the results of operating on 183 acromegalics at the Mayo Clinic.[136,137] The results confirm findings of others; that the smaller tumors have a higher cure rate, and that preoperative GH levels less than 40 ng/ml have a better prognosis than those greater than 40 ng/ml. All these reports emphasize an exceedingly low rate of recurrence after successful transsphenoidal surgery, that is, less than 1 percent per year.

Despite the general increasing enthusiasm for transsphenoidal surgery, Schuster and coworkers[216] reported 8 of 11 patients undergoing transsphenoidal surgery who were not cured. Importantly, 4 of 7 acromegalics showed recurrence of clinical symptoms several months after they were thought to have been cured (although, in fact, none of these 4 patients had GH lowered to 5 ng/ml). Unfortunately, tumor grade, a most important determinant of cure, is not mentioned in their article.

Relief of headache and sweating, two prominent complaints in acromegaly, is frequently noted immediately after the operation. Symptoms of carpal-tunnel compression often clear during the first postoperative week, and a reduction in soft-tissue thickening is evident within a month. The resolution of signs and symptoms correlates closely to GH levels (that is, reduction to less than 5 ng/ml). In the Williams[264] series, carbohydrate tolerance improved in all patients when GH was reduced to normal levels. The majority of patients operated on via the transsphenoidal approach recover without deficit of other anterior pituitary hormones. We believe that this is due primarily to the fact that hypothalamic-pituitary connections are preserved and that even small amounts of residual pituitary tissue can return to normal function under normal hypothalamic drive.

As transsphenoidal microsurgery has advanced technically, we have almost uniformly recommended this form of surgery as the initial approach in patients even if complete removal is unlikely.

PHARMACOLOGIC TREATMENT

Estrogens

The earliest pharmacologic treatment for acromegaly was estrogen therapy, which produces in some cases a decrease in the severity of the metabolic disturbance. The basis of this treatment has been shown to be suppression of the formation of somatomedin C and an interference with its effects on cartilage and connective tissue. Estrogen therapy does not depress the secretion of GH, and, in fact, may increase GH secretion, presumably owing to direct stimulation of somatotrope cell function. Estrogen administration sensitizes the pituitary gland to GHRH and, after prolonged administration in experimental animals, may induce mammotropic-somatotropic pituitary tumors. The use of estrogen therapy in treatment of acromegaly fell into disrepute following the observation that there seemed to be an excess number who developed pituitary apoplexy. The possibility that estrogens may stimulate the tumor directly, and the modest benefits of the treatment, have led clinicians away from estrogen therapy.

Progesterone

A number of workers have studied the effects of progesterone derivatives on GH secretion. In particular, medroxyprogesterone acetate (MPA) has been shown in some cases to reduce GH levels. In the early report of Lawrence and Kirsteins,[133] 10 of 12 patients had a decline in plasma GH levels after six days of treatment, together with a blunting of the GH response to arginine. In later studies of Malarkey and Daughaday[148] and of Jackson and Ormston,[112] less than 50 percent of cases had a lowering of GH levels, and in most cases, the GH concentration failed to fall to the normal range. Medroxyprogesterone acetate, like estrogen therapy, has been discarded as primary therapy. A trial of combined estrogen and progesterone has not, as far as we know, been reported.

Chlorpromazine

In 1971, Kolodny and coworkers[121] reported that treatment of one patient with chlorpromazine led to a reduction in plasma GH levels from 18 to 4 ng/ml. Unfortunately, other workers have failed to confirm this finding. There has been no systematic study of single and combined neuroleptic agents designed to inhibit all three of the biogenic amines thought to be involved in physiologic GH regulation of GH secretion, that is, dopaminergic, serotonergic, and catecholaminergic factors.

Bromocriptine

Bromocriptine is the first drug shown to have significant and meaningful effects in reducing GH secretion in a proportion of acromegalics.[19,62,107,138,175,179] This drug initially gained notice by virtue of its potent and sustained suppression of prolactin in patients with galactorrhea. Several recent investigations have provided unequivocal evidence that 30 to 60 percent of acromegalic patients show suppression in response to bromocriptine; improvement in clinical symptoms in a minority is dramatic. Bromocriptine is used widely in patients in whom surgical or radiation treatment has failed to produce a definitive cure. In some clinics such as that of Besser at St. Bartholomew's Hospital, London, most acromegalic patients are treated simultaneously with large doses of bromocriptine and conventional x-ray therapy, the rationale being that the drug will lower GH levels during the lag time for radiation effects. This would be a preferred approach if the patient refuses surgery, or when expert neurosurgical services are not available (see chapter 7 for discussion of treatment with bromocriptine).

Somatostatin Analogs

The development of potent, long-acting somatostatin analogs has provided a highly successful backup treatment for acromegalic patients. The majority of patients will show a marked reduction in GH levels after a single intravenous dose,[192] and sustained decreases in GH are observed in the majority of patients given twice-daily injections of the Sandoz long-acting analog SMS 201-995.[47,129] This drug now is being used with success in worldwide clinical trials in patients who have failed surgical and x-ray therapies. Shrinkage of tumors has been observed in several cases. Except for mild glucose intolerance, this therapy is well tolerated. As experience is gained with this agent, it is likely that it will be evaluated as a first-line treatment alternative to radiotherapy or surgery in a few special cases.

OVERVIEW OF THERAPEUTIC OPTIONS IN ACROMEGALY

We currently recommend that all patients with acromegaly be treated initially by transsphenoidal adenomectomy if feasible. There is a chance for a cure if the tumor is small, and even if complete removal is not possible, debulking of the tumor reduces the risk of optic nerve involvement and decreases the mass of secreting tissue. Suprasellar extension is not a contraindication because the transsphenoid route allows the residual tumors to drop down into the sella unless it is growing in a "dumbbell" fashion through an intact dorsum sella. If the tumor has not been removed completely and GH levels are consistently above 5 ng/ml, the patient should be given a course of x-ray therapy, 4500 rads total in divided doses. We believe that x-ray therapy alone is also feasible, but the many drawbacks (see above) make this a procedure for only those who cannot or will not undergo surgical resection or in whom surgery has failed.

If the tumor has invaded the sphenoid sinus or the cavernous sinus, with or without suprasellar invasion, transsphenoidal hypophysectomy is indicated as a debulking procedure followed by postoperative radiation.

If hypersecretion of GH persists after transsphenoidal hypophysectomy, reoperation is sometimes warranted. This procedure will increase the likelihood of cerebrospinal fluid rhinorrhea and of panhypopituitarism (because the surgeon will be more aggressive in removing questionable tissue). If GH levels are normal after surgery, there is no need to institute radiation therapy immediately. If relapse occurs after transsphenoidal hypophysectomy, it usually happens within a few months.

The most distressing therapeutic problem in acromegaly, seen in an uncomfortably large proportion of cases (about 15 percent), is persistent hypersecretion following surgery and radiation therapy. Such patients either have locally invasive tumors in the sphenoid sinus, in the lining dura, or even the temporal lobe, or have intrasellar tumors so large and extensive that ablation is impossible. Repeated courses of radiation therapy carry the risk of inducing brain necrosis or sarcoma.

Bromocriptine is the first line of treatment of cases with persistent elevation of GH levels. Somatostatin analogs are the backup therapy now shown to be effective in a high proportion of cases.

REFERENCES

1. ABE, H, MOLITCH, ME, VAN WYK, JJ, ET AL: *Human growth hormone and somatomedin C suppress the spontaneous release of growth hormone in unanesthetized rats.* Endocrinology 113:1319–1324, 1983.
2. ABRAMS, RL, GRUMBACH, MM, KAPLAN, SL: *The effect of administration of human growth hormone on the plasma growth hormone, cortisol, glucose, and free fatty acid response to insulin: Evidence for growth hormone autoregulation in man.* J Clin Invest 50:940–950, 1971.
3. ADAMS, EF, BRAJKOVICH, IE, MASHITER, K: *Hormone secretion by dispersed cell cultures of human pituitary adenomas: Effects of theophylline, thyrotropin-releasing hormone, somatostatin and 2-bromo-a-ergocryptine.* J Clin Endocrinol Metab 49:120–126, 1979.
4. ALFORD, FP, BAKER, HW, BURGER, HG: *The secretion of human growth hormone. 1. Daily secretion rates, effect of posture and sleep.* J Clin Endocrinol Metab 37:515–520, 1973.
5. ALPERT, LC, BRAWER, JR, PATEL, YC, ET AL: *Somatostatinergic neurons in anterior hypothalamus: Immunohistochemical localization.* Endocrinology 98:255–258, 1976.
6. ANTHONY, GJ, VAN WYK, JJ, FRENCH, JS: *Influence of pituitary stalk section on growth hormone, insulin and TSH secretion in women with metastatic breast cancer.* J Clin Endocrinol Metab 29:1238–1250, 1969.
7. ANTONI, FA, KANYICSKA, B, MEZEY, E, MAKARA, GB: *Neonatal treatment with monosodium-L-glutamate: Differential effects on growth hormone and prolactin release induced by morphine.* Neuroendocrinology 35:231–235, 1982.
8. ARIMURA, A, SMITH, W, SCHALLY, AV: *Blockade of the stress-induced decrease in blood GH by anti-somatostatin serum in rats.* Endocrinology 98:540–543, 1976.
9. ARNOLD, MA, REPPERT, SM, RORSTAD, OP, SAGAR, SM, KEUTMAN, HT, PERLOW, MJ, MARTIN, JB: *Temporal patterns of somatostatin immunoreactivity in the cerebrospinal fluid of the Rhesus monkey: Effect of environmental lighting.* J Neurosci 2:225–231, 1982.
10. AROSIO, M, GIOVANELLI, MA, RIVA, E, NAVA, C, AMBROSI, B, FAGLIA, G: *Clinical use of pre- and postsurgical evaluation of abnormal GH responses in acromegaly.* J Neurosurg 59:402–408, 1983.
11. ASA, SL, KOVACS, K, THORNER, MO, LEONG, DA, RIVIER, J, VALE, W: *Immunohistological localization of growth hormone-releasing hormone in human tumors.* J Clin Endocrinol Metab 60:423–427, 1985.
12. ASA, SL, SCHEITHAUER, BW, BILBAO, J, HORVATH, E, RYAN, N, KOVACS, K, RANDALL, RV, LAWS, ER, SINGER, W, LINFOOT, JA, THORNER, MO, VALE, W: *A case for hypothalamic acromegaly: A clinicopathological study of six patients with hypothalamic gangliocytomas producing growth hormone-releasing factor.* J Clin Endocrinol Metab 58:796–803, 1984.
13. AUDHYA, T, MANZIONE, MM, NAKANE, T, KANIE, N, PASSARELLI, J, RUSSO, M, HOLLANDER, CS: *Levels of human and rat hypothalamic growth hormone-releasing factor as determined by specific radioimmunoassay systems.* Proc Natl Acad Sci USA 82:2970–2974, 1985.

14. BARINAGA, M, YAMANOTO, G, RIVIER, G, VALE, W, EVANS, R, ROSENFELD, MG: *Transcriptional regulation of growth hormone gene expression by growth hormone-releasing factor.* Nature 306:84–86, 1983.

15. BENOIT, R, BOHLEN, P, LING, N, BRISKIN, A, ESCH, F, BRAZEAU, P, YING, SY, GUILLEMIN, R: *Presence of somatostatin-28-(1-12) in hypothalamus and pancreas.* Proc Natl Acad Sci USA 79:917–921, 1982.

16. BERELOWITZ, M, SZABO, M, FROHMAN, L, ET AL: *Somatomedin-C mediates growth hormone negative feedback by effects on both the hypothalamus and the pituitary.* Science 212:1279–1281, 1981.

17. BERGER, G, TROUILLAS, J, BLOCK, B, SASSOLAS, G, BERGER, F, PARTENSKY, C, CHAYVAILLE, JA, BRAZEAU, P, CLAUSTRAT, B, LESBROS, F, ET AL: *Multihormonal carcinoid tumor of the pancreas secreting growth hormone-releasing factor as a cause of acromegaly.* In *Laboratoire d'Anatoie Pathologique, Universite de Lyon, France.* Cancer 54:2097–2108, 1984.

18. BESSER, GM, MORTIMER, CH, McNEILLY, AS, ET AL: *Long-term infusion of growth hormone release inhibiting hormone in acromegaly: Effects on pituitary and pancreatic hormones.* Br Med J 4:622–627, 1974.

19. BESSER, GM, AND WASS, JAH: *The medical management of acromegaly.* In BLACK, PM, ZERVAS, NT, RIDGWAY, EC, MARTIN, JB (EDS): *Secretory Pituitary Tumors.* Raven Press, New York, 1984, pp 155–168.

20. BICKNELL, RJ, AND SCHOFIELD, JG: *Inhibition by somatostatin of bovine growth hormone secretion following sodium channel activation.* J Physiol 316:85–96, 1981.

21. BILEZIKJIAN, LM, AND VALE, WW: *Stimulation of adenosine 3',5'-monophosphate production by growth hormone-releasing factors and its inhibition by somatostatin in anterior pituitary cells in vitro.* Endocrinology 113:1276–1731, 1983.

22. BIVENS, CH, LEBOVITZ, HE, FELDMAN, JM: *Inhibition of hypoglycemia-induced growth hormone secretion by the serotonin antagonists cyropheptadine and methysergide.* N Engl J Med 289:236–239, 1973.

23. BLATT, J, BERCU, BB, GILLIN, JC, MENDELSON, WB, POPLACK, DB: *Reduced pulsatile growth hormone secretion in children after therapy for acute lymphoblastic leukemia.* J Pediatr 104:182–186, 1984.

24. BLOOD, B, AND KARMER, S: *Conventional radiation therapy in the management of acromegaly.* In BLACK, PM, ZERVAS, NT, RIDGWAY, EC, MARTIN, JB (EDS): *Secretory Pituitary Tumors.* Raven Press, New York, 1984, pp 179–190.

25. BOHLEN, P, BRAZEAU, P, BLOCK, B, LING, N, GAILLARD, R, GUILLEMIN, R: *Human hypothalamic growth hormone releasing factor (GRF): Evidence for two forms identical to tumor derived GRF-44-NH2 and GRF-40.* Biochem Biophys Res Commun 114:930–936, 1983.

26. BLOCK, B, BRAZEAU, P, BLOOD, F, LING, N: *Topographical study of the neurons containing hpGRF immunoreactivity in monkey hypothalamus.* Neurosci Lett 37:23–28, 1983.

27. BLOCK, B, BRAZEAU, P, LING, N, BOHLEN P, ESCH, F, WEHRENBERG, WB, BENOIT, R, BLOOM, F, GUILLEMIN, R: *Immunohistochemical detection of growth hormone-releasing factor in brain.* Nature 301:607–608, 1983.

28. BLOCK, B, LING, N, BENOIT, R, WEHERENBERG, WB, GUILLEMIN, R: *Specific depletion of growth hormone-releasing factor by monosodium glutamate in rat median eminence.* Nature 307:272–273, 1984.

29. BLOOM, S (ED): *Somatostatin Symposium.* (In press).

30. BOSTICK, DG, QUAN, R, HOFFMAN, AR, WEBB, RJ, CHANG, JK, BENSCH, KG: *Growth-hormone-releasing factor immunoreactivity in human endocrine tumors.* Am J Pathol 117:167–170, 1984.

31. BORGES, JL, BLIZZARD, RM, EANS, WS, ET AL: *Stimulation of growth hormone (GH) and somatomedin C in idiopathic GH-deficient subjects by intermittent pulsatile administration of synthetic human pancreatic tumor GH-releasing factor.* J Clin Endocrinol Metab 59:1–6, 1984.

32. BORGES, JL, BLIZZARD, RM, GELATO, MC, FURLANETTO, R, ET AL: *Effects of human pancreatic tumour growth hormone releasing factor on growth hormone and somatomedin C levels in patients with idiopathic growth hormone deficiency.* Lancet 2:119–124, 1983.

33. BORGES, JL, USKAVITCH, DR, KAISER, DL, CRONIN, MJ, EVANS, WS, THORNER, MO: *Human pancreatic growth hormone-releasing factor-40 (hpGRF-40) allows stimulation of GH release by TRH.* Endocrinology 113:1519–1521, 1983.

34. BOYD, AE, LEBOVITZ, HE, PFEIFFER, JB: *Stimulation of growth hormone secretion by L-dopa.* N Engl J Med 283:1425–1429, 1970.

35. BRAZEAU, P, VALE, W, BURGUS, R, ET AL: *Hypothalamic polypeptide that inhibits the secretion of immunoreactive pituitary growth hormone.* Science 179:77–79, 1973.

36. BRAZEAU, P, LING, N, ESCH, F, BOHLEN, P, BENOIT, R, GUILLEMIN, R: *High biological activity of the synthetic replicates of somatostatin-28 and somatostatin-25.* Reg Peptides 1:255–264, 1981.

37. BRESSON, JL, CLAVEQUIN, MC, FELLMAN, D, BUGNON, C: *Ontogeny of the neuroglandular system revealed with HPGRF 44 antibodies.* Neuroendocrinology 39:68–73, 1984.

38. BROWN, GM, AND REICHLIN, S: *Psychologic and neural regulation of growth hormone secretion.* Psychosom Med 34:45–61, 1972.

39. BROWN, GM, SCHALCH, DS, REICHLIN, S: *Hypothalamic mediation of growth hormone and adrenal stress response in the squirrel monkey.* Endocrinology 89:694–703, 1971.

40. BROWN, P, GAJDUSEK, DC, GIBBS, CJ, JR, ASNER, DM: *Potential epidemic of Creutzfeldt-Jakob disease from human growth hormone therapy.* N Engl J Med 313:728–731, 1985.

41. BROWNSTEIN, MJ, ARIMURA, A, FERNANDEZ-DURANGO, R, SCHALLY, AV, PALKOVITS, M, KIZER, JS: *The effect of hypothalamic deafferentation on somatostatin-like activity in the rat brain.* Endocrinology 100:246–249, 1977.

42. BROWNSTEIN, M, ARIMURA, A, SATO, H, ET AL: *The regional distribution of somatostatin in the rat brain.* Endocrinology 96:1456–1461, 1975.

43. BUCHER, H, ZAPF, J, TORRESANI, T, PRADER, A, FROESCH, E, ILLIG, R: *Insulin-like growth factors I and II, prolactin, and insulin in 19 growth hormone-deficient children with excessive, normal, or decreased longitudinal growth after operation for craniopharyngioma.* N Engl J Med 309:1142–1146, 1983.

44. CHAMBERS, JW, AND BROWN, GM: *Neurotransmitter regulation of growth hormone and ACTH in the rhesus monkey: Effects of biogenic amines.* Endocrinology 98:420–428, 1976.

45. CHIHARA, K, KAJI, HJ, MINAMITANI, N, KODAMA, H, KITA, T, GOTO, B, CHIBA, T, COY, DH, FUJITA, T: *Stimulation of growth hormone by vasoactive intestinal polypeptide in acromegaly.* J Clin Endocrinol Metab 58:81–86, 1984.

46. CHIHARA, K, KATO, Y, MAEDA, K, ET AL: *Effects of thyrotropin-releasing hormone on sleep and sleep-related growth hormone release in normal subjects.* J Clin Endocrinol Metab 4:1094–2000, 1977.

47. CHNG, LJ, SANDLER, LM, KRAENZLIN, ME, BURRIN, JM, JOPLIN, GF, BLOOM, SR: *Long term treatment of acromegaly with a long acting analogue of somatostatin.* Br Med J 290:284–285, 1985.

48. CHIODINI, PG, LIUZZI, A, DALLABONZANA, D, OPPIZZI, G, VERDE, GG: *Changes in growth hormone (GH) secretion induced by human pancreatic GH releasing hormone-44 in acromegaly: A comparison with thyrotropin-releasing hormone and bromocriptine.* J Clin Endocrinol Metab 60:48–52, 1985.

49. CLEMENTS, D, AND ELIAS, E: *Regression of metastatic vipoma with somatostatin analogue SMS 201–995.* Lancet 1:874–875, 1985.

50. CLEMMONS, DR, VAN WYK, JJ, RIDGWAY, EC, KLIMAN, B, KJELLBERG, RN, UNDERWOOD, LE: *Evaluation of acromegaly by radioimmunoassay of somatomedin-C.* N Engl J Med 301:1138–1142, 1979.

51. COBB, WE, REICHLIN, S, JACKSON, IMD: *Growth hormone secretory status is a determinant of the thyrotropin response to thyrotropin releasing hormone (TRH) in euthyroid patients with hypothalamic-pituitary disease.* J Clin Endocrinol Metab 52:324–329, 1981.

52. CHRISTOFIDES, ND, STEPHANOU, A, SAZUKI, H, YIANGOU, Y, BLOOM, SR: *Distribution of immunoreactive growth hormone-releasing hormone in human brain and intestine and its production by tumors.* J Clin Endocrinol Metab 59:747–751, 1984.

53. CRITCHLOW, V, RICE, RW, ABE, K, VALE, W: *Somatostatin content of the median eminence in female rats with lesion-induced disruption of the inhibitory control of growth hormone secretion.* Endocrinology 103:817–825, 1978.

54. CROWLEY, WR, AND TERRY, LC: *Biochemical mapping of somatostatinergic system in rat brain: Effects of periventricular hypothalamic and medial basal amygdaloid lesions on somatostatin-like immunoreactivity in discrete brain nuclei.* Brain Res 200:283–291, 1980.

55. DAUGHADAY, WH, HERINGTON, AC, PHILLIPS, LS: *The regulation of growth by endocrines.* Annu Rev Physiol 37:211–244, 1975.

56. DAUGHADAY, WH, LARON, Z, PERTZELAN, A, HEINS, JN: *Defective sulfation factor generation: A possible etiologic link in dwarfism.* Tran Assoc Am Physic 82:129–140, 1969.

57. DAWSON-HUGHES, B, STERN, D, GOLDMAN, J, REICHLIN, S: *Regulation of growth hormone and somatomedin-C secretion in postmenopausal women. Effect of estrogen therapy.* J Clin Endocrinol Metab 63:424–434, 1986.

58. DAYAL, Y, LIN, HD, TALLBERT, K, REICHLIN, S, DELELLIS, RA, WOLFE, HJ: *Immunocytochemical demonstration of growth hormone releasing factor in gastrointestinal and pancreatic endocrine tumors.* Amer J Clin Pathol 85:13–20, 1986.

59. DAYAL, Y, LIN, HD, REICHLIN, S, ET AL: *Immunoreactivity for growth hormone-releasing factor (GRF) in endocrine tumors of the GEP axis.* Lab Invest 1:14A, 1984.

60. DIEREICKX, K, AND VANDESANDE, F: *Immunocytochemical localization of somatostatin-containing neurons in the rat hypothalamus.* Cell Tiss Res 201:349–359, 1979.

61. DELITALA, G, GROSSMAN, A, BESSER, GM: *Opiate peptides control growth hormone through a cholinergic mechanism in man.* Clin Neuroendocrinol 18:401–405, 1983.

62. DOLECEK, R, KUBIS, M, SAJNAR, J, ZAVADA, M: *Bromocriptine and glucose tolerance in acromegalics.* Pharmacotherapeutica 3:100–106, 1982.

63. Drobny, EC, Amburn, K, Baumann, G: *Circadian variation of basal growth hormone in man.* J Clin Endocrinol 57:524–528, 1983.

64. Drobny, EC, Martin, JB, Brazeau, P: *Evidence for a role of α-adrenergic mechanism in regulation of episodic growth hormone secretion in the rat.* Endocrinology 100:722–728, 1977.

65. Eastman, RC, Gorden, P, Roth, J: *Conventional supervoltage irradiation is an effective treatment for acromegaly.* J Clin Endocrinol Metab 48:931–940, 1979.

66. Eddy, RL, Gillilard, PF, Ibarra, JD, Jr, McMurray, JF, Thompson, IQ: *Human growth hormone release: Comparison of provocative test procedures.* Am J Med 56:179–185, 1974.

67. Enjalbert, A, Epelbaum, J, Aranciba, S, Tapia-Arancibia, M, Bluet-Pajot, M, Kordon, C: *Reciprocal interactions of somatostatin with thyrotropin-releasing hormone and vasoactive intestinal peptide on prolactin and growth hormone secretion in vitro.* Endocrinology 111:42–47, 1982.

68. Epelbaum, J, Willoughby, JO, Brazeau, P, Martin, JB: *Effects of brain lesions and hypothalamic deafferentation on somatostatin distribution in the rat brain.* Endocrinology 101:1495–1502, 1977.

69. Evans, WS, Borges, JL, Kaiser, DL, Vance, ML, Sellers, RP, MacLeod, RM, Vale, W, Rivier, J, Thorner, MO: *Intranasal administration of human pancreatic tumor GH-releasing factor-40 stimulates GH release in normal men.* J Clin Endocrinol Metab 57:1081–1083, 1983.

70. Faglia, G, Beck-Peccoz, P, Ambrosi, B, et al: *Plasma growth hormone response to thyrotropin-releasing hormone in patients with active acromegaly.* J Clin Endocrinol Metab 36:1259–1262, 1973.

71. Feek, CM, McLelland, J, Seth, J, et al: *How effective is external pituitary irradiation for growth hormone-secreting pituitary tumors.* Clin Endocrinol 20:401–408, 1984.

72. Finkelstein, JW, Boyar, RM, Roffwarg, HP, et al: *Age-related change in the twenty-four-hour spontaneous secretion of growth hormone.* J Clin Endocrinol Metab 35:665–70, 1972.

73. Finley, JWC, Maderchut, JL, Roger, LJ, Petrusz, P: *The immunocytochemical localization of somatostatin-containing neurons in the rat central nervous system.* Neuroscience 6:2173–2192, 1981.

74. Frasier, SD: *Human pituitary growth hormone (hGH) therapy in growth hormone deficiency.* Endo Rev 4:155–170, 1983.

75. Frasier, SD: *Pediatric Endocrinology.* Grune & Stratton, New York, 1980.

76. Friesen, HG, Dean, HJ, Kaspar, S, et al: *A perspective on growth hormone and growth. A tribute to Maurice Raben.* In Raiti, S, and Tolman, RA (eds): *Human Growth Hormone.* Plenum, New York, 1986, pp 21–28.

77. Frohman, LA, Bernardis, LL, Kant, KJ: *Hypothalamic stimulation of growth hormone secretion.* Science 162:580–582, 1968.

78. Frohman, LA, Szabo, M, Berelowitz, M, et al: *Partial purification and characterization of a peptide with growth hormone-releasing activity from extrapituitary tumors in patients with acromegaly.* J Clin Invest 65:43–54, 1980.

79. Garfinkel, PE: *Anorexia nervosa: An overview of hypothalamic-pituitary function.* In Brown, GM, Koslow, SH, Reichlin, S (eds): *Neuroendocrinology and Psychiatric Disorder.* Raven Press, New York, 1984, pp 301–314.

80. Gelato, MC, Pescovitz, O, Cassorla, F, Loriaux, DL, Merriam, GR: *Effects of a growth hormone releasing factor in man.* J Clin Endocrinol Metab 57:674–676, 1983.

81. Gelato, MC, Merriam, GR, Vance, ML, Rock, J, Oldfield, EH, Molitch, ME, Rivier, J, Goldman, JA, Webb, C, Evans, WS: *Effects of growth hormone-releasing factor on growth hormone secretion in acromegaly.* J Clin Endocrinol Metab 60:251–257, 1985.

82. Gerich, JE: *Somatostatin.* In Brownlee, M (ed): *Handbook of Diabetes Mellitus,* vol. 1. Garland STPM Press, New York, 1978, pp 297–354.

83. Gertner, JM, Genel, M, Gianfredi, SP, et al: *Prospective clinical trial of human growth hormone in short children without growth hormone deficiency.* J Pediatr 104:172–176, 1984.

84. Gibbs, CJ, Jr, Joy, A, Heffner, R, Franko, M, Miyazaki, M, Asher, DM, Parisi, JE, Brown, PW, Gajdusek, DC: *Clinical and pathological features and laboratory confirmation of Creutzfeldt-Jakob disease in a recipient of pituitary-derived human growth hormone.* N Engl J Med 313:734–738, 1985.

85. Giustina, G, Reschini, E, Peracehi, M, Cantalamessa, L, Cauagnini, F, Pinto, M, Bulgheroni, P: *Failure of somatostatin to suppress thyrotropin releasing actor and luteinizing hormone releasing factor-induced growth hormone release in acromegaly.* J Clin Endocrinol Metab 38:906–909, 1974.

86. Gold, PW, Kellner, CH, Rubinow, DR, Altemus, M, Post, RM: *Abnormal Growth Hormone Responses to Corticotropin Releasing Factor in Patients with Primary Affective Disorder.* Endocrine Society, 1983, 191 (abstract).

87. Golde, DW, Bersch, N, Kaplan, SA, Rimoin, DL, Li, CH: *Peripheral unresponsiveness to human growth hormone in Laron dwarfism.* N Engl J Med 1156–1159, 1980.

88. Goldman, JA, Molitch, ME, Thorner, MO, Rivier, J, Vale, W. Reichlin, SR: *Growth Hor-*

mone Releasing Hormone I-40-OH (GHRH) is a Prolactin (PRL)-Releasing Factor. Endo Society, 1984, p 606.

89. GOLDSMITH, SJ, AND GLICK, SM: *Rhythmicity of human growth hormone secretions.* Mt Sinai J Med NY 37:501–509, 1970.

90. GOMEZ-PAN, A, AND RODRIGUEZ-ARNAO, MD: *Somatostatin and growth hormone releasing factor: Synthesis, location, metabolism and function.* In SCANLON, MF (ED): *Clinics in Endocrinology and Metabolism.* Saunders, London, 1983, pp 469–508.

91. GOODMAN, RH, JACOBS, JW, CHIN, WW, LUND, RK, DEE, PC, HABENER, JF: *Nucleotide sequences of a cloned structural gene coding for a precursor of pancreatic somatostatin.* Proc Natl Acad Sci USA 77:5869–5873, 1980.

92. GOURMELEN, M, PHAM-HUU-TRUNG, MT, GIRARD, F: *Transient partial hGH deficiency in prepubertal children with delayed growth.* Pediat Res 13:221–224, 1979.

93. GREEN, WH, CAMPBELL, M, DAVID, R: *Psychosocial dwarfism: A critical review of the evidence.* J Am Acad Child Psychiatry 1:39–48, 1984.

94. GROSSMAN, A, LYTRAS, N, SAVAGE, MO, WASS, JAH, COY, DH, REES, LH, JONES, AE, BESSER, GM: *Growth hormone releasing factor: Comparison of two analogues and demonstration of hypothalamic defect in growth hormone release after radiotherapy.* Br Med J 288:1785–1787, 1984.

95. GROSSMAN, A, SAVAGE, MO, WASS, JA, LYTRAS, N, SUEIRAS-DIAZ, J, COY, DH, BESSER, GM: *Growth-hormone-releasing factor in growth hormone deficiency: Demonstration of a hypothalamic defect in growth hormone release.* Lancet 2:137–138, 1983.

96. GUBLER, U, MONAHAN, JJ, LOMEDICO, PT, BHATT, RS, COLLIER, KJ, HOFFMAN, BJ, BOHLEN, P, ESCH, F, LING, N, ZEYTIN, F, BRAZEAU, P, POONIAN, MS, GAGE, LP: *Cloning and sequence analysis of cDNA for the precursor of human growth hormone-releasing factor, somatocrinin.* Proc Natl Acad Sci USA 80:4311–4314, 1983.

97. GUILLEMIN, R: *A summary of current studies with somatostatin, growth hormone releasing factors.* Clin Res 31:338–341, 1983.

98. GUIOT, G: *Transsphenoidal approach in surgical treatment of pituitary adenomas: General principles and indications in non-functioning adenomas.* In KOHLER, PO, AND ROSS, GT (EDS): *Diagnosis and Treatment of Pituitary Tumors.* American Elsevier, New York, 1973, pp 159–178.

99. GUIOT, G, AND THIBAUT, BL: *L'extirpation des adenomes hypohysaires pare voie trans-sphenoidale.* Neurochirugia (Stuttg) 1:133–150, 1959.

100. GUILLEMIN, R, BRAZEAU, P, BOHLEN, P, ESCH, F, LIN, N, WEHRENBERG, WB: *Growth hormone-releasing factor from a human pancreatic tumor that caused acromegaly.* Science 218:585–587, 1982.

101. GUILLEMIN, R, BRAZEAU, P, BOHLEN, P, ET AL: *Somatocrinin, the growth hormone releasing factor.* Recent Prog Horm Res 40:233–299, 1984.

102. GUNOZ, H, NEYZ, O, SENCER, E, ET AL: *Growth hormone secretion in protein energy malnutrition.* Acta Paediatr Scand 70:521–536, 1981.

103. HARDY, J, AND WIGSER, SM: *Trans-sphenoidal surgery of pituitary fossa tumors with televised radiofluoroscopic control.* J Neurosurg 23:612, 1965.

104. HARDY, J: *Transsphenoidal surgery of hypersecreting pituitary tumors.* In KOHLER, PO, AND ROSS, GT (EDS): *Diagnosis and Treatment of Pituitary Tumors.* American Elsevier, New York, 1973, pp 179–194.

105. HEIDINGSFELDER, SA, AND BLACKARD, WG: *Adrenergic control mechanism for vasopressin-induced plasma growth hormone response.* Metabolism 17:1019–24, 1968.

106. HIMSWORTH, RL, CARMEL, PW, FRANTZ, AG: *The location of the chemoreceptor controlling growth hormone secretion during hypoglycemia in primates.* Endocrinology 91:217–226, 1972.

107. HIZUKA, N, HENDRICKS, CM, ROTH, J, GORDON, P: *Failure of bromocriptine to alter the qualitative characteristics of human growth hormone in acromegaly.* Metabolism 33:582–584, 1984.

108. HOFFMAN, GE, AND HAYES, TA: *Somatostatin neurons and their projections in dog diencephalon.* J Comp Neurol 186:271–297, 1979.

109. HOYTE, KM, AND MARTIN, JB: *Recovery from paradoxical growth hormone responses in acromegaly after transphenoidal selective adenomectomy.* J Clin Endocrinol Metab 41:656–659, 1975.

110. IMURA, H, NAKAI, Y, YOSHIMI, T: *Effect of 5-hydroxytryptophan (5-HTP) on growth hormone and ACTH release in man.* J Clin Endocrinol Metab 36:204–206, 1973.

111. IMAKI, T, SHIBASAKI, T, SHIZUME, K, MASUDA, A, HOTTA, M, KIYOSAWA, Y, JIBIKI, K, DEMURA, H, TSUSHIMA, T, LING, N: *The effect of free fatty acids on growth hormone (GH)-releasing hormone-mediated GH secretion in man.* J Clin Endocrinol Metab 60:290–292, 1985.

112. JACKSON, IMD, AND ORMSTON, BJ: *Lack of beneficial response of serum GH in acromegaly patients treated with medroxyprogesterone acetate (MPA).* J Clin Endocrinol Metab 35:413–415, 1972.

113. JACOBWITZ, DM, SCHULTE, H, CHROUSOS, GP, LORIAUX, DL: *Localization of GRF-like immunoreactive neurons in the rat brain.* Peptides 4:521–524, 1983.

114. JACOBS, LS, SNEID, DS, GARNAND, JT, LARON, Z, DAUGHADAY, WH. *Receptor-active growth hormone in Laron dwarfism.* J Clin Endocrinol 42:403–406, 1976.

115. JADRESIC, A, BANKS, LM, CHILD, DF, ET AL: *The acromegaly syndrome: Relation between clinical features, growth hormone values and radiologic characteristics of the pituitary tumor.* Q J Med 51:189–204, 1982.

116. JADRESIC, A: *Recent developments in acromegaly: A review.* J Roy Soc Med 76:947–956, 1983.

117. KANNAN, V: *Diazepam test of growth hormone secretion.* Horm Metab Res 13:390–393, 1981.

118. KAPLAN, SL, AND GRUMBACH, MM: *Development of hormonal secretion by the human fetal pituitary gland.* In MARTINI, L, AND GANONG, WF (EDS): *Frontiers in Neuroendocrinology,* vol 4. Raven Press, New York, pp 255–276.

119. KITA, T, CHIHARA, K, ABE, H, MINAMITANI, N, KAJI, H, KODAMA, H, KASNIO, Y, OKIMURA, Y, FUJITA, T, LING, N: *Regional distribution of rat growth hormone releasing factor-like immunoreactivity in rat hypothalamus.* Endocrinology 116:259–262, 1985.

120. KLIMAN, B, KJELLBERG, RN, SWISHER, B, BUTLER, W: *Proton beam therapy of acromegaly: A 20-year experience.* In McBLACK, P, ET AL (EDS): *Secretory Tumors of the Pituitary Gland.* Raven Press, New York, 1984.

121. KOLODNY, HD, SHERMAN, L, SINGH, A, KIM, S, BENJAMIN, F: *Acromegaly treated with chlorpromazine. A case study.* N Engl J Med 284:819–822, 1971.

122. KOCH, TK, BERG, BO, ARMOND, SJ, DE GRAVINA, DF: *Creutzfeldt-Jakob disease in a young adult with idiopathic hypopituitarism.* N Engl Med 313:731–738, 1985.

123. KOVACS, K, HORVATN, E, THORNER, MO, ROGOL, AD: *Mammosomatotroph hyperplasia associated with acromegaly and hyperprolactinemia in a patient with McCune-Albright syndrome.* Virchows Archiv A 403:77–87, 1985.

124. KRIEGER, DT, GLICK, S, SILVERBERG, A, ET AL: *A comparative study of endocrine tests in hypothalamic disease. Circadian periodicity of plasma 11-OHCS and growth hormone response to insulin hypoglycemia and metyrapone responsiveness.* J Clin Endocrinol Metab 28:1589–1598, 1968.

125. KRULICH, L, ILLNER, P, FAWCETT, CP, QUIJADA, M, McCANN, SM: *Dual hypothalamic regulation of growth hormone secretion.* In PECILE, A, AND MÜLLER, EE (EDS): *Growth and Growth Hormone.* Excerpta Medica Foundation, Amsterdam, 1972, pp 306–316.

126. KVOLS, L, MARTIN, JK, MARSH, HM, MOERTEL, CG: *Rapid reversal of carcinoid crisis with a somatostatin analogue.* N Engl J Med 313:1229–1230, 1985.

127. LAL, S, MARTIN, JB, DE LA VEGA, CE, ET AL: *Comparison of the effect of apomorphine and L-dopa on serum growth hormone levels in normal men.* Clin Endocrinol (Oxf):4:277–95, 1975.

128. LAL, S, TOLIS, G, MARTIN, JB, ET AL: *Effect of clonidine on growth hormone, prolactin, luteinizing hormone, follicle-stimulating hormone, and thyroid-stimulating hormone in the serum of normal men.* J Clin Endocrinol Metab 41:827–32, 1975.

129. LAMBERTS, SW, OOSTEROM, R, NEUFELD, M, DEL POZO, E: *The somatostatin analog SMS 201–995 induces long-acting inhibition of growth hormone secretion without rebound hypersecretion in acromegalic patients.* J Clin Endocrinol Metab 60:1161–1165, 1985.

130. LARON, Z: *Syndrome of familial dwarfism and high plasma immunoreactive growth hormone.* Isr J Med Sci 10:1247–53, 1974.

131. LARON, Z, GIL-AD, T, TOPPER, E, KAUFMAN, H, JOSEFSBERG, Z: *Oral dose of clonidine: An effective screening test for growth hormone deficiency.* Acta Paediat 71:847–848, 1982.

132. LARON, Z, TOPPER, E, GIL-AD, I: *Oral clonidine—a simple, safe and effective test for growth hormone secretion.* In *Evaluation of Growth Hormone Secretion: Physiology and Clinical Application.* Pediatr Adolesc Endocrinol 12:103–115, 1983.

133. LAWRENCE, AM, AND KIRSTEINS, L: *Progestins in the medical management of active acromegaly.* J Clin Endocrinol Metab 30:646–652, 1970.

134. LAWRENCE, JH, TOBIAS, CA, LINFOOT, JA, BORN, JL, LYMAN, JT, CHONG, CY, MANOVGIAN, E, WET, WC: *Successful treatment of acromegaly. Metabolic and clinical studies in 145 patients.* J Clin Endocrinol Metab 31:180–203, 1970.

135. LAWRENCE, JH: *Heavy particle irradiation of intracranial lesions.* In WILKINS, RH AND RENGACHARY, SS (EDS): *Neurosurgery.* McGraw Hill, New York, 1984.

136. LAWS, ER, JR: *The neurosurgical management of acromegaly.* In BLACK PM, ZERVAS, NT, RIDGWAY, EC, MARTIN, JB (EDS): *Secretory Pituitary Tumors.* Raven Press, New York, 1984, pp 169–174.

137. LAWS, ER, PIEPGRAS, DG, RANDALL, RV, ABBOUD, CP: *Neurosurgical management of acromegaly.* J Neurosurg 50:454–461, 1979.

138. LIUZZI, A, CHIODINI, PG, BOTALLA, L, ET AL: *Decreased plasma growth hormone (GH) levels in acromegalics following CB 154 (2-Br-alpha-ergocryptine) administration.* J Clin Endocrinol Metab 338:910–912, 1974.

139. LIUZZI, A, CHIODINI, PG, BOTALLA, L, ET AL: *Growth hormone (GH)-releasing activity of TRH and GH-lowering effect of dopaminergic drugs in acromegaly: Homogeneity in the two responses.* J Clin Endocrinol Metab 39:871–876, 1974.

140. LECHAN, RM, MOLITCH, ME, JACKSON, IMD: *Distribution of immunoreactive human growth*

hormone-like material and thyrotropin-releasing hormone in the rat central nervous system: Evidence for their coexistence in the same neurons. Endocrinology 112:877–884, 1983.

141. LEWIN, MJ, REYL-DESMARS, F, LIND, N: Somatostatin receptor coupled with cAMP-dependent protein kinase on anterior pituitary granules. Proc Natl Acad Sci USA 80:6538–6541, 1983.

142. LEWIS, UJ, SINGH, RNP, TUTWILER, GF, SIGEL, MB, VANDERLAAN, ER, VANDERLAAN, WP: Human growth hormone: A complex of proteins. Recent Prog Horm Res 36:477–508, 1980.

143. LIN, HD, BOLLINGER, J, LING, N, REICHLIN, S: Immunoreactive growth hormone-releasing factor in human stalk median eminence. J Clin Endocrinol Metab 58:1197–1199, 1984.

144. LING, N, ESCH, R, BOHLEN, P, BRAZEAU, P, WEHRENBERG, WB, GUILLEMIN, R: Isolation, primary structure, and synthesis of human hypothalamic somatocrinin: Growth hormone-releasing factor. Proc Natl Acad Sci USA 81:4302–4306, 1984.

145. LUMPKIN, MD, NEGRO-VILAR, A, McCANN, SM: Paradoxical elevation of growth hormone by intraventricular somatostatin: Possible ultrashort-loop feedback. Science 211:1072–1074, 1980.

146. MADSEN, K, FRIBERG, U, ROOS, P, EDEN, S, ISAKSSON, O: Growth hormone stimulates the proliferation of cultured chondrocytes from rabbit ear and rabbit rib growth cartilage. Nature 304:545–547, 1983.

147. MAEDA, K, KATO, Y, CHIHARA, K, OHGO, S, IWASAKI, Y: Suppression by thyrotropin-releasing hormone (TRH) of growth hormone release induced by arginine and insulin-induced hypoglycemia in man. J Clin Endocrinol Metab 43:453–456, 1976.

148. MARLARKEY, WB, AND DAUGHADAY, WH: Variable response of plasma GH in acromegalic patients treated with medroxyprogesterone acetate. J Clin Endocrinol Metab 33:424–431, 1971.

149. MALACARA, JM, VALVERDE, C, REICHLIN, S: Elevation of plasma radioimmunoassayable growth hormone in the rat induced by porcine hypothalamic extract. Endocrinology 91:1189–98, 1972.

150. MARSHALL, PE, MARTIN, JB, MILLARD, WJ, SAGAR, SM, LANDIS, DMD: The distribution of growth hormone releasing factor (GRF) in the human hypothalamus. Abstract 1513, Presented at the 7th International Congress of Endocrinology, Quebec City, July 1984.

151. MARTIN, JB: Plasma growth hormone (GH) response to hypothalamic or extrahypothalamic electric stimulation. Endocrinology 91:107–115, 1972.

152. MARTIN, JB: Neural regulation of growth hormone secretion. Medical progress report. N Engl J Med 228:1384–1393, 1973.

153. MARTIN, JB: The role of hypothalamic and extrahypothalamic structures in the control of GH secretion. In RAITI, S (ED): Advances in Human Growth Hormone Research. DHEW publication no. (NIH)74-612, Washington, DC, 1974.

154. MARTIN, JB: Brain regulation of growth hormone secretion. In MARTINI, L, AND GANONG, WF (EDS): Frontiers in Neuroendocrinology, vol 4. Raven Press, New York, 1976, pp 129–168.

155. MARTIN, JB: Pathophysiology of growth hormone regulation. In TOLIS, G, LABRIE, F, MARTIN, JB, ET AL (eds): Clinical Neuroendocrinology: A Pathophysiological Approach. Raven Press, New York, 1979, pp 269–277.

156. MARTIN, JB: Functions of central nervous system neurotransmitters in regulation of growth hormone secretion. Fed Proc 39:2902–2906, 1980.

157. MARTIN, JB: Hypothalamic regulation of growth hormone secretion. In BLACK, PM, ZERVAS, NT, RIDGWAY, EC, MARTIN, JB: (EDS): Secretory Pituitary Tumors. Raven Press, New York, 1984, pp 109–134.

158. MARTIN, JG, BRAZEAU, P, TANNENBAUM, GS: Neuroendocrine organization of growth hormone regulation. In REICHLIN, S AND BALDESSARINI, RJ (EDS): The Hypothalamus, vol. 56. Raven Press, New York, 1978, pp 329–357.

159. MARTIN, JB, KONTOR, J, MEAD, P: Plasma GH responses to hypothalamic, hippocampal and amygdaloid electrical stimulation: Effects of variation in stimulus parameters and treatment with α-methyl-p-tyrosine (α-MT). Endocrinology 92:1354–1361, 1973.

160. MASUDA, A, SHIBASAKI, T, NAKAHARA, M, IMAKI, T, KIYOSAWA, Y, JIBIKI, K, DEMURA, H, SHIZUME, K, LING, N: The effect of glucose on growth hormone (GH)-releasing hormone-mediated GH secretion in man. J Clin Endocrinol Metab 60:523–526, 1985.

161. MATON, PN, O'DORISO, TM, HOWE, BA, MacARTHUR, KE, HOWARD, JM, CHERNER, JA, MALARKEY, TB, COLLEN, MJ, GARDNER, JD, JENSEN, RT: Effect of a long-acting somatostatin analogue (SMS 201-995) in a patient with pancreatic cholera. N Engl J Med 312:17–21, 1984.

162. MAYO, KE, VALE, W, RIVIER, J, ROSENFELD, MG, EVANS, RM: Expression-cloning and sequence of a cDNA encoding human growth hormone-releasing factor. Nature 306:86–88, 1983.

163. MELMED, S, BRAUNSTEIN, GD, HORVATH, E, EZRIN, C, KOVACS, K: Pathology of acromegaly. Endocrine Rev. 4:271–290, 1983.

164. MELMED, S, EZRIN, C, KOVACS, K, GOODMAN, RS, FROHMAN, LA: Acromegaly due to secretion of growth hormone by an ectopic pancreatic islet-cell tumor. N Engl J Med 312:9–17, 1985.

165. MERCHENTHALER, I, VIGH, S, SCHALLY, AV, PETRUSZ, P: Immunocytochemical localization of

growth hormone releasing factor in the rat hypothalamus. Endocrinology, 114:1082–1085, 1984.

166. MERIMEE, TJ, ZAPF, J, FROESCH, ER: *Dwarfism in the pygmy.* N Engl J Med 305:965–968, 1981.

167. MICHEL, D, LEFEVRE, G, LABRIE, F: *Interactions between growth hormone-releasing factor, prostaglandin E$_2$ and somatostatin on cyclic AMP accumulation in rat adenohypophysial cells in culture.* Mol Cell Endocrinol 33:255–264, 1983.

168. MILLARD, WJ, MARTIN, JB, JR, AUDET, J, SAGAR, SM, MARTIN, JB: *Evidence that reduced growth hormone secretion observed in monosodium glutamate-treated rats is the result of a deficiency in growth hormone-releasing factor.* Endocrinology 110:540–550, 1982.

169. MILLER, JD, TANNENBAUM, GS, COLLE, E, ET AL: *Daytime pulsatile growth hormone secretion during childhood and adolescence.* J Clin Endocrinol Metab 55:989–994, 1982.

170. MILLER, WL, EBERHARDT, WL: *Structure and evolution of the growth hormone gene family.* Endocrine Rev 4:97–103, 1983.

171. MOLITCH, ME: *Growth hormone hypersecretory states.* In RAITI, S, AND TOLMAN, RB (EDS): *Human Growth Hormone.* Plenum, New York, 1986, pp 29–50.

172. MONEY, J, ANNECILLO, C, KELLEY, JF: *Growth of intelligence: Failure and catchup associated respectively with abuse and rescue in the syndrome of abuse dwarfism.* Psychoneuroendocrinology 8:309–319, 1983.

173. MONTMINY, MR, GOODMAN, RH, HOROVITCH, SJ, HABENER, JF: *Primary structure of the gene encoding rat pre-prosomatostatin.* Proc Natl Acad Sci USA 81:3337–3340, 1984.

174. MORETTI, C, FABRI, A, GNESSI, L, CAPPA, M, CALZOLARI, A, FRAIOLI, F, GROSSMAN, A, BESSER, GH: *Naloxone inhibits exercise-induced release of PRL and GH in athletes.* Clin Endocrinol (Oxford) 18:135–138, 1983.

175. MOSES, AC, MOLITCH, ME, SAWIN, CT, JACKSON, IM, BILLER, BJ, EVRLANETTO, R, REICHLIN, S: *Bromocriptine therapy in acromegaly. Use in patients resistant to conventional therapy and effect on serum levels of somatomedin C.* J Clin Endocrinol Metab 53:752–758, 1981.

176. MOSHANG, T JR, PARKS, JS, VAIDYA, V, BONGIOVANNI, AM: *Recovery from probable, acquired growth hormone deficiency.* Am J Dis Child 127:397–399, 1974.

177. NORTIER, JW, CROUGHS, RJ, THIJSSEN, JH, SCHWARTZ, F: *Plasma growth hormone suppressive effect on bromocriptine in acromegaly. Evaluation by plasma GH day profiles and plasma GH concentrations during oral glucose tolerance tests.* Clin Endocrinol 20:565-571, 1984.

178. NUTT, RF, VEBER, DR, CURLEY, PE, ET AL: *Somatostatin analogs which define the role of the lysine-9 amino group.* Int J Pept Protein Res 21:66–73, 1983.

179. OPPIZZI, G, LIUZZI, A, CHIODINI, P, ET AL: *Dopaminergic treatment of acromegaly: Different effects of hormone secretion and tumor size.* J Clin Endocrinol Metab 58:988–992, 1984.

180. PALKOVITS, M, KOBAYASHI, RM, BROWN, M, VALE, W: *Changes in hypothalamic, limbic and extrapyramidal somatostatin levels following various hypothalamic transections in rat.* Brain Res 195:499–505, 1980.

181. PANDOL, SJ, SEIFERT, H, THOMAS, MW, RIVIER, J, VALE, W: *Growth hormone-releasing factors stimulates pancreatic enzyme secretion.* Science 225:326–328, 1984.

182. PARKER, DC, AND ROSSMAN, LG: *Human growth hormone release in sleep: Nonsuppression by acute hyperglycemia.* J Clin Endocrinol Metab 32:65–69, 1971.

183. PATEL, YC, AND TANNENBAUM, GS (EDS): *Somatostatin.* Adv Exp Med Biol 188, 1985.

184. PATEL, YC, RAO, K, REICHLIN, S: *Somatostatin in human cerebrospinal fluid.* N Engl J Med 296:529–533, 1977.

185. PATEL, YC, REICHLIN, S: *Somatostatin in hypothalamus, extrahypothalamic brain and peripheral tissues of the rat.* Endocrinology 102:523–530, 1978.

186. PELLETIER, G: *Immunohistochemical localization of somatostatin.* Prog Histochem Cytochem 12, 1–40, 1980.

187. PELLETIER, F, LECLERC, G, DUBE, R, LABRIE, F, PUVIANI, R, ARIMURA, A, SCHALLY, AV: *Localization of growth hormone-release-inhibiting hormone (somatostatin) in the rat brain.* Am J Anat 142:397–400, 1975.

188. PHILLIPS, LS, AND VASILOPOULOU-SELLIN, R: *Somatomedins, parts 1 and 2.* N Engl J Med 302:371–438, 1980.

189. PIETERS, GFFM, HERMUS, ARMM, SMALS, AGH, KLOPPENBORG, PWC: *Paradoxical responsiveness of growth hormone to corticotropin-releasing factor in acromegaly.* J Clin Endocrinol Metab 58:560–562, 1984.

190. PINTO, C, CELLA, SG, CORDA, R, LOCATELLI, V, PUGGIONI, R, LOCHE, S, MÜLLER, EE: *Clonidine accelerates growth in children with impaired growth hormone secretion.* Lancet 1482–1484, 1985.

191. PINTOR, C, CELLA, S, CORDA, R, LOCATELLI, V, PUGGIONI, R, LOCHE, S, MILLER, E: *Clonidine accelerates growth in children with impaired growth hormone secretion.* Lancet 1482–1484, 1985.

192. PLEWE, G, BEYER, J, KRAUSE, U, NEUFELD, M, DEL POZO, E: *Long-acting and selective suppression of growth hormone secretion by somatostatin analogue SMS 201-995 in acromegaly.* Lancet 782–784, 1984.

193. Powell, GF, Brasel, JA, Blizzard, RM: *Emotional deprivation and growth retardation simulating idiopathic hypopituitarism. II. Endocrinologic evaluation of the syndrome.* N Engl J Med 276:1279–1283, 1967.

194. Pritchard, PB, Wanamaker, BB, Sagel, J, Nair, R, DeVillier, C: *Endocrine function following complex partial seizures.* Ann Neurol 14:27–32, 1983.

195. Raptis, S, Rosenthal, J, Gerich, JE: *2nd International Symposium on Somatostatin, Athens (Greece).* Attempto Verlag Tubingen GMBH, Germany, 1984.

196. Reichlin, S: *Growth and hypothalamus.* Endocrinology 67:760–773, 1960.

197. Reichlin, S: *Regulation of somatotrophic hormone secretion.* In Harris, GW, and Donovan, BT (eds): *The Pituitary Gland,* vol 2. Butterworth, London, 1966, pp 270–298.

198. Reichlin, S: *The physiology of growth hormone regulation: Pre- and postradioimmunoassay.* Metabolism 22:987–994, 1973.

199. Reichlin, S: *Regulation of somatotrophic hormone secretion.* In Greep, RO, and Astwood, EB. (eds): *Handbook of Physiology, Section 7: Endocrinology,* vol. 4, part 2. American Physiological Society. Williams & Wilkins, Baltimore, 1975, pp 405–447.

200. Reichlin, S: *Somatostatin.* N Engl J Med 309:1495, 1983.

201. Reichlin, S: *Somatostatin.* In Krieger, DT, Brownstein, M, Martin, JB (eds): *Brain Peptides.* John Wiley & Sons, New York, 1983.

202. Reichlin, S (ed): *Fourth International Conference on Somatostatin.* Plenum, New York (in press).

203. Rivier, J, Spiess, J, Thorner, M, Vale W: *Characterization of a growth hormone-releasing factor from a human pancreatic islet tumor.* Nature 300:276–278, 1982.

204. Rodman, E, Dayal, T, Adelman, LS, Shucart, W, Reichlin, S: *Micronodular pituitary hyperplasia in acromegaly with polyostotic fibrous dysplasia* (submitted).

205. Rogol, AD, Blizzard, RM, Johanson, AJ, et al: *Growth hormone release in response to human pancreatic tumor growth hormone-releasing hormone-40 in children with short stature.* J Clin Endocrinol Metab 59:580–586, 1984.

206. Romshe, CA, Zipf, WB, Miser, A, Miser, J, Sotos, JF, Newton, WA: *Evaluation of growth hormone release and human growth hormone treatment in children with cranial irradiation-associated short stature.* J Pediatr 104:177–181, 1984.

207. Rosenthal, SM, Schriock, EA, Kaplan, SL, Guillemin, R, Grumbach, MD: *Synthetic human pancreas growth hormone-releasing factor (hpGRF 1-44-NH2) stimulates growth hormone secretion in normal men.* J Clin Endocrinol Metab 57:677–679, 1983.

208. Roth, J, Glick, SM, Yalow, RS, Berson, S: *Hypoglycemia: A potent stimulus to secretion of growth hormone.* Science 10:987–988, 1963.

209. Rudman, D, Kunter, MH, Goldsmith, MA, Blackston, RD: *Predicting the response of growth hormone-deficient children to long term treatment with human growth hormone.* J Clin Endocrinol Metab 48:472–477, 1979.

210. Rudman, D, Kutner, MH, Blackston, RD, Cushman, RA, Bain, RP, Patterson, JH: *Children with normal-variant short stature: Treatment with human growth hormone for six months.* N Engl J Med 305:123–131, 1981.

211. Sachar, EJ, Mushrush, G, Perlow, M, et al: *Growth hormone responses to L-dopa in depressed patients.* Science 178:1304–1305, 1972.

212. Schaff-Blass, E, Burstein, S, Rosenfield, RL: *Advances in diagnosis and treatment of short stature, with special reference to the role of growth hormone.* J Pediatr 104:801–813, 1984.

213. Schaison, G, Couzinet, B, Moatti, N, Pertuiset, B: *Critical study of the growth hormone response to dynamic tests and the insulin growth factor assay in acromegaly after microsurgery.* Clin Endocrinol (Oxford) 18:541–549, 1983.

214. Scheithauer, BW, Kovacs, K, Randall, RV, et al: *Hypothalamic neuronal hamartoma and adenohypophysial neuronal choristoma: Their association with growth hormone adenoma of the pituitary gland.* J Neuropathol Exp Neurol 42:648–663, 1983.

215. Schriock, EA, Lustig, RH, Rosenthal, SM, Kaplan, SL, Grumbach, MM: *Effect of growth hormone (GH)-releasing hormone (GRH) on plasma GH in relation to magnitude and duration of GH deficiency in 26 children and adults with isolated GH deficiency or multiple pituitary hormone deficiencies: Evidence for hypothalamic GRH deficiency.* J Clin Endocrinol Metab 58:1043–1049, 1984.

216. Schuster, LD, Bantle, JP, Oppenheimer, JH, Seljeskog, EL: *Acromegaly: Reassessment of long-term therapeutic effectiveness of transsphenoidal pituitary surgery.* Ann Int Med 95:172–174, 1981.

217. Sheline, GE: *Radiation therapy of pituitary tumors.* In Givens, JR (ed): *Hormone-Secreting Pituitary Tumors.* Year Book Medical Publishers, Chicago, 1982, pp 121–144.

218. Shen, LP, and Rutter, WJ: *Sequence of human somatostatin I gene.* Science 224:168–171, 1984.

219. Shibasaki, T, Shizume, K, Masuda, A, Nakahara, M, Hizuka, N, Miyakawa, M, Takano, K, Demura, H, Wakabayashi, I, Ling, N: *Plasma growth hormone response to growth hormone-releasing factor in acromegalic patients.* J Clin Endocrinol Metab 58:215–217, 1984.

GROWTH HORMONE SECRETION AND ITS DISORDERS   291

220. SHIBASAKI, T, SHIZUME, K, NAKAHARA, M, MASUDA, A, JIBIKI, K, DEMURA, H, WAKABAYASHI, I, LING, N: *Age-related changes in plasma growth hormone response to growth hormone-releasing factor in man.* J Clin Endocrinol Metab 58:212–214, 1984.

221. SHIBASAKI, T, KIYOSAWA, Y, MASUDA, A, ET AL: *Distribution of growth hormone-releasing hormone-like immunoreactivity in human tissue extracts.* J Clin Endocrinol Metab 59:263–268, 1984.

222. SLOW IN: *Ostogenic sarcoma arising in a preexisting fibrous dysplasia: Report of case.* J Oral Surg 29:126–129, 1971.

223. SMITH, RM, HOWE, PRC, OLIVER, JR, WILLOUGHBY, JO: *Growth hormone releasing factor immunoreactivity in rat hypothalamus.* Neuropeptides 4:109–115, 1984.

224. SPIESS, J, RIVIER, J, VALE, W: *Characterization of rat hypothalamic growth hormone-releasing factor.* Nature 303:532–535, 1983.

225. SPILER, IJ, AND MOLITCH, ME: *Lack of modulation of pituitary hormone stress response by neural pathways involving opiate receptors.* J Clin Endocrinol Metab 50:516–520, 1980.

226. SPILIOTIS, BE, AUGUST, GP, HUNG, W, SONIS, W, MENDELSON, W, BERCU, B: *Growth hormone neurosecretory dysfunction.* JAMA 251:2223–2230, 1984.

227. SRIKANT, CB, AND PATEL, YC: *Somatostatin analogs. Dissociation of brain receptor binding affinities and pituitary actions in the rat.* Endocrinology 108:341–343, 1981.

228. SRIKANT, CB, AND PATEL, YC: *Receptor binding of somatostatin-28 is tissue specific.* Nature 294:259–260, 1981.

229. SRIKANT, CB, AND PATEL, YC: *Somatostatin receptors: Identification and characterization in rat brain membranes.* Proc Natl Acad Sci USA 78:3930–3934, 1981.

230. SRIKANT, CB, AND PATEL, YC: *Characterization of pituitary membrane receptors for somatostatin in the rat.* Endocrinology 110:2138–2144, 1982.

231. SPEISS, J, RIVIER, J, VALE W: *Characterization of rat hypothalamic growth hormone-releasing factor.* Nature 303:532–535, 1983.

232. STEWART, C, CASTRO-MAGANA, M, SHERMAN, J, ET AL: *Septo-optic dysplasia and median cleft face syndrome in a patient with isolated growth hormone deficiency and hyperprolactinemia.* Am J Dis Child 137:484–487, 1983.

233. STRYKER, TD, CONLON, T, REICHLIN, S: *Influence of a benzadiazephine, madazolam and Gaba on basal somatostatin secretion from cerebral and diencephalic neuron in dispersed cell culture.* Brain Res 362:339–343, 1986.

234. STRYKER, T, GREENBLATT, D, REICHLIN, S: *Somatostatin suppression as possible cause of GH and TSH secretory response to benzodiazepines.* 7th International Congress of Endocrinology, September 1984.

235. TAKAHASHI, Y., KIPNIS, DM, DAUGHADAY, WH: *Growth hormone secretion during sleep.* J Clin Invest 47:2079–2090, 1968.

236. TAKANO, K, HIZUKA, N, SHIZUME, K, ET AL: *Plasma growth hormone (GH) response to GH-releasing factor in normal children with short stature and patients with pituitary dwarfism.* J Clin Endocrinol Metab 58:236–241, 1984.

237. TANNENBAUM, GS: *Growth hormone-releasing factor: Direct effects on growth hormone, glucose, and behaviour via the brain.* Science 226:464–466, 1984.

238. TANNENBAUM, GS, AND MARTIN, JB: *Evidence for an endogenous ultradian rhythm governing growth hormone secretion in the rat.* Endocrinology 98:562–570, 1976.

239. TANNENBAUM, GS, EPELBAUM, J, COLLE, E, ET AL: *Antiserum to somatostatin reverses starvation-induced inhibition of growth hormone but not insulin secretion.* Endocrinology 102:1909–1914, 1978.

240. TANNENBAUM, GS, GUYDA, HJ, POSNER, BI: *Insulin-like growth factors: A role in growth hormone negative feedback and body weight regulation via brain.* Science 220:77–79, 1983.

241. TANNENBAUM, G, MARTIN, JB, COLLE, E: *Ultradian growth hormone rhythm in the rat: Effects of feeding, hyperglycemia and insulin-induced hypoglycemia.* Endocrinology 99:720–727, 1976.

242. TANNENBAUM, GS, VAN DER REST, M, FRONMAN, LA, DOWNS, TR: *Identification of a putative GH releasing factor (GRF) batch as predominantly ovine CRF with a small quantity of human GRF.* Endocrinology 118:1246–1248, 1986.

243. TATEMOTO, K, AND MUTT, V: *Isolation and characterization of the intestinal peptide porcine PHI (PHI-27), a new member of the glucagon—secretin family.* Proc Natl Acad Sci USA 78:6603–6607, 1981.

244. TERRY, LC, WILLOUGHBY, JO, BRAZEAU, P, ET AL: *Antiserum to somatostatin prevents stress-induced inhibition of growth hormone secretion in the rat.* Science 192:565–567, 1976.

245. TERRY, LC, CROWLEY, WR, LYNCH, C, LONGSERRE, C, JOHNSON, MD: *Role of central epinephrine in regulation of anterior pituitary hormone secretion.* Peptides 3:311–318, 1982.

246. THORNER, MO, AND CRONIN, MJ: *Growth hormone-releasing factor: Clinical and basic studies.* MILLER, EE, AND FROHMAN, LA (EDS): *Neuroendocrine Perspectives.* Elsevier, Amsterdam, 1985, pp 95–114.

247. THORNER, MO, FROHMAN, LA, LEONG, DA, ET AL: *Extrahypothalamic growth-hormone-releas-*

ing factor (GRF) secretion is a rare cause of acromegaly: Plasma GRF levels in 177 acromegalic patients. J Clin Endocrinol Metab 59:846–849, 1984.

248. THORNER, MO, PERRYMAN, RL, CRONIN, MJ, ET AL: *Somatotroph hyperplasia: Successful treatment of acromegaly by removal of a pancreatic islet tumor secreting a growth hormone-releasing factor.* J Clin Invest 70:965–977, 1982.

249. THORNER, MO, RESCHKE, J, CHITWOOD, J, ROGOT, AD, FURLANETTO, R, RIVIER, J, VALE, W, BLIZZARD, RM: *Acceleration of growth in two children treated with human growth hormone-releasing factor.* N Engl J Med 312:3–9, 1985.

250. THORNER, MO, RIVIER, J, SPIESS, J: *Human pancreatic growth hormone-releasing factor selectively stimulates growth hormone secretion in man.* Lancet 1:24–28, 1983.

251. TINDALL, GT, AND TINDALL, SC: *Transsphenoidal surgery for acromegaly: Long-term results in 50 patients.* In BLACK, PM, ZERVAS, NT, RIDGWAY, EC, MARTIN, JB (EDS): *Secretory Pituitary Tumors.* Raven Press, New York, 1984, pp 175–178.

252. TOIVOLA, PTK, AND GALE, CC: *Stimulation of growth release by microinjection of norepinephrine into hypothalamus of baboons.* Endocrinology 90:895–902, 1972.

253. TOLIS, G, KOUTSILIERIS, M, BERTRAND, G: *Endocrine diagnosis of growth hormone-secreting pituitary tumors.* In BLACK, PM, ZERVAS, NT, RIDGWAY, EC, MARTIN, JB (EDS): *Secretory Pituitary Tumors.* Raven Press, New York, 1984, pp 145–154.

254. TRYGSTAD, O: *Transitory growth hormone deficiency successfully treated with human growth hormone.* Acta Endocrinologica 84:11–22, 1977.

255. TUCKER, HSG, GRUB, SR, WIGAND, JP, WATLINGTON, CO, BLACKARD, WG, BECKER, DP: *The treatment of acromegaly by transsphenoidal surgery.* Arch Intern Med 140:795–802, 1980.

256. VALENTA, LJ, SIGEL, MB, LESNIAK, MA, ET AL: *Pituitary dwarfism in a patient with circulating abnormal growth hormone polymers.* N Engl J Med 312:214–217, 1985.

257. VAN VLIET, G, STYNE, DM, KAPLAN, SL, GRUMBACH, MM: *Growth hormone treatment for short stature.* N Engl J Med 309:1016–1022, 1983.

258. VEBER, DF, FREIDINGER, RM, PERLOW, DS, PALEVEDA, WJ, HOLLY, FW, STRACHAN, RG, NUTT, RF, ARISON, BH, HOMRICK, RANDALL, WC, GLITZER, MS, SAPERSTEIN, R, HIRSCHMANN, RA: *A potent cyclic hexapeptide analog of somatostatin.* Nature 292:55–58, 1981.

259. WASS, JAH: *Growth hormone neuroregulation and the clinical relevance of somatostatin.* In SCANLON, MF (ED): *Clinics in Endocrinology and Metabolism.* WB Saunders, Philadelphia, 1983, pp 695–724.

260. WEHRENBERG, WB, BAIRD, A, LING, N: *Potent interaction between glucocorticoids and growth hormone-releasing factor in vivo.* Science 221:556–558, 1983.

261. WEHRENBERG, WB, BRAZEAU, P, LUBEN, R, BÖHLEN, P, GUILLEMIN, R: *Inhibition of the pulsatile secretion of growth hormone by monoclonal antibodies to the hypothalamic growth hormone releasing factor (GRF).* Endocrinology 111:2147–2151, 1982.

262. WEHRENBERG, WB, LING, H, BOHLEN, P, ET AL: *Physiological roles of somatocrinin and somatostatin in the regulation of growth hormone secretion.* Biochem Biophys Res Commun 109:562–567, 1982.

263. WHITTEN, CF, AND PETIT, MG: *Evidence that growth failure from maternal deprivation is secondary to undereating.* JAMA 209:1675–1682, 1969.

264. WILLIAMS, RA, JACOBS, HS, KURTZ, AB, MILLAR, JG, OAKLEY, NW, SPATHIS, GS, SULWAY, MJ, NABANO, JD: *The treatment of acromegaly with special reference to transsphenoidal hypophysectomy.* Q J Med 64:79–98, 1975.

265. WILLIAMS, T, BERELOWITZ, M, JOFFE, SN, THORNER, MO, RIVIER, J, VALE, W, FROHMAN, LA: *Impaired growth hormone response to growth hormone-releasing factor in obesity.* N Engl J Med 311:1403–1407, 1984.

266. WILLOUGHBY, JO, TERRY, LC, BRAZEAU, P, MARTIN, JB: *Pulsatile growth hormone, prolactin and thyrotropin secretion in rats with hypothalamic deafferentiation.* Brain Res 127:137–152, 1977.

267. WOOD, SM, CHNG, JL, ADAMS, EF, WEBSTER, JD, JOPLIN, GF, MASHITER, K, BLOOM, SR: *Abnormalities of growth hormone release in response to human pancreatic growth hormone releasing factor (GRF(1–44)) in acromegaly and hypopituitarism.* Br Med J Clin Res 286:1687–1691, 1983.

268. WRIGHT, AD, HILL, DM, LOWY, C, FRASER, TR: *Mortality in acromegaly.* Q J Med 39:1–16, 1970.

269. ZIMMERMAN, EA, CARMEL, PW, HUSAIN, MK, ET AL: *Vasopressin and neurophysin: High concentrations in monkey hypophyseal portal blood.* Science 182:925–927, 1973.

270. ZIMMERMAN, EA, DEFENDINI, R, FRANTZ, AG: *Prolactin and growth hormone in patients with pituitary adenomas: A correlative study of hormone in tumor and plasma by immunoperoxidase technique and radioimmunoassay.* J Clin Endocrinol Metab 38:577–585, 1974.

271. RAITI, S, AND TOLMAN, RA (EDS): *Human Growth Hormone.* Plenum, New York, 1986.

272. ATKINSON, PR, WEIDMAN, ER, BHAUMICK, B, BALA, RM: *Release of somatomedin-like activity by cultured WI-38 human fibroblasts.* Endocrinology 106:2006–2012, 1980.

273. CASANUEVA, FF, VILLANUEVA, L, CABRANES, JA, ET AL: *Cholinergic mediation of growth hormone secretion elicited by arginine, clonidine, and physical exercise in man.* J Clin Endocrinol Metab 59:526–529, 1984.

274. CASANUEVA, FF, VILLANUEVA, L, DIEGUEZ, C, ET AL: *Atropine blockade of growth harmone (GH) releasing hormone-induced GH secretion in man is not exerted at pituitary level.* J Clin Endocrinol Metab 62:186–191, 1986.

275. RICHARDSON, SB, HOLLANDER, CS, DE' LETTO, R: *Acetylcholine inhibits the release of somatostatin from rat hypothalamus in vitro.* Endocrinology 107:122–129, 1980.

276. ROBBINS, RJ, SUTTON, RE, REICHLIN, S: *Effects of neurotransmitters and cyclic AMP on somatostatin release from cultured cerebral cortical cells.* Brain Res 234:377–386, 1982.

277. PETERFREUND, R, VALE, GR: *Muscarinic cholinergic stimulation of somatostatin secretion from long-term dispersed cell cultures of fetal rat hypothalamus—inhibition by gamma-amino-butyric acid and serotonin.* Endocrinology 112:526–534, 1983.

278. BENOIT, R, BEHLEM, P, LING, N, ET AL: *Somatostatin-28$_{1-12}$-like peptides.* In PATEL, YC, AND TANNENBAUM, GS (EDS): *Somatostatin.* Adv Exp Biol Med 188:89–108, 1985.

279. SCHÖNBRUNN, A, DORFLINGER, LJ, KOCH, BD: *Mechanisms of somatostatin action in pituitary cells.* In PATEL, YC, AND TANNENBAUM, GS (EDS): *Somatostatin.* Adv Exp Biol Med 188:305–324, 1985.

280. COY, DH, MURPHY, WA, LANCE, VA, ET AL: *Somatostatin agonists and antagonists—peptide control of growth hormone secretion.* In PATEL, YC, AND TANNENBAUM, GS (EDS): *Somatostatin.* Adv Exp Biol Med 188:325–337, 1985.

281. MARBACH, P, NEUFELD, M, PLESS, J: *Clinical applications of somatostatin analogues.* In PATEL, YC, AND TANNENBAUM, GS (EDS): *Somatostatin.* Adv Exp Biol Med 188:339–353, 1985.

282. MACGILLIVRAY, MH: *Clinical features, tests, and causes of growth hormone deficiency.* In RAITI, S, AND TOLMAN, R (EDS): *Human Growth Hormone.* Plenum, New York, 1986, pp 51–65.

283. FROHMAN, LA, THOMINET, JL, SZABOR, M: *Ectopic growth hormone-releasing factor synclromes.* In RAITI, S, AND TOLMAN, RA (EDS): *Human Growth Hormone.* Plenum, New York, 1986, pp 347–360.

284. BERCU, BB, SHULMAN, D, ROOT, AW, ET AL: *Growth hormone (GH) provocative testing frequently does not reflect endogenous GH deficiency.* J Clin Endocrinol Metab 63:709–716, 1986.

285. MECHANICK, JI, HOCHBERG, FH, LA ROCQUE, A: *Hypothalamic dysfunction following whole-brain irradiation.* J Neurosurg 65:490–494, 1986.

286. YOKOTA, M, TANI, E, MAEDA, Y, ET AL: *Acromegaly associated with suprasellar and pulmonary hemangiopericytomas.* J Neurol Surg 63:767–771, 1985.

Chapter 9

NEUROENDOCRINOLOGY OF REPRODUCTION

Perpetuation of the species requires that maturation of eggs in the ovary and sperm in the testes be correlated with mating behavior. These functions are integrated by complex neuroendocrine mechanisms involving the brain, the pituitary gland, and the sex steroid hormones. Neural factors determine the onset of puberty and the initiation and maintenance of lactation. That neural control is involved in human pituitary-gonad function is clear from the clinical effects of disease of the hypothalamus, emotional stress, and psychopharmacologic drugs.

HORMONES INVOLVED IN PITUITARY-GONAD REGULATION

PITUITARY HORMONES

The two hormones of the pituitary responsible for regulation of the gonads are follicle-stimulating hormone (FSH) and luteinizing hormone (LH).[19,22,52,71,120,123] Together they are termed *gonadotropins*. The luteinizing hormone has also been called interstitial cell stimulating hormone (ICSH), because in the male subject it stimulates the secretion of interstitial cells (Leydig cells) of the testes, the cellular source of the secretion of testosterone. Today, only the term luteinizing hormone (LH) is used to describe the hormones secreted by both sexes.

Both FSH and LH are glycoproteins, that is, they contain an appreciable amount of carbohydrate, a component that is responsible for the characteristic basophilic staining of the anterior pituitary gonadotrope cells. The two pituitary gonadotropins are chemically related to a third, human chorionic gonadotropin (HCG). Human chorionic gonadotropin is secreted by the placenta as early as the ninth day of pregnancy and is the basis of the common pregnancy tests. In its biologic actions HCG closely resembles LH, and in fact is used clinically to induce ovulation in anovulatory women. It is important in clinical medicine also because of the occasional abnormal (ectopic) secretion of HCG by hydatidiform mole and choriocarcinoma, both derived from placenta. Tumors of the testes and teratomas of the lung, hypothalamus, and the pineal gland (cells of germ cell lines) also may secrete HCG,[61] as may other parenchymal tumors including bronchogenic carcinoma and pancreatic carcinoma. In some

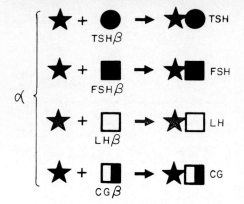

FIGURE 1. The subunit nature of the glycoprotein hormones is shown here. Each glycoprotein hormone consists of two different glycopeptide subunits called α and β, which are products of separate genes. The common α-subunit (shown here as a star) associates with a specific β-subunit in a noncovalent fashion to yield the biologically active dimer. The four hormones in this family are TSH, FSH, LH, and CG. (From Chin, WW,[22] with permission.)

nonendocrine tumors the abnormal secretion may serve as a marker of cancer.

Human menopausal gonadotropin (HMG), a slightly altered mixture of pituitary gonadotropins (mainly FSH-like), is excreted in large amounts by menopausal and castrated women.

> The immunoassayable form of gonadotropins may not correspond completely to the biologically active form, and values may vary markedly from minute to minute, particularly in patients with high levels, thus reflecting the pulsatile release of gonadotropins. By agreement, the potency of LH and FSH is related to an international reference preparation (IRP) of partially purified urinary menopausal gonadotropin, maintained in the Biologic Standards Laboratory of the National Research Council in Mill Hill, England. The National Hormone Distribution Committee of the National Institutes of Health has provided an immunoassay reference preparation from human pituitary extract which has been standardized by bioassay, using the IRP as reference. Values for immunoassayable LH and FSH now appearing in current literature usually are related to equivalents of the IRP and are given as international units (IU).

All the gonadotropic hormones (both pituitary and placental) and thyrotropin (thyroid-stimulating hormone, TSH) are composed of two chains, termed α and β, which are dissociable under relatively mild conditions. The α chains of all four hormones are virtually identical in chemical behavior and amino acid sequence. Specificity is a function of the β chain, which is different for each hormone (Fig. 1). Immunoassays can now use this property to measure the characteristic β chain of each hormone and thus provide specific measurements. The molecular biology of biosynthesis of α and β chains has been elucidated.[22]

GONADAL HORMONES

Under control of the two gonadotropins the gonads form germ cells and secrete sex steroids.[52,120] There are three main classes of sex steroids: estrogens, progestins, and androgens (Fig. 2). The etymologic derivations of the names of these hormones provide an excellent clue to their key actions. Estrogens (*oistros,* mad desire + *gennan,* to produce) are substances that bring about estrus, that is, sexual receptivity in the female sex. The term has been extended to mean a hormone that brings about characteristic female

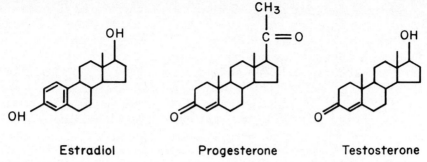

| Estradiol | Progesterone | Testosterone |

FIGURE 2. Structural formulae of principal sex steroids are shown here. The three classes of steroids involved in sexual function are estrogens, progestogens (gestagens), and androgens. Estradiol-17β, progesterone, and testosterone are the most important steroids of these classes. The ovary secretes other related estrogens and progestins as well as testosterone. The testis secretes testosterone and small amounts of estradiol-17β. Some conversion of testosterone to estrogenic hormones can take place in peripheral tissues, including fat and brain.

changes, such as growth of the uterus and breasts, female type of skeletal structure, and female pattern of fat distribution of buttocks, thighs, and abdomen. Progestins (*pro*, before + *gestare*, to bear) prepare the uterus for implantation of a fertilized egg and maintain gestation. Hormones of this type also are involved in the differentiation of the breast. Androgens (*andros*, man + *gennan*, to produce) stimulate the development of characteristic male features, such as hair on face and chest, growth of the accessory sex organs (penis, prostate, seminal vesicles), skeleton and muscle development, deepening of the voice (growth of the larynx), and regression of scalp hair in genetically susceptible individuals.

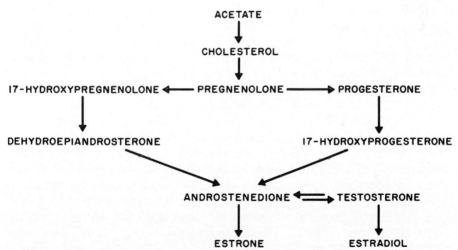

FIGURE 3. Pathways of enzymatic synthesis of gonadal steroids are shown here. The biosynthetic pathway of sex steroids in both ovary and testis is outlined. Many intermediate steps up to pregnenolone are omitted. From acetate as precursor the steroid nucleus is synthesized by way of cholesterol. In both ovary and testis, testosterone is a precursor of estradiol. Thus in tumors or synthetic defects of the ovary, excessive testosterone may be synthesized, thus causing virilization; tumors of the testis may produce estrogens. Dehydroepiandrosterone and androstenedione are synthesized and secreted chiefly by the adrenal cortex. These are precursors of both estrogens and androgens.

All three classes of steroid hormones are synthesized from acetate through cholesterol by a series of enzymatic transformations in both the cytosol and the mitochondria of hormone-producing cells in the gonads. Analogous syntheses take place in the adrenal cortex: hence the occasional abnormal estrogen or androgen production by adrenal tumors, the abnormal production of estrogens by testicular tumors, or the secretion of testosterone by the ovary. A schematic outline is shown in Figure 3. It is important to recognize that particular steps in hormone biosynthesis can be blocked in certain genetic diseases of the adrenal gland, or by certain drugs.

Of the hormones secreted by the ovary, estradiol 17β is the most important of the estrogens, and progesterone is the most important of the progestins. The principal androgen secreted by the testis is testosterone, but in certain target glands such as male accessory structures, testosterone is converted to dihydrotestosterone, a tissue-active form of the hormone. The adrenal glands of both men and women secrete hormones that can be converted in peripheral tissues to weekly androgenic compounds that are less potent than testosterone. If secreted in increased amounts, these steroids may bring about mild or even severe masculinization. The adrenal androgens are necessary for maintaining libido in women.

HYPOTHALAMIC HYPOPHYSIOTROPIC HORMONES

The third hormonal link in pituitary-gonad regulation is the hypothalamic gonadotropin releasing hormone (GnRH).[27] This substance, originally isolated from the porcine hypothalamus by Matsuo and collaborators[88] and Schally,[126] is a linear decapeptide (Fig. 4) that has all the hormonal properties of the native hormone isolated from porcine, ovine, and human hypothalamic tissue. It also is called luteinizing hormone releasing hormone (LHRH) because of its potent effects on LH secretion. The injection of the GnRH brings about the release of both of the gonadotropic hormones, LH and FSH (Fig. 5),[11,48,66,96] and for this reason, most workers now believe that this material is the principal hypophysiotropic factor regulating gonadotropin release.[152] It has been proposed that there is a second FSH-releasing factor distinct from GnRH, but the chemical evidence on which this claim is based is not extensive; evidence supporting this view has been summarized by McCann and colleagues.[91] All the known effects of the hypothalamus on both FSH and LH can be explained by variations in dose, timing, and steroid hormone interaction at the pituitary level with a single GnRH; furthermore, gonadotropic hormone-releasing effects of hypothalamic extracts are blocked by antibody to the GnRH decapeptide. In addition, the ovary and testis secrete a peptide designated *inhibin* (also termed folliculostatin) which acts relatively specifically to inhibit FSH secretion.[4,158] The ovary also secretes a follicle-stimulating peptide that is structurally related to inhibin.[160,161] Its function is unknown. The pituitary-stimulating effects of GnRH are specifically restricted to changes in gonadotropic hormone

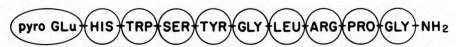

FIGURE 4. The amino-acid sequence of gonadotropin-releasing hormone (GnRH).

REGULATION OF THE PITUITARY GLAND

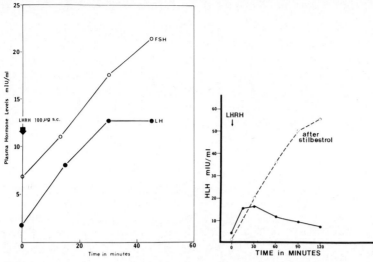

FIGURE 5. (*Left*) Effect of intravenous injection of GnRH on serum LH and FSH levels in a woman with galactorrhea-amenorrhea owing to prolactinoma. (*Right*) Response of LH in a normal woman during the follicular phase of the menstrual cycle. Treatment with stilbestrol for 5 days sensitized the response. (Left figure from Reichlin, S: *The control of anterior pituitary secretion.* In Beeson, PB, and McDermott, W (eds): *Textbook of Medicine.* WB Saunders, Philadelphia, 1975, p 1671, with permission.)

secretion, none of the other anterior pituitary hormones being released in response to injection of this hypothalamic hormone. One exception to this generalization is the finding that GnRH releases GH in some patients with acromegaly.[37] GnRH has been shown to be different in several species of birds and fish.[6,67,132] Its molecular biology has been elucidated using human placenta as starting material[129] (see chapter 18).

The pattern of administration of GnRH is of crucial importance to pituitary secretory responses. As shown in the rhesus monkey subjected to arcuate nucleus lesions (which renders them GnRH deficient) and confirmed in the human being, sustained high secretion of LH and FSH requires pulsatile doses of GnRH administered at approximately the same intervals that correspond to the normal pulse in blood gonadotropic level, that is, approximately 60 to 90 minutes[8,71,85] (Fig. 6). If GnRH (or analogs) is given continuously, gonadotropin secretion is suppressed (see Figure 6). These properties are the basis of the clinical use of GnRH in treatment of anovulation, infertility, precocious puberty, and prostatic carcinoma, among other disorders (see below). The timing of pulsation determines the ratio of FSH to LH. Within certain limits, infrequent pulses raise FSH/LH ratios.[86] The gonadal steroids also interact with GnRH in gonadotropic control (see below).

The mechanism of GnRH action on gonadotropic cells has been defined.[28,162]

> GnRH binds to a specific class of membrane receptors localized to patches on cells (indicating segregation of receptors), gathers into a "cap," and is internalized. The GnRH receptor is internalized, but internalization is not necessary for action. Following binding, changes in membrane enzyme activity lead to the increase of phosphoinositide turnover with an increase in the formation of inositol phosphate 3

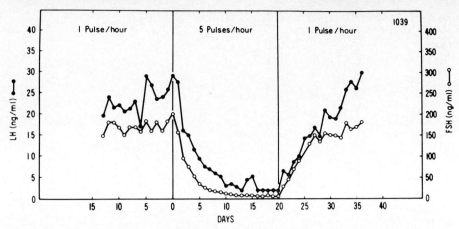

FIGURE 6. Gonadotropin secretion is maintained in a monkey with a large hypothalamic lesion by the pulsatile administration of GnRH at 1 pulse per hour. Infusion of GnRH at 5 pulses per hour leads to suppression of LH and FSH secretion.

and diacyl glycerol in a manner analogous with the changes produced in thyrotropes by TRH. In addition, calcium uptake is stimulated, and intracellular calcium is mobilized from intracellular compartments. Through a series of phosphorylations of regulatory proteins the release process is activated, and activated complexes bind to specific gene sequences to stimulate new hormone production.

LEVELS OF HYPOTHALAMIC FUNCTION IN PITUITARY-GONAD CONTROL

Secretion of GnRH by GnRH-peptidergic neurons constitutes the final common pathway of gonadotropin control. The function of these neurons is involved in many aspects of gonadotropin regulation. These aspects include the maintenance of "basal" levels of secretion, generation of the phasic release of gonadotropins responsible for ovulation, determination of the time of onset of puberty, and integration of mating behavior with gonadal readiness.[8]

Under basal conditions in both men and women, pituitary secretion of LH and FSH is episodic, one secretory burst occurring approximately each hour (Fig. 7).[16,17,20] The amplitude of the bursts is greater in castrated or hypogonadal individuals. Based on studies in monkeys, who manifest similar secretory bursts,[18] it seems likely that the spiking of secretion is due to changes in hypothalamic secretion of GnRH. In sexually mature women, the "ovulatory surge" of gonadotropin secretion is imposed upon the basal secretion pattern.[9] The occurrence of an ovulatory surge is widely considered to be characteristic of the "female" pattern of gonadotropin secretion, whereas the tonic phase (with minor spiking) is considered typical of the "male" gonadotropin pattern.[51] Most workers believe that the ability to release gonadotropins in an ovulatory surge pattern means that the hypothalamic-pituitary axis has a positive-feedback capacity, but the exact site of the positive-feedback receptor(s) is still under study (see below). The rise in LH that precedes ovulation is composed of a series of progressively larger surges.

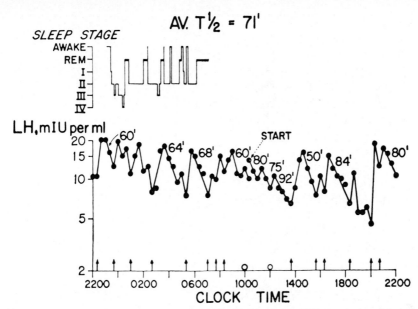

FIGURE 7. Plasma LH concentration sampled every 20 minutes for 24 hours in an adult male. In the mature subject, cyclic changes in plasma gonadotropic hormones occur throughout the day and night and are unrelated to cyclic brain activity. (From Boyar, R,[16] with permission.)

The hypothalamus also is involved in determining the time of onset of puberty.

Finally, the hypothalamus, at a still higher level of function, is responsible for integrating sexual behavior with the function of the gonads. Patterned sexual behavior, so readily induced in lower forms by sex hormones, facilitates mating so that insemination can occur when the egg is ripe. The far more complex nature of the hormonal control of human sexual behavior will be discussed in chapter 20.

NEURAL PATHWAYS OF CONTROL OF GONADOTROPIN SECRETION

In human beings, as in vertebrates, GnRH in nerve endings is found in highest concentration in the median eminence of the hypothalamus in the portal-vessel contact zone. These fibers reach the median eminence by two routes, a lateral one which parallels the base of the brain, and a periventricular one which parallels the third ventricle.[68,69] Cells of origin of these pathways are dispersed in the preoptic area and basal hypothalamus (Fig. 8). Studies using antisera specific for processed and precursor forms of GnRH indicate that the peptide is processed in transit presumably by specific enzymes in granules during transport toward the terminal. In the human being, GnRH fibers also terminate in the neurophysis (Fig. 9).

Most GnRH neurons are bipolar. In rats one terminal is in the median eminence and the other in the organum vasculosum of the lamina terminalis (OVLT).

Electrical stimulation studies of the hypothalamus confirm that regions in which GnRH neurons are present release LH and FSH into the blood (Figs. 10,11)

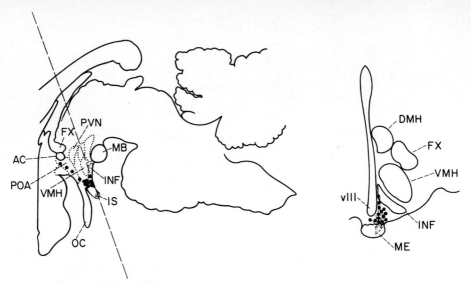

FIGURE 8. Anatomic localization of GnRH in the human brain. (From Riskind, P, and Martin, JB,[166] with permission.)

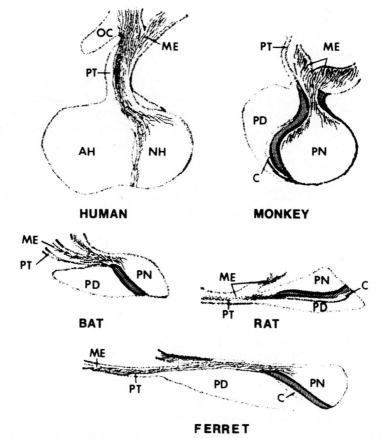

HUMAN　　　**MONKEY**

BAT　　　**RAT**

FERRET

FIGURE 9. Comparative anatomic studies of distribution of GnRH-staining nerve fibers in hypothalmus and pituitary gland. In all species studied, GnRH terminals are found in the median eminence. In several species, including the human being (but not the rat), GnRH fibers also terminate in the neural lobe. (From King, JC, and Anthony, ELP,[68] with permission.)

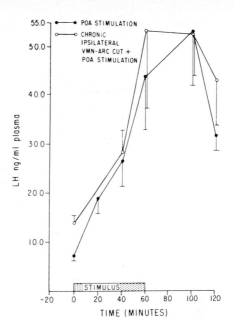

FIGURE 10. Effect of electrical stimulation of the preoptic area (POA) of the hypothalamus on plasma LH in the rat is shown here. This experiment illustrates the presence of electrically excitable neurons in the POA that regulate secretion of GnRH. Hemisections in the region of the ventromedial nucleus (VMN-ARC) failed to interfere with ipsilateral preoptic simulations: Evidently fibers from the POA to the median eminence do not cross anterior to this region. On the other hand, there is evidence from other transection studies for crossover between the VMN-arcuate complex and the median eminence itself. (From Cramer, OM, and Barraclough, CA: *Effects of preoptic electrical stimulation on pituitary LH release following interruption of components of the preoptico-tuberal pathway in rats.* Endocrinology 93:369–376, 1973, with permission.)

Some GnRH positive terminals can be shown to end on other nuclei in the hypothalamus and limbic system,[68] suggesting a nonpituitary regulating function. They also terminate on other GnRH cells,[70] suggesting an autofeedback function previously postulated as an ultra short-loop feedback by Motta and associates,[99] based on their studies of intrahypothalamic injections. Gonadotropin-releasing hormone neurons are found in the olfactory system,[153] where they may be important in mediating sexual behavior in rodents.

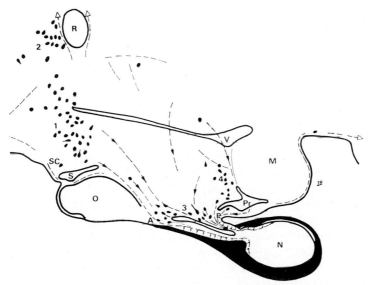

FIGURE 11. Localization of sites in rat hypothalmus electrically excitable for LH release (From Clemens, JA, et al: *Areas of the brain stimulatory to LH and FSH secretion.* Endocrinology 88: 180, 1971, with permission.)

NEUROENDOCRINOLOGY OF REPRODUCTION   303

Neurotransmitters and Gonadotropin Regulation

The secretion of GnRH is influenced by neural inputs — catecholaminergic, serotonergic, cholinergic, and peptidergic.[7,65,131,145] The relative importance of these pathways and substantial differences among species have made this subject somewhat difficult to interpret. The classical studies of Sawyer and colleagues,[124] among the first to demonstrate that ovulation was under neuropharmacologic control, showed that reflex ovulation in the rabbit could be blocked by treatment with high doses of atropine, an acetylcholine blocker, or with dibenzyline, an α-adrenergic antagonist. In the rabbit, ovulation can be induced regularly by the intrahypothalamic injection of norepinephrine. In rats, gonadotropin secretion at midcycle is blocked by inhibitors of α-adrenergic receptors, and partially blocked by agents that inhibit the synthesis of either norepinephrine or epinephrine. If both are inhibited, ovulation is completely blocked. Administration of α-adrenergic blockers, moreover, inhibits the spontaneous pulsatile secretion of LH in monkeys and in rats. It is clear from these data that central catecholamines play an important role in regulation of the ovulatory surge in laboratory animals. Inasmuch as hypothalamic catecholaminergic pathways arise, for the most part, from ascending noradrenergic pathways originating in the locus coeruleus and neighboring nuclei, it would seem evident that neural inputs from this region must impinge upon GnRH neurons. Moreover, both inhibitory and excitatory adrenergic impulses also have been described. In the human being, depletion of hypothalamic catecholamines by reserpine can cause anovulation. In keeping with the idea that central catecholamines are important in gonadotropin regulation is the extensive evidence that gonadal state markedly changes the rate of synthesis of dopamine and norepinephrine in the brain (see Fuxe and others[49] for review).

Even the feedback effects of gonadal steroids, so important in regulation of gonadotropins, may be exerted by way of catecholaminergic pathways because inhibition of catecholamine synthesis blockers prevents estrogen-induced ovulation,[1] and a detailed study has failed to show estrogen receptors on GnRH cells,[133] thus implying that the steroid target must be directed at a more remote target.

Having drawn this generalization, we must admit that the role of catecholamines in human gonadotropin regulation is not well worked out in comparison with data available in laboratory animals.

Other neurotransmitters also have been implicated in gonadotropin regulation.[110] A large and contradictory literature on the role of serotonergic stimuli has been published, with reports of either inhibition or stimulation. An anatomic basis for serotonergic control has been established by demonstration of serotonin-containing nerve endings terminating on GnRH-containing hypothalamic cells.[70] Dopamine also has been implicated in the regulation of gonadotropin secretion, especially in the human female. L-dopa (the precursor to dopamine) has been reported to inhibit LH secretion, and metoclopramide, a dopamine antagonist, to increase LH secretion. Under certain conditions, the pulsatile pattern of PRL secretion is paralleled exactly by pulsatility of LH.[20] L-dopa administration inhibits LH secretion.[107]

A number of endogenous peptidergic pathways have been implicated in gonadotropin regulation at the hypothalamic level. Most data available concern the endogenous opioid peptides.[23,39,40,53,106] Morphine inhibits gonadotropin secretion in both men and women (causing infertility, anovulation, and low testosterone levels), and in a number of women with stress-induced amenorrhea, the administration of naloxone (an opiate antagonist) has led to gonadotropin release. These findings are taken to mean that stress-induced amenorrhea may be due to excess endogenous opioid activity. Endogenous opioids appear to play a physiologic role in regulation of the menstrual cycle. Infusion of naloxone raises LH levels when administered during the second half of the menstrual cycle[138] (and at least one group has reported that naloxone raises LH during the first half of the cycle also). Ferrin[38] has proposed that the opioid effect is primarily a change in the frequency of GnRH pulses; slowing pulse frequency causes a relatively greater inhibition of LH than of FSH.

But the opioids are not the only hypothalamic peptides that affect gonadotropin secretion. At the level of the hypothalamus, vasoactive intestinal peptide (VIP) and substance P bring about LH release.[90] Central actions of corticotropin-releasing factor (CRF) and neuropeptide Y[92] have been reported to inhibit gonadotropin secretion, and α-MSH also increases LH release.[113]

NEGATIVE FEEDBACK CONTROL OF GONADOTROPIC HORMONE SECRETION

Deficiency of gonad secretion — whether occurring "spontaneously" as in menopausal women, after castration in men and women, or developmentally as in certain chromosomal disorders — leads to increased secretion of both LH and FSH. Administration of estrogens or androgens leads to a fall in plasma gonadotropin levels (Fig. 12). These observations indicate that sex steroids regulate gonadotropic hormones through negative-feedback mechanisms.

There are two components of the feedback effect of estrogens. Brief exposure to estrogens diminishes the sensitivity of the pituitary gland to GnRH (Fig. 13). Longer-term exposure to estrogens sensitizes the pituitary gland to GnRH (see Figure 5). The bulk of evidence suggests that long-term suppression of gonadotropins by estrogens is exerted at the hypothalamic level. In men, long-term exposure to estrogens suppresses pituitary responsiveness to GnRH.[130] Testosterone also causes long-term suppression of gonadotropins in men but does so by acting on the hypothalamus. In the sexually mature woman, a "positive-feedback" control system develops which is responsible for inducing the midcycle ovulatory surge (see below). The various elements of hypothalamic-pituitary gonadal control are summarized in Figures 14 and 15.

Self-priming Action of GnRH

Before we discuss the regulation of the normal menstrual cycle, another property of GnRH should be emphasized. In addition to the finding that pulsatile GnRH can maintain normal gonadotropin secretion, and that

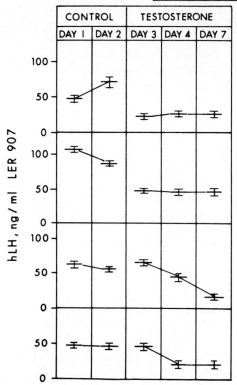

EFFECT OF TESTOSTERONE, 300 mg I.M.
ON hLH LEVELS IN 4 MEN

FIGURE 12. Inhibitory effects of sex steroids on LH secretion are illustrated here. The administration of testosterone to men results in a fall in plasma hLH demonstrating the negative-feedback control.

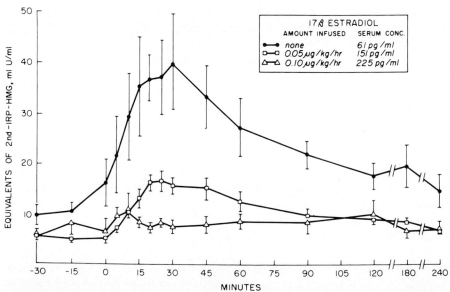

FIGURE 13. Modulation of pituitary gonadotropin response to GnRH by estradiol infusions. Estradiol was infused intravenously to maintain levels of hormone within the physiologic range. Increasing levels of estradiol were found to inhibit pituitary responses to GnRH. This illustrates the negative-feedback component of estrogen effect on the pituitary gland. If given for longer periods of time, estradiol sensitizes the pituitary gland to exogenous GnRH (see Figure 5). (From Keye, WR, Jr, and Jaffe, RB: *Modulation of pituitary gonadotropin response to gonadotropin-releasing hormone by estradiol.* J Clin Endocrinol Metab 38:805, 1974, with permission.)

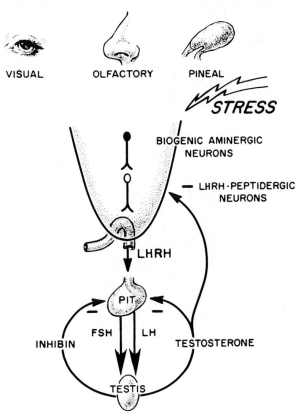

VISUAL   **OLFACTORY**   **PINEAL**

STRESS

BIOGENIC AMINERGIC NEURONS

LHRH-PEPTIDERGIC NEURONS

LHRH

PIT

FSH   LH

INHIBIN   TESTOSTERONE

TESTIS

FIGURE 14. This is a schematic diagram of the gonadotropin control system in men, showing the interactions of neural and hormonal feedback controls. Pituitary gland and testis are connected by a negative feedback link. Secretion of testosterone by the testis is stimulated by LH; maturation and growth of the tubule cells, by FSH. The secretion of testosterone in turn inhibits the secretion of LH. It is likely that the major target of negative feedback is the hypothalamus; long-term testosterone administration in men does not interfere with the effectiveness of LHRH (pituitary sensitivity is relatively unaltered). A newly discovered peptide secretion of the testis, "inhibin," is believed to be secreted by tubular epithelium and to exert a direct inhibitory effect on FSH secretion. It is not known whether inhibin affects the hypothalamus directly. The LHRH-peptidergic neurons are in turn regulated by a biogenic amine neural system that links gonadotropin regulation to the remainder of the brain. Through this system a wide variety of impulses can be brought to bear on reproductive function. Stimuli affecting male gonadotropic function have been well demonstrated in experimental animals, though they are not as well worked out in the human being. Visual influences include light-induced changes in seasonal breeders such as domestic cattle, deer, and birds. Olfactory signals in male rats influence gonadal function. The pineal gland in many species of animals inhibits gonadotropin secretion by a direct effect of a pineal secretion either on the hypothalamus or on the pituitary gland.

sustained GnRH inhibits gonadotropin secretion (see above), it has also been shown that exposure of the pituitary gland to pulsatile GnRH sensitizes it to further injections of GnRH. This is illustrated in Figure 16, which shows that the first response to GnRH is less than the second response. It has been postulated that this effect is due to stimulation of GnRH receptors on the pituitary gland. This phenomenon has important clinical implications. In the patient with long-standing deficiency of GnRH (as, for example, in anorexia nervosa) initial responses to GnRH are very small or absent; they increase with continued pulsatile exposure.

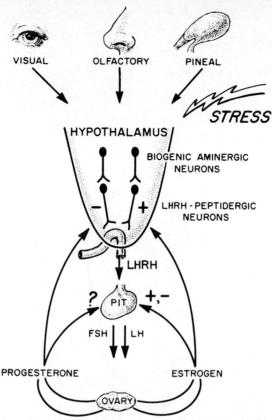

FIGURE 15. This is a schematic diagram of gonadotropin control system in women, showing the interactions of neural and hormonal feedback controls. The development of the ovarian follicle is largely under control of the follicle-stimulating hormone (FSH). Secretion of estrogens by the developing follicle is both FSH- and LH-dependent. Ovulation is brought about by the luteinizing hormone (LH), which stimulates the secretion of progesterone in addition to estrogenic hormones. Estrogenic hormones have complex effects on the feedback control mechanism of LH and FSH secretion. Depending upon dose, time course, and prior hormonal status, estrogens can either inhibit or stimulate the secretion of LH through effects at both hypothalamic and pituitary levels. Thus, there is evidence for both negative and positive feedback control. Progesterone also can either stimulate or inhibit LHRH secretion, depending upon the setting in which it is given, but its effects at the pituitary level are relatively insignificant. Secretions of the LHRH peptidergic neurons are in turn regulated by the biogenic-aminergic system through which a variety of nonhormonal signals can influence reproductive function. Visual stimuli in many lower animals can influence onset of sexual function (as in seasonal breeders). Olfactory signals through "pheromones" influence estrus cycles in many rodents, and may do so in women. Pineal factors in lower animals delay onset of puberty.

REGULATION OF THE MENSTRUAL CYCLE

Normal women menstruate regularly at approximately 28-day intervals and ovulate on the fourteenth day of the cycle (the first day of bleeding is designated day 1). The menses are due to the loss of the endometrium-stimulating effects of estrogens and progesterone, the plasma levels of which drop dramatically toward the end of the cycle.

Plasma levels of the pituitary and gonad secretions follow a characteristic pattern through a normal cycle (Fig. 17). During the menses, plasma levels of progesterone and 17 β-estradiol are at the lowest levels of the

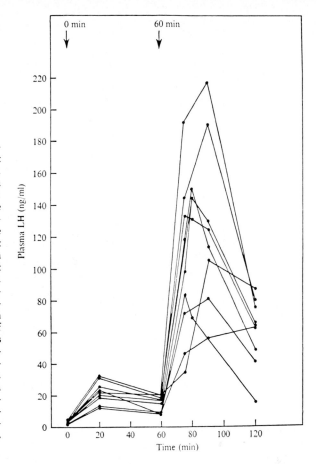

FIGURE 16. The "priming" effect of GnRH on subsequent response to GnRH in the rat. Female rats were injected with two equal doses of GnRH at 1 hour intervals. Note that the response to the second injection is much greater than to the first. It has been proposed that due to the continuing secretion of modestly increased GnRH at the time of the midcycle surge, there is an accelerating secretory responsiveness contributing to the ovulatory increase in LH secretion characteristic of midcycle. Similar experiments in humans indicate that estrogens must be present to produce this effect. (From Aiyer, MS, Chiappa, SA, Fink, G: *A priming effect of luteinizing hormone releasing factor on the anterior pituitary gland in the female rat.* J Endocrinol 62:573, 1974, with permission.)

cycle. During the first half of the cycle the follicle grows and matures under the influence of FSH and LH. Early in this follicular phase, the hormonal secretion of the ovary is quite modest, but toward the middle of the cycle a burst of estrogen secretion occurs, accompanied by a modest increase in 20α-progesterone, a progesterone analog. This hormonal secretion comes from the follicle itself and appears to be due to a continuing secretion of FSH and an increasingly responsive follicular cell. This time course of sensitization is programmed genetically in the ovary and is not due to increasing stimulation by FSH. The spurt of estrogen appears to be crucial in triggering the neuroendocrine mechanisms which bring about ovulation. This was shown by giving a bolus injection of estrogen to women during the follicular phase which brings about a normal gonadotropin surge (Fig. 18). Detailed studies by Hoff and coworkers[59] and Liu and associates[78] have clarified the hormonal events around the midcycle. They have shown that the secretion of progesterone that precedes the onset of ovulatory gonadotropin surge, though quite small, is crucial to the development of a normal ovulatory pattern. They reconstruct the events at midcycle as follows (Fig. 19):

"Incremental E_2 (estradiol) is the ovarian signal that triggers the onset of the LH-FSH surge and P_4 (progesterone) in the levels found during the preovulatory

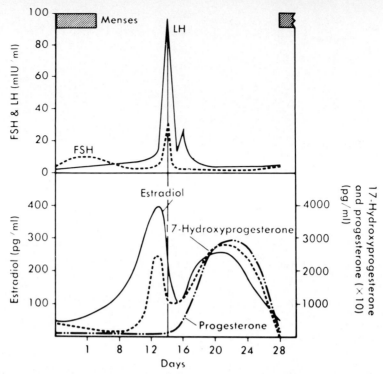

FIGURE 17. Pattern of secretion of sex steroids and gonadotropins during the reproductive cycle in women is illustrated here. The complex hormonal events leading to ovulation involve interaction among two classes of ovarian hormones, two pituitary hormones, and a hypothalamic hormone (LHRH). Early development of the follicle during the first half (follicular stage) of the menstrual cycle is stimulated by the secretion of FSH. At midcycle there is surge of secretion of LH, which is responsible for ovulation. The accompanying less marked surge of FSH secretion does not have a clearly defined function. The follicular phase is associated with developing ovarian function. Immediately preceding the ovulatory surge, there is a rise in plasma estradiol and 17-hydroxyprogesterone. The preovulatory estradiol secretion is mainly responsible for triggering the release of LH, but progesterone may be needed for this response to occur. Following ovulation the luteinized follicle secretes progesterone (luteal phase of the cycle). The crucial event for neuroendocrine control of ovulation is believed to be the trigger to hypothalamus and pituitary gland from the rising estrogen level. (From Odell, WD, Moyer, DL: *Physiology of Reproduction.* CV Mosby, St Louis, 1971, p 66, with permission.)

phase of the cycle, amplifies the duration of the surge and augments the effect of E_2 rather than serving an obligatory role. Thus preovulatory levels of P_4 may be required for the full expression of the surge in women."[78]

The precise timing of ovulation is now clinically important in attempts to carry out *in vitro* fertilization. Ovulation occurs approximately 10 to 12 hours after the LH peak and 24 to 36 hours after the estradiol peak.

Estrogen and progesterone bring about the LH surge by a complex neuroendocrine mechanism. Chronic long-term estrogen sensitizes the pituitary gland to the action of GnRH (see Figure 5). It also induces the appearance of progesterone receptors in both hypothalamus and pituitary gland. Crucial to the positive-feedback signal is the rapid pulse of estrogen immediately prior to ovulation, which produces an acute sensitization to GnRH. There is some controversy as to whether there is also an increase in GnRH secretion at midcycle under the influence of the estrogen surge. In

REGULATION OF THE PITUITARY GLAND

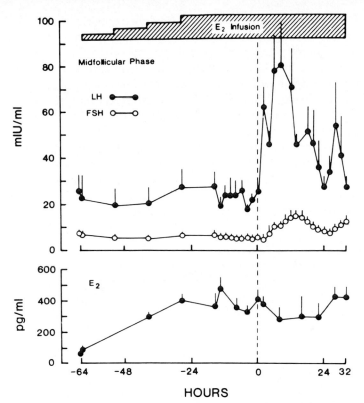

FIGURE 18. Illustration of the *positive* feedback effects of estrogen on gonadotropin secretion. In this experiment, carried out in normal women during the midfollicular phase, the infusion of estradiol-17β was followed after 64 hours by the appearance of a typical midcycle ovulatory surge of LH and FSH. In other studies (for example, see Figure 5), it was shown that estrogen sensitizes the pituitary to GnRH. Thus the positive feedback is exerted, at least in part, by sensitization of the pituitary gland to hypothalamic influences (From Liu and Yen,[78] with permission.)

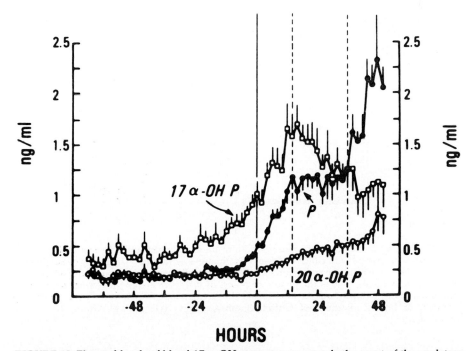

FIGURE 19. Elevated levels of blood 17 α-OH progesterone precede the onset of the ovulatory surge of gonadotropins (designated 0). From substitution experiments, Yen and colleagues have shown that this secretion is in part responsible for the stimulation of gonadotropin secretion at midcycle. (From Hoff JD,[59] with permission.)

favor of this argument is the demonstration of increased GnRH levels in hypophysial-portal blood of monkeys at midcycle,[38] and controversial data concerning the appearance in peripheral blood of GnRH in the human being.[35] On the other hand, female monkeys and humans with complete deficiency of GnRH will ovulate when treated with pulsatile GnRH at a fixed dose level (Fig. 20). A GnRH pulse possibly may be induced during the midcycle in human being and monkey, but it is not essential for the ovulatory surge.

The estrogen and progesterone surge regulated by a genetically regulated ovarian program (that requires FSH for its expression) is the crucial triggering factor. Knobil[71] has epitomized these relationships by saying that the clock that times ovulation is located in the pelvis. Neurogenic menstrual disorders are due to abnormal GnRH secretion.

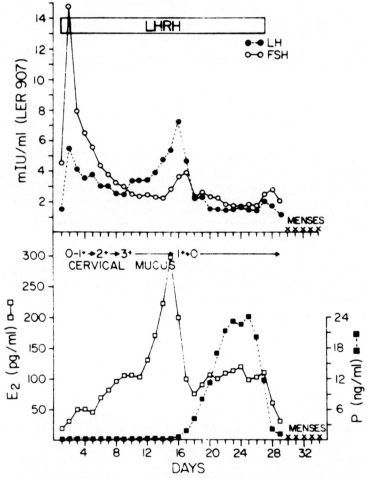

FIGURE 20. Ovulation induced by pulsatile administration of GnRH utilizing a portable pump in an amenorrheic patient with GnRH deficiency (Kallmann's syndrome). The timing of administration is crucial to the response and mimics the spontaneous fluctuations in gonadotropin secretion in normal individuals. One of the important points of this work is that the normal sequence of hormonal changes throughout the month, and thus ovulation, can be induced by a nonvarying program of hourly injections of GnRH. (From Crowley, WF, and McArthur, JW,[29] with permission.)

Following the release of LH at midcycle (accompanied by FSH release), the developed egg leaves the ovary. The remaining follicular cells in the ovary, under the influence of LH, undergo luteinization, the conversion to the corpus luteum, a progesterone-secreting structure. The corpus luteum involutes after about 12 days of secretion. The consequent fall in plasma estrogens and progesterone leads to uterine bleeding, and the cycle begins again. In the rat, the life of the corpus luteum is regulated by still another pituitary hormone, prolactin (PRL), which in this species has a luteotropic function. Under experimental conditions, the rat corpus luteum, which ordinarily involutes in 48 hours, may persist for up to 16 days in a condition called pseudopregnancy. Some of the stimuli that can cause this reaction are mating (with a sterile male rat), severe stress, and mechanical or direct electrical stimulation of the cervix of the uterus. Pseudopregnancy is believed to be due to increased PRL secretion.[93]

It has long been suspected that an analogous reaction might be responsible for certain cases of false pregnancy (pseudocyesis), but evidence that PRL is luteotropic (maintains corpus luteum function) in human beings or in primates has been lacking. However, PRL is luteotropic in rhesus monkeys, and women with pseudocyesis may have high prolactin levels (see below).

REGULATION OF GONADOTROPIN SECRETION IN MEN

Unlike the phasic pattern of gonadotropin secretion in the woman, which is induced by the intrinsic ovarian cyclic rhythm, the function of the testes develops under the influence of tonic LH and FSH secretion. The maturation of spermatozoa requires sustained gonadotropin stimulation over a 70-day period.[52] Spermatozoa form from primitive spermatogonia in the testicular tubules; these divide all through reproductive life. This is in contrast to the eggs of the ovary which are all formed by the time of birth (primordial follicles) and remain dormant until stimulated by the pituitary.

Testosterone, an androgenic hormone, is secreted by the interstitial cells of the testis (Leydig cells) under the influence of LH. The maturation of the spermatozoa requires stimulation by both FSH and LH. Androgenic hormones play a role in sperm maturation as well, and under certain well-defined experimental conditions, androgen administration can maintain spermatogenesis even after hypophysectomy. It has been proposed that the effects of LH and FSH on spermatogenesis are mediated in part through changes in testicular androgen economy. Luteinizing hormone stimulates the secretion of androgen by Leydig cells, and FSH stimulates the secretion of an androgen-binding protein by one of the components of the testicular tubule, the Sertoli cell, which has a sustaining function in the maintenance of the maturing sperm cell. The androgen-binding protein, it is believed, brings about extremely high local concentrations of testosterone in the immediate vicinity of the sperm, stimulating their development.

Although castration leads to elevation of both FSH and LH, and testosterone administration leads to a depression of both LH and FSH, there is good evidence that the negative-feedback control of gonadotropins by the testes is not mediated soley by an androgenic hormone. It has been shown that selective destruction of the tubules (for example, by the antitumor agent cyclophosphamide) leads to selective increase in FSH secretion. Occasionally, a similar syndrome develops in patients with isolated testicular tubular disease. The nature of the tubular component responsible for feedback regulation of FSH was unknown for many years, although the biologic activity had been suspected, and it had been given the name "inhibin." Recently a number of laboratories have found that inhibin is a polypeptide, a nonsteroid substance, and intense efforts to isolate this material and to determine its amino acid sequence are underway.[4] One structure has already been claimed,[109] but this report has not been confirmed. The structure of porcine inhibin deduced from chemical and recombinant DNA analysis indicates that it is a peptide consisting of an α and β chain of approximately 32,000 daltons.[158] Through its selective suppression of FSH, inhibin can inhibit maturation of the germinal element of the testes without affecting its secretory function.

Studies of response to GnRH injection suggest that inhibin inhibits FSH secretion through action at the level of the pituitary gland. Inhibin-like activity has been identified in ovarian cyst fluid and probably plays a role in female reproduction as well (see above).

NEUROENDOCRINOLOGY OF PUBERTY

By the time of birth, all of the structures needed to maintain adult levels of sexual function have been developed, but in normal infants and children, puberty is delayed until adolescence. The mechanisms responsible for timing are predominantly neural and require the appearance of adolescent patterns of pulsatile GnRH secretion.[54,62,101,102,114,142]

Precocious puberty has been observed in children as early as the time of birth, and infantile monkeys can be stimulated to show pubertal changes by the administration of GnRH. Because selective lesions of the anterior hypothalamus in rats, and posterior hypothalamic lesions in the human being[160] and monkey,[144] can bring on precocious puberty, it has been generally recognized that the predominant effect of the brain in timing the onset of puberty is in the loss of a tonic restraining influence. It has been proposed that the neural change is due to a decrease in sensitivity of the hypothalamus to the negative-feedback effects of gonadal steroids, and in fact the prepubertal rat and human being can be shown to have exquisite sensitivity to gonadal steroid feedback inhibition of gonadotropins. However, this view has been modified by studies of the course of pubertal development in experimental animals and humans who lack gonadal secretions (for example, congenital absence of the testicle, or Turner's syndrome). In such individuals, gonadotropins increase at puberty in the absence of any steroid secretion. Hence, it can be concluded that loss of feedback inhibition is not the driving factor in timing of puberty. It appears, instead, that the appearance of pulsatile GnRH secretion is part of a programmed pattern of brain development analogous to changes in other brain function seen in human development.

The neuroendocrine events occurring at the time of puberty in female subjects have been summarized by Ojeda and colleagues[101] (Fig. 21).

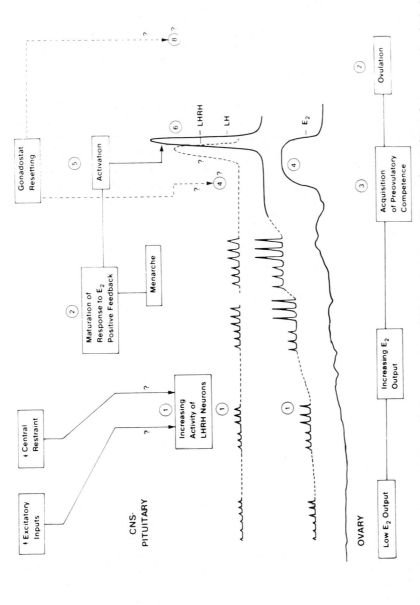

FIGURE 21. Proposed sequence of events leading to the first preovulatory LH surge in primates. The numbers indicate the sequence in which the events may occur. Present evidence does not permit a firm conclusion as to the timing of gonadostat resetting. It may occur shortly before the first ovulation or after it. A preovulatory GnRH surge may or may not be necessary for the preovulatory gonadotropin surge to occur. Although the magnitude of GnRH pulses may increase during development an increase in baseline is not necessary. (From Ojeda et al,[101] with permission.)

"The onset of puberty can be considered as the climax of a cascade of changes that occur harmoniously during reproductive immaturity. In primates, the onset of puberty is signaled by nocturnal rises in circulating gonadotropin levels which are more pronounced than in childhood and also by the accentuation of pulsatile LH release. As the diurnal pattern of LH release becomes more prominent, the ovary is driven to secrete more estradiol, the levels of which increase in a gradual but fluctuating manner as puberty progresses. By midpuberty and about the time of menarche, the hypothalamic-pituitary unit acquires the ability to release LH in response to estradiol, but the ovary is still immature and thus cannot produce estrogen levels of magnitude and duration sufficient to elicit an LH surge. Within a year after menarche, and under persistent gonadotropin stimulation, the secretory activity of the ovary increases sufficiently to produce preovulatory levels of estradiol. The first LH surge is then evoked, but the ovary may still fail to ovulate for variable periods after the first gonadotropin discharge."

A feature of gonadal development not generally appreciated is that the male and female fetuses have appreciable secretions of testosterone and estradiol and that the fetal gonad shows histologic evidence of gonadotropin effects. Gonadal secretion falls at the time of birth but is activated again during the first few months of infancy, only to decline and to remain extremely low (but not absent) during most of childhood. It is reasonable to infer that these sequential changes in gonadal secretion are crucial to the development of the genitalia, and perhaps of the brain at critical stages.

Although a case can be made that the timing of puberty is an intrinsically programmed brain developmental pattern, there is evidence that extrinsic factors are also important. The two factors that have received the most study are body weight and exercise.

That extrinsic factors can influence puberty is demonstrated by the secular trend to an earlier age of menarche which has been demonstrated by Frisch[44-46] (Fig. 22). Analysis of historical data indicates that there has been a trend toward an earlier menarche of about three or four months per decade in Europe for the past 100 years, although the trend in Europe now seems to be slackening off. In 1800, average age of menarche was just over 16.5 years of age, and in 1970 12.9 ± 0.1 year. This secular change has been correlated to the age at which a "critical" weight has been achieved. The delayed puberty of earlier generations is attributed to poorer nutrition, more infections, environmental crowding, and other stresses. The feature of body weight, which is crucial, has not been determined precisely because the evidence is correlational. However, the most convincing hypothesis is that there is a critical mass of fat tissue which is correlated with normal gonadotropin status, and that is associated with a mean weight at menarche of 47.8 ± 0.5 kg. Frisch has argued from a teleologic point of view that this represents fat storage sufficient to maintain a pregnancy (50,000 added calories, and lactation, 1000 additional calories per day), an absolute requirement for successful childbearing in an era of alternating feast and famine of primitive humankind.

The influence of weight is not only secular. In individuals who are grossly malnourished, menstrual disturbances are common, and in anorexia nervosa, normal menses do not reappear unless the critical mass is regained. In most cases more than the critical mass is required.

Delayed puberty also occurs in women who exercise intensely, for example, competitive swimmers, runners, and ballet dancers. Menses fre-

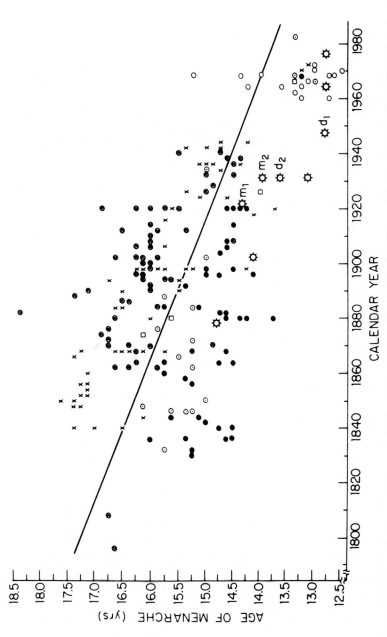

FIGURE 22. Secular trend in the age of onset of puberty in northern European countries and the United States. Mean age at menarche has fallen from approximately 17.2 years in 1800 to 15.2 years in 1900, with continued decline up to 1980. Frisch and colleagues found that this trend has correlated with the mean weight at onset of puberty, which has remained relatively constant throughout the same time period. This relationship has been interpreted to mean that puberty begins when a "critical weight" has been achieved, and that some metabolic factor associated with fat stores determines the timing of puberty. (From Frisch, RE,[44] with permission.)

quently are absent until normal weight is regained. Frisch[44,45] reported that the mean age of menarche of 38 college swimmers and runners was 13.9 ± 0.3 years, significantly later than that of 12.8 ± 0.05 of the general population. If training began prior to menses, mean age was 15.1 ± 0.5 years. It is not entirely clear whether the change is due to excessive exercise or to the fact that such women are always much more lean, that is, have much less fat than those who menstruate.

Intensive exercise in men can similarly cause impaired gonadal function.

The consequences of impaired gonadal secretion in intensely exercising women is not trivial. Several workers[77,84] have shown that trabecular bone mass was significantly reduced (spine density 151 ± 8 versus 182 ± 5 mg/cm^3) in one study of women runners, but not as low as that of amenorrheic women who did not run. Thus, running did protect the women somewhat, but not fully, from the consequences of induced estrogen deficiency. Stress fractures of the lower extremities were reported by 6 of 11 amenorrheic runners, and only 1 of 6 cyclic women.

NEUROENDOCRINE CONTROL OF LACTATION

Almost all the hormones of the pituitary gland and its target glands are involved in one way or another in the development of the breast, the control of milk production, and the delivery of milk at the nipple.[43,55,81,93,146] This richness of endocrine control may reflect the evolutionary fact that the differentiation of sebaceous glands into an apocrine milk-producing gland is characteristic only of mammals. Early breast development requires normal amounts of glucocorticoids and growth hormone and the added effects of estrogen (from the adolescent ovaries). These three hormones are essential for the growth of the breast bud, characteristic of early puberty, due largely to the formation of ducts and stroma. The lobular alveoli of the breast develop under the influence of progesterone and PRL. During pregnancy, the increased secretion of estrogens and progestins, as well as increased secretion of the PRL-like hormone of the placenta (human placental lactogen, HPL), lead to the characteristic breast growth. Lactation is initiated at the time of delivery by the sudden decline in plasma levels of placental estrogens, which during pregnancy have suppressed milk production by direct action on breast acinar membranes.

The continued manufacture of milk requires the repetitive suckling stimulus, which initiates a neuroendocrine reflex leading to release of prolactin (see chapter 7). The afferent arc of this reflex is carried to the upper thoracic segment of the spinal cord through the midbrain to hypothalamus, where it activates the paraventricular and supraoptic nuclei. Frequent nipple stimulation also can cause milk production excess in nonpuerperal women, a reflex that has been exploited by foster mothers so that they can nurse their adopted child. Prolactin release also follows stimulation of the breast in men but requires a particular psychologic "set." For example, self-stimulation fails to release PRL, but stimulation of the subject by his wife is effective.[60] This observation suggests a "gating" phenomenon permitting the nipple stimulation reflex to occur.

Nipple stimulation also is involved in the milk "let-down" reflex.[13] If one observes the nursing process closely in humans or in animals, it is apparent that the initial sucking of the infant is not followed immediately by the appearance of milk at the nipple. There is a delay of twenty to thirty seconds before quantities of milk can be removed from the nipple. This response is due to the contraction of specialized myoepithelial cells that surround the terminal acinar lobules of the breast and expel contained milk through the lobular ducts. The let-down is attributable to the release of oxytocin through a reflex arc involving the hypothalamus and the neurohypophysis. If blocked (for example, by lesions of the hypothalamus), the nursling may be unable to get milk from the breast. In the rat, this leads to death of the litter. Oxytocin release also can be conditioned; in nursing women the first cries of the hungry baby can trigger oxytocin secretion (Fig. 23). Let-down can be duplicated by oxytocin injection, which has been used in women who are having difficulty in providing milk to their infants.[21]

Oxytocin release is probably mediated by cholinergic pathways, impinging on a population of neurons in both the supraoptic-hypophysial and the paraventricular-hypophysial pathways. Emotional stress can block this response, as can the administration of epinephrine. In part this is due to the inhibitory effect of catecholamines on the myoepithelial cells of the breast, and in part to central inhibitory adrenergic effects at the hypothalamic level.

An important accompaniment of nursing is anovulation, which lasts for up to eight or more months after delivery. From a teleologic point of view, this protects the mother from another pregnancy while the child is

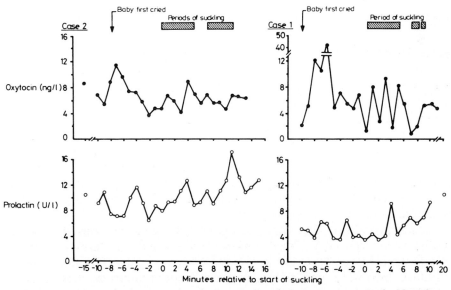

FIGURE 23. Patterns of oxytocin and prolactin secretion during a nursing episode. Note that a burst of oxytocin release occurred in each of these women in response to the sound of her baby's cries, indicating that this is a conditioned response. There were, in addition, bursts of oxytocin secretion during the suckling episode. On the other hand, PRL responses were not conditioned and rose only during suckling. (From McNeilly, AS, Robinson, ICAF, Houston, MJ, Howie, PW: *Release of oxytocin and prolactin in response to suckling.* Br Med J 286:257–259, 1983, with permission.)

still an infant. It has a profound effect on population dynamics in that it spaces pregnancies and is a natural form of birth control.[134] Of course, the birth control offered is only relative, because prevention of conception is not complete and the recovery of ovulatory cycles is variable. The suppression of ovulation by suckling is attributable to neurogenic inhibition of release of GnRH. High plasma PRL levels suppress gonadotropin secretion through an action at the hypothalamic level, and there are probably additional direct hypothalamic effects on GnRH secretion independent of PRL.[125] The intensity of suckling-induced PRL release gradually declines in the months after delivery, roughly paralleling the return of menses.

The act of breastfeeding has for most women a strong psychologic effect associated with enhanced maternal feelings and tranquility. This phenomenon is striking in many individuals and is emphasized as one of the personal rewards of nursing. The nature of this response is not fully understood. There are erotic components in some women, and nipple stimulation in the nursing setting also may have a central tranquilizing effect through the release of central biogenic amines or other transmitters. On the other hand, it is possible that the PRL released during suckling has a direct effect on the affective state, by mechanisms analogous to its short-loop-feedback hypothalamic effect on dopamine and gonadotropin release. From animal studies it might be anticipated that PRL would have behavioral effects. In lower forms, PRL induces maternal behavior (broodiness in hens, nest building and pup recovery in rats, and egg-guarding behavior in fish; see chapter 7). Unfortunately, this question has not been subjected to critical inquiry. The possible central effect of PRL and peptides is a promising area for psychosomatic research. The incidence of depression is higher than normal in hyperprolactinemic women.[163]

DISEASES OF GONADOTROPIN REGULATION

HYPOGONADISM

From an historic point of view, the 1901 description by Fröhlich[47] of adiposogenital dystrophy in a young boy with a pituitary tumor must be looked upon as a landmark in the recognition of the role of the pituitary gland in the control of human sex function[112] (Fig. 24). In 1904, by careful pathologic study of a suprasellar cyst Erdheim[36] determined that hypogonadism could result from damage to the regions of the hypothalamus controlling gonadotropin secretion. Today this all seems very simple, but for a long time the claim that hypogonadism could be produced by selective hypothalamic damage was controversial.

The clinical endocrinologist recognizes two general types of hypogonadism: one, caused by local disease of the gonad, is termed primary hypogonadism; the other is secondary to disease of the hypothalamus or pituitary. Intrinsic gonad disease with consequent failure of steroid secretion leads to secondary activation of pituitary gonadotropin secretion through the operation of the negative-feedback control system (see above). This group is termed *hypergonadotropic hypogonadism*. Secondary hypogonadism is recognized when gonadotropic secretion is inappropriately low in the face of gonadal steroid deficiency *(hypogonadotropic hypogonadism)*.

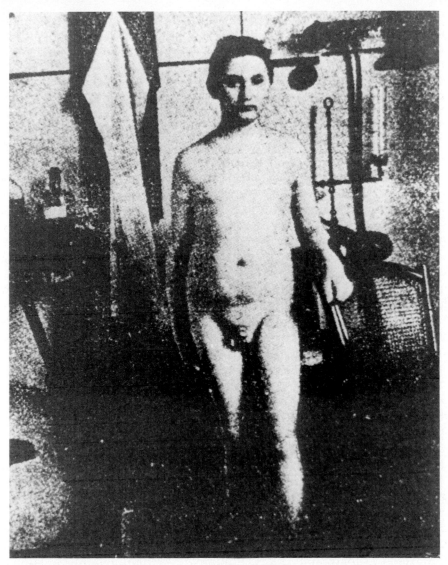

FIGURE 24. Fröhlich's patient at age 14 years. This case report, published in 1901 under the title (translation: "A case of tumor of the hypophysis without acromegaly") first described the association of obesity and hypogonadism (adiposogenital dystrophy). At first obesity was thought to be due to the pituitary dysfunction. Subsequently it became clear that obesity is usually due in such cases to hypothalamic involvement, and still later it was recognized that hypogonadism could arise strictly from hypothalamic disease. (Illustration reprinted from *The Hypothalamus.* Proc Assoc for Res in Nervous and Mental Diseases, 1940. Facsimile edition reprinted by Hafner Publishing Company, New York, 1960. Case discussion in Reichlin, S.[112])

Hypogonadotropic hypogonadism caused by hypothalamic disorder is also termed hypophysiotropic hypogonadism. Primary and secondary hypogonadism are readily differentiated by measurement of plasma gonadotropins (see below). In the absence of clear-cut evidence of local pituitary or hypothalamic disease, the differentiation of pituitary from hypothalamic failure is often difficult.[5,96] GnRH deficiency in hypothalamic disease leads to loss of pituitary sensitivity to GnRH; in cases of hypothalamic failure, the pituitary gland becomes abnormal. In this chapter only the hypogonadotropic disorder is discussed, because intrinsic gonad disease properly relates to endocrine rather than neuroendocrine disease. See Table 1 for normal values of gonadotropic hormones.

Hypogonadotropic Hypogonadism in Women

Of all pituitary functions, gonadotropin secretion is second only to growth hormone secretion in its vulnerability to lesions of the hypothalamic-pituitary unit. Preservation of normal menstrual cycles or male gonadal function, therefore, usually indicates normal pituitary function, although there may be occasional exceptions. All the known causes of disease in this region (see chapter 11) cause amenorrhea and hypogonadism. Of greater numeric importance are the far more common instances of abnormalities in ovulatory control in the absence of clinically evident structural abnormality.

It must be emphasized that intrinsic pituitary disease may rarely cause relatively isolated deficiency of gonadotropin secretion. Isolated FSH deficiency has been described, thought to be due to congenital absence or deficiency of this group of cells.[108]

Secondary Amenorrhea. Secondary amenorrhea (defined as amenorrhea occurring after normal menstrual cycles have been established in nonpregnant women) is by far the most common symptom attributable to disordered pituitary function.[5,155,156] In the great majority of cases, the amenorrhea is unaccompanied by evident deficiency of other pituitary hormones, and careful study will not show structural abnormality of ovary, pituitary gland, or hypothalamus. The amenorrhea usually is temporary, and its spontaneous regression indicates that significant structural disease was not the cause of the illness. Amenorrhea of this type is commonly termed "functional," "psychogenic," or "hypothalamic." Psychogenic amenorrhea occurs in several clearly defined clinical settings as the sole manifestation of pituitary insufficiency. If the pituitary disorder begins before menarche, delayed puberty may result. It commonly occurs in young women undergoing relatively minor stresses such as going away to school.

Many psychotropic drugs, including reserpine and the phenothiazines, can cause amenorrhea. In general, any agent that interferes with central catecholamine function can have this effect. These drugs probably act on the biogenic amine control of GnRH and PRL secretion (chapter 3). Drug-induced amenorrhea is almost always accompanied by elevated levels of PRL, and sometimes by galactorrhea. Amenorrhea can be a sign of severe depressive illness and can also be precipitated by a course of electroshock therapy for psychosis. Systemic disease and hypothyroidism must be excluded.

Pseudocyesis. Pseudocyesis is one of the forms of "grand hysteria." Recognized since the time of Hippocrates, it is now uncommon, as are other manifestations of gross conversion states. In its full-blown form, the affected woman complains of amenorrhea and numerous sensations commonly associated with pregnancy and believes herself to be pregnant. Patients commonly desire strongly to be pregnant or, conversely, fear being

TABLE 1. Serum Gonadotropins in Children and Adults: Radioimmunoassay

Sexual Stage and Age (yr)	FSH*	LH*	Sexual Stage and Age (yr)	FSH*	LH*
Prepubertal (5–11)	4.5 ± 0.2	3.9 ± 0.2	Prepubertal (2–12)	4.2 ± 0.2	2.9 ± 0.4
Adult	7.4 ± 0.7	10.9 ± 1.4	Adult†	8.3 ± 0.3	12.8 ± 1.0
Prepubertal (>5)	2.4 ± 0.1	9.6 ± 0.2	Prepubertal (>5)	3.0 ± 0.1	8.8 ± 0.4
Adult	9.6 ± 0.2	12.2 ± 0.4	Adult†	7.1 ± 0.8	11.8 ± 0.7
Prepubertal (8)	3.2 ± 0.2	1.1 ± 0.3	Prepubertal (8)	4.4 ± 0.3	1.9 ± 0.1
Adult (age 15)	9.1 ± 0.5	4.0 ± 0.5	Adult†	12.5 ± 0.6	13.6 ± 1.1
Prepubertal (1–10)	4.6 ± 0.2	2.8 ± 0.2	Prepubertal (1–10)	5.4 ± 0.3	2.7 ± 0.2
Adult	11.0 ± 0.3	11.1 ± 0.3		12.3 ± 0.3	9.2 ± 0.3
Prepubertal (0.2 ± 12)	4.9 ± 0.2	7.7 ± 0.5			
Adult	8.3 ± 0.3	18.0 ± 0.9			

*X ± SE in mIU/ml 2nd IRP/HMG, immunoassay.
†Follicular phase of cycle.
(Adapted from Kulin, HE, and Reiter, EO.: *Gonadotropins during childhood and adolescence: A review.* Pediatrics 51:260, 1973.)

pregnant. Some of the manifestations include enlargement and bloating of the abdomen, sensation of fetal movements, engorgement and tenderness of the breasts (sometimes with galactorrhea), nausea, morning sickness, and even labor pains. Although an apparent misnomer, pseudocyesis has been reported to occur even with normal periods. At one time, pseudocyesis was apparently not uncommon, and one series reported as many as 1 case in 250 maternity clinic admissions, many of which had misled one or more unwary obstetricians. The precise pathogenesis of pseudocyesis is unknown, though it is clearly psychogenic. By analogy with the syndrome of pseudopregnancy in the rat, which is brought on by stress or cervical stimulation, it has been proposed that the crucial feature of the condition is persistence of the corpus luteum secondary to inappropriate PRL secretion. In fact, a persistent corpus luteum has been observed in a few human cases at laparotomy, and recently several cases with elevated plasma levels of PRL have been reported.[141] Levels have not been reported to exceed 47 ng/ml, but experience with PRL assays in this condition is limited.

Pseudocyesis and the galactorrhea-amenorrhea syndrome have common endocrine changes (see chapter 7). Indeed, some cases of pseudocyesis may represent examples of the galactorrhea-amenorrhea syndrome, perhaps brought on by psychic stress and interpreted by suggestable, hysterical, or unsophisticated women as being due to pregnancy because of their need for or fear of pregnancy. The psychiatric treatment of pseudocyesis, like that of hysteria, is relatively unsuccessful. In one series of patients, 27 individuals were informed that they were not pregnant. More than half refused to accept the diagnosis. Even those who did usually developed pseudocyesis again in a few months. There is no generally applicable way of handling these cases, but psychiatric intervention is advised.

Anorexia Nervosa. Amenorrhea is almost always found in active anorexia nervosa, but it does not dominate the clinical picture as does the marked wasting and disturbed eating behavior. See chapter 21 for complete discussion.

Psychogenic Amenorrhea. Anorexia nervosa and pseudocyesis are the clearest examples of neurogenic (psychogenic) amenorrhea. But these make up the minority of cases of functional amenorrhea or oligomenorrhea. Amenorrhea may occur as a response to relatively trivial events (even ones with generally pleasant associations), such as going away to college or to summer camp, and is also seen after profoundly disturbing stress, such as an automobile accident, rape, or incarceration in a concentration camp. In the famous series of cases observed during the London blitz, each of four women who had stopped menstrual cycling in response to a bombing attack was shown by endometrial biopsy to have endocrine arrest at the stage of the cycle present at the time of the emotional stress.

Unfortunately for the diagnostician, many cases of hypothalamic amenorrhea do not fit the categories of psychic disorder mentioned above. These women are not apparently different psychologically from comparable groups of normal women, and the diagnosis is usually made by exclusion and by prolonged followup. We have had the experience in about one fifth of these women of observing resumption of normal periods soon after careful medical evaluation.

Diagnosis and Management of Hypothalamic Amenorrhea

The GnRH secretory reserve test is not a powerful discriminatory tool and hence seldom is used.[97,120,121,157] The administration of clomiphene will bring about an ovulatory LH surge with or without subsequent menses in 50 to 80 percent of cases of functional amenorrhea, and it is a useful diagnostic aid because it will be effective only in the presence of an intact hypothalamic-pituitary-gonad axis. Even if clomiphene is ineffective, if other pituitary functions (including PRL) and CAT scans are normal, it is our recommendation to do no further diagnostic procedures but to observe the patient for prolonged periods of time. It is important to reassure the patient that in great likelihood this is a self-limited condition and that the use of drugs such as clomiphene, gonadotropins, or GnRH will permit the induction of ovulation (with subsequent pregnancy) in up to 80 percent of cases when pregnancy is desired. The plan of treatment depends on the patient's needs. If she is severely hypogonadal secondary to the gonadotropin deficiency, substitution therapy is indicated, as is also the case if the patient wants to have regular menses. Drugs to induce ovulation are indicated if the patient wishes to become pregnant. The decision regarding psychotherapy is determined by psychologic evaluation and criteria. Psychologic distress and malfunction are the indications for therapy, and not anovulation per se, because the latter is not closely correlated with the severity of psychic disturbance.

Hypogonadotropic Hypogonadism in Men

Deficiency of GnRH secretion in men, as in women, results in hypogonadism. Acquired structural disease of the hypothalamus and stalk can be the cause of GnRH deficiency, and there appears to be at least one type of isolated congenital hypophysiotropic-hormone failure.[2,14,52,76,100] Specific causes of acquired disease include craniopharyngioma, internal hydrocephalus (of any cause), neoplasms of many types including leukemia, granuloma (eosinophilic granuloma, histiocytosis X, sarcoidosis, tuberculosis), encephalitis, microcephaly, Freidreich's ataxia, olivopontocerebellar atrophy, and demyelinating disorders.

Although any of these conditions can cause isolated gonadotropin failure, usually other pituitary deficiencies are present or develop in time. On the other hand, isolated hypogonadotropic hypogonadism is usually a congenital developmental problem and is permanent.

Primary neurogenic hypogonadism has been recognized for a long time. With the benefit of modern knowledge, one can review early case reports of neurologic developmental abnormalities accompanied by hypogonadism such as this case quoted in *Psychopathia Sexualis* by Krafft-Ebbing:[72]

"A case mentioned by Heschl ("Wiener Zeitschrift f. pract. Heilkunde," 22d March, 1861) is remarkable, where the absence of both olfactory lobes was accom-

sity. So common, in fact, is the association of obesity and delayed puberty that is has been considered that hypogonadism may be caused by the obesity or that both are manifestations of the same functional hypothalamic disorder.[87,127,135,142] The endocrinologist always should determine whether the apparent small size of the penis is due to a large pubic fat pad. A very small penis is suggestive evidence of extremely marked hypogonadism of long standing and suggests that the disorder is true gonadotropin deficiency and not delayed puberty. Growth hormone deficiency also can be responsible for inadequate penile growth; GH administration in such cases restores penile growth.

Because delayed puberty must be differentiated from the more serious causes of hypogonadism, and because of the severe psychologic consequences of prolonged infantilism in adolescent-age boys, efforts should be made before age 15 to establish the diagnosis with certainty and to initiate some form of treatment.[34] It is important to treat testosterone deficiency at an early age, because normal psychosocial development in the man requires testosterone at a critical period. Late replacement (for example, after the age of 20) is generally unsatisfactory in restoring normal sexual vigor and a normal male aggressive personality (see chapter 20).

Some believe that treatment may trigger the onset of normal sexual maturation by stimulating maturation of the hypothalamus, but, in any case, it does not prevent the normal process if it is to occur. Testes development is clear evidence of onset of gonadotropic function, but treatment must be stopped for a month every year up to the age of 20 to determine whether normal sexual function has begun. Of course, neurologic status and other pituitary functions should also be evaluated. It is generally assumed that if sexual maturity does not occur by age 20 to 22, normal spontaneous gonadotropic functions will never develop.

Delayed Puberty in Women

Many of the considerations discussed above for boys also govern the diagnosis and management of girls with delayed onset of sexual development. Age 16 is commonly taken as the criterion of delay, even though the normal age range for this development is from age 11 to age 13 in healthy Caucasian girls. Nutrition plays an even greater role in the girl than in the boy, either obesity or extreme inanition delaying the onset of menses. In both girls and boys, gonadal failure and hypothalamic-pituitary failure readily can be differentiated because at the normal time of puberty, children with gonadal failure show an increased secretion of gonadotropic hormones.

PRECOCIOUS PUBERTY

The term precocious puberty is used when otherwise normal pituitary-gonad function appears at an abnormally early age.[12,33,63,75,104,114] In boys this means onset of androgen secretion and spermatogenesis, and in girls onset of estrogen secretion and cyclic ovarian activity. In primary disease of testis or ovary, causing early hypersecretion of androgens and estrogens (in boys and girls, respectively), physical sex characteristics develop prematurely; but in contrast to the situation in true precocious puberty, gametogenesis does not develop similarly. Examples are the adrenogenital syndrome owing to enzymatic defects of the adrenal cortex, or tumors of ovary or testis. These disorders are classified as pseudoprecocious puberty.

True precocious puberty always arises from disturbed neural function, which may or may not have an identifiable structural basis. Only this form of neurogenic disorder is considered in this text; pseudoprecocious puberty is classified here as a primary endocrine problem.

Normal Age of Onset of Puberty

The mean age at menarche in the United States was estimated as 12.6 ± 1.1 years (SD). In the studies of Tanner,[143] the mean onset of the growth spurt in girls was 10.7 years; of breast development, 10.8 years; of the appearance of pubic hair, 11.3 years; and of menarche, 10.5 to 15.5 years (see Tables 2 and 3). The diagnosis of precocity usually is made if the age at menarche is under 8 years. Partial puberty is not uncommon in girls. Precocious thelarche refers to premature development of breast unaccompanied by other signs of puberty, and precocious pubarche (adrenarche) refers to premature development of pubic hair. The mechanisms underlying these partial forms of puberty have not been elucidated. They do not have the same clinical significance as does precocious menstruation.

In boys, testes growth begins at a mean age of 11.8. In Tanner's series, the age of normal onset of testes growth was as low as 9.5 years; of penis growth, 10.5 to 14.5 years; and of the growth spurt, 10.5 to 16 years (see Table 2). It is common to use the term precocious puberty if spermatogenesis is present before the age of 10 years, but it is obvious that in the age range 9 to 10 the diagnosis of precocity may be ambiguous.

Incidence and Causes of Precocious Puberty

True precocious puberty is at least twice as common in girls as in boys. In girls this diagnosis is less serious than in boys because less than 10 percent

---

TABLE 2. Sequence of Appearance of Sexual Characteristics in Normal Puberty

Onset	Mean (yr)	Range (yr)
Male		
Testes growth	11.5	9.5–13.5
Pubic hair	12.0	10.5–14.5
Penis growth	12.5	10.5–14.5
Growth spurt	12.7	10.5–16.0
Female		
Growth spurt	10.7	
Breast development	10.8	8.0–13.0
Pubic hair	11.3	
Menarche	12.7	10.5–15.5

(Adapted from Tanner, JM: *Growth and Endocrinology of the Adolescent.* In Gardner, LI (ed): *Endocrine and Genetic Diseases of Childhood and Adolescence,* ed 2. WB Saunders, Philadelphia, 1975.)

TABLE 3. Representative Ages at Menarche in Various Groups

Country	Year	Age at Menarche
England	1965	13.0 ± 0.2 (S.E.M.)
United States	1968	
Whites		12.8 ± 0.04
Blacks		12.5 ± 0.11
Istanbul	1965	
Rich		12.3 ± 0.15
Average		12.8 ± 0.11
Poor		13.2 ± 0.10
Hong Kong (Chinese)	1962	
Rich		12.5 ± 0.18
Average		12.8 ± 0.20
Poor		13.3 ± 0.19

(Adapted from Tanner, JM: *Growth and Endocrinology of the Adolescent.* In Gardner, LI (ed): *Endocrine and Genetic Diseases of Childhood and Adolescence,* ed 2. WB Saunders, Philadelphia, 1975.)

TABLE 4. Differential Diagnosis of Precocious Puberty

Central precocious puberty
1. Idiopathic
2. Hypothalamic hamartoma
3. Other CNS lesions: astrocytoma, optic glioma, 3rd ventricle cysts, Arnold-Chiari malformation, neuroblastoma, hydrocephalus, etc.

Peripheral precocious puberty
1. Premature adrenarche*
2. Exogenous/factitious ingestion of sex steroids
3. Adrenal
    enzymatic defects: CAH (21-hydroxylase or 11-hydroxylase deficiency)
4. Ovary
    cysts
    tumors—virilizing or feminizing
    McCune-Albright syndrome (MAS)
5. Testis
    tumors: dysgerminoma, Leydig-Sertoli cell
    familial male precocious puberty (FMPP)
6. hCG-secreting tumors: hepatoblastoma, dysgerminoma
7. Increased peripheral aromatization

Combined precocious puberty
1. CAH and central precocious puberty
2. Adrenal tumor and central precocious puberty
3. Ovarian tumor and central precocious puberty
4. McCune-Albright syndrome and central precocious puberty

Mechanism unknown
1. Hypothyroidism†
2. Premature thelarche*

*Sex steroid levels in premature adrenarche and thelarche remain below the adult range. There is little or no growth acceleration, and the bone age remains within the normal range (less than 2 years above chronologic age).
†The only form of precocious puberty in which the bone age may be retarded.
Modified from Pescovitz, et al.[104]

of the cases have organic structural intracranial lesions, whereas 20 to 40 percent of cases in boys have significant intracranial lesions. A comprehensive list of causes was compiled by Pescovitz et al[104] (Table 4).

Idiopathic Sexual Precocity. This is the largest category of true precocity. There is a hereditary form, largely confined to boys, but familial occurrence is uncommon. In the studies of Liu and coworkers,[79] girls with true precocity were found to have a high incidence of abnormal electroencephalograms and behavioral disturbance, suggesting the presence of an underlying brain disturbance. Bierich[12] disputes this contention and claims that precocious puberty is unaccompanied by even occult brain damage. The recent studies by Pescovitz and colleagues[104] indicate that hypothalamic hamartomas (see below) make up a much higher proportion of so-called idiopathic puberty than previously recognized.[165] In their study of 129 cases, 14 out of 95 girls, and 10 out of 34 boys, had hamartomas detectable by CAT scanning. Nevertheless, idiopathic precocity was still the largest cause of the disorder in girls but was rare in boys (6%). The pathogenesis of this disorder therefore remains a matter of controversy.

Neurogenic Precocious Puberty. The site of hypothalamic lesions that influence the timing of puberty are not well localized in the human, because most cases coming to autopsy have relatively widespread disease. In the classic compilation of Weinberger and Grant,[150] approximately two thirds of the cases in which anatomic correlations could be made had destruction of the posterior hypothalamus. This is in contrast to the situation in the rat, in which localized lesions in the preoptic hypothalamus induce precocious puberty. However, posterior hypothalamic lesions in monkeys cause precocious puberty; the effect of anterior lesions has not been determined.[144] Invasive lesions that have been recognized to cause precocity include craniopharyngioma (although delayed puberty is more common), hamartoma, astrocytoma, pineal lesion (see below), encephalitis, miliary tuberculosis, tuberous sclerosis, Sturge-Weber syndrome, porencephaly, craniostenosis, microcephaly, hydrocephalus, and Tay-Sachs disease.[52]

Hypothalamic Hamartoma. One category of neoplasms of the hypothalamus that merits special mention is the hamartoma.[58,64,116] This lesion is an exception to the generalization that tumors of the brain cause precocious puberty by destructive effects on the regions that normally suppress gonadotropin secretion. A hamartoma may be defined neuropathologically as a tumor-like collection of normal nerve tissue lodged in an abnormal location. One type of hypothalamic hamartoma consists of a sharply encapsulated nodule of nerve tissue attached to the posterior hypothalamus at a point between the anterior portion of the mammillary body and the posterior region of the tuber cinereum. These differ from glial tumors that may occupy the same region but that are invasive.

The hypothalamic hamartoma grows into the cisternal space between the cerebral peduncles, often adapting itself to the pyramidal shape of the cisternal space, and may produce signs of early puberty before other neural effects occur. Tumors of this type were long considered to be quite rare; less than 50 cases were reported in the literature up to 1972. But the recent studies of Pescovitz and colleagues (see above), using high resolution CAT scanning, indicate that they occur in a much higher frequency; they were found in 14 of 95 cases in girls and in 10 of 34 cases in boys. Many hypothalamic hamartomas are small and asymptomatic, and it has been proposed that precocious puberty occurs when the tumor has specific connections to the median eminence, thus serving as an "accessory hypothalamus" as proposed by Richter.[116] That the tumor may secrete GnRH was proposed by Bierich,[12] who found GnRH in the spinal fluid of three such patients. Neurosecretory cells that contained GnRH demonstrable by immunohistochemical study have been described in two hamartomas.[58,64]

The clinical presentation in patients with hamartoma is not different from other known cerebral causes of precocity but tend to occur earlier. Hamartomas occur in either sex, have been seen as early as 3 months of age, and are usually fatal before age 20. These tumors are said to be radioresistant, and the surgical removal can be hazardous.

Hypothyroidism. The association of sexual precocity with juvenile hypothyroidism, though rare, is well known and is reversed by treatment with thyroxine.[147,154] In a small proportion of cases, the precocity is associated with galactorrhea. Van der Werff ten Bosch[147] compiled a series of 14 girls and 3 boys with a combination of thyroid deficiency and precocious puberty. In the case reported by Sadeghi-Nejad and Senior,[122] the disorder was induced by propylthiouracil treatment of hyperthyroidism. A few patients with hypothyroidism (with or without galactorrhea) may have elevated plasma PRL levels,[48] and other patients with hypothyroidism also may show elevation of plasma gonadotropins. The syndrome of hypothyroidism, galactorrhea, and precocious puberty must require a special susceptibility, because it is an uncommon manifestation of the hypothyroid state. Rarely, the pituitary fossa is enlarged and hyperpigmentation occurs. Pituitary enlargement is probably due to hyperplasia and hypertrophy of thyrotrope cells. The cause of the pigmentation is unknown.

Various theories of pathogenesis have been proposed to explain the association between sexual maturation and hypothyroidism. That proposed by Van Wyck and Grumbach[148] suggests that there is cross-specificity in feedback control of TSH, LH, and FSH, all glycoprotein hormones secreted by basophil cells and now known to have a common α-subunit. An alternative theory has been proposed that hypothyroidism causes hypothalamic encephalopathy, which in turn interferes with brain regions that normally suppress GnRH secretion. The high PRL levels sometimes seen in this syndrome might be due to a similarly produced deficiency of prolactin-inhibiting factor (PIF).

The importance of early recognition of this disease lies in the fact that it is completely benign and readily treated by thyroid hormone replacement. Occasionally an ovarian cyst may mimic an estrogen-secreting ovarian tumor. Treatment with thyroid hormone leads to a regression of the ovarian mass.

Sexual Precocity with Polyostotic Fibrous Dysplasia. A number of endocrine disturbances are noted in association with the bone lesion polyostotic fibrous dysplasia. This disorder, called the Weil-Albright-McCune-Sternberg syndrome (more commonly the McCune-Albright syndrome) includes precocious puberty in one third of the cases and smooth-margined pigmented skin areas in most.[73,118,128] Other endocrine disturbances seen in this condition include the rare occurrence of thyrotoxicosis, Cushing's syndrome, acromegaly, hyperprolactinemia, and gynecomastia. This syndrome commonly is listed as a cause of true precocious puberty because in one case a 6½-year-old boy showed testes development to the point of spermatogenesis and in another case one female patient showed ovulatory levels of LH. Another clue to a hypothalamic-pituitary etiology is the occasional thickening of the basal skull. On theoretic gounds Hall and Warrick[56] have proposed that there may be hypersecretion of the hypothalamic releasing hormones in this condition. The condition is much more common in girls than in boys.

However, the bulk of evidence now available indicates that this condition is not true precocity but, rather, at least in the female, is a primary disease of the ovary. Ovulation has not been demonstrated; upon surgical exploration, luteinized corpora were not found, which is evidence that ovulation had not taken place. In four patients with sexual precocity studied at the Massachusetts General Hospital by Danen and Crawford,[32] plasma estrogens were elevated and gonadotropin levels depressed, findings that point to primary hypersecretion of the ovary. In a similar case the patient, in addition, had a prepubertal rather than pubertal type of response to injections of GnRH.[41] Uterine bleeding is of the characteristic breakthrough type. The supposition that the disorder is not primary in the hypothalamic-pituitary unit has been proven by administering GnRH agonists. In contrast to patients with true precocity, this treatment (which desensitizes gonadotropin cells) does not reverse the precocious puberty.[26]

A rare form of primary testicular hypersecretion causing precocious puberty in boys has been described. The disorder appears to be inherited as an autosomal dominant in most cases. In contrast to true precocious puberty, these children do not have pulsatile gonadotropin secretion, and their disease is not reversed by treatment with GnRH superagonists.[119] The primary testicular nature of this condition has been emphasized by Grumbach and colleagues who refer to the disease as "familial testotoxicosis." Several large kindreds have been reported. The pineal gland in precocious puberty is discussed in chapter 10.

Clinical Approach to the Diagnosis of Precocious Puberty

In the child with precocious development of secondary sex characteristics, the first requirement is to determine whether mature germ cells are being formed.[104] If spermatogenesis and ovulation are taking place, the diagnosis of true precocity is evident, and the problem then becomes a neurologic one in evaluating the presence of anatomic damage to the hypothalamus. Polyostotic fibrous dyplasia, a rare cause of pseudoprecocity in boys but more common in girls, can be considered on the basis of characteristic bone cysts on roentgenograms of the long bones, pelvis, and skull, and by the finding of smoothly marginated brown-pigmented spots on the skin. Factitious precocious development caused by ingestion of hormone pills may cause precocity, but it is much more likely to be seen in girls than in boys. Family history is a clue to "familial testotoxicosis."

Boys. Clues to normal testes development in boys include testis enlargement to adult size, the appearance of sperm in overnight voided urine specimens after seminal vesicle and prostate massage and, if necessary, biopsy of the testicle. Excessive secretion of androgenic hormone by adrenal or other tumors usually leads to small prepubertal-size testes. Rarely, however, they may appear to be of normal adult size because they contain adrenal rest tumors or familial testotoxicosis. Congenital adrenal hyperplasia occasionally can cause true precocious puberty as well.[103] Other reasons testes size may appear normal in pseudoprecocious puberty are tumors producing testosterone and testes growth due to excessive HCG from a teratoma located elsewhere (mediastinum, pineal region). The laboratory is helpful in distinguishing these forms of abnormality. The precocious boy with true cerebral precocity will show hormonal values similar to those of a normal adult male. In cases owing to excessive adrenal androgens, urinary 17-ketosteroid excretion will be markedly and diagnostically elevated; if owing to excessive HCG secretion, plasma radiommunoassays of HCG or the specific β-chain of HCG will be grossly abnormal. If caused by a testosterone-producing testicular or adrenal tumor, plasma testosterone will be elevated to or above the normal male adult level, unaccompanied by evidence of spermatogenesis.

Once the diagnosis of cerebral precocity is made in the male patient, the high frequency with which intracranial disease is found (94%) requires full neurologic evaluation, including CAT and MRI scans because small hypothalamic tumors can be missed. Close followup is indicated. It is important to recognize that in pineal teratomas, pineal calcification occurs earlier than normal. Pineal lesions occur almost exclusively in male subjects.

Girls. The appearance of regular menses is evidence for a normal gonadotropin-ovarian axis. The best confirmation of normal ovulatory function by noninvasive methods is the demonstration of a midcycle elevation of plasma LH and FSH by immunoassay. Ovarian cysts can be diagnosed by ultrasound examination. However, more or less regular periods may result from "breakthrough" owing to sustained estrogen effect. This can be due to intrinsic ovarian disease or to estrogen secretion by an adrenal tumor or by a teratoma. In all such cases, however, plasma estradiol levels will be persistently elevated to the normal adult range, and plasma gonadotropin concentrations will be in the adult normal range and will not show the characteristic elevation at 12, 13, or 14 days prior to the menses. One possible source of confusion is the occurrence, even in normal puberty, of anovulatory cycles so that irregular and scanty periods may appear for one to three years before periods become normal. Hence, there may be some confusion in differentiating a mild hyperestrogenic state from the early pubertal state accompanying precocious puberty. It may take a period of observation, pelvic ultrasound, or even colposcopy to evaluate the state of ovarian function. Demonstration of a corpus luteum is adequate evidence that ovulation has taken place. Plasma progesterone measurements or aspiration endometrial biopsy can indicate the presence of a luteinized ovary. Because a relatively conservative neurologic approach is indicated in true precocity in girls, the main condition to identify early is an estrogen-secreting tumor. This can be done readily by measurement of plasma estradiol and gonadotropins by immunoassay. In estrogen hypersecretion, estradiol is adult normal or higher and gonadotropins (LH and FSH) are decreased.

In girls with true precocity, neurologic evaluation should include CAT and MRI scans and electroencephalogram. If there are no abnormal neurologic findings, and if pituitary function is otherwise normal, including tests for diabetes insipidus and growth hormone secretory reserve (see chapter 14), invasive neurologic diagnostic procedures usually are not indicated.

Management

In true precocity with demonstrable neurologic lesions, management usually requires biopsy because many lesions that are not curable surgically may respond to roentgenotherapy (see also chapter 10). Special diagnostic consideration must be given to hamartomas and to ectopic seminomatous pinealomas. As emphasized by the NIH group (G.B. Cutler, Jr., personal communication, 1986), biopsy for diagnosis of hamartoma is rarely indicated. The CAT scan appearance is quite typical, the response to GnRH superagonist therapy (see below) quite favorable, and the natural history of the disease much less aggressive than previously believed. For example, in the NIH series, 24 cases "encountered between 1979 and 1983 have had no progression by CAT scan over what is now a mean followup of 4 years." They report one case which, following biopsy, suffered hemiparesis, seizures, and mental retardation as a result of postoperative bleeding. Early postoperative death due to cerebral edema occurred in a patient following removal of a large hamartoma.[58] There is very little experience with the use of x-ray therapy for this condition.

HCG-secreting pineal tumors found *in situ,* or arising from the hypothalamus, can be diagnosed successfully by measurements of the β HCG subunit either in blood and/or in CSF or by identification of HCG immunopositive cells in the CSF. Such findings are sufficient proof of the nature of the lesion to make biopsy unnecessary. The traditional hormonal therapy used for treatment of precocious puberty has been medroxyprogesterone, which usually inhibits ovulation and causes a regression of breast hypertrophy and menses. However, this therapy usually does not delay the progressive skeletal maturation; the child still continues to show accelerated growth when young but ultimately becomes a short adult because of early closure of the epiphyses.

The most dramatic advance in therapy of precocious puberty has been the introduction of superagonist GnRH therapy by Crowley and colleagues[30,83] and Loriaux and colleagues.[24,25,104] These workers have shown successful suppression of gonadotropins and sex steroids, reversal in sexual maturation, and a return to normal growth rates (Fig. 26). Approximately 100 patients thus far have been treated, of which several have achieved the normal pubertal age and are menstruating normally. As a diagnostic tool superagonist inhibition of precocity proves that one is dealing with a cen-

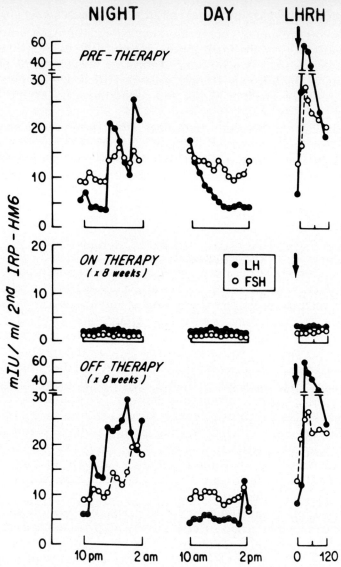

FIGURE 26. Administration of superagonists of GnRH selectively suppress the secretion of the gonadotropins. Shown here is the response in a child with idiopathic precocious puberty, treated with the analog D-Trp6-Pro9-NEt-LHRH (LHRH a) 4 μg/kg/day subcutaneously. During administration of the medication, gonadal cycling returned to normal. Larger series of cases have confirmed these findings. (From Crowley, WR, et al,[30] with permission.)

tral defect in sexual maturation. This approach has still not been approved for general use by the Food and Drug Administration.

The use of this approach has been criticized on theoretic grounds by MacGillivray.[82] She pointed out that degenerative changes have been observed in the testes of rats given GnRH agonist doses, that sufficient primate toxicity studies have not been completed, that antibody to GnRH has been reported to occur in at least one person, and that antisera to GnRH can cause gonadal insufficiency in experimental animals. She also pointed out that at least two thirds of untreated children with precocious puberty reach the height of 5 feet.

Criticism of this kind forces one to conclude that the general safety of GnRH superagonists has not been completely established as yet. However, sufficient information now is being accumulated to permit an adequate judgment. Should it prove to be a safe therapy, it will certainly be the treatment of choice for neurogenic precocious puberty.

Psychologic management is of great importance in precocious puberty. This aspect of management has been emphasized.[34,94,95] Fortunately, almost all girls and most boys do not show precocious sex drive and interests.

Steroids and Meningioma

A number of findings have suggested that sex steroids have an influence on the course of meningioma (see Reiter and coworkers[115] for review). Meningiomas are rarely diagnosed before puberty and rarely after the age of 75. They occur more frequently in women than in men (female : male ratio of 2.5 : 1 for intracranial meningioma, 9 : 1 for spinal cord meningiomas). The ratio is 1 : 1 in elderly patients. "In some cases meningiomas were found to have a relapsing course in relation to pregnancy. The oculomotor and visual signs usually developed during the last 4 months of pregnancy and regressed just after delivery." These changes may be due to hormone-induced edema of the cells. Obesity in women is significantly correlated with the incidence of meningioma, and the incidence of breast cancer is also associated with meningioma. Both these findings possibly are related to the increased conversion of the adrenal androgen, androstenedione, to estrone in fatty tissue. Meningiomas have steroid receptors. In the series reported by Poisson,[105] of 25 meningiomas in 23 individuals, estrogen receptors were found in 33 percent, progesterone receptors in 96 percent, androgen receptors in 92 percent, glucocorticoid receptors in 83 percent, mineralocorticoid receptors in 18 percent. Because fibroblasts in connective tissue outside the brain also are steroid dependent, it is not surprising that meningiomas derived from connective tissue elements of the meninges are also steroid dependent. It is probable that meningiomas would be susceptible to stimulation by fibroblast growth factor, but we are not aware of studies of this question. Meningiomas also have somatostatin receptors whose functions are unknown.

GONADOTROPIN-SECRETING TUMORS

Clinical aspects of gonadotropin-secreting tumors have been reviewed in detail by Ridgway,[117] whose paper is quoted extensively in this section (see also chapter 12). The tumors are exceedingly rare, accounting for 3.5 percent of tumors in one large series. According to this author 42 cases reported in the literature are authenticated by either immunologic or bioassay techniques. Most cases occur in older men and are relatively large by the time that they are discovered, reflecting their subtle endocrine effects.

Ridgway divides these tumors into three groups, those that produce LH alone, those that produce FSH and LH, and those that produce FSH alone.

Only one case of isolated LH excess has been reported, 5 cases of combined gonadotropins, and the remainder were predominantly FSH secretors. The high LH syndrome is manifested as high androgen, normal libido, but reduced sperm production, reflecting the importance of FSH for testicular maturation. In the single reported male patient with LH deficiency, testosterone production was reduced, and the patient was impotent. In the other cases, testosterone ranged from deficient to increased levels. Serum levels of the β-chain of LH or FSH are elevated relative to the α-chain, which is quite different from the normal pattern in eugonadal or hypogonadal individuals. Of cases that have been studied, 16 of 20 responded to injections of GnRH with release of FSH and/or LH. About one half of cases appropriately tested show suppression with exogenous estrogens. More than half of the cases show paradoxical FSH release to the injection of TRH. Because the diagnosis of these tumors is usually quite late, they are generally treated as mass lesions by partial removal and x-irradiation.

Mention should be made of tumors that secrete only the α-chain of the gonadotropins (see chapter 12). Most are macroadenomas. Some also secrete PRL and less frequently GH, although at least two cases have been reported who had no abnormalities other than isolated α-chain excess, and who would have, except for this finding, been classified as chromophobe adenomas.

Diagnosis of Disorders of Gonadotropin Secretion

Primary gonadotropin hypersecretion occurs in patients with gonadotropin-secreting tumors (see above). Precocious puberty is not associated with abnormally increased gonadotropins but, rather, with normal adult values presenting prematurely. Decreased gonadotropin secretion is a common manifestation of hypothalamic-pituitary disease and is observed frequently as a functional disturbance as in "hypothalamic amenorrhea," anorexia nervosa, and in the equivalent disorders in the male patient.

The diagnosis of gonadal failure can usually be made on clinical grounds by the failure to develop normal secondary sex characteristics in adolescence, and by loss of established sexual function in adults. Gonadotropin failure is graded depending upon the extent of the loss. In women, shortening of the luteal phase may be the first evidence of minimal gonadotropin failure. Loss of the ovulatory patterns of LH and FSH secretion can give rise to irregular, scant periods (oligomenorrhea), or prolonged, irregular periods (menometrorrhagia) owing to breakthrough bleeding secondary to persistent unopposed estrogen effect. When basal levels of FSH and LH are reduced, varying degrees of estrogen deficiency ensue, ranging from partial to complete.

Estrogen deficiency causes amenorrhea; atrophy of the breasts, uterus, and genitalia; decrease in body hair growth; and premature osteoporosis. In men, loss of potency is probably the earliest manifestation of testosterone deficiency, followed by low sperm count, loss of libido, decrease in growth of facial and body hair, decrease in muscle strength and mass, and general loss of vigor.

The determination of plasma gonadal steroids (testosterone in men,

17-β-estradiol in women) confirms the diagnosis of gonadal deficiency. Normal testosterone values in men are 300 to 1000 ng/ml. Estradiol in normal women ranges from 20 to 60 pg/ml in the follicular phase, 330 to 700 pg/ml during midcycle, and 100 to 200 pg/ml in the luteal phase. Primary gonadal failure can be distinguished from hypothalamic-pituitary disease by measurement of plasma gonadotropins. If gonadotropins are elevated, the disease lies in the gonad; if low or in the normal range in the face of testosterone or estrogen deficiency, this inappropriately low level indicates gonadotropin deficiency, permitting the diagnosis of *hypogonadotropic hypogonadism*. Normal values for FSH and LH in men are 5 to 25 mIU/ml and 6 to 30 mIU/ml, respectively. Normal values for LH in women are 5 to 30 mIU/ml in the follicular phase, 40 to 200 mIU/ml midcycle, and 5 to 40 mIU/ml in the luteal phase. Normal values for FSH in women range from 5 to 40 mIU/ml during various phases of the cycle. Clinicians should be aware of the diagnostic standards in the laboratory that they use because there is some variability.

Luteinizing hormone and FSH are secreted episodically, with a periodicity of about 1 to 1.5 hours; the fluctuations are particularly great in hypogonadal individuals who may show, at times, values within the normal range. For this reason, it may be necessary to collect repeated samples at intervals of 15 to 30 minutes. A valid method is to collect three separate samples at 15-minute intervals and to pool them for immunoassay.

Urine gonadotropin hormones traditionally have been measured by bioassay, but this procedure has been outmoded by modern diagnostic methods for plasma measurement. Urine methods by immunoassay have been utilized in experimental studies of children and provide useful information.

Hypogonadotropic Hypogonadism

The finding of hypogonadotropic hypogonadism requires further testing to determine whether the disease is hypothalamic or pituitary in origin, and whether it is due to structural abnormalities, or is "functional."

Delayed Puberty. Puberty normally occurs between the ages of 10 and 15 in girls and between 11 and 16 in boys. If growth is otherwise normal and the plasma GH reserve is normal, isolated gonadotropic hormone deficiency must be considered as the cause of delayed puberty. Family history of delayed puberty, abnormal growth patterns such as seen in Prader Willi syndrome or Laurence-Moon Biedl syndrome (see chapter 11), osteodystrophy, presence of chromosomal abnormalities (Turner's syndrome in the girl, Kleinfelter's syndrome in the boy), and the finding of hyposmia or anosmia (Kallmann's syndrome) give clues to the diagnosis. If one of these is present, the differential diagnosis lies between "constitutional" delayed puberty and organic disease of the hypothalamus or pituitary gland. Hypothalamic primary amenorrhea can be caused by prepubertal hyperprolactinemia. If all other pituitary functions are normal and there are no localizing neurologic findings, normal CAT and MRI scans are usually (but not always) sufficient to exclude structural neurologic disease. Tests of gonadotropic secretory reserve (clomiphene, GnRH) do not help to differentiate delayed puberty from organic hypothalamic-pituitary disease, because clomiphene cannot stimulate LH release unless hypothalamic mechanisms for LH control have matured; GnRH is only marginally effective in normal prepubertal children. In normal prepubertal children, FSH responses to GnRH are relatively greater than are LH responses. The appearance of LH and FSH responses suggests that puberty is imminent.[52] The PRL response to TRH has been reported to be useful in differentiating delayed development from hypothalamic hypogonadism.[140] This may prove to be of value in differential diagnosis. We recommend careful followup in such cases, with special emphasis on hypothalamic-pituitary function. Puberty may commence as late as age 18 in girls and 20 in boys, although this is rare.

The recommendation of prolonged observation does not imply that no treatment is indicated. Because of the severe psychologic effects of hypogonadism, and the crucial requirement of sex hormones for normal brain development (including psychosocial maturation), it is advisable in most cases to commence substitution therapy in either sex by age 15. In boys, treatment with HCG for 1 to 2 years to stimulate testes development is indicated, followed by testosterone maintenance. In girls, cyclic estrogen-progesterone therapy is indicated periodically; the therapy should be discontinued to permit the evaluation of pituitary-gonad function. In boys, testes growth during the course of testosterone therapy usually means that normal gonadotropic function has returned and that replacement therapy need not be continued. The use of GnRH for the treatment of adult male and female infertility has been successful in cases of hypothalamic disease.[29,31,80,136,137] It is likely that this approach may prove to be successful for delayed development and hypothalamic disease in the young.

Evaluation for Amenorrhea. In the evaluation of amenorrhea, it is essential to determine that the uterus and vagina are normal and responsive to sex steroids. In practice, persistent amenorrhea (defined as absence of menses for at least three months in a nonpregnant woman) initially is evaluated by administering a progesterone compound such as progesterone acetate 100 to 150mg intramuscularly or medroxyprogesterone 10mg daily by mouth for 5 days. Menstruation within 2 to 7 days after commencing therapy indicates that the uterus has been previously stimulated by estrogen and that the uterus and vagina are probably normal. Because progesterone and its derivatives may be harmful to the developing fetus, the test should be done after laboratory tests show that the patient is not pregnant. If bleeding fails to occur, the patient should be treated for one or two months with an estrogen (1.25 or 2.5mg daily for 24 days) plus medroxyprogestrone 10mg daily on days 20 to 24 of each cycle. If menstruation ensues, uterine-response capacity is intact; if it does not, the disorder is most likely in the uterus, but definitive diagnosis may require endometrial biopsy. If bleeding occurs, then further testing of hypothalamic, pituitary, and ovarian functions is required. Primary ovarian failure can be excluded as a cause of amenorrhea by measurement of plasma gonadotropins. If they are low, attention is drawn to disorder of hypothalamic-pituitary function. Head CAT and MRI scanning and evaluation of other endocrine functions are indicated.

Clomiphene as a Diagnostic and Therapeutic Tool. Approximately 60 to 80 percent of women with "functional amenorrhea" respond to the administration of clomiphene, which acts as an "antiestrogen" at estrogen receptor sites in hypothalamus and pituitary gland to bring about a functional estrogen-deficiency state. The block of negative-feedback effects of estrogen triggers gonadotropin release. The criterion of response to clomiphene is a normal menstrual period approximately 12 days after administration of the drug, or evidence of ovulation as reflected in change in body temperature. A positive response is assumed to mean that functional abnormality of hypothalamic gonadotropin regulation was present. Clomiphene effects can be demonstrated also by measurement of plasma LH 5 to 10 days after the first day of administration of clomiphene. Plasma LH levels should be in the ovulatory range.

For therapeutic induction of ovulation, the usual starting dose of clomiphene is 50mg daily for 5 days followed by no therapy for 25 days. If two consecutive months of therapy are ineffective, the dose is increased to 100mg daily for 5 days for a further two months. Some recommend doses as high as 150 or 200mg daily if lower doses are ineffective. In addition to establishing a diagnosis of "functional amenorrhea," clomiphene therapy commonly leads to ovulation in women who want to become pregnant. It is believed that some patients with intrinsic pituitary disease also may respond to clomiphene. The efficacy of treatment is greater in women with relatively normal basal estrogen levels, but some relatively estrogen-deficient women also may release LH in response to the drug.

Differential diagnosis of causes of amenorrhea includes disease of the ovary such as the polycystic ovary syndrome, virilizing disorders of ovarian medullary tissue such as hyperthecosis and thecoma, and adrenal disorders such as the adrenogenital syndrome (which may be due to enzymatic defects in the adrenal cortex) or tumor of endocrine tissue (adenoma or carcinoma). Cushing's disease is also a cause of amenorrhea. Usually disorders of this general type are accompanied by clinical evidence of virilization or hirsutism which may include excessive hair growth on face and body, acne, increased muscle mass, and in severe cases, clitoral enlargement. Differentiation of primary gonadotropin failure from disorders due to excessive production of androgenic hormones is therefore usually made on clinical grounds, but in questionable cases, workup should include a study of urinary and plasma adrenal and ovarian steroids. Details of this approach are found in textbooks of clinical or gynecologic endocrinology.

REFERENCES

1. ADLER, BA, JOHNSON, MD, LYNCH, CO, CROWLEY, WR: *Evidence that norepinephrine and epinephrine systems mediate the stimulatory effects of ovarian hormones on luteinizing hormone and luteinizing hormone-releasing hormone.* Endocrinology 113:1431–1438, 1983.
2. ANTAKI, A, SOKMA, M, WYMAN, H, VAN-CAMPENHOUT, J: *Hypothalamic-pituitary function in the olfacto-genital syndrome.* J Clin Endocrinol Metab 38:1083–1089, 1974.
3. ANTHONY, ELP, KING, JC, STOPA, EG: *Immunocytochemical localization of LHRH in the median eminence, infundibular stalk, and neurohypophysis.* Cell Tissue Res 236: 5–14, 1984.
4. BAKER, HWG, EDDIE, LW, HIGGENSON, RE, HUDSON, B, NIALL, HD: *Clinical context, neuroendocrine relationshps, and nature of inhibin in males and females.* In BESSER, GM, AND MARTINI, L (EDS): *Clinical Neuroendocrinology,* vol 2. Academic Press, New York, 1982, pp 283–331.

5. BARNEA, ER, NAFTOLIN, F, TOLIS, G, DE CHERNEY, A: *Hypothalamic amenorrhea syndromes.* In GIVENS, JR (ED): *The Hypothalamus.* Year Book Medical Publishers, Chicago, 1984, pp 147–170.

6. BARNETT, FH, SOHN, J, REICHLIN, S, JACKSON, IMD: *Three luteinizing hormone-releasing hormone like substances in a teleost fish brain; none identical with the mammalian LH-RH decapeptide.* Biochem Biophys Res Commun 105:209–216, 1982.

7. BARRACLOUGH, CA, AND WISE, PM: *The role of catecholamines in the regulation of pituitary luteinizing hormone and follicle-stimulating hormone secretion.* Endocrine Revs 3:91–119, 1982.

8. BELCHETZ, PE, PLANT, TM, NAKAI, Y, KEOUGH, EJ, KNOBIL, E: *Hypophysial responses to continuous and intermittent delivery of hypothalamic gonadotropin-releasing hormone.* Science 202:631–633, 1978.

9. BELCHETZ, PE: *Gonadotropin regulation and clinical applications of GnRH.* In SCANLON, MF (ED): *Clinics in Endocrinology and Metabolism.* WB Saunders, Philadelphia, 1983, pp 619–640.

10. BERKOVIC, SF, BLADIN, PF, VAJDA, FJE: *Temporal lobe epilepsy in hyposexual men* (letter). Lancet March 17, 622–623, 1984.

11. BESSER, GM, MCNEILLY, AS, ANDERSON, DC, MARSHALL, JC, HARSOULIS, P, HALL, R, ORMSTON, BJ, ALEXANDER, L, COLLINS, WP: *Hormonal responses to synthetic luteinizing hormone and follicle stimulating hormone-releasing hormone in man.* Br Med J 3:267–271, 1972.

12. BIERICH, JR: *Sexual precocity.* In BIERICH, JR (ED): *Clinics in endocrinology and metabolism,* vol 4, no 1. WB Saunders, Philadelphia, 1975, pp 107–142.

13. BISSETT, GW: *Milk ejection.* In KNOBIL, E, AND SAWYER, WH (EDS): *Handbook of Physiology, sect 7. Endocrinology, vol IV Part I. The Pituitary Gland and Its Neuroendocrine Control.* American Physiological Society, Washington DC, 1974, pp 493–520.

14. BOYAR, RM: *The effect of clomiphene citrate in anosmic hypogonadotrophism.* Ann Int Med 71:1127–1131, 1969.

15. BOYAR, RM: *Sleep-related endocrine rhythms.* In REICHLIN, S, BALDESSARINI, RJ, MARTIN, JB, (EDS): *The Hypothalamus, vol 56.* Raven Press, New York, 1978, pp 373–386.

16. BOYAR, RM, PERLON, M, HILLMAN, N, KAPAN, S, WEITZMAN, E: *Twenty-four hour pattern of luteinizing hormone secretion in normal men with sleep stage.* J Clin Endocrinol Metab 35:73–81, 1972.

17. BOYAR, RM, FINKELSTEIN, J, ROFFWARG, H, ET AL: *Synchronization of augmented lutenizing hormone secretion with sleep during puberty.* New Engl J Med 287:582–586, 1972.

18. CARMEL, PW, ARAKI, S, FERIN, M: *Pituitary stalk portal blood collection in Rhesus monkeys; evidence for pulsatile release of gonadotropin-releasing hormone (Gn-RH).* Endocrinology 99:243–248, 1976.

19. CATT, KJ, AND PIERCE, PG: *Gonadotropic hormones of the adenohypophysis (FSH, LH, and prolactin).* In YEN, SSC, AND JAFFE, RB, (EDS): *Reproductive Endocrinology.* WB Saunders Company, Philadelphia, 1978, 34–62.

20. CATEL, NS, AND YEN, SSC: *Concomitant pulsatile release of prolactin and luteinizing hormone in hypogonadal women.* J Clin Endocrinol Metab. 56:1313–1315, 1983.

21. CHART, T: *Oxytocin.* In MARTINI, L, BESSER, GM (EDS): *Clinical Neuroendocrinology.* Academic Press, New York, 1977, pp 569–583.

22. CHIN, WW: *Biosynthesis of the glycoprotein hormones.* In Secretory tumors of the pituitary gland. BLACK, P McL, ZERVAS, NT, RIDGWAY, EC, MARTIN, JB (EDS): Raven Press, New York, 1984, pp 327–342.

23. CLEMENT-JONES, V, REES, L: *Neuroendocrine correlates of the endorphins and enkephalins.* In *Clinical Neuroendocrinology,* vol 2. Academic Press, 1982, pp 139–203.

24. COMITE, F, PESCOVITZ, HO, REITH, K, DWYER, A. McNEMAR, A, CUTLER, GB, JR, LORIAUX, DL: *Luteinizing hormone releasing hormone analogue treatment of boys with hypothalamic hamartoma and true precocious puberty.* J Clin Endocrinol Metab 58:857–861, 1984.

25. COMITE, F, CUTLER, GB, JR, RIVIER, J, VALE, WW, LORIAUX, DL, CROWLEY, WF, JR: *Short-term treatment of idiopathic precocious puberty with a long-acting analogue of luteinizing hormone-releasing hormone.* New Engl J Med 305:1546–1550, 1981.

26. COMITE, F, SHAWKER, TH, PESCOVITZ, OH, LORIAUX, DL, CUTLER, GB, JR: *Cyclic ovarian function resistant to treatment with an analogue of luteinizing hormone releasing hormone in McCune-Albright syndrome.* New Engl J Med 311:1032–1036, 1984.

27. CONN, PM, HSUEH, AJW, CROWLEY, WF, JR: *Gonadotropin-releasing hormone: Molecular and cell biology, physiology and clinical applications.* Fed Proc 43:2351–2361, 1984.

28. CONN, PM, MARIAN, JM, MCMILLIAN, M, STERN, J, ROGERS, D, HAMBY, M, PENNA, A, GRANT, E: *Gonadotropin-releasing hormone action in the pituitary: A three step mechanism.* Endocrine Rev 2:174–185, 1981.

29. CROWLEY, WF, MCARTHUR, JW: *Simulation of the normal menstrual cycle in Kallman's syndrome by pulsatile administration of luteinizing hormone-releasing hormone (LHRH).* J Clin Endocrinol Metab 51:173–175, 1980.

30. CROWLEY, WF, COMITE, F, VALE, W, RIVIER, J, LORIAUX, DL, CUTLER, GB, JR: *Therapeutic use of pituitary desensitizition with a long-acting LHRH agonist: A potential new treatment for idiopathic precocious puberty.* J Clin Endocrinol 52:370–372, 1981.

31. CUTLER, GB, JR, HOFFMAN, AR, SWERDLOFF, RS, SANTEN, RJ, MELDRUM, DR, COMITE, F: *Therapeutic applications of luteinzing hormone-releasing hormone and its analogs.* Ann Int Med 102:643–657, 1985.

32. DANEN, M, CRAWFORD, JD: *Peripheral endocrinopathy causing sexual precocity in Albright's syndrome.* Pediatr Res 8:368A, 1964.

33. DONOVAN, BT, VAN DER WERFF TEN BOSCH, JJ: *Physiology of Puberty.* Williams & Wilkins, Baltimore, 1965.

34. EHRHARDT, AA, AND MEYER-BAHLBURG, JFL: *Psychological correlates of abnormal pubertal development.* In BIERICH, JR (ED): *Clinics in Endocrinology and Metabolism,* vol 4, no 1. WB Saunders, Philadelphia, 1975, pp 207–222.

35. ELKIND-HIRSCH, K, RAVNIKAR, V. TULCHINSKY, D, ET AL: *Episodic secretory patterns of immunoreactive luteinizing hormone-releasing hormone (IR-LH-RH) in the systemic circulation of normal women throughout the menstrual cycle.* Fertil Steril 41:56–61, 1984.

36. ERDHEIM, J: *Uber Hypophysenganggeschwulste and Hirncholesteratome.* Akad Wiss Wien, Sitzber, 113:537–726, 1904.

37. FAGLIA, G, BECK-PECCOZ, P, TRAVAGLINI, P, PARACCHI, A, SPADA, A, LEWIN, A: *Elevations in plasma growth hormone concentration after luteinizing hormone-releasing hormone (LRH) in patients with active acromegaly.* J Clin Endocrinol Metab 37:338–340, 1973.

38. FERIN, M: *Endogenous opioid peptides and the menstrual cycle.* Trends in Neurosciences 7:194–196, 1984.

39. FERIN, M: *Neuroendocrine control of ovarian function in the primate.* J Reprod Fertil 69:369–381, 1983.

40. FINK, G, STANLEY, HF, WATTS, AG: *Central nervous control of sex and gonadotropin release: Peptide and nonpeptide transmitter interactions.* In KRIEGER, DT, BROWNSTEIN, MJ, MARTIN, JB (EDS): *Brain Peptides.* John Wiley & Sons, New York, 1983, pp 423–435.

41. FOSTER, CM, ROSS, JL, SHAWKER, T, PESCOVITZ, OH, LORIAUX, DL, CUTLER, GB, JR, COMITE, F: *Absence of pubertal gonadotropin secretion in girls with McCune-Albright syndrome.* J Clin Endocrinol Metab 58:1161–1165, 1984.

42. FRANCHIMONT, P, BECKER, H, ERNOULD, C, THYS, C, DEMOULIN, A, BOURGUIGNON, JP, LEGROS, JJ, VALCKE, JC: *The effect of hypothalamic luteinizing hormone—releasing hormone (LH-RH) on plasma gonadotropin levels in normal subjects.* Clin Endocrinol (Oxf) 3:27–39, 1974.

43. FRANTZ, AG, WILSON, JD: *Endocrine disorders of the breast.* In WILSON, JD, AND FOSTER, DW, (EDS): *Williams Textbook of Endocrinology.* WB Saunders, Philadelphia, 1985, pp 402–421.

44. FRISCH, RE: *Body fat, puberty and fertility.* Biol Rev 59:161–188, 1984.

45. FRISCH, RE: *Fatness, menarche, and female fertility.* Perspectives in Biology and Medicine 28:611–633, 1985.

46. FRISCH, RE: *Population, food intake and fertility: Historical evidence for a direct effect of nutrition on reproductive ability.* Science 199:22–30, 1978.

47. FROHLICH, A: *Ein Fall von Tumor der Hypophysis cerebrie ohne Acromegalle.* Wein Klin Rdsch 15:883–886, 1901.

48. FUTTERWEIT, W, AND GOODSELL, CH: *Galactorrhea in primary hypothyroidism: Report of two cases and review of the literature.* Mt Sinai J Med NY 37:584–589, 1970.

49. FUXE, K, HOKFELT, T, LOFSTROM, A, JOHANSSON, O, AGNATI, L, EVERITT, B, GOLDSTEIN, M, JEFFCOATE, S, WHITE, N, ENEROTH, P, GUSTAFSSON, JA, SKETT, P: *On the role of neurotransmitters and hypothalamic hormones and their interactions in hypothalamic and extrahypothalamic control of pituitary function and sexual behavior.* In NAFTOLIN, F, RYAN, KJ, DAVIES, J (EDS): *Subcellular Mechanisms in Reproductive Neuroendocrinology.* Elsevier, Amsterdam, 1976, pp 193–246.

50. GORSKI, RA: *Sexual differentiation of the brain.* In KRIEGER, DI, HUGHES, JC (EDS): *Neuroendocrinology.* Sinauer Associates, Sunderland, MA, 1980, pp 215–222.

51. GORSKI, RA: *Steroid-induced sexual characteristics in the brain.* In MÜLLER, EE, AND MACLEOD, RM (EDS): *Neuroendocrine perspectives,* vol 2. Elsevier, Amsterdam, 1983, pp 1–35.

52. GRIFFIN, JE, AND WILSON, JD: *Disorders of the testes and male reproductive tract.* In WILSON, JD, AND FOSTER, D (EDS): *Textbook of Endocrinology,* ed 7. WB Saunders, Philadelphia, 1985, pp 259–311.

53. GROSSMAN, A, CLEMENT-JONES, V, BESSER, GM: *Clinical implications of endogenous opioid peptide.* In MÜLLER, EE, MACLEOD, RM, FROHMAN LA (EDS): *Neuroendocrine Perspectives,* vol 4. Elsevier, Amsterdam, 1985, pp 243–294.

54. GRUMBACH, MM: *The neuroendocrinology of puberty.* In KRIEGER, DT, HUGHES, JC (EDS): *Neuroendocrinology.* Sindauer Associates, Sunderland, MA, 1980, pp 249–258.

55. GUNNETT, JW AND FREEMAN, ME: *The mating-induced release of prolactin: A unique neuroendocrine response.* Endocr. Rev. 4:44–61, 1983.

56. HALI, R, AND WARRICK, C: *Hypersecretion of hypothalamic releasing hormones: A possible*

explanation of the endocrine manifestations of polyostotic fibrous dysplasia (Albrights' syndrome). Lancet 1:1313–1316, 1972.

57. HEATH, H, III: *Athletic women, amenorrhea, and skeletal integrity.* Ann Int Med 102:258–260, 1985.

58. HOCHMAN, HI, JUDGE, DM, REICHLIN, S: *Precocious puberty and hypothalamic hamartoma.* Pediatrics 67:236–244, 1981.

58. HOFF, JD, GUIGLEY, ME, YEN, SSC: *Hormonal dynamics at midcycle: A reevaluation.* J Clin Endocrinol Metab 57:792–796, 1983.

60. JACOBS, LS: *The role of prolactin in mammogenesis and lactogenesis.* Adv Exp Med Biol 80:173–91, 1977.

61. JENNINGS, MT, GELMAN, R, HOCHBERG, F: *Intracranial germ-cell tumors: Natural history and pathogenesis.* J Neurosurg 63:155–167, 1985.

62. JOB, JC: *The neuroendocrine system and puberty.* In MARTINI, I, AND BESSER, GM (EDS): *Clinical Neuroendocrinology.* Academic Press, New York, 1978, pp 488–501.

63. JOLLY, H: *Sexual Precocity.* Charles C Thomas, Springfield, IL, 1955.

64. JUDGE, DM, KULIN, HE, PAGE, R, SANTEN, R, TRAPUKDI, S: *Hypothalamic hamartoma — a source of luteinizing-hormone-releasing factor in precocious puberty.* New Engl J Med 296:7–10, 1977.

65. KALRA, SP, AND KALRA, PS: *Neural regulation of luteinizing hormone secretion in the rat.* Endocr Rev 4:311–351, 1983.

66. KASTIN, AJ, GUAL, C, SCHALLY, AV: *Clinical experience with hypothalamic releasing hormones. Part 2. Lutenizing hormone-releasing hormone and other hypophysiotropic releasing hormone.* Recent Progr Horm Res 28:201–217, 1972.

67. KING, JA, AND MILLAR, RP: *Comparative aspects of luteinizing hormone-releasing hormone structure and function in vertebrate phylogeny.* Endocrinology 106:707–717, 1980.

68. KING, JC, AND ANTHONY, ELP: *LHRH neurons and their projections in humans and other mammals: Species Comparisons.* Peptides 5 (Suppl 1):195–207, 1984.

69. KING, JC, ANTHONY, ELP, FITZGERALD, DM, STOPA, EG: *Luteinizing hormone-releasing hormone neurons in human preoptic/hypothalamus; differential intraneuronal localization of immunoreactive forms.* J Clin Endocrinol Metab 60:88–97, 1985.

70. KISS, J, AND HALASZ, B: *Demonstration of serotoninergic axons terminating on luteinizing hormone-releasing hormone neurons in the preoptic area of the rat using a combination of immunocytochemistry and high resolution autoradiography.* Neuroscience 14:69–78, 1985.

71. KNOBIL, E: *The neuroendocrine control of the menstrual cycle.* Recent Prog Horm Res 35:53–88, 1980.

72. KOVACS, K, HORVATH, E, THORNER, MO, ROGOL, AD: *Mammosomatotroph hyperplasia associated with acromegaly and hyperprolactinemia in a patient with the McCune-Albright syndrome. A histologic, immunocytologic and ultrastructural study of the surgically-removed adenohypophysis.* Virchows Arch 403:77–86, 1984.

73. KRAFT-EBBING, R VON: *Psychopathia Sexualis* (first English edition of the seventh German edition). Physicians and Surgeons Book Company, New York, 1927, p 32.

74. KULIN, HE, AND REITER, EO: *Gonadotropins during childhood and adolescence: A review.* Pediatrics 51:260–271, 1973.

75. KULIN, HE, AND SANTEN, RJ: *Normal and aberrant pubertal development in man.* In VAITUKAITIS, JL (ED): *Clinical Reproductive Neuroendocrinology.* Elsevier, Amsterdam, 1982, pp 19–68.

76. LIEBLICH, JM, ROGOL, AD, WHITE, BJ, ET AL: *Syndrome of anosmia with hyperogonadotropic hypogonadism (Kallman syndrome). Clinical and laboratory studies in 23 cases.* Am J Med 73:506–519, 1982.

77. LINDBERG, JS, FEARS, WB, HUNT, MM, POWELL, MR, BOLL, D, WADE, CE: *Exercise-induced amenorrhea and bone density.* Ann Intern Med 101:647–648, 1984.

78. LIU, JH, AND YEN, SSC: *Induction of midcycle gonadotropin surge by ovarian steroids in women: A critical evaluation.* J Clin Endocrinol Metab 57:797–802, 1983.

79. LIU, N, GRUMBACH, MM, DE NAPOLI, RA: *Prevalence of electroencephalographic abnormalities in idiopathic precocious puberty and premature pubarche: Bearing on pathogenesis and neuroendocrine regulation of puberty.* J Clin Endocrinol Metab 25:1296–1308, 1965.

80. LYENDECKER, G, WILDT, L, HANSMAN, M: *Pregnancies following chronic intermittent (pulsatile) administration of GnRH by means of a portable pump ("Zyklomat") — a new approach to the treatment of infertility in hypothalamic amenorrhea.* J Clin Endocrinol Metab 51:1214–1216, 1980.

81. LYONS, WR, LI, CH, JOHNSON, RE: *The hormonal control of mammary growth and lactation.* Recent Progr Horm Res 14:219–254, 1958.

82. MACGILLIVRAY, MH: *Treatment of idiopathic precocious puberty* (letter). New Engl J Med 306:1109–1110, 1982.

83. MANSFIELD, MJ, BEARDSWORTH, DE, LOUGHLIN, JS, CRAWFORD, JD, BODE, HH, RIVIER, I, VALE, W, KRUSHNER, DC, CRIGUR, JF, JR, CROWLEY, WF, JR: *Long-term treatment of central precocious*

REGULATION OF THE PITUITARY GLAND

puberty with a long-acting analogue of luteinizing hormone releasing hormone. N Engl J Med 309:1286–1290, 1983.

84. MARCUS, R, CANN, C, MADVIG, P, MINKOFF, J, GODDARD, M. BAYER, M, MARTIN, M, GAUDIANI, L, HASKELL, W. GENANT, H: *Menstrual function and bone mass in elite women distance runners.* Ann Int Med 102:158–163, 1985.

85. MARSHALL, JC, KELCH, RP, SAUDER, SE, BARKAN, A, REAME, NE, KHOURY, S: *Pulsatile gonadotropin-releasing hormone (GnRH)—studies of puberty and the menstrual cycle.* In LABRIE, F, AND PROUIX, L (EDS): *Proceedings of the seventh International Congress of Endocrinology.* Quebec City 1–7, July 1984. Excerpta Medica, Amsterdam, 1984, pp 25–32.

86. MARSHALL, JC, CASE, GD, VALK, TW, CORLEY, KP, SAUDER, SE, KELCH, RP: *Selective inhibition of follicle-stimulating hormone secretion by estradiol. Mechanism for modulation of gonadotropin responses to low dose pulses of gonadotropin-releasing hormone.* J Clin Invest 71:248–257, 1983.

87. MARSHALL, WA: *Growth and sexual maturation in normal puberty.* In BIERICH, JR (ED): *Clinics in Endocrinology and Metabolism,* vol 4, no 1. WB Saunders, Philadelphia, 1975.

88. MATSUO, H, BABA, Y, NAIR, RM, ARIMURA, A, SCHALLY, AV: *Structure of the porcine LH- and FSH-releasing hormone. The proposed amino acid sequence.* Biochem Biophys Res Commun 43:1334–1339, 1971.

89. McCANN, SM: *Regulation of secretion of follicle-stimulating hormone and lutenizing hormone.* In GREEP, RO, AND ASTWOOD, EB (EDS): *Handbook of physiology, Section 7: Endocrinology,* vol 4, part 1. American Physiological Society, William & Wilkins, Baltimore, 1974, pp 489–517.

90. McCANN, SM: *The role of brain peptides in the control of anterior pituitary hormone secretion.* In MÜLLER, EE, AND MacLEOD, RM, (EDS): *Neuroendocrine Perspectives,* vol 1. Elsevier, Amsterdam, 1982, pp 1–22.

91. McCANN, SM, MIZUNUMA, H, SAMSON, WK: *Differential hypothalamic control of FSH secretion: A review.* Psychoneuroendocrinology 8:299–308, 1983.

92. McDONALD, JK, LUMPKIN, MD, SAMSON, WK, McCANN, SM: *Neuropeptide Y affects secretion of luteinizing hormone and growth hormone in ovariectomized rats.* 82:561–564, 1985.

93. MEITES, J: *Control of mammary growth and lactation.* In MARTINI, L, AND GANONG, WF (EDS): *Neuroendocrinology.* Academic Press, New York, 1966, pp 669–707.

94. MONEY, J, AND HAMPSON, JG: *Idiopathic sexual precocity in the male: Management; Report of a case.* Psychosom Med 17:1–15, 1955.

95. MONEY, J, AND ALEXANDER, D: *Psychosexual development and absence of homosexuality in males with precocious puberty: Review of 18 cases.* J Nerv Ment Dis 148:111–123, 1969.

96. MORTIMER, CH: *Gonadotropin-releasing hormone.* In MARTINI, L, AND BESSER, GM (EDS): *Clinical Neuroendocrinology.* Academic Press, New York, 1977, pp 213–236.

97. MORTIMER, CH, BESSER, GM, McNEILLY, AS, MARSHALL, JC, HARSOULIS, P, TUNBRIDGE, WMG, GOMEZ-PAN A, HALL, R: *Luteinizing hormone and follicle stimulating hormone-releasing hormone test in patients with hypothalamic-pituitary-gonadal dysfunction.* Br Med J 4:73–77, 1973.

98. MORTIMER, CH, McNEILLY, AS, MURRAY, MAF, FISHER, RAF, BESSER, GM: *Gonadotrophin-releasing hormone therapy in hypogonadal males with hypothalamic or pituitary dysfunction.* Br Med J. 4:617–621, 1974.

99. MOTTA, M, FRASCHINI, F, MARTINI, L: *"Short" feedback mechanisms in the control of anterior pituitary function.* In GANONG, WF, AND MARTINI, L. (EDS): *Frontiers in Neuroendocrinology.* Oxford University Press, London, 1969, pp 211–254.

100. NOWAKOWSKI, H. AND LENZ, W: *Genetic aspects of male hypogonadism.* Recent Progr Horm Res 17:53–95, 1961.

101. OJEDA, SR, ANDREWS, WW, ADVIS, JP, SMITH, SS: *Recent Advances in the endocrinology of puberty.* Endocr Rev 1:228–257, 1980.

102. OJEDA, SR, SMITH, (WRIGHT) SS, URBANSKI, HF, AGUADO, LI: *Onset of female puberty: Underlying neuroendocrine mechanisms.* In MÜLLER, EE, AND MacLEOD, RM (EDS): *Neuroendocrine Perspectives,* vol 3. Elsevier, Amsterdam, 1984, pp 225–278.

103. PESCOVITZ, OH, COMITE, F, CASSORIA, F, DWYER, AJ, POTH, MA, SPERLING, M, HENCH, K, McNEMAR, A, SKERDA, M, LORIAUX, DL, CUTLER, GB, JR: *True precocious puberty complicating congentical adrenal hyperplasia: treatment with a luteining hormone releasing hormone analogue.* J Clin Endocrinol Metab 58:857–861, 1984.

104. PESCOVITZ, OH, CUTLER, GB, JR, LORIAUX, DL: *Precocious puberty.* In MÜLLER, EE, MACLEOD, RM, FROHMAN, LA (EDS): *Neuroendocrine Perspectives,* vol 4. Elsevier, Amsterdam, 1985, pp 73–93.

105. POISSON, M: *Sex steroid receptors in human meningiomas.* Clin Neuropharmacology 7:320–324, 1984.

106. QUIGLEY, ME, AND YEN, SSC: *The role of endogenous opiates on LH secretion during the menstrual cycle.* J Clin Endocrinol Metab 51:179–81, 1980.

107. QUIGLEY, ME, RAKOFF, JS, YEN, SS: *Increased luteinizing hormone sensitivity to dopamine inhibition in polycystic ovary syndrome.* J Clin Endocrinol Metab 52:234–234, 1981.

108. RABIN, D, SPITZ, I, BERCOVICI, B, BELL, J, LAUFER, A, BENVENISTE, R, POLISHUK, W: *Isolated deficiency of follicle-stimulating hormone. Clinical and Laboratory Features.* N Engl J Med 287:1313, 1972.

109. RAMASHARMA, K, SAIRAM, MR, SEIDAH, NG, CHRETIEN, M, MANJUNATH, P, SCHILLER, PW, YAMASHIRO, D, LI, CH: *Isolation, structure, and synthesis of a human seminal plasma peptide with inhibin-like activity.* Science 223:1199–1202, 1984.

110. RAMIREZ, VD, FEDER, HH, SAWYER, CH: *The role of brain catecholamines in the regulation of LH secretion: A critical inquiry.* In MARTINI, L, AND GANONG, WR (EDS): *Frontiers in Neuroendocrinology,* vol 8. Raven Press, New York, 1984, pp 27–84.

111. REICHLIN, S: *Neuroendocrine aspects of human reproduction.* In MACK, HC, AND SHERMAN, AI (EDS): *The neuroendocrinology of human reproduction.* Charles C Thomas, Springfield, IL, 1971, pp 3–5.

112. REICHLIN, S: *Overview of the anatomical and physiological basis of anterior-pituitary regulation.* In TOLIS, G, LABRIE, F, MARTIN, JB, NAFTOLIN, F (EDS): *Clinical Endocrinology.* Raven Press, New York, 1979, pp 1–14.

113. REID, RL, LING, N, YEN, SSC: *Gonadotropin-releasing activity of a-melanocyte-stimulating hormone in normal subjects and in subjects with hypothalamic-pituitary dysfunction.* J Clin Endocrinol Metab 58:773–777, 1984.

114. REITER, EO, AND GRUMBACH, MM: *Neuroendocrine control mechanisms and the onset of puberty.* Annu Rev Physiol 44:595–613, 1982.

115. REITER, EO, BROWN, RS, LONGCOPE, C, BEITINS, IZ: *Male-limited familial precocious puberty in three generations.* New Engl J Med 311:515–519, 1984.

116. RICHTER, RB: *True hamartoma of the hypothalamus associated with pubertal praecox.* J Neuropath Exp Neurol 10:368–373, 1951.

117. RIDGWAY, EC: *Glycoprotein hormone production by pituitary tumors.* In BLACK, PM, ZERVAS, NT, RIDGWAY, EC, MARTIN, JB (EDS): *Secretory pituitary tumors.* Raven Press, New York, 1984, pp 343–364.

118. RODMAN, E, DAYAL, Y, ADELMAN, L, SHUCART, L, REICHLIN, S: *Acromegally due to nodular hyperplasia of the pituitary in polyostotic fibrous dysplasia.* (In preparation.)

119. ROSENTHAL, SM, GRUMBACH, MM, KAPLAN, SL: *Gonadotropin-independent familial sexual precocity with premature Leydig and germinal cell maturation (familial testotoxicosis): Effects of a potent luteinzing hormone-releasing factor agonist and medroxyprogesterone acetate therapy in four cases.* J Clin Endocrinol Metab 57: 571–579, 1983.

120. ROSS, GT: *Disorders of the ovary and female reproductive tract.* In WILSON, JD, AND FOSTER, DW (EDS): *Textbook of Endocrinology,* WB Saunders, Philadelphia, 1985, pp 206–258.

121. ROTH, JC, KELCH, RP, KAPLAN, SL, GRUMBACH, MM: *FSH and LH response to luteinizing hormone-releasing factor in prepubertal and pubertal children, adult males and patients with hypogonadotropic and hypertropichypogonadism.* J Clin Endocrinol Metab 35:926–930, 1972.

122. SADEGHI-NEJAD, A, AND SENIOR, B: *Sexual precocity: An unusual complication of propylthiouracil therapy.* J Pediatr 79:833–837, 1971.

123. SAIRAM, MR, AND PAPKOFF, H: *Chemistry of pituitary gonadotrophins.* In *Handbook of Physiology, Section7: Endocrinology, vol IV. The pituitary gland and its neuroendocrine control, part 2.* American Physiological Society, Washington, DC, 1974, pp 111–132.

124. SAWYER, CH, MARKEE, JE, TOWNSEND, BF: *Cholinergic and adrenergic components in the neurohumoral control of the release of LH in the rabbit.* Endocrinology 44:18–37, 1949.

125. SCHALLENBERGER, E, RICHARDSON, DW, KNOBIL, E: *Role of prolactin in the lactational amenorrhea of the rhesus monkey (Macaca mulatta).* Biol Reprod 25:370–374, 1981.

126. SCHALLY, AV: *Aspects of hypothalamic regulation of the pituitary gland. Its implications for the control of reproductive processes (Nobel lecture).* Science 202:18–28, 1978.

127. SCHONBERG, D: *Dynamics of hypothalamic-pituitary function during puberty.* In BEIRICH, JR (ED): *Clinics in Endocrinology and Metabolism,* vol 4, no 1. WB Saunders, Philadelphia, 1975, pp 57–88.

128. SCULLY, RE, GALDABINI, JJ, MCNEELY, BU: *Case Records of the Massachusetts General Hospital. Clincopathological exercises,* case 33-1975. N Engl J Med 293:394–399, 1975.

129. SEEBURG, PH, ADELMAN, JP: *Characterization of cDNA for precursor of human luteinizing hormone releasing hormone.* Nature 311:666–668, 1984.

130. SEYLER, LE, JR, GRAZE, K, CANALIS, E, SPARE, S, REICHLIN, S: *Effects of sex-steroid priming on pituitary responses to LH-RH.* In BELING, CG, AND WENTZ, AC (EDS): *The LH-releasing Hormone.* Masson, 1980, pp 87–100.

131. SHARP, PJ, AND FRASER, HM: *Control of reproduction.* In JEFFCOATE, SL, AND HUTCHINSON, JSM (EDS): *The Endocrine Hypothalamus.* Academic Press, London, 1978, pp 271–332.

132. SHERWOOD, N, EIDEN, L, BROWNSTEIN, M, ET AL: *Characterization of a teleost gonadotropin-releasing hormone.* Proc Natl Acad Sci USA 80:2794–2798, 1983.

133. SHIVERS, BD, HARLAN, RE, MORRELL, JI, ET AL: *Absence of oestradiol concentration in cell nuclei of LHRH-immunoreactive neurons.* Nature 304:345–347, 1983.

134. SHORT, RV: *Breastfeeding.* Sci Am 250:35–41, 1984.

REGULATION OF THE PITUITARY GLAND

135. SIZONENKO, PA: *Endocrine laboratory findings in pubertal disturbances.* In BEIRICH, JR (ED): *Clinics in Endocrinology and Metabolism,* vol 4, no 1. WB Saunders, Philadelphia, 1975, pp 173–206.

136. SKARIN, G, NILIUS, SJ, WIBELL, L, WIDE, L: *Chronic pulsatile low-dose GnRH therapy for induction of testosterone production and spermatogenesis in a man with secondary hypogonadotropic hypogonadism.* J Clin Endocrinol Metab 55:723–726, 1982.

137. SKARIN, G, NILIUS, SJ, WIDE, L: *Pulsatile low dose luteinizing hormone releasing hormone treatment for induction of follicular maturation and ovulation in women with amenorrhea.* Acta Endocrinol 101:78–86, 1982.

138. SNOWDEN, EU, KHAN-DAWOOD, FS, DAWOOD, MY: *The effect of naloxone on endogenous opioid regulation of pituitary gonadotropins and prolactin during the menstrual cycle.* J Clin Endocrinol Metab 59:298–302, 1984.

139. SPARK, RF, WILLS, CA, ROVAL, H: *Hypogonadism, hyperprolactinemia, and temporal lobe epilepsy in hyposexual men.* Lancet Feb 25, 1984, 413–416.

140. SPITZ, IM, HIRSCH, HJ, TRESTIAN, S: *The prolactin response to thyrotropin-releasing hormone differentiates isolated gonadotropin deficiency from delayed puberty.* New Engl J Med 308:575–579, 1983.

141. STARKMAN, MN, MARSHALL, JC, LAFERLA, J, KELCH, RP: *Pseudocyesis: Psychologic and neuroendocrine interrelationships.* Psychosomatic Med 47:46–57, 1985.

142. STYNE, DM, GRUMBACH, MM: *Puberty in the male and female: Its physiology and disorders.* In YEN, SSC, AND JAFFE, RB (EDS): *Reproductive Endocrinology.* WB Saunders, Philadelphia, 1978, pp 189–240.

143. TANNER, JM: *Growth and endocrinology of the adolescent.* In GARDNER, LI (ED): *Endocrine and Genetic Diseases of Childhood and Adolescence,* ed 2. WB Saunders, Philadelphia, 1975, 14–64.

144. TERASAWA, E, NOONAN, JJ, NASS, TE, LOOSE, MD: *Posterior hypothalamic lesions advance the onset of puberty in the female rhesus monkey.* Endocrinology 115:2241–2250, 1984.

145. TERRY, LC: *Neuropharmacologic regulation of anterior pituitary hormone secretion in man.* In GIVENS, JR (ED): *Hormone-secreting Pituitary Tumors.* Year Book Medical Publishers, Chicago, 1982, pp 27–44.

146. TINDAL, JS: *Control of prolactin secretion.* In JEFFCOATE, SL, HUTCHINSON, JSM (EDS): *The Endocrine Hypothalamus.* Academic Press, New York, 1978, pp 333–361.

147. VAN DER WERFF TEN BOSCH, JJ: *Isosexual precocity.* In GARDNER, LI (ED): *Endocrine and Genetic Diseases of Childhood and Adolescence,* ed 2. WB Saunders, Philadelphia, 1975, pp 619–639.

148. VAN WYCK, JJ, AND GRUMBACH, MM: *Syndrome of precocious menstruation and galactorrhea in juvenile hypothyroidism: An example of hormonal overlap in pituitary feedback.* J Pediatr 57:416–435, 1960.

149. VELDHUIS, JD, BEITINS, IZ, JOHNSON, ML, SERABIAN, MA, DUFAU, ML: *Biologically active luteinizing hormone is secreted in episodic pulsations that vary in relation to stage of the menstrual cycle.* J Clin Endocrinol Metab 58:1050–1058, 1984.

150. WEINBERGER, LM, AND GRANT FC: *Precocious puberty and tumors of the hypothalamus.* Arch Int Med. 67:762–792, 1941.

151. WINTERS, SJ: *Clinical male reproductive neuroendocrinology.* In VAITUKAITUS, JL (ED): *Clinical Reproductive Endocrinology.* Elsevier, Amsterdam, 1982, pp 69–104.

152. WISE, PM, RANCE, N, BARR, GD: *Further evidence that luteinizing hormone-releasing hormone also is follicle-stimulating hormone-releasing hormone.* Endocrinology 104:940–947, 1979.

153. WITKIN, JW, AND SILVERMAN, AJ: *Luteinizing hormone-releasing hormone (LHRH) in rat olfactory systems.* J Comp Neurol 218:426–432, 1983.

154. WOOD, LC, OLICHNEY, M, LOCKE, H, CRISPELL, KR, THORNTON, WN, KITAY, JI: *Syndrome of juvenile hypothyroidism associated with advanced sexual development: Report of two new cases and comment of the management of an associated ovarian mass.* J Clin Endocrinol 25:1289–1308, 1965.

155. YEN, SSC: *Neuroendocrine regulation of gonadotropin and prolactin secretion in women: Disorders in reproduction.* In VAITUKAITIS, JL (ED): *Clinical Reproductive Neuroendocrinology.* Elsevier, New York, 1982, pp 137–176.

156. YEN, SSC: *Chronic anovulation due to CNS-hypothalamic-pituitary dysfunction.* In YEN, SSC, AND JAFFE, RB (EDS): *Reproductive Endocrinology.* WB Saunders, Philadelphia, 1978, pp 341–372.

157. YEN, SSC, REBAR, R, VANDEN BERG, G, JUDD, H: *Hypothalamic amenorrhea and hypogonadotropinism: Responses to synthetic LRF.* J Clin Endocrinol Metab 36:811–816, 1973.

158. MASON, AJ, HAYFLICK, JS, LING, N, ESCH, F, VENO, N, YING, S-Y, GUILLEMIN, R, NIALL, H, SEEBURG, PH: *Complementary DNA sequences of ovarian follicular fluid inhibin show precursor structure and homology with transforming growth factor β.* Nature 318:659–663, 1985.

159. KOLODNY, RC, JACOBS, LS, DAUGHADAY, WH: *Mammary stimulation causes prolactin secretion in nonlactating women.* Nature 238:284–286, 1972.

160. LING, N, YING, SY, UENO, N, SHIMASAKI, S, ESCH F, HOTTA, M, GUILLEMIN, R: *Pituitary FSH is*

released by a heterodimer of the beta-subunits from the two forms of inhibin. Nature 321 (6072): 779–782, 1986.

161. VALE, W, RIVIER, J, VAUGHAN, J, MCCLINTOCK, R, CORRIGAN, A, WOO, W, KARR, D, SPIESS, J: *Purification and characterization of an FSH releasing protein from porcine ovarian follicular fluid.* Nature 321 (6072): 776–779, 1986.

162. NAOR, Z: *Phosphoinositide turnover, Ca^{2+} mobilization, protein kinase C activation and leukotriene action in pituitary signal transduction: Effect of gonadotropin releasing hormone.* In *Advances in Prostaglandin, Thromboxane and Leukotriene research.* ZOR, U, KOHEN, F, NAOR, Z, (EDS): Raven Press, New York, (in press).

163. MATTOX, JH, BUCKMAN, MT, BERNSTEIN, J, ET AL: *Dopamine agonists for reducing depression associated with hyperprolactinemia.* J Reprod Med 31:694–698, 1986.

164. KALLMAN, FJ, SCHOENFELD, WA: *The genetic aspects of primary eunuchoidism.* Am J Ment Deficiency 48:203–236, 1944.

165. PESCOVITZ, OH, COMITE, F, HENCH, K, BARNES, K, MCNEMAR, A, FOSTER, C, KENIGSBERG, D, LORIAUX, DL, CUTLER, GB, JR: *The NIH experience with precocious puberty: Diagnostic subgroups and response to short-term luteinizing hormone releasing hormone analogue therapy.* J Pediatr 108:47–54, 1986.

166. RISKIND, P, AND MARTIN, JB: *Functional anatomy of the hypothalamic-anterior pituitary complex.* In DEGROOT, LJ (ED): *Endocrinology,* ed 2. Grune & Stratton, Orlando (in press).

PART 3

Pineal and Periventricular Organs

Chapter 10

THE PINEAL GLAND AND PERIVENTRICULAR ORGANS

Although readily overlooked in dissections of the brain because of its small size (100 to 150 mg) and its relatively inaccessible position (attached to the posterior roof of the third ventricle, under the corpus callosum), the pineal gland (Latin *pinea*, pine cone) has been recognized for many centuries, and its function has been the subject of much speculation. Galen believed that it served as a valve controlling thoughts flowing in the brain ventricles, and Descartes, quite reasonably "observing that the pineal gland is the only part of the brain that is single was determined by this to make that gland the soul's habitation." The function of the pineal gland in the human is still unknown, but the vast amount of recent research on the pineal gland in lower mammals makes it virtually certain that it plays a role in neuroendocrine control of the pituitary gland. And its secretion, melatonin, is a marker of circadian rhythms. In this chapter, the evidence relating the pineal gland to neuroendocrine function in the human is reviewed, and pineal function as known from the experimental literature is summarized. Many comprehensive reviews and monographs have been published.[4,10,12,18,25,38,41,43,50,62,84,86,93,112,130]

ANATOMY AND DEVELOPMENT

The pineal gland of the human being and other vertebrates arises from modified ependymal cells of the epithalamic region of the third ventricle as one of a family of circumventricular secretory organs which includes the *subcommissural organ,* the *area postrema,* the *subfornical organ,* the *median eminence,* and *neurohypophysis.*[36–38] In lower animals (amphibians and certain fishes), the pineal cells have characteristics of photoreceptors, displaying photosensitivity and electric activity suggestive of a "third eye";[40,129] in higher vertebrates, the eye-like features of the pineal gland give way to the glandular-secretory characteristics of the pineal cell (pinealocyte). In this evolutionary change the primitive afferent nerve connections which are analogous to an optic nerve are lost; instead, a new efferent (sympathetic secretomotor) nerve supply reaches the pineal gland from the superior cervical ganglia. These fibers pass by way of paired nervi conarii, which penetrate the dome of the organ from the tentorium of the cerebellum. Additional sympathetic innervation also may reach the pineal gland within the walls of the veins of the region. There is also evidence that a parasym-

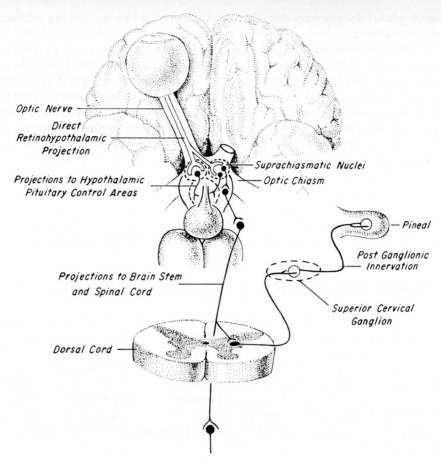

FIGURE 2. This is a schematic diagram of neural structures underlying circadian rhythms. Light impinging on the retina is transduced into neural signals which reach the brain to give both visual and nonvisual activation. This diagram outlines the nonvisual component. Those involved in endocrine regulation are conducted mainly by the direct retinohypothalamic projection to the suprachiasmatic nuclei (located in the hypothalamus). From the suprachiasmatic nuclei, nerve pathways project to the hypophysiotropic control areas of the hypothalamus and also to the spinal cord, where they influence the primary neurons of the sympathetic nerve outflow tract that terminates in the superior cervical ganglia. From the superior cervical ganglia, postganglionic sympathetic nerves (noradrenergic in function) accompanying the venous drainage of the pineal gland enter the gland to innervate the pineal parenchymal cells. Suprachiasmatic nuclei are responsible for endogenous rhythms as well as those influenced by external lighting. (From Reichlin, S: *The Pineal*. In Wyngaarden, JM, and Smith, LH [eds]: *Cecil Textbook of Medicine*. WB Saunders, Philadelphia, 1982, pp 1199–1201, with permission.)

tion in quadriplegics (who do not show normal circadian rhythms) is evidence that the sympathetic innervation is also important in the human being.[45]

Pineal parenchymal cells contain the enzymes that mediate the synthesis of serotonin from tryptophan (see Figure 3).

> This occurs through conversion of 5-hydroxytryptophan (5-HT) to serotonin and subsequently to N-acetylserotonin, the latter regulated by the enzyme N-acetyltransferase (NAT). Melatonin is finally formed by the enzyme hydroxyindole-O-methyltransferase (HIOMT). The N-acetyltransferase enzyme is rate limiting for melatonin formation.

PINEAL AND PERIVENTRICULAR ORGANS

The melatonin-forming enzyme, HIOMT, has served as a highly specific marker for the site of formation of melatonin, both in pineal and extrapineal sites, and also as a marker for human pineal tumors.[20] Outside the pineal gland, which is the richest source of the enzyme, small amounts are found in the retina, the Harderian gland (a modified lachrymal gland) of rodents, and in the choroid plexus. This last site presumably reflects the ependymal-cell origin of both the choroid plexus and pineal gland. One of the most valuable aspects of the study of pineal enzymes is that it has permitted accurate study of the factors that regulate pineal function.

Melatonin has been localized by immunohistologic methods in the outer nuclear layer of the retina, the optic chiasm and optic nerve, and the suprachiasmatic nucleus.[17] It also has been found outside the central nervous system in secretory cells throughout the gastrointestinal tract, namely, in the esophagus, stomach, duodenum, cecum, colon, and rectum.[16] Melatonin crosses the placenta[92] and appears in milk.[95] By these routes, the maternal pineal gland conceivably could influence fetal and sexual functions. These findings, taken together with the presence of synthesizing enzymes in various nonpineal tissues, suggest that melatonin may have

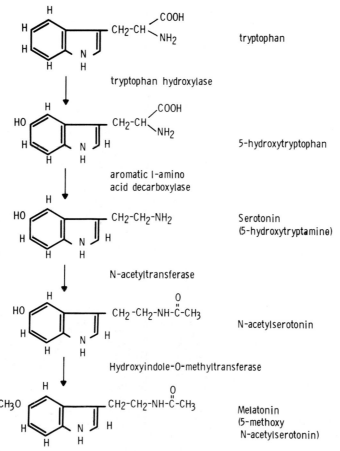

FIGURE 3. Shown here is the metabolic pathway for synthesis of serotonin, N-acetylserotonin, and melatonin.

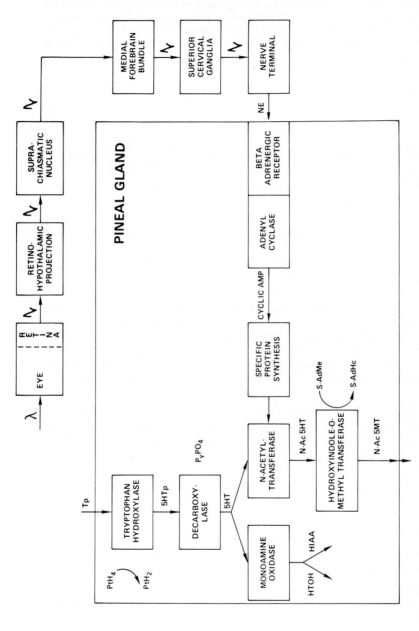

FIGURE 6. This is a diagram of pineal innervation. Norepinephrine (NE) released from nerve terminals combines with β-adrenergic receptor to activate adenyl cyclase. Increased cyclic AMP stimulates specific protein synthesis which leads to increase in N-acetyltransferase activity and formation of melatonin. (From Klein, DC, and Parfitt, A: *Ouabain blocks the adrenergic-cyclic AMP stimulation of pineal N-acetyltransferase activity.* In Weiss, B (ed): *Cycle AMP in Disease.* University Park Press, Baltimore, 1976, p 36, with permission.)

PINEAL AND PERIVENTRICULAR ORGANS

The details of this interaction have been documented extensively.[43,50] During initial exposure to darkness, sympathetic nerve terminals within the pineal gland liberate more norepinephrine. The released catecholamine acts on β-adrenergic receptors located on the pinealocyte plasma membrane to increase adenyl cyclase activity and the subsequent formation of cyclic AMP. Cyclic AMP, in turn, increases the activity of the rate-limiting enzyme, NAT, which results in increased melatonin synthesis (Fig. 6). The decline in serotonin content during the night reflects enhanced synthesis of melatonin. The sympathetic input seems to control virtually all aspects of enzyme function in the pineal gland, including nucleic acid metabolism.

Effects of Melatonin on the Brain

Radioactive melatonin is taken up from the blood by brain tissue, particularly by the hypothalamus and brainstem, and these regions may be specific target areas for melatonin action.[6] Melatonin cannot be detected in the blood following pinealectomy, indicating that most brain melatonin is of pineal origin.[49] A number of effects on human brain function follow administration of melatonin in "pharmacologic doses." These include amelioration of the tremor and rigidity of Parkinson's disease,[5] sleep-inducing effects, and an increase in the proportion of REM sleep. A relative increase in sleep stages 3 and 4 was noted in patients taking melatonin chronically.

Although *lights out* leads to increased melatonin secretion, there is still uncertainty as to whether melatonin plays a role in physiologic sleep. This uncertainty arises because the levels achieved spontaneously are much lower than those required to cause drowsiness following administration of the hormone.[52,123] The potential significance of the peptides TRH, GnRH, and somatostatin, which are present in the pineal gland, in relation to these electrophysiologic and behavioral effects has not been investigated.

TRH, but not GnRH or somatostatin, blocks β-receptor stimulation of cyclic AMP formation in the pineal gland.[116] The sedative effects of melatonin have been attributed to ability to inhibit spontaneous neuronal activity in the mesencephalic reticular formation.[72] Melatonin receptors have been demonstrated in brain tissue and in the pineal gland.[21,22,117] In brain, melatonin increases the concentration of the second messenger cyclic guanidine methyl phosphate (CGMP)[136] and inhibits β-adrenoreceptor-stimulated cyclic AMP accumulation in rat astroglial cell cultures.[117]

In lower animal forms such as the frog, melatonin lightens skin color by aggregating melatonin granules. The underlying mechanism of this response is contraction of microtubules in the cytoskeleton.[18,19,28] Ehrlich and Apuzzo[25] summarize the evidence that suggests that melatonin might affect nerve function by interacting with microtubules:

"Melatonin causes an ultrastructural decrease in microtubules in frog sciatic nerve, and has a colchicine-like effect in preventing microtubular reassembly during temperature recovery. Melatonin treatment *in vivo* decreases hypothalamic microtubule protein content." "Melatonin impairs axonal transport in the sciatic nerve and in the visual pathway." The microtubular binding hypothesis is elaborated fully by Cardinali.[18,19]

around the time of puberty, it has been suggested that the pineal gland may have a role in producing puberty and then cease to function. In fact, this is not the case. Calcification can be detected in autopsied cases before puberty, and the ground-substance matrix for calcification is present as early as one year of life. No difference in enzyme activity is found between heavily calcified glands from aged subjects and lightly calcified ones from young subjects.[130] Normal structure and weight of the pineal gland are preserved into old age, supporting the concept of a functional role of the gland during one's entire life. A lower incidence of calcification occurs in subjects in Japan and Nigeria than in Europe and America. In Europe and in the United States the incidence of calcification ranges from 33 to 97 percent.

HYPOPLASIA AND APLASIA

Hypoplasia and aplasia of the pineal gland are rare. A high proportion of patients with primary hypoplasia are reported to have genital precocity, and many of these patients have associated pituitary lesions.

TUMORS

Tumors of the pineal gland are rare, making up less than 1 percent of intracranial neoplasms, and are seen almost exclusively in young men. As defined by Russell,[100,101] the term *pinealoma* refers to a tumor of the pineal parenchymal cell, called *pineoblastoma* or *pineocytoma*, according to its immaturity. In the series of 53 cases classified as tumors of the pineal gland by DeGirolami and Schmidek[23] (Table 1) at the Massachusetts General Hospital, only nine fitted this category. Glial tumors of the pineal gland such as astrocytomas and glioblastomas were more common, accounting for 13 cases. The most common tumor of the pineal region is best termed germinoma because it apparently arises from undifferentiated germ cells.[32] Approximately one half of the cases in the DeGirolami series were classified as germinomas. Germinomas also are called ectopic pinealomas or seminomatous pinealomas. Although the pineal gland is the site of origin of these tumors, they do not arise from pineal parenchymal cells. Identical types of tumors are found in the testis, the anterior mediastinum, and in the suprasellar region. The pathogenesis of the germinomas, as described by Scully,[105] is that "during early embryonic development, germ cells, which arise in the yolk sac and migrate to the gonadal ridges of the male and female embryo, may be aberrant, wandering into atypical sites where the anterior mediastinum and pineal gland eventually lie. Isolated germ cells have been found within the head of the embryo." Scully also points out that "in addition to germinomas, most other types of germ-cell tumors seen in the testis and ovary, including the endodermal sinus tumor, the choriocarcinoma and benign and malignant teratomas have arisen in the pineal gland and anterior mediastinum." Approximately 10 percent of intracranial germinomas metastasize via the CSF to the meninges of the spinal cord. Germinomas can arise in the pineal gland and then infiltrate the third ventricle and the floor of the hypothalamus or arise in the ventral hypothalamus.[32] In the suprachiasmatic region they produce a characteristic

PINEAL AND PERIVENTRICULAR ORGANS

TABLE 1. Classification of Tumors of Pineal Region

A. Germ Cell Tumors
   1. Germinoma
      a. Posterior third ventricle and pineal
      b. Anterior third ventricle, suprasellar or intrasellar
      c. Combined lesions in anterior and posterior third ventricle, apparently noncontiguous, with or without foci of cystic or solid teratoma
   2. Teratoma
      a. Evidencing growth along two or three germ lines in varying degrees of differentiation
      b. Dermoid and epidermoid cysts with or without solid foci of teratoma
      c. Histologically malignant forms with or without differentiated foci of benign, solid, or cystic teratoma—teratocarcinoma, chorioepithelioma, embryonal carcinoma (endodermal-sinus tumor or yolk-sac carcinoma), combinations of these with or without foci of germinoma, chemodectoma
B. Pineal Parenchymal Tumors
   1. Pineocytes
      a. Pineocytoma
      b. Pineoblastoma
      c. Ganglioglioma and chemodectoma
      d. Mixed forms exhibiting transitions between these
   2. Glia
      a. Astrocytoma
      b. Ependymoma
      c. Mixed forms and other less frequent gliomas (glioblastoma, oligodendroglioma, etc.)
C. Tumors of Supporting or Adjacent Structures
   1. Meningioma
   2. Hemangiopericytoma
D. Non-neoplastic Conditions of Neurosurgical Importance
   1. Degenerative cysts of pineal lined by fibrillary astrocytes
   2. Arachnoid cysts
   3. Cavernous hemangioma

(From DeGirolami, U. In Schmidek, HH (ed): *Pineal Tumors.* Masson, New York, 1977, pp 1–19.)

triad: diabetes insipidus, hypogonadism, and visual field defects. Although these tumors usually produce severe damage to the hypothalamus before bone is destroyed, at least two rare cases have been observed in which the germinoma grew within the pituitary fossa and mimicked completely an expanding intrasellar tumor. True pinealomas also can spread to the floor of the third ventricle and can produce various degrees of compression and destruction of the hypothalamus. About one third of germinomas may synthesize human chorionic gonadotropin (HCG) and secrete the hormone into either the CSF or blood.[134] Radioimmunoassay determination of elevated levels of HCG (or of the β-subunit of HCG) can provide the clue to the histologic nature of the tumor. Germinomas are relatively radiosensitive.

A small porportion of tumors in the pineal region are true teratomas believed also to arise from ectopic germ cells. Teratomas contain cell types originating from each of the three germinal layers that differentiate to form somatic structures. Pineal teratomas are identical with those of testis and mediastinum and can give rise to choriocarcinoma which is also capable of secreting HCG. The CSF in such cases has elevated HCG levels. In one case of a male patient, the nuclei of a typical pineal teratoma were chromatin-positive, whereas the normal epidermal nuclei were chromatin-negative. Scully[105] suggests "that in that case, the tumor arose from a germ cell that had undergone meiotic division, so that each new cell contained either an X or a Y chromosome, and that after a subsequent division, two haploid cells with an X chromosome reunited to form a cell with female sex chromatin which differentiated to form the tumor."

Other rare tumors in this region are spongioblastomas, ependymomas, choroid-plexus papillomas, and chemodectomas related to the carotid sinus-type cell. Familial pineoblastoma has been reported rarely,[49] and the association with retinoblastoma also has been reported. A case of apoplexy of the pineal gland has been reported[7] in a patient receiving radiation therapy.

The natural history and pathogenesis of intracranial germ-cell tumors (GCTs) have been comprehensively reviewed by Jennings and colleagues.[32]

> From a study of 389 cases culled from the literature they report that, "65 per cent were germinomas, 18 per cent teratomas, 5 per cent embryonal carcinomas, 7 per cent endodermal sinus tumors and 5 per cent choriocarcinomas. Intracranial GCT's display specificity in site of origin. Ninety-five per cent arise along the midline from the suprasellar cistern (37 per cent) the pineal gland (48 per cent), and an additional 6 per cent involve both sites. The majority of germinomas (57 per cent) arise in the suprasellar cistern, while most nongerminomatous GCT's (68 per cent) preferentially involve the pineal gland. Prolonged symptomatic intervals prior to diagnosis are common in germinomas, in suprasellar GCT's and among females. Parasellar germinomas commonly present with diabetes insipidus, visual field defects, and hypothalamic-pituitary failure. Nongerminomatous GCT's present as posterior third ventricular masses with hydrocephalus and midbrain compression. Germ cell tumors may infiltrate the hypothalamus (11 per cent), or disseminate to involve the third ventricle (22 per cent) and spinal cord (10 per cent)."
>
> Two factors were of prognostic significance: "(1) histological diagnosis: germinomas were associated with significantly longer survival than nongerminomatous GCT's; and (2) staging of the extent of the disease; this emphasizes the ominous character of involvement of the hypothalamus, third ventricle or spinal cord."
>
> These authors further suggest that "the abrupt rise in age distribution at 10 to 12 years suggests that the neuroendocrine events of puberty are an "activating" influence in the malignant expression of these embryonal tumors.

The Pineal Gland and Precocious Puberty

In 1898, Huebner[31] reported a case of precocious puberty in a boy with a tumor of the pineal gland. This clinical observation, subsequently reported in a number of other patients, has stimulated much investigation of the role of the pineal gland in sexual maturation, but it also has led to an exaggerated view of the importance of pineal tumors as the cause of true sexual precocity. In the three large series of patients with cerebral precocious puberty assembled by Wilkins,[128] Jolly,[33] and Thamdrup[115] no cases of pineal disease were identified, and Van der Werff ten Bosch[118] estimated in 1975 that only about 50 cases altogether had been described in the literature. Although both precocity and delayed puberty have been recorded in pineal tumors, such sexual disturbance is not a common finding. In a series of 65 pineal tumors recorded by Ringertz and others,[96] only seven occurred in children under age 11, and in none did sexual precocity occur. In Bing and associates'[11] series of 177 patients, 56 were under age 15, and of these, one third had sexual precocity. In their series, precocious puberty occurred only when the tumor had extended well beyond the pineal region. Clinical evidence of hypothalamic involvement such as diabetes insipidus, hyperphagia, somnolence, obesity, or behavioral disturbance was found in 71 percent of the cases.

These complications have led some workers, such as Bing and coworkers,[11] to the view that when pineal tumors produce precocious puberty, they do so by the same mechanism that other brain tumors do, that is, by physical destruction of the regions of the brain that tonically inhibit gonadotropin secretion. This view is further supported by a consideration of the histologic nature of pineal neoplasms. Most tumors arising from the pineal gland are probably not derived from pineal cells but are germ cell tumors.

On the other hand, there is some evidence that at least a proportion of pineal tumors have endocrine function. In an extensive review of all published cases of pineal tumor, Kitay[42] noted that nonparenchymal tumors were three times as likely to produce precocity as were parenchymal tumors. He therefore postulated that the high incidence was due to pineal destruction; the loss of a pineal secretion believed to inhibit development of sexual maturity. At least one pineal parenchymal tumor has been reported to contain hydroxyindole-0-methyltransferase (HIOMT) enzyme activity, a marker enzyme which signifies the presence of a biochemical mechanism for the formation of melatonin from its precursor N-acetylserotonin, a characteristic pineal function.

From a theoretic point of view, it is reasonable to predict that some pineal tumors would cause disease by excessive secretion of the puberty-delaying pineal hormone melatonin or another, as yet unidentified, hormone. Although delayed puberty or hypogonadism has been reported by Puschett and Goldberg[80] to occur in cases of pineal tumor, all have been teratomas rather than true pinealomas, and most have had anatomic evidence of invasion of the third ventricle and damage to surrounding structures, including vision loss and diabetes insipidus.[11] In two of Puschett and Goldberg's cases, there was no clinical evidence of basal hypothalamic destruction, but they correctly emphasize the observation of Horrax[29] that "in some cases in which gross evidence of hypothalamic involvement is absent, careful sectioning of the pathologic specimen may reveal microscopic infiltration by tumor in the floor of the third ventricle."

A final opinion as to the mechanism of precocious puberty in pineal tumors cannot be given at this time, but we believe that most likely the bulk of such cases are due to direct hypothalamic damage and not to pineal hormonal effects.

It should be recognized that germinomas and choriocarcinomas of the pineal region, arising as teratomas, have secreted sufficient amounts of HCG hormones to stimulate testes growth and mimic true puberty.[12] This is, however, a rare occurrence.

The most important manifestation of pineal neoplasms relates to their propensity to invade the third ventricle and hypothalmus and to produce neurologic symptoms through local pressure on the quadrigeminal plate of the midbrain.[103,104] An enlarging mass in the pineal region compresses the aqueduct of Sylvius and distorts the upper brainstem. Internal hydrocephalus gives rise to characteristic headache, vomiting, papilledema, and disturbed consciousness. Pressure on the pretectal area causes paralysis of conjugate upward gaze and disturbances of pupillary reactions to light (Parinaud's syndrome). Gait also may be disturbed owing to either hydrocephalus or pressure on the cerebellum or brainstem.

Diagnosis and Management of Pineal and Third Ventricular Tumors

Diagnosis of Tumors of the Floor of the Third Ventricle. Pinealoma and other tumors of the floor of the third ventricle are relatively safe to approach surgically for biopsy, which is generally recommended unless a tissue diagnosis can be made by demonstrating elevated blood or cerebrospinal fluid levels of human chorionic gonadotropin (HCG) and/or of α-fetoprotein. If one or both of these tumor markers are positive, it is not necessary to obtain a surgical biopsy, and one can proceed directly to treat by local irradiation.[104,108]

If the diagnosis of parasellar pinealoma cannot be made by tumor markers, it should be approached as any other parasellar lesion in which a tissue specimen is essential for proper management.

Diagnosis of Tumors of the Pineal Region. The management of tumors of the pineal region is somewhat complex because the surgical approach to the pineal gland is far more complicated. Prior to the introduction of microsurgery under dissecting microscopic control, it also carried a high risk. As in the case of hypothalamic germinomas, if the tumor markers HCG, or α-fetoprotein, or HCG immunopositive cells are detectable in CSF, this is adequate diagnostic evidence of a germ cell tumor to justify x-irradiation or chemotherapy. Occasionally, only blood tests (and not CSF) are positive for the tumor markers. If these markers are absent, surgical biopsy is indicated because of the wide variety of lesions encountered in this region (see Table 1), because some can be completely removed surgically[104] and because some are radioresistant. If the patient presents with internal hydrocephalus, a shunt procedure may be a necessary first step, but it should be recalled that tumor implants may be carried into the spinal cord by such shunts.

"Radiotherapy has achieved 5-year survival rates of 60 to 88 per cent among a group of patients with heterogeneous pineal tumors."[32] Local recurrence rates have been reduced even further by increasing radiation dosage to 5000 to 5500 rads. Pineal germinomas are more common in Japan than in the United States. In Japan it is current practice to first irradiate the tumor with 2000 rads, and if a favorable response is observed, to continue radiotherapy. However, radiation response may not be indicative of curability.

For many years surgical treatment of pineal tumors was associated with extremely high mortality, but with the introduction of microsurgery, operative mortality has fallen dramatically. For example, in a series of 128 cases subjected to direct surgical approach (summarized by Schmidek and Waters[104]) there were only two operative deaths; one from hemorrhage into a glioblastoma occurring 1 week after surgery, and the other related to a large infiltrating tumor of the midbrain. It appears, therefore, that these rare tumors are best treated surgically in a center with much experience in this approach. The advantages and disadvantages of the various surgical approaches have been summarized by these authors.

Chemotherapy should be considered in cases that fail to respond to x-irradiation or that relapse after an initial good response.

There is extensive experience comparing various chemotherapeutic protocols for therapy of testicular choriocarcinoma; the cure rate is encouragingly high—between 60 and 90 percent.

This experience has led to similar approaches in treatment of central germ-cell tumors.[32] The combined experience in 21 cases is summarized in Table 2. In this group, treated with a variety of drugs, 9 were dead between 13 days and 11 months after starting therapy, and the remainder were still living when reported between 4 months and 114 months after starting therapy.

Prognosis. Survival curves of patients with intracranial germ-cell tumors of patients receiving conventional therapy are shown in Figure 7. Choriocarcinomas have the worst prognosis, and germinomas, the best.

TABLE 2. Chemotherapeutic Experience with Primary Intracranial Germ-cell Tumors

Tumor Type & Chemotherapy	Survival Period & Outcome
germinoma	
MTX, CyP, ActD	13 days, dead
MTX, CyP, ActD	114 mos, alive
BCNU	1 mo, dead
CyP	12 mos, alive
Vbl, Pbz, CCNU	4 mos, alive
c-Pl, Ble, Vbl	12 mos, alive
c-Pl, Ble, Vbl	24 mos, alive
Vcr, NM	38 mos, alive
c-Pl, Ble, Vbl	8 mos, dead
embryonal carcinoma	
Ble	4 mos, dead
Ble	11 mos, dead
CyP, ActD, Vcr	9 mos, alive
endodermal sinus tumor	
CyP, ActD, Vcr	12 mos, alive
Pbz, Vcr, DHGC	9 mos, dead
CyP, ActD, c-Pl, Chl, Vbl, Ble	
MTX, Ble, Vcr	8 mos, dead
choriocarcinoma	
Ble	1 mo, dead
MTX, BCNU, Vcr	30 mos, alive
MTX, ActD, Ble, Vbl	20 mos, alive
MTX, ActD	48 mos, alive
MTX	20 mos, alive
MTX	3 mos, dead

*Abbreviations: GCT = germ-cell tumors; ActD = actinomycin D; BCNU = 1,3-bis(2-chloroethyl)-1-nitrosourea; Ble = bleomycin; Chl = chlorambucil; c-Pl = cis-platinum; CyP = cyclophosphamide; CCNU = 1-(2-chloroethyl)-3-cyclohexyl-1-nitrosourea; DHGC = dianhydrogalactitol; MTX = methotrexate; NM = nitrogen mustard; Pbz = procarbazine; Vbl = vinblastine; and Vcr = vincristine. (Reproduced with permission from Jennings MT, Gelman R, Hochberg F: Intracranial germ cell tumors: Natural history and pathogenesis. J Neurosurg 63:155–167, 1985.)

vessels from the pia covering the external wall of the lamina form arching loops directed toward the ventricular lumen. Nerve endings in the interstitial space of the OVLT conceivably could transmit secretory products to capillaries in this region. There is no evidence of a "portal system" analogous to that for anterior pituitary regulation, nor of an anatomic basis for direct transport of secretory product to the pituitary.

The function of the OVLT is unknown, but recent studies have modified speculations as to its function. Nerve fibers of the OVLT are rich in LHRH, somatostatin, and several other peptides.[75] The LHRH fibers arise from bipolar neurons in the anterior hypothalamus; one process is directed to the OVLT and the other to the median eminence. The anatomic relationships of the other peptidergic innervations are not as well delineated. Because there is no direct relationship to the pituitary, it would appear likely that if LHRH is liberated at nerve endings in the OVLT, the peptide would enter the general circulation via the capillary loops or be transported by ependyma either into the lumen of the third ventricle or into the cisternal space. At present, evidence is insufficient to support any of these possibilities. A clue to the function of the OVLT is the finding that destruction of this region in the rat leads to loss of the mechanism for cyclic gonadotropin secretion,[79,127] but it is not clear whether this function involves the OVLT or adjacent nerve fibers. There is also evidence that perikarya in the region of the OVLT may project to the median eminence.[40] On the basis of the finding by Moss and McCann[63] and Pfaff[78] that intraventricular injection of LHRH stimulates sexual activity in the rat, and previous demonstrations that lesions of the preoptic hypothalamus interfere with sexual function, it is also possible that this structure is involved in some way with sexual behavior, possibly by a hormonal factor borne in CSF.

Subfornical Organ (SFO)

The subfornical organ is a neurohemal structure found at the junction between the lamina terminalis and the tela choroidea of the third ventricle.[1] Its name is derived from its location under the fornices of the hippocampus. It consists of both neurosecretory neurons and modified ependymal cells. Cells are oriented so that secretion into the lumen of the ventricle is at least a theoretic possibility, although it has not been demonstrated. Neurons of the SFO are reported to receive a cholinergic innervation from cells in the midbrain. Morphology of the SFO cells is modified by stress of various kinds, by hypertonic salt injection, and by estrogen administration.

A role for the SFO in salt and water regulation is supported by recent studies of the effects of injection of angiotensin II in the region of the SFO (although the localization of effect cannot be regarded as being entirely specific).[106] Such injections lead to the release of ADH and the stimulation of drinking behavior. The effects are enhanced by the addition of hypertonic saline. The endothelium of this region (as well as most other endothelia of the brain) contains enzymes capable of converting angiotensin I to angiotensin II.[82] Moreover, circulating angiotensin II might activate receptors in this region.[82]

It is clear that the function of the ependymal glands is still uncertain. It is fascinating to consider that the secretion of unknown hormones, especially peptides, into the fluid bathing the cerebral hemispheres may exert behavioral effects.

REFERENCES

1. AKERT, K: *The mammalian subfornical organ.* J Neurovisceral Relations (Suppl) 9:78–94, 1969.
2. AHMED, SR, SHALET, SM, PRICE, DA, PEARSON, D: *Human chorionic gonadotrophin secreting pineal germinoma and precocious puberty.* Arch Dis Child 58(9):743–745, 1983.
3. ALBERS, HE, FERRIS, CF, LEEMAN, SE, GOLDMAN, BO: *Avian pancreatic polypeptide phase shifts hamster circadian rhythms microinjected into the suprachiasmatic region.* Science 223:833–835, 1984.
4. ALTSCHULE, MD: *Frontiers of Pineal Physiology.* MIT Press, Cambridge, MA, 1975, pp 1–4.
5. ANTON-TAY, F, DIAZ, JL, FERNANDEZ-GUARDIOLA, A: *On the effect of melatonin upon human brain. Its possible therapeutic implications.* Life Sci 10:841–850, 1971.
6. ANTON-TAY, F, WURTMAN, RJ: *Regional uptake of ³H-melatonin from blood or cerebrospinal fluid by rat brain.* Nature 221:474–476, 1969.
7. APUZZO, MIJ, DAVEY, LM, MANUELIDIS, EE: *Pineal apoplexy associated with anticoagulant therapy.* Case Report J Neurosurg 45:223–226, 1976.
8. ASCHOFF, J: *The circadian rhythms in man.* In KRIEGER, DT (ED): *Endocrine Rhythms.* Raven Press, New York, pp 1–61, 1979.
9. ASCHOFF, J: *The circadian system in man.* In KRIEGER DT, HUGHES, JC (EDS): *Neuroendocrinology.* Sinauer Associates, Sunderland, MA, 1980, pp 85–92.
10. AXELROD, J: *The pineal gland: A neurochemical transducer.* Science 184:1341–1348, 1974.
11. BING, JF, ET AL: *Pubertas praecox: A survey of the reported cases and verified anatomical findings.* J Mt Sinai Hosp 4:935–965, 1938.
12. BLASK, DE: *The pineal: An oncostatic gland.* In REITER, RJ (ED): *The Pineal Gland.* Raven Press, New York, 1984, pp 253–284.
13. BLASK, DE, VAUGHN, MK, REITER, RJ: *Pineal peptides and reproduction.* In RELKIN, R (ED): *The Pineal Gland.* Elsevier Biomedical, New York, 1983, pp 201–224.
14. BRAMMER, GL, MORLEY, JE, GELLER, E, YUWILER, A, HERSHMAN, JM: *Hypothalamus-pituitary-thyroid axis interactions with pineal gland in the rat.* Am J Physiol 236:E416–E420, 1979.
15. BUBENIK, GA, BROWN, GM, UHLIR, I, GROTA, LI: *Immunohistological localization of N-acetylindolealkylamines in pineal gland, retina and cerebellum.* Brain Res 81:233–242, 1974.
16. BUBENIK, GA, BROWN, GM, GROTA, LJ: *Immunohistological localization of melatonin in the rat digestive system.* Experientia 33:662–663, 1977.
17. BUBENIK, GA, BROWN, GM, GROTA, LJ: *Differential localization of n-acetylated indolealkylamines in CNS and the Harderian gland using immunohistology.* Brain Res 118:417–427, 1976.
18. CARDINALI, DP: *Molecular biology of melatonin: Assessment of the microtubule hypothesis of melatonin action.* In BIRAU, N, SCHLOOT, W (EDS): *Melatonin: Current Status and Perspectives.* Pergamon Press, New York, 1981, pp 247–256.
19. CARDINALI, DP: *Melatonin. A mammalian pineal hormone.* Endocr Res 2:327–346, 1981.
20. CARDINALI, DP, AND WURTMAN RJ: *Hydroxyindole-O-methyltransferases in rat pineal, retina and harderian gland.* Endocrinology 91:247–252, 1972.
21. CARDINALI, DP, AND VACAS, MI: *Molecular endocrinology of melatonin: Receptor sites in brain and peripheral organs.* In BIRAU, N, AND SCHLOOT, W (EDS): *Melatonin: Current Status and Perspectives.* Pergamon Press, New York, 1981, pp 237–246.
22. COHEN, M, ROSELLE, D, CHABNER, B, ET AL: *Evidence for a cytoplasmic melatonin receptor.* Nature 274:894–895, 1978.
23. DEGIROLAMI, U, AND SCHMIDEK, HH: *Clinicopathological study of 53 tumors of the pineal region.* J Neurosurg 39:455–462, 1973.
24. EHRENKRANZ, JR, TAMARKIN, L, COMITE, F, ET AL: *Daily rhythms of plasma melatonin in normal and precocious puberty.* J Clin Endocrinol Metab 55:307–310, 1982.
25. EHRLICH, SS, AND APUZZO, MLJ: *The pineal gland: Anatomy, physiology, and clinical significance.* J Neurosurg 63:321–341, 1985.
26. FOLDVARA, IP, AND PALKOVITS, M: *Effect of sodium and potassium restriction on the functional morphology of the subcommissural organ.* Nature 202:905–906, 1964.
27. FRASCHINI, F, CULLO, R, MARTINI, L: *Mechanisms of inhibitory action of pineal principles on gonadotropin secretion.* In WOLSTEINHOLME, GEW, AND KNIGHT, J (EDS): *The Pineal Gland.* Churchill, London, 1971, p 259.
28. GERN, WA, GORELL, TA, OWENS, DW: *Melatonin and pigment cell rhythmicity.* In BIRAU, N, AND SCHLOOT, W (EDS): *Melatonin: Current Status and Perspectives.* Pergamon Press, New York, 1981, pp 223–233.

29. Horrax, G: *The role of pinealomas in the causation of diabetes insipidus.* Ann Surg 126:725–739, 1947.

30. Hsu, LL, and Mandell, AJ: *Multiple N-methyltransferases for aromatic alkylamines in brain.* Life Sci 13:847–858, 1973.

31. Huebner, O: *Tumor der glandula pinealis.* Deutsch Med Wochenschr 24:214, 1898.

32. Jennings, MT, Gelman, R, Hochberg, F: *Intracranial germ-cell tumors: Natural history and pathogenesis.* J Neurosurg 63:155–167, 1985.

33. Jolly, H: *Sexual Precocity.* Charles C Thomas, Springfield, IL, 1955.

34. Kafka, MD: *Central nervous system control of mammalian circadian rhythms.* Fed Proc 42:2782–2782, 1983.

35. Kamberi, IA, Mical, RS, Porter, JC: *Effects of melatonin and serotonin on the release of FSH and prolactin.* Endocrinology 88:1288–1299, 1971.

36. Kappers, JA: *The mammalian pineal organ.* J Neurovisceral Relations (Suppl) 9:140 (review), 1969.

37. Kappers, JA: *The pineal organ: An introduction.* In Wolstenholme, GEW, and Knight, J (eds): *The Pineal Gland.* Churchill, London, 1971, p 3.

38. Kappers, JA, Smith, AR, DeVries, RAC: *The mammalian pineal gland and its control of hypothalamic activity.* In Swaab, DF, and Schade, JP (eds): *Progress in Brain Research,* vol. 41. Elsevier, Amsterdam, 1974, pp 149–174.

39. Kelly, DE: *Developmental aspects of amphibian pineal systems.* In Wolstenholme, GEW, and Knight, J (eds): *The Pineal Gland.* Churchill, London, 1971, p 53.

40. King, JC, and Anthony, ELP: *LHRH neurons and their projections in humans and other mammals: Species comparisons.* Peptides (Suppl 1) pp 195–207, 1984.

41. Kitay, JI, and Altschule, MD: *The Pineal Gland.* Harvard University Press, Cambridge, 1954.

42. Kitay, JI: *Pineal lesions and precocious puberty: A review.* J Clin Endocrinol Metab 14:622–625, 1954.

43. Klein, DC: *The pineal gland: A model of neuroendocrine regulation.* In Reichlin, S, and Baldessarini, RJ (eds): *The Hypothalamus,* vol. 56. Raven Press, New York, 1978, pp 303–327.

44. Klein, DC: *Melatonin and puberty.* Science 224:6, 1984.

45. Kneisly, LW, Moskowitz, MA, Lynch, HJ: *Cervical spinal cord lesions disrupt the rhythm in human melatonin excretion.* J Neural Transm 13 (Suppl):311–323, 1978.

46. Korf, HW, and Wagner, U: *Evidence for a nervous connection between the brain and the pineal organs in the guinea pig.* Cell Tissue Res 209:505–510, 1980.

47. Krieger, D (ed): *Endocrine Rhythms.* Raven Press, New York, 1979.

48. Lapin, V: *Pineal influence on tumor.* Progr Brain Res 52:523–533, 1979.

49. Lesnick, JE, Chayt, KJ, Bruce, DA, Roorke, LB, Trojanowski, J, Savino, PJ, Schatz, NJ: *Familial pineoblastoma.* J Neurosurg 62:930–932, 1985.

50. Lewy, AJ: *Biochemistry and regulation of mammalian melatonin production.* In Relkin R (ed): *The Pineal Gland.* Elsevier Biomedical, New York, 1983, pp 77–128.

51. Lewy, AJ, and Newsome, DA: *Different types of melatonin circadian secretion rhythms in some blind subjects.* J Clin Endocrinol Metab 56:1103–1107, 1983.

52. Lieberman, HR, Waldhauser, F, Garfield, G, Lynch, HJ, Wurtman, RJ: *Effects of melatonin on human mood and performance.* Brain Res 323:201–207, 1984.

53. Lincoln, G: *Melatonin as a seasonal time-cue: A commercial story.* Nature 302:755, 1983.

54. Lukaszyk, A, and Reiter, RJ: *Histopathological evidence for the secretion of polypeptides by the pineal gland.* Am J Anat 143:451–464, 1975.

55. Lynch, HJ: *Assay methodology.* In Relkin, R (ed): *The Pineal Gland.* Elsevier, New York, 1983, pp 129–150.

56. Martin, JE, and Klein, DC: *Melatonin inhibition of the neonatal pituitary response to luteinizing hormone-releasing factor.* Science 191:301–302, 1976.

57. Martin, JE, and Sattler, C: *Developmental loss of the acute inhibitory effect of melatonin on the in vitro pituitary LH and FSH response to LH-releasing hormone.* Endocrinology 105:1007–1012, 1979.

58. Mazzi, V: *L'Organe-Sous-Commissural.* Scientia, Italy, 1969, p 1.

59. Moore, RY: *Organization and function of a central nervous system circadian oscillator: The suprachiasmatic hypothalamic nucleus.* Fed Proc 42:2783–2789, 1983.

60. Moore, RY: *Central neural control of circadian rhythms.* In Ganong, WF, and Martini, L (eds): *Frontiers in Neuroendocrinology,* vol. 5. Raven Press, New York, 1978, pp 185–206.

61. Moore-Ede, MC: *The circadian timing system in mammals: Two pacemakers preside over many secondary oscillators.* Fed Proc 42:2802–2808, 1983.

62. Moskowitz, MA, and Wurtman, RJ: *Pathological states involving the pineal.* In Martini, L, and Besser, GM (eds): *Clinical Neuroendocrinology.* Academic Press, New York, 1977, pp 503–526.

63. Moss, RL, and McCann, SM: *Action of luteinizing hormone-releasing factor (lrf) in the initiation of lordosis behavior in the estrone-primed ovariectomized female rat.* Neuroendocrinology 17(4):309–318, 1975.

64. Niles, LP, Brown, GM, Grota, LJ: *Effects of pineal and indoleamines on adrenocortical function.* Clin Res 23:617A, 1975.

65. Oksche, A: *The subcommissural organ.* J Neurovisceral Relations 9(Suppl):111, 1969.

66. Palkovits, M, Monos, E, Fachet, J: *The effect of subcommissural-organ lesions on aldosterone production in the rat.* Acta Endocrinol 48:169–176, 1965.

67. Pavel, S: *Arginine vasotocin release into cerebrospinal fluid of cats induced by melatonin.* Nature (New Biol) 246:183–184, 1973.

68. Pavel, S: *Arginine vasotocin as a pineal hormone.* J Neural Transm 13(Suppl):135–155, 1978.

69. Pavel, S: *Pineal vasotocin and sleep: Involvement of serotonin containing neurons.* Brain Res Bull 4:731–734, 1979.

70. Pavel, S, Goldstein, R, Popoviciu, L, et al: *Pineal vasotocin: REM sleep dependent release into cerebrospinal fluid of man.* Waking Sleeping 3:347–352, 1979.

71. Pavel, S, Psatta, D, Goldstein, R: *Slow-wave sleep induced in cats by extremely small amounts of synthetic and pineal vasotocin injected into the third ventricle of the brain.* Brain Res Bull 2:251–254, 1977.

72. Pazo, JH: *Effects of melatonin on spontaneous and evoked neuronal activity in the mesencephalic reticular formation.* Brain Res Bull 4:725–730, 1979.

73. Pazo, JH: *Electrophysiological study of evoked electrical activity in the pineal gland.* J Neural Trans 52:137–148, 1981.

74. Peat, F, and Kinson, GA: *Testicular steroidogenesis in vitro in the rat in response to blinding, pinealectomy and to the addition of melatonin.* Steroids 17:251–264, 1971.

75. Pelletier, G: *Immunohistochemical localization of somatostatin.* Progr Histochem Cytochem 12:1–41, 1980.

76. Penny, R: *Melatonin excretion in normal males and females: Increase during puberty.* Metabolism 8:816–823, 1982.

77. Pévet, P: *Anatomy of the pineal gland of mammals.* In Relkin, R (ed): *The Pineal Gland.* Elsevier Biomedical, New York, 1983, pp 1–76.

78. Pfaff, DW: *Luteinizing hormone releasing factor potentiates lordosis behavior in hypophysectomized ovariectomized female rats.* Science 182:1148–1149, 1973.

79. Piva, F, Limonta, P, Martin, L: *Role of the organum vasculosum laminae terminalis in the control of gonadotrophin secretion in rats.* J Endocrin 93:355–364, 1982.

80. Puschett, JB, Goldberg, M: *Endocrinopathy associated with pineal tumor.* Ann Int Med 69:203–219, 1968.

81. Ralph, CL, Mull, D, Lynch, HJ, Hedlund, L: *A melatonin rhythm persists in rat pineals in darkness.* Endocrinology 89:1361–1366, 1971.

82. Ramsay, DJ: *Effects of circulating angiotensin II on the brain.* In Ganong, WF, and Martini, L (eds): *Frontiers in Neuroendocrinology,* vol 7. Raven Press, New York, 1982, pp 263–285.

83. Reiter, RJ: *The pineal gland: An intermediary between the environment and the endocrine system.* Psychoneuroendocrinology 8:31–40, 1983.

84. Reiter, RJ: *The pineal and its hormones in the control of reproduction in mammals.* Endocr Rev 1:109–131, 1980.

85. Reiter, RJ, Blask, DE: *Melatonin: Its inhibition of pineal antigonadotrophic activity in male hamsters.* Science 185:1169–1171, 1974.

86. Reiter, RJ: *The Pineal Gland.* Raven Press, New York, 1984.

87. Reiter, RJ, Welsh, MG, Vaughn, MK: *Age-related changes in the intact and sympathetically denervated gerbil pineal gland.* Am J Anat 146:427–432, 1976.

88. Reiter, RJ, Richardson, BA, King, TS: *The pineal gland and its indole products: Their importance in the control of reproduction in mammals.* In Relkin, R (ed): *The Pineal Gland.* Elsevier Biomedical, New York, 151–200, 1983.

89. Relkin, R: *Pineal-hormone Interactions.* In Relkin, R (ed): *The Pineal Gland.* Elsevier Biomedical, Amsterdam, 1983, pp 225–246.

90. Relkin, R: *Effects of pinealectomy and constant light and darkness on thyrotropin levels in the pituitary and plasma of the rat.* Neuroendocrinology 10:46–52, 1972.

91. Relkin, R (ed): *The Pineal Gland.* Elsevier Biomedical, New York, 1983.

92. Reppert, SM, Chez, RA, Anderson, A, et al: *Maternal-fetal transfer of melatonin in the nonhuman primate.* Pediatr Res 13:788–791, 1979.

93. Reppert, SM, and Klein, DC: *Mammalian pineal gland. Basic and clinical aspects.* In Motta, M (ed): *The Endocrine Functions of the Brain.* Raven Press, New York, 1980, pp 327–372.

94. Reppert, SM, Perlow, MJ, Tamarkin, L, Klein, DC: *A diurnal melatonin rhythm in primate cerebrospinal fluid.* Endocrinology 104(2):295–301, 1979.

95. Reppert, SM, Klein, DC: *Transport of maternal [³H]melatonin to suckling rats and the fate of [³H]melatonin in the neonatal rat.* Endocrinology 102:582–588, 1978.

96. RINGERTZ, N, NORDENSTAM, H, FLYGER, G: *Tumors of the pineal region.* J Neuropath Exp Neurol 13:540–561, 1954.

97. RONNEKLIEV, OK, McCANN, SM: *Effects of pinealectomy, anosmia and blinding on serum and pituitary prolactin in intact and castrated male rats.* Neuroendocrinology 17:340–353, 1975.

98. ROWE, JW, REICHERT, JR, KLEIN, DC, REICHLIN, S: *Relation of the pineal gland and environmental lighting to thyroid function in the rat.* Neuroendocrinology 6:247–254, 1970.

99. RUDMAN, D, DEL RIO, AE, HOLLINS, B, HOUSER, DH, SUTIN, J, MOSTELLER, RC: *Comparison of lipolytic and melanotropic factors in bovine choroid plexus and in bovine pineal gland.* Endocrinology 90(5):1139–1146, 1972.

100. RUSSELL, DS: *The pinealoma: Its relationship to teratoma.* J Pathol Bacteriol 56:145–150, 1944.

101. RUSSELL, DS, RUBINSTEIN, LJ: *Pathology of tumors of the nervous system.* Edward Arnoid, London, 1963.

102. SADUN, AA, SCHAECHTER, JD, SMITH, LE: *A retinohypothalamic pathway in man: Light mediation of circadian rhythms.* Brain Res. 302(2):371–377, 1984.

103. SCHMIDEK, HH: *Surgical management of pineal region tumors.* In SCHMIDEK, HH (ED): *Pineal Tumors.* Masson Publishing, New York, 1977, pp 99–113.

104. SCHMIDEK, HH, AND WATERS, A: *Pineal masses: Clinical features and management.* In Neurosurgery, 1985.

105. SCULLY, RE: *Discussion in case records of the Massachusetts General Hospital.* N Engl J Med 284:1427–1434, 1971.

106. SIMPSON, JB, AND ROUTTENBERG, A: *Subfornical organ: Site of drinking elicitation by angiotensin-II.* Science 173:1172–1175, 1973.

107. SORRENTINO, S, JR, REITER, RJ, SCHALCH, DS: *Pineal regulation of growth hormone synthesis and release in blinded and blinded-anosmic male rats.* Neuroendocrinology 7(4):210–218, 1971.

108. SPIEGEL, AM, DiCHIRO, G, GORDEN, P, OMMAYA, AK, KOLINS, J, POMEROY, TC: *Diagnosis of radiosensitive hypothalamic tumors without craniotomy. Endocrine and neuroradiologic studies of intracranial atypical teratomas.* Ann Intern Med 85:290–294, 1976.

109. STEIN, BM: *Supracerebellar-infratentorial approach to pineal tumors.* Surg Neurol 11:331–337, 1979.

110. STOPA, EG, KING, JC, LYDIC, R, SCHOENE, WC: *Human brain contains vasopressin and vasoactive intestinal polypeptide neuronal subpopulations in the suprachiasmatic region.* Brain Res. 297(1):159–163, 1984.

111. TAMARKIN, L, DANFORTH, D, DeMOSS, E, LICHTER, A, COHEN, M, CHABNER, B, LIPPMAN, M: *Decreased nocturnal plasma melatonin peak in patients with estrogen receptor positive breast cancer.* Science 216:1003–1005, 1982.

112. TAMARKIN, L, BAIRD, CJ, ALMEIDA, OFX: *Melatonin: A coordinating signal for mammalian reproduction.* Science 227:714–720, 1985.

113. TAPP, E: *The pineal gland in malignancy.* In REITER, RJ (ED): *The Pineal Gland,* vol 3. CRC Press, Boca Raton, FL, 1981, pp 171–188.

114. TETSUO, M, POTH, M, MARKEY, SP: *Melatonin metabolite excretion during childhood and puberty.* J Clin Endocrinol Metab 55:311–313, 1982.

115. THAMDRUP, E: *Precocious sexual development, a clinical study of 100 children.* Dan Med Bull 8:140–142, 1961.

116. TSANG, D, MARTIN, JB: *Effect of hypothalamic hormones on the concentration of adenosine 3.5' -monophosphate in incubated rat pineal glands.* Life Sci 19:911–917, 1976.

117. VACAS, MI, BERRIA, MI, CARDINALI, DP, ET AL: *Melatonin inhibits α-adrenoceptor-stimulated cyclic AMP accumulation in rat astroglial cell cultures.* Neuroendocrinology 38:176–181, 1984.

118. VANDER WERFF TEN BOSCH, JJ: *Isosexual precocity.* In GARDNER, LI (ED): *Endocrine and genetic diseases of childhood and adolescence,* ed 2. WB Saunders, Philadelphia, 1975, p 619.

119. VAUGHAN, MK, RICHARDSON, BA, PETTERBORG, LJ, HOLTORF, AP, VAUGHAN, GM, CHAMPNEY, TH, REITER, RJ: *Effects of injections and/or chronic implants of melatonin and 5-methoxytryptamine on plasma thyroid hormones in male and female Syrian hamsters.* Neuroendocrinology. 39(4):361–366, 1984.

120. VAUGHN, MK: *Pineal peptides an overview.* In REITER, R (ED): *The Pineal Gland.* Raven Press, New York, 1984, 39–82.

121. VOLLRATH, L: *Functional anatomy of the human pineal gland.* In REITER, R (ED): *The Pineal Gland.* Raven Press, New York, 1984, pp 285–322.

122. WALDHAUSER, F, WEISZENBACHER, G, FRISCH, H, ZEITLHUBER, U, WALDHAUSER, M, WURTMAN, R: *Fall in nocturnal serum melatonin during prepuberty and pubescence.* Lancet 1:362–365, 1984.

123. WALDHAUSER, F, WALDHAUSER, M, LIEBERMAN, HR, DENG, M-H, LYNCH, HJ, WURTMAN, RJ: *Bioavailability of oral melatonin in humans.* Neuroendocrinology 39:307–313, 1984.

124. WEINDL, A: *Neuroendocrine aspects of circumventricular organs.* In GANONG, WF, AND MARTINI, L (EDS): *Frontiers in Neuroendocrinology.* Oxford University Press, London, 1973, pp 3–32.

PINEAL AND PERIVENTRICULAR ORGANS

125. WEINDL, A, SCHWINK, A, WETZSTEIN, R: Der Feinbau des Gefässorgans der Lamina terminalis beim Kaninchen. I. Die Gerfässe. Z Zellforschung 79:1–48.

126. WEINDL, A, AND SOFRONIEW, MV: *Relation of neuropeptides to mammalian circumventricular organs.* Adv Biochem Psychopharmacol 28:303–320, 1981.

127. WENGER, T, KERDELHUE, B, HALASZ, B: *Does the organum vasculosum of the lamina terminalis play a role in the regulation of reproduction.* Acta Physioloica Academiae Scientarium Hungaricae, Tomas 58:257–267, 1981.

128. WILKINS, L: *The diagnosis and treatment of endocrine disorders in childhood and adolescence.* Charles C Thomas, Springfield, IL, 1965.

129. WURTMAN, RJ, AXELROD, J, KELLY, DE: *The Pineal.* Academic Press, New York, 1968.

130. WURTMAN, RJ, AND MOSKOWITZ, MA: *The pineal organ.* N Engl J Med 296:1329–1333, 1383–1386, 1977.

131. YAMASHITA, K, MIENO, M, SHIMIZU, T, YAMASHITA, E: *Inhibition by melatonin of the pituitary response to luteinizing hormone releasing hormone in vivo.* J Endocrinol 76:487–491, 1978.

132. YOUNG, SN, GAUTHIER, S, KIELY, ME, LAL, S, BROWN, GM: *Effect of oral melatonin administration on melatonin. 5-hydroxyindoleacetic acid, indoleacetic acid and cyclic nucleotides in human cerebrospinal fluid.* Neuroendocrinology 39:87–92, 1984.

133. ZUCKER, I: *Light, behavior, and biological rhythms.* In KRIEGER, DR, AND HUGHES, JC (EDS): Neuroendocrinology, Sinauer Associates, Sunderland, MA, 93–101, 1980.

134. KASPER, CS, SCHNEIDER, NR, CHILDERS, JH, WILSON, JD: *Suprasellar germinoma: Unresolved problems in diganosis, pathogenesis, and management.* Am J Med 75:705–711, 1983.

PART 4

Clinical Approach to Hypothalamic-Pituitary Disease

Chapter 11

NEUROLOGIC MANIFESTATIONS OF HYPOTHALAMIC DISEASE

In addition to its role in the regulation of the anterior and posterior pituitary, the hypothalamus controls water balance through thirst;[3] regulates food ingestion and body temperature;[14] and influences consciousness,[99] sleep,[78] emotion, and behavior[48] (Table 1). Many of the insights into hypothalamic function came first from the careful observation of patients with diencephalic disease—as detailed, for example, in the classic reviews by Fulton and Bailey[43] in 1929 of the effects of third-ventricle tumors and by Bauer[10] in 1954 on manifestations of hypothalamic lesions (Table 2). However, clinical-pathologic correlations have not been very useful in precise analysis of hypothalamic function.[97] Its relatively small size and inaccessibility make it difficult to analyze deficits except at autopsy, by which time lesions are often large and the primary areas of involvement obscured.[29] Moreover, manifestations of hypothalamic disease depend in part upon the time course of their development. For example, relatively trivial trauma to the anterior hypothalamus, if inflicted acutely, can cause fatal hyperthermia, but massive destruction of this region is compatible with almost normal function if the disease has developed gradually over many years, as can occur with a slowly growing craniopharyngioma or meningioma. The capacity for compensation of function is rather striking and not fully explained, although it has been shown that certain groups of neurons in the hypothalamus (central catecholaminergic and neurosecretory neurons), unlike other central nervous system (CNS) neurons, can regenerate after damage. Some clues to hypothalamic function have been derived from hereditary disorders that affect the development of this region of brain, for example, de Morsier's syndrome and Kallmann's syndrome (see chapters 8 and 9).

It is recognized that vegetative and affective functions are not mediated solely by the hypothalamus acting as an isolated, distinct functional or anatomic entity.[102] Rather, the hypothalamus forms but one important component of an extensive and complex brain network comprising the limbic system. Because this system functions as an integrated whole, it is frequently difficult or impossible to determine the functions of the hypothalamus itself as opposed to its involvement as part of the larger system. Loss or disturbance of function when lesions are placed in the hypothalamus does not prove that these functions reside in the hypothalamus. For example, a lesion in the anterolateral hypothalamus of several species of

TABLE 1. Neurologic Manifestations of Nonendocrine Hypothalamic Disease

Disorders of Temperature Regulation
  Hyperthermia
  Hypothermia
  Poikilothermia
Disorders of Food Intake
  Hyperphagia (bulimia)
  Anorexia, aphagia
Disorders of Water Intake
  Compulsive water drinking
  Adipsia or hypodipsia
  Essential hypernatremia
Disorders of Sleep and Consciousness
  Somnolence
  Sleep-rhythm reversal
  Akinetic mutism
  Coma
Disorders of Psychic Function
  Rage behavior
  Hallucinations

Periodic Disease of Hypothalamic Origin
  Diencephalic epilepsy
  Kleine-Levin syndrome
  Periodic discharge syndrome of Wolff
  Narcolepsy
Disorders of the Autonomic Nervous System
  Pulmonary edema
  Cardiac arrhythmias
  Sphincter disturbance
Hereditary Hypothalamic Disease
  Laurence-Moon-Biedl syndrome
  de Morsier's syndrome
  Kallmann's syndrome
Miscellaneous
  Prader-Willi syndrome
  Diencephalic syndrome of infancy
  Cerebral gigantism

animals is followed by fatal aphagia.[2] Although this finding suggests that a "feeding center" exists in the lateral hypothalamus, it cannot be taken as final proof that this part of the hypothalamus is the only, or even the primary, region involved in the regulation of feeding. Such a lesion not only destroys neurons located in the lateral hypothalamus but also interrupts numerous axons that pass through this area in the medial forebrain bundle, the main rostral-caudal pathway of the limbic system connecting the amygdala, hippocampus, and mesencephalon.

Even when the hypothalamus has been shown to be important in the regulation of a particular behavior or homeostatic mechanism, the possibility is not excluded that other areas of the brain can mediate similar functions.[59] An example can be taken from experimental work by Chi and coworkers,[7,25] in which hypothalamic islands that disconnected the hypothalamus from the rest of the brain in the cat were shown to permit fully

TABLE 2. Symptoms and Signs of Hypothalamic Disease (From a Review of 60 Autopsy-proven Cases)

Symptoms and Signs	Number of Cases
Sexual abnormalities (hypogonadism or precocious puberty)	43
Diabetes insipidus	21
Psychic disturbance	21
Obesity or hyperphagia	20
Somnolence	18
Emaciation, anorexia	15
Thermodysregulation	13
Sphincter disturbance	5

(Adapted from Bauer, HG.[10])

integrated responses to painful stimuli. Aggressive responses (a behavior classically attributed to the hypothalamus) persisted in such animals. Moreover, the animals were able to stalk and to kill in a relatively normal manner and to eat and to drink when presented with food and water. However, the animals showed a striking general lethargy and lack of interest in the environment, manifested by a marked diminution in spontaneous activity. In this context, the hypothalamus appeared to act as an amplifier of certain behavioral responses organized elsewhere in the brain, rather than as the "center" for these responses.

TEMPERATURE REGULATION

The first evidence of a role of the brain in temperature regulation was obtained by Aronsohn and Sachs[4] when they observed that large puncture lesions in the brain of the rabbit resulted in a rise in body temperature. In 1912, Isenschmid and Krehl[63] demonstrated that posterior hypothalamic lesions prevented normal adaptive responses to cold exposure, providing evidence that the hypothalamus functions to protect against cold.

In the 1930s and 1940s Ranson[99] showed that anterior hypothalamic lesions in cats and monkeys resulted in a tendency to hyperthermia with defective defense against heat, whereas posterior hypothalamic lesions caused hypothermia or poikilothermia. (Poikilothermia, the normal temperature regulating mode in amphibia and fishes, is defined as a disorder of temperature regulation in which body core temperature follows that of the environment.) In a poikilothermic animal exposure to cold results in hypothermia and exposure to warmth leads to hyperthermia. Subsequent studies have clarified the mechanisms of neural control of body temperature.

Hypothalamic regulation of temperature is achieved by a complex, multi-integrated system that determines autonomic, behavioral, and hormonal responses to variations in central or environmental temperature. The maintenance of a constant core temperature requires the integration of several inputs, a comparison of this information with a predetermined setpoint, and the coordination of the various effector systems.

The essential components of the temperature regulatory system are diagrammed in Figure 1. Specific temperature-sensitive neurons located in the anterior hypothalamus and preoptic area alter their firing rates in response to local changes in hypothalamic temperature.[14,56,57] The responsivity of such cells varies diurnally with the circadian temperature rhythm and is altered by afferent impulses from peripheral thermoreceptors. Few, if any, temperature-sensing cells are located in the posterior hypothalamus. Lesions in the anterior hypothalamus and preoptic area interfere with heat-loss mechanisms, including sweating and vasodilatation. Because heat production in normal persons exceeds need in most ambient temperature settings, active heat dissipation is usually required under temperate environmental conditions; anterior lesions may therefore result in severe *hyperthermia*. The extent of hyperthermia that occurs in such circumstances depends upon the acuteness, location, and size of the lesion. Acute destruction of the preoptic area may result in severe, even fatal, fever.

Lesions in the posterior hypothalamus may cause *hypothermia* by interference with shivering and vasoconstrictive mechanisms. If the lesions

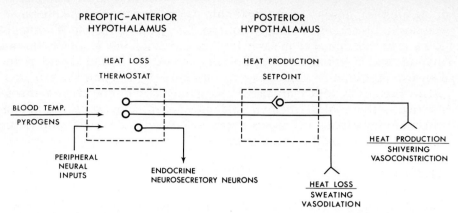

FIGURE 1. This diagram outlines hypothalamic temperature regulation mechanisms. The preoptic-anterior hypothalamic area functions as a thermostat and contains mechanisms for regulation of heat loss. The posterior hypothalamus integrates heat production mechanisms. Lesions of the preoptic-anterior hypothalamic area result in hyperthermia; lesions of the posterior hypothalamus cause hypothermia or poikilothermia.

are large enough to damage both anterior and posterior hypothalamic efferent systems, poikilothermia results. Anterior hypothalamic lesions also have been shown to interfere with shivering, suggesting that facilitatory inputs may reach the posterior hypothalamus from anterior hypothalamic areas.

The mechanism by which the hypothalamus senses environmental temperature and how this information is transduced into neural signals of a type appropriate to initiate temperature adaptation has been extensively studied.[14,56,57] Two major inputs control temperature, one central via temperature-sensitive neurons in the anterior hypothalamus and the other peripheral from cold or warmth receptors in the skin and internal organs. Local warming of the anterior hypothalamic-preoptic area induces sweating and vasodilatation; local cooling has opposite effects—shivering, vasoconstriction, and thyroid activation. The anterior hypothalamic-preoptic area alone appears to subserve this function. Changes in local temperature in the posterior hypothalamus and in other brain areas are without effect. Studies of single-neuron activity confirm that nerve cells in the anterior region of the hypothalamus can transduce temperature changes into varying rates of cell firing.

Units that show an increased rate of activity with warming have been identified in several species and are labeled as warmth receptors. Units with increasing activity on cooling are less readily demonstrated but also exist. However, data obtained from recording of units in relation to temperature changes must be interpreted with caution, because it is not generally possible to distinguish between primary-receptor neurons and secondary interneurons affected by primary temperature-sensing neurons at a separate site.

The relative importance in caloric homeostasis of thermosensitive hypothalamic neurons as compared with peripheral skin receptors has been extensively investigated. Core-temperature recordings from the hypothalamus show little fluctuation with changes in environmental temperature, and changes in hypothalamic blood flow are probably the result rather than the cause of body temperature regulatory adjustments. Peripheral inputs are believed to be of greater physiologic significance than local effects in temperature regulation.

HYPOTHALAMIC-PITUITARY DISEASE

In addition to adjustments in heat-loss and heat-maintenance mechanisms which are mediated via the autonomic nervous system, the hypothalamus also integrates behavioral and neuroendocrine responses appropriate for homeostasis. The behavioral responses include seeking warmer or colder environments, and altered food intake. The neuroendocrine control response includes the sympathoadrenal system, the pituitary-thyroid axis, and the pituitary-adrenal axis.[44] Rats with lesions in the anterior hypothalamic-preoptic area, for example, demonstrate abnormalities of feeding behavior when thermally stressed. Normal rats reduce food intake when the ambient temperature is raised and eat more in the cold. In contrast, anterior hypothalamic-preoptic-lesioned animals fail to reduce food intake in warm environments, and exposure to cold fails to increase food intake. Local hypothalamic cooling in goats stimulates food intake. These data would indicate a strong influence of thermoregulatory functions on food intake. These connections are believed to be mediated through descending pathways from the anterior hypothalamic-preoptic region to ventromedial and lateral hypothalamic areas. In lower poikilotherms body temperature homeostasis is guarded mainly by behavioral changes.

As emphasized by Hardy,[56] there is a striking correlation between skin temperature and the sensation of comfort or discomfort (Fig. 2).

> Two components of conscious perceptual experience relate to changes in environmental temperature. As skin temperature is reduced during cold exposure, the human being perceives increasing sensations of both cold and discomfort. It is evident that warm/cold sensation and comfort/discomfort motivation can be consciously distinguished as two separate aspects of thermal experience. When placed in a warm environment, a sense of warmth increases with the rise in skin temperature, and the feeling of thermal discomfort correlates more closely to sweat rate (and evaporative loss). Such studies indicate the importance of peripheral receptors in the control of both autonomic responses for temperature regulation and the perception of discomfort associated with deviations from the norm.

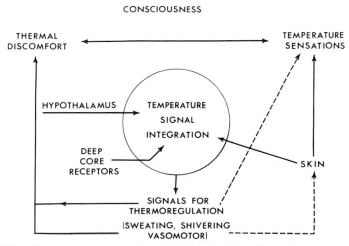

FIGURE 2. This diagram shows the relationship of thermal discomfort and temperature sensation. Although both sensations reach consciousness, they result in differing subjective experiences. The emotional feelings do not reflect the activity of peripheral thermoreceptors alone but, rather, an integrated state of the themoregulatory system. (Courtesy of J.D. Hardy.)

TABLE 4. Effects of Neuropeptides on Temperature Regulation

Neuropeptide	Effects of Central Administration	Pharmacologic Alteration of Response
Neurotensin	Lowers body temperature	Enhanced by DA depletion Suppressed by DA agonists Antagonists of NE, 5HT, ACh, and opioids do not affect.
TRH	Elevates body temperature in rat Decreases body temperature in cat (↑respiration)	Reverses hypothermia caused by neurotensin, bombesin, opioids and ETOH Depends on prostaglandins because effect is prevented by indomethacin and ASA.
Opioids	Low doses cause hyperthermia High doses cause hypothermia	Hypothermic effects blocked by naloxone Hyperthermia effects are not blocked by naloxone Stress-induced hypothermia is blocked by naloxone. Naloxone awakens hibernating animals. Antagonized by TRH
Bombesin	Hypothermia in animals exposed to low environmental temp. No effect on animals at normal environmental temp. Hyperthermia in animals exposed to high environmental temp.	Reversed by TRH Prostaglandins, somatostatin, naloxone (partially); DA and ACh blockers have no effect
Somatostatin	Hypothermia (very large doses) Hyperthermia — analogs of somatostatin	Prevents hyperthermia caused by bombesin neurotensin, ACh, DA. Does not affect β-endorphin ↓ temp. Not influenced by PG inhibitors (unlike TRH).
Vasopressin CRH	Hypothermia (sheep) Slight hyperthermia	VP into septum blocks pyrogen-induced fever. ↑plasma E + NE.

Abbreviations: DA, dopamine; NE, norepinephrine; 5HT, serotonin; ACh, acetylcholine; ETOH, ethyl alcohol; E, epinephrine; ASA, acetylsalicylic acid; TRH, thyrotropin releasing hormone; PG, prostaglandins; CRH, corticotropin releasing hormone.

HYPOTHALAMIC-PITUITARY DISEASE

Thyrotropin-releasing Hormone. Thyrotropin-releasing hormone placed into brains of rats or rabbits causes a dose-dependent rise in core temperature.

> Its effects are greater when given at high ambient temperature than when given at low ambient temperature. Thyrotropin-releasing hormone reduces hypothermia caused by bombesin, neurotensin, β-endorphin, and ethanol. It induces behavioral effects, including increased motor activity, and neuroendocrine effects, including increased TSH secretion. TRH causes hypothermia in the cat, presumably secondary to its stimulation of respiration (tachypnea). Hyperthermia induced by TRH is prevented by indomethacin and salicylates, suggesting that its effects are mediated through endogenous prostaglandins. The sites of action of TRH in causing hyperthermia are the hypothalamus and medial preoptic area. Passive immunization against endogenous TRH with antibodies placed into the lateral ventricles results in a decrease in core body temperature. In summary, TRH appears to have multiple central effects, including increased motor activity, enhanced sympathetic nervous system activity, behavioral thermoregulatory responses, increased body temperature, and increased pituitary TSH secretion.

Neurotensin. Neurotensin *lowers* body temperature in several species, including monkey.

> This occurs only when animals are placed in lowered environmental temperature; however, the peptide has no effects on central temperature in animals placed in a warm environment. Its site of action includes the medial preoptic area, the inferior dorsal and medial hypothalamus, and the periaqueductal gray. Neurotensin-induced hypothermia is enhanced by depletion of brain dopamine and is blocked by administration of dopamine agonists. Blockers of norepinephrine, serotonin, acetylcholine, and the opioids do not alter neurotensin-induced hypothermia. Antibodies to neurotensin placed into the lateral ventricle cause elevation of rectal temperature in rats.

Opioid Peptides. Morphine and its peptide congeners influence body temperature regulation in several species. The effects are dose dependent and species dependent. Low doses of morphine and β-endorphin produce *hyperthermic* effects, whereas high doses of these substances elicit *hypothermia.*

> It has been proposed by Clark[26] that β-endorphin fits into that category of substances which interferes with thermoregulatory efferent mechanisms rather than alters the hypothalamic setpoint or affects afferent mechanisms. The hypothermic effects of β-endorphin are blocked by naloxone, whereas its hyperthermic effects are not. Naloxone does not reverse the hypothermia induced by the enkephalins. These observations suggest that the enkephalins and endorphins may act through separate receptors. Other evidence suggests a function of endorphins in aberrations of body temperature regulation. Stress-induced hyperthermia is blocked by the administration of naloxone. Animals exposed to cold or hot environments reduce or increase their body temperatures, respectively, following the administration of naloxone. As emphasized by Brown,[19] these results suggest that endogenous opiates may be involved in adaption to extremes of thermal environment. Hence, administration of naloxone may result in a disorder of thermal regulation at these extremes. Administration of naloxone awakens animals from hibernation.

Bombesin. Intraventricular administration of bombesin or local injection in the anterior hypothalamic-preoptic area produces a decrease in body temperature in animals exposed to low thermal environment but has no

conversion of thyroxine to the metabolically more active triiodothyronine.[128] The thyroid gland is not activated in response to cold in the adult human (unlike most lower animal forms), but its normal function is nevertheless important in body heat regulation.[44,77] In the absence of thyroid function (as in myxedema), body heat production is reduced, the peripheral vascular system is constricted, and the patient may develop hypothermia. Patients with hyperthyroidism respond poorly to increased environmental temperature and may develop hyperthermia if the mechanisms for heat dissipation fail to work, if the heat load is too great, or if environmental temperatures are too high. This situation is characteristic of thyrotoxic "storm." The possible exception to the generalization that exposure to cold does not activate thyroid function in the human is the response of the newborn. Within a few hours of delivery, human babies develop a surge in TSH and thyroid-hormone secretion which can be blocked in part by warming. Cellular conversion of thyroxine to the more potent thyroid hormone analog triiodothyronine also may play a role in thyroid adaptation to cold in adults.

Exposure to cold also leads to activation of the pituitary-adrenal axis, as made evident by adrenal hypertrophy and elevated circulating levels of cortisol.[44]

DISORDERS OF THERMOREGULATION IN THE HUMAN BEING

Disturbance of temperature regulation in the human being is a rather common manifestation of hypothalamic disease. A few decades ago, it was considered that hyperthermia was the most common, because acute lesions or pressure on the anterior hypothalamus could result in intense vasoconstriction, tachycardia, and hyperthermia. Careful testing of patients in recent years has demonstrated that hypothermia is more common.

CENTRAL TYPES OF HYPOTHERMIA

Chronic Hypothermia

Central hypothermia states may be either chronic or periodic. Patients with the chronic form suffer from a disturbance of thermoregulation that is persistent or demonstrates only slow change. The CNS defect predisposes to hypothermia under conditions in which a normal subject would maintain normal body temperature. The lesion usually affects other neurologic functions as well. The majority of such patients have a structural lesion of the posterior or entire hypothalamus; several pathologic lesions have been described (Table 5). The predominance of lesions involving the posterior hypothalamus is compatible with experimental evidence indicating that this region functions to integrate thermoregulatory cold-defense mechanisms. Paradoxically, in the case reported by Fox and coworkers,[40] scarring and neuronal damage were observed in the anterior hypothalamus; the posterior hypothalamus was intact. Endocrinologic studies in this patient, a 26-year-old man, showed that he had lost normal diurnal variation of

TABLE 5. Neuropathologic Abnormalities in Chronic Disorders of Central Thermoregulation

Neoplasm	Metabolic
Craniopharyngioma	Wernicke's encephalopathy
Glioblastoma multiforme	Degenerative
Neuroblastoma	Glial scarring, anterior hypothalamus
Angioma, third ventricle	Parkinson's disease with reduction and
Facial hemangioma involving the	shrinkage of neurons in posterior
hypothalamus	hypothalamus
Infectious	Developmental
Poliomyelitis	Hydrocephalus
Syphilitic endarteritis	Encephalocele
Vascular	Traumatic
Infarction	Postneurosurgical
Granulomatous	Head trauma
Sarcoidosis	

plasma cortisol and was hypothyroid, but had preserved cortisol and growth hormone (GH) responses to metyrapone, glucose, and insulin. Periventricular lesions such as those in Wernicke's encephalopathy may lead to severe hypothermia.[121]

Several drugs, including barbiturates and alcohol, also contribute to defective heat-maintenance mechanisms. Sustained hypoglycemia may result in hypothermia, and this effect can be mimicked by 2-deoxyglucose (which blocks glucose metabolism by the cell), suggesting that the hypothermia is induced by intracellular glucopenia. Exclusion of glucose from CNS sites appeared to be the mechanism of this hypothermia, which is present despite markedly increased excretion of catecholamines. Hypothermia is recognized to occur in hypothyroidism.

Episodes of hypothermia in elderly, nonalcoholic patients may be more common than usually is appreciated.[65,66] Such patients, it is suggested, have defective central thermoregulatory mechanisms. Similar defects are seen in anorexia nervosa.

Spontaneous Periodic Hypothermia

In 1907, Gowers[49] described two patients, a 28-year-old woman and a 30-year-old man, with periodic excessive autonomic activity associated with icy coldness of the extremities. Temperatures were not measured in Gowers's cases, but the similarity of their clinical features to later reports suggests that he should receive recognition for first description of the disorder now called spontaneous periodic hypothermia. In 1929, Penfield[95] reported a 41-year-old woman with periodic vasodilatation, sweating, lacrimation, and hypothermia associated with a cholesteatoma of the third ventricle. The periodic symptoms were attributed to seizure activity, and the descriptive term "diencephalic autonomic epilepsy" was applied.

Various authors have applied the descriptions "spontaneous periodic hypothermia," "diencephalic epilepsy," or "intermittent hypothermia with disabling hyperhidrosis" to this syndrome.[40,54,113] The term spontaneous periodic hypothermia adequately characterizes the clinical syndrome.

The literature contains several reports of this condition occurring in association with intracranial abnormalities.

The syndrome presents as periodic hypothermia with normal body temperature regulation present during the intervals between attacks. Symptoms of profound autonomic nervous system activity such as sweating, vasodilatation, nausea, vomiting, salivation, lacrimation, and bradycardia may occur. Often dulling of mentation is noted, and shivering may coincide with return of the body temperature to normal. Neurologic deficits usually are absent between paroxysms. The episodes are short-lived, lasting minutes or hours. The rectal temperature may drop below 30°C. In some patients a moderate degree of hypothermia persists between episodes. In most patients normal thermoregulatory responses to either cold or warm exposure can be demonstrated during attack-free periods.[74] Seizures may occur, probably related to other common associated developmental abnormalities (heterotopias, hamartomas, and so forth).

Sixteen cases of spontaneous periodic hypothermia have been reported, ten of which had agenesis of the corpus callosum. Gliosis of the arcuate nucleus and premammillary area was observed in a patient with agenesis of the corpus callosum associated with spontaneous periodic hypothermia.[91] This finding supports the concept that lesions of the hypothalamus may coexist with agenesis of the corpus callosum and cause the manifestations of spontaneous periodic hypothermia. The majority of patients with agenesis of the corpus callosum, however, do not develop spontaneous periodic hypothermia.

Few endocrine disorders have been reported to occur in patients with spontaneous periodic hypothermia. Guihard and associates[54] described a 9-year-old boy with precocious puberty, diabetes insipidus, and GH deficiency associated with agenesis of the corpus callosum. Noel and co-workers[91] noted hypogonadism but did not measure gonadotropins. Assays of serum T_4 and GH were normal, as was the cortisol response to metyrapone administration. Extensive neuroendocrine testing in one patient reported by deWitt and colleagues[74] showed no abnormalities. Biochemical assessments of anterior pituitary function in seven other patients (including one with agenesis of the corpus callosum) were normal.

HYPERTHERMIA

Acute Hyperthermia

Acute lesions of the anterior hypothalamus and preoptic area secondary to trauma or neurosurgical damage may produce profound, fulminant hyperthermia. The fever so induced rarely persists for more than a few hours or days. Treatment is supportive, using measures to reduce body temperature and brain swelling.

Hyperthermia also may occur postanesthesia in patients with the malignant hyperthermia syndrome, owing to a defect in skeletal muscle associated with sensitivity to muscle relaxants.[24,89] The malignant neuroleptic syndrome occurs as an idiosyncratic reaction in patients receiving butyrophenones or phenothiazines.[6,24]

HYPOTHALAMIC-PITUITARY DISEASE

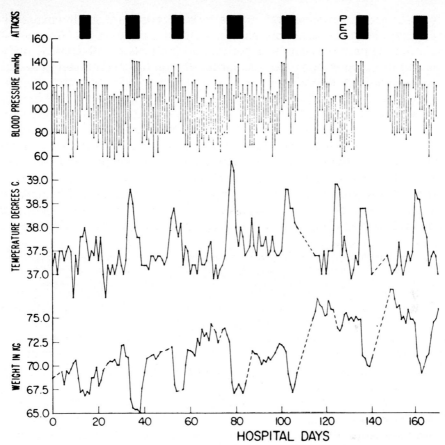

FIGURE 4. Shown here are recurrent episodes of hypertension, hyperthermia, and weight loss in a 14-year-old boy. Clinical attacks occurred at approximately three-week intervals. Pneumoencephalogram (PEG) was associated with fever only. (From Wolff, SM et al,[124] with permission.)

Spontaneous Periodic Hyperthermia (Wolff's Syndrome)

A case of an interesting periodic discharge syndrome has been described by Wolff and colleagues.[124] The patient presented with recurrent episodes of fever, hypertension, vomiting, and weight loss, associated with increased excretion of glucocorticoids (Fig. 4). Treatment with chlorpromazine was successful in ameliorating the symptoms. After 22 years, the patient still requires chlorpromazine to control symptoms. No localizing neurologic defect has appeared in this case (S.M. Wolff, personal communication, 1985).

CARDIOVASCULAR MANIFESTATIONS OF HYPOTHALAMIC DISEASE

Neural Regulation of the Cardiovascular System

Maintenance of constant arterial blood pressure and heart rate depends on the coordination of cardiac output by the sympathetic and parasympathetic nervous systems.[61,72] Reflex arcs arising in the baroreceptors, volume receptors, and chemoreceptors of the heart, lungs, and great vessels are relayed to medullary centers via input of the ninth and tenth cranial nerves terminating in the nucleus of the tractus solitarius (NTS). A detailed analysis and description of cardiovascular regulation has been given in several recent reviews.[111,112,116]

ELECTRICAL STIMULATION

Cardiovascular changes are readily elicited by stimulation of the hypothalamus and of other regions of the limbic system (amygdala, prefrontal and cingulate cortexes). These responses are inseparable in many instances from more generalized behavioral responses. Hence, increased alertness and manifestations of agitation or of rage may be observed together with elevation of blood pressure and tachycardia.

Smith and coworkers[111,112] have investigated the localization of emotional and cardiovascular responses by using a paradigm of the "conditioned emotional response" (CER), in which the animal is conditioned to elicit an emotional response with specific cardiovascular accompaniments. The major anatomic loci of the hypothalamic area controlling emotional responses include the perifornical region and the medial portion of the lateral hypothalamus. The afferents and efferents of this system "include the amygdala, the septal nuclei, the preoptic area and the diagonal band of Broca, all of which have been implicated as being involved in emotional behavior." There are also connections with the central gray, the zona incerta, paraventricular hypothalamus, locus coeruleus, raphe nuclei, the nucleus of the tractus solitarius, and the dorsal motor nucleus of the vagus.

The hypothalamus projects *directly* to the intermediolateral cells of the spinal cord and *indirectly* to other structures of the CNS that project to the intermediolateral column (Fig. 5). Hence, it is apparent that this region of the hypothalamus can be operationally and anatomically defined as a "center" for autonomic nervous system regulation, exerting effects via both the sympathetic and parasympathetic components.

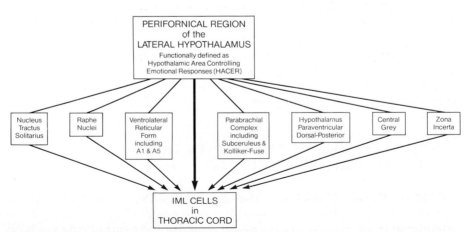

FIGURE 5. The anatomic basis for the integrative role of the hypothalamic area controlling emotional responses (HACER) is illustrated here. Projections are shown to the intermediolateral cells and also to every other region that projects to them.

Functions of Central Noradrenergic and Vasopressinergic Systems in Blood Pressure Control

It is a well-known clinical observation that acute lesions at virtually any site in the CNS can elicit a dramatic, even fulminant, elevation of arterial blood pressure. Experimental studies show that hypertension follows lesions placed in several sites in the medulla oblongata and hypothalamus. Chemical substances or destructive lesions in the NTS cause hypertension by disinhibition of the afferents from peripheral baroreceptors.[35] Experimental animals with such lesions have persistent labile blood pressure. Similar lesions in the region of the NTS in humans have been shown to cause hypertension.

The classic response to increased intracranial pressure described by Cushing, which consists of bradycardia, hypertension, and apnea, can be produced experimentally by distortion or compression of the floor of the fourth ventricle overlying the dorsal medulla. Whether hypothalamic compression or stimulation alone can elicit the Cushing response is not known.

> Bilateral lesions of the A_1 noradrenergic cell group (see chapter 3) cause hypertension, which seems to be dependent on release of vasopressin resulting from disinhibition of a noradrenergic-hypothalamic pathway.[13] Circulating levels of vasopressin are high, and the hypertension can be reversed by antibodies against vasopressin. Whether a similar mechanism of hypertension exists in the human being remains to be shown.

Hypertension occurring with a lesion near the hypothalamus was described in a human subject by Penfield in the well-known case of "diencephalic epilepsy" (see page 391). Experimental hypothalamic lesions can produce hypertension that is dependent on adrenal medullary hypersecretion of catecholamines.[116] Thyrotropin-releasing hormone causes hypertension and tachycardia after local hypothalamic injection.[34] In the human being, lumbar intrathecal injection of TRH leads to hypertension, shivering, sweating, and a sense of warmth.[130]

Brain lesions that cause *hypotension* seem to be confined to the medulla or spinal cord (interfering with the descending regulation of the intermediolateral cell column).

Central Nervous System Lesions, Electrocardiographic Changes, and Cardiac Arrhythmias

Acute lesions of the brain, particularly subarachnoid hemorrhage, are commonly associated with cardiac disturbances. Supraventricular tachycardia, ectopic ventricular contractions, multifocal ventricular tachycardias, ventricular flutter, and ventricular fibrillation all have reported in patients with subarachnoid hemorrhage, and less commonly after cerebral ischemia, cerebral tumors, and during neurosurgical procedures.[116] Electrocardiographic (ECG) changes that occur include prolonged QT intervals, depressed ST segments, flat or inverted T waves, peaked or notched T waves, elevated ST segments, and increased QRS voltages. These have been described after subarachnoid hemorrhage, intracerebral hemorrhage, head trauma, brain tumors, meningitis, multiple sclerosis, and during neurosurgical procedures involving the forebrain. Forty to 70 percent of patients with subarachnoid hemorrhage may show one or more of these changes. Severe ECG changes, like ST segment depression, are associated with a poorer prognosis.[58]

Cardiac arrhythmias also can result from CNS lesions. As emphasized by Talman,[116] "the importance of these complicating cardiac arrhythmias to the overall prognosis of subjects with intracranial disease is profound. They presumably are a major cause of sudden death in patients with subarachnoid hemorrhage, which alone accounts for 4 to 5 percent of all nonviolent sudden deaths."

Pathophysiology of Cardiac Abnormalities

Focal myocytolysis, myofibrillar degeneration, and histiocytic infiltration, independent of any coronary artery disease, can result from CNS alterations of sympathetic nervous system regulation. Focal subendocardial necrosis and hemorrhages have been found after hypothalamic stimulation in the monkey.[15] It is speculated, without direct experimental proof, that release of catecholamines from sympathetic nerve fibers in the heart causes the damage.

There seems little doubt that these arrhythmias result from central sympathetic nervous system activation, but the exact mechanism remains obscure. Treatment with β-receptor agonists is usually effective, suggesting a role of β-receptors, but this is not likely the sole mechanism. Ranson and colleagues reported in their classic studies that only sympathetic responses are elicited by hypothalamic stimulation, but Evans and Gillis[38] showed in anesthetized cats that stimulation of the hypothalamus consistently caused increases in blood pressure and heart rate, accompanied by arrhythmias that were prevented by vagotomy or cholinergic blockers, suggesting a vagal-cholinergic mechanism.

NEURAL CONTROL OF FOOD INTAKE

In 1901, Fröhlich[41] described a case of hypogonadism with obesity in a 14-year-old boy with a pituitary tumor. Originally obesity was attributed to pituitary dysfunction, but Erdheim[131] later showed that an identical syndrome could be caused by lesions of the hypothalamus. Subsequently, Hetherington and Ranson[60] showed that obesity could be induced by localized injury to the hypothalamus. The association of obesity with hypogonadism in hypothalamic disease is now a commonly recognized, although not invariable, association; hypogonadism of hypothalamic origin may occur as an isolated disorder, and hypothalamic obesity may occur without hypogonadism. Disturbance of affect frequently accompanies the hypothalamic form of obesity, particularly when it occurs in the adult. This is characterized by unprovoked rages, overt aggression, and antisocial behavior. The precise hypothalamic area involved in the human being has been documented only infrequently. Lesions of the tuberal and median eminence areas of the hypothalamus usually are described, which accounts for the frequent association of diabetes insipidus with obesity and hypogonadism. Lesions in the human being are usually too extensive to provide a useful anatomic correlation.

A case described in some detail by Reeves and Plum[100] has contributed a great deal to the understanding of the precise localization of such lesions in producing this syndrome in the human. The patient was a 28-year-old obese woman with a one-year history of excessive eating, polyuria, polydypsia, and amenorrhea (Fig. 6). Neurologic examination was normal; pneumoencephalography showed a filling defect in the anterior third ventricle, but nothing abnormal was found on surgical exploration. Two years later the patient returned with a two-month history of behavioral abnormality characterized by intermittent withdrawal, unprovoked laughing, crying, and at times uncontrolled rages and aggression. On examination, the patient was intermittently confused and appeared to have hallucinations. She was even more obese and was extremely uncooperative and at times physically aggressive, especially when food was restricted. These episodes alternated with periods during which she was cooperative and even apologetic for her behavior. The endocrine studies of the patient were not extensive but indicated borderline-low thyroid and adrenal function. Caloric intake ranged from 8,000 to 10,000 per day. The patient died of a pulmonary embolus. Autopsy showed a pale mass that protruded from the basal hypothalamus extending from the posterior optic chiasm to the anterior region of the mammillary bodies. The mass, a hamartoma, was found to have invaded the ventromedial nucleus bilaterally, destroying the me-

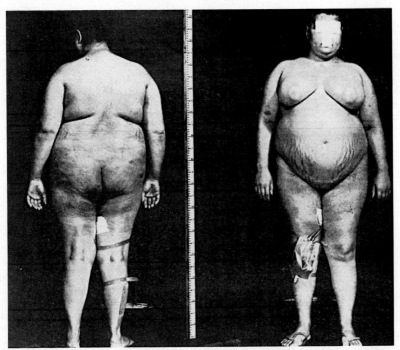

FIGURE 6. Obesity in a 28-year-old woman with a hypothalamic lesion. Catheter had been inserted for metabolic balance studies. (From Reeves, AG, and Plum, F,[100] with permission.)

MANIFESTATIONS OF HYPOTHALAMIC DISEASE   397

dian eminence but sparing the lateral hypothalamus (Fig. 7). The lesion extended anteriorly into the anterior hypothalamic-preoptic area.

The clinical-pathologic correlation in this case was remarkable. The symptom complex of excessive appetite, hyperphagia with obesity, diabetes insipidus, amenorrhea, and grossly disordered emotional reactivity was correlated with a lesion destroying the median eminence and the ventromedial hypothalamic nuclei but sparing the lateral zones of the hypothalamus. Few other clinical reports of patients with hypothalamic obesity have shown as precise a localization of the hypothalamic lesion.

Hypothalamic disorders reported to occur in association with obesity have been summarized in a comprehensive review by Bray and Gallagher,[16] which includes eight cases of their own. The most common causes were solid tumors, leukemia, inflammatory disease, external head trauma, and surgical intervention for various tumors or vascular lesions involving the base of the brain. Craniopharyngioma was the most common solid tumor; others included pituitary adenoma, angiosarcoma, glioma, cysts, cholesteatoma, hamartoma, ganglioneuroma, epithelioma, meningioma,

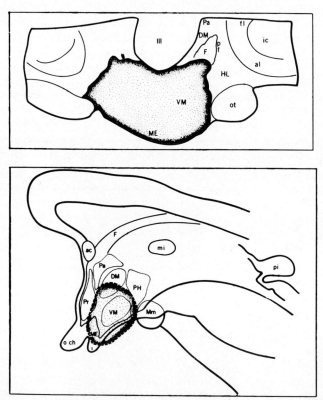

FIGURE 7. A hypothalamic lesion producing hyperphagia and obesity is illustrated. The lesion destroyed the ventromedial (VM) nucleus bilaterally and invaded the median eminence (ME). Abbreviations: ac, anterior commissure; al, ansa lenticularis; DM, dorsomedial nuclear regions, F, fornix; fl, fasciculus lenticularis; HL, lateral hypothalamus; i, infundibular stalk; ic, internal capsule; mi, massa intermedia; Mm, mammillary body; ME, median eminence; o ch, optic chiasm; ot, optic tract; Pa, paraventricular nucleus; ph, pallidohypothalamic tract; pf, perifornical region; PH, posterior hypothalamus; pi, pineal body; Pr, preoptic region; so, supra optic nucleus; t, thalamus; VM, ventromedial nuclear region; zi, zonia incerta; III, third ventricle. (From Reeves, AG, and Plum, F,[100] with permission.)

and chordoma. Inflammatory diseases included sarcoidosis, tuberculosis, arachnoiditis, and encephalitis. In approximately half of these cases endocrine function was abnormal, the most common finding being impaired gonadotropin secretion and diabetes insipidus.

The vastness of the literature on regulation of food intake indicates the complexity of the regulatory process, as well as its importance.[2,53,69,70,105] Under normal conditions, animals and human beings eat appropriately for caloric balance and growth and in maturity achieve a relatively stable body weight. On a short-term basis, cyclic eating behavior is initiated, then stopped in response to some form of satiety signal. On a long-term basis, food intake is adjusted to maintain a constant depot of calories in the form of triglyceride stored in fat tissues. Neural factors are involved in both kinds of homeostatic response, and they are integrated with each other.

Physiologic Sensors of Caloric State

Short-Term Regulation

Extensive ablation studies carried out in the classic era of physiology indicated that afferent stimuli from mouth, throat, and gastrointestinal tract all contribute to the sense of satiety in animals.[69,70] The physiologic constructs that underlie short-term and long-term regulation are summarized succinctly by Schneider and coworkers.[105] "The short-term system regulates periods of feeding, or meal patterns, throughout the day. Investigation of animal and human feeding behavior has demonstrated that meals are highly structured events, with very typical meal sizes, inter-meal intervals, and satiety-associated behaviors. It is likely that these short-term feeding parameters are individually regulated and can be individually affected by various pharmacological and nutritional manipulations. In addition, it appears highly probable, although not definitely proved, that mammalian fuel reserve stored within adipocytes as neutral triglyceride is also subject to long term regulation, by modulations in both food intake and basal energy consumption."

The regulation of feeding behavior is the result of an integrated homeostatic system comprising a series of interacting circuits (Fig. 8). By an unknown mechanism, after food ingestion the amount of nutrient consumed is rapidly quantified and transduced into neural or humoral signals that are processed by the CNS to terminate the meal. An important element of this response is the regulation of rate of gastric emptying by cholecystokinin (CCK) effects on the pyloric sphincter mechanism.[79] Gastric sensation is mediated by vagal afferents. There is evidence to indicate that short-term, preabsorption satiety signals originate in the gastrointestinal tract during a meal and result in rapid succession of feeding. For long-term regulation, the amount of stored triglyceride also may be monitored. It is speculated that by some unknown mechanism the global nutritional status of the animal is continually assessed and compared against an ideal reference or "setpoint" for body weight. The ability of humans and animals to maintain fairly stable body weights over long periods of time when fed *ad libitum* and to restore normal body weights following periods of over or under nutrition is quite remarkable. However, as reviewed by Schneider

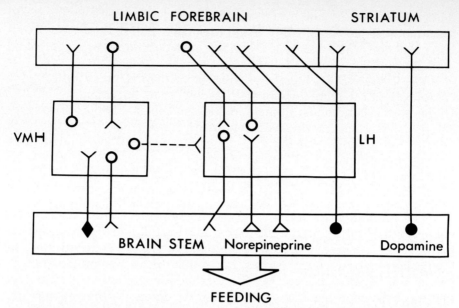

FIGURE 8. This is a diagram of the role of the hypothalamus in feeding. Noradrenergic fibers from brainstem project to both lateral hypothalamus (LH) and limbic forebrain. Lesions of these fibers interfere with normal feeding; chemical stimulation via α-receptors stimulates feeding. The ventromedial hypothalamus (VMH) is interconnected with the limbic forebrain and the brainstem. Interactions between a LH "feeding center" and a VMH "satiety center" may thus be indirect via either limbic or brainstem connections. The dotted line between LH and VMH indicates that anatomic connections between these areas do exist. The dopaminergic system to the basal ganglia has been implicated in the motor control of feeding, rather than in the "motivational" aspects.

and colleagues, we currently have little information about the chemical, physical, or neuroanatomic composition of the setpoints. It is evident that the level of setpoint can be altered by a variety of conditions including physical activity, temperature, and the palatability of the diet. Thus animals with ventromedial hypothalamic lesions demonstrate an initial phase of hyperphagia and rapid weight gain until a new plateau is achieved and maintained. On the other hand, lateral hypothalamic lesions yield opposite results with hypophagia, weight loss, and the maintenance of a lower body weight. Setpoints for long-term control of body weight may exist but are capable of changing in response to internal or external perturbations.

> "Whatever the nature of such short term or long term homeostasis, the existence of a regulated system or set of systems necessitates some mechanism of information exchange among multiple loci, including adipose tissue, the gastrointestinal tract, and the central nervous system. In hypothetical terms, this homeostatic system could be regulated at any of three levels: an afferent loop (with signals originating from the gastrointestinal tract, adipose tissue, liver); an integrated center within the central nervous system; and an efferent loop comprising the neurophysiological events that initiate or constitute a behavioral or metabolic change relevant to nutrition."[105]

The factors that regulate short-term satiety are incompletely understood. Mayer[78] emphasized the "glucostat" hypothesis in which he proposed that glucosensitive hypothalamic neurons monitor blood glucose, rate of change of blood glucose, or rate of glucose utilization. Experimental findings that support the Mayer hypothesis include the demonstration of neurons in the ventromedial area of the hypothalamus which increase their firing rate in response to increases in blood glucose, and the phenomenon of gold thioglucose-induced obesity. In this experimental model of obesity, glucose conjugated with gold, a neurotoxin, is selectively concentrated in the ventromedial nucleus (VMN), where it causes both neural destruction and hyperphagia. Gold salts, which are not chemical analogs of glucose, are not toxic; the effect of the agent is increased by insulin administration which increases gold thioglucose uptake, and the extent of the damage is decreased by diabetes (insulin deficiency), which reduces uptake. Localization of this reaction in the ventromedial nucleus is indicated by the observation that electrolytic destruction of this region (or of adjacent fibers) causes obesity, and electric stimulation of the VMN inhibits eating.

The possibility has been considered that glucoreceptors exist in other regions of the brain, or in the gastrointestinal tract. Russek[103] has proposed that glucose-sensitive hepatocytes can monitor glucose concentrations in the portal vein of the liver. He has shown that the transmembrane potentials of the hepatocyte increase after local administration of glucose and that these detectors signal central regulatory centers via the vagus or the sympathetic nerves. Also, surgical section of the vagi in rats partially prevents the development of hypothalamic obesity.

Long-Term Regulation

The precision of long-term control of appetite is remarkable. Humans gain, on the average, 15 pounds in weight between the ages of 20 and 40, representing a daily excess intake of only 16 calories (equivalent to 1 teaspoon of sugar). Over this period, each individual will have ingested a total of approximately 1.5×10^7 calories, and thus will have adjusted intake to need with an accuracy of 0.8 percent per year, or 0.001 percent per meal. Most investigators do not believe that any short-term monitoring system such as receptor afferents from the gastrointestinal tract, or a central glucoreceptor, could possibly provide this extraordinary precision. Moreover, detailed balance studies in the human show that most people have rather wide short-term swings in food intake, but on a longer timescale, intake is quite constant. In experimental animals it is easy to show that forced feeding, which leads to increased fat deposition, is followed by sustained periods of decreased food intake, indicating that the animals adjust to the total fat stores. Forced feeding experiments in the human being have shown similar results. Even in obesity owing to hypothalamic lesions in rats, food intake ceases after a certain weight has been reached. Starvation of such animals followed by free access to food is followed by restitution of the prior (though excess) weight.

On the basis of these observations, Kennedy[69,70] has proposed that long-term caloric balance is primarily mediated by a "lipostatic" mechanism, that is, an appetite sensory mechanism responsive to total fat mass. In support of this hypothesis is the experimental finding that rats with hypothalamic hyperphagia and obesity when joined parabiotically to a normal animal cause the normal partner to stop eating and finally to die from cachexia. Moreover, animals whose fat depots have been removed soon

indicate that the effect is a true effect on satiety and not a food aversive or nauseating effect. Even after the demonstration that a given dose of peptide is capable of affecting ingestive behavior, questions predictably arise about the interpretation of the results: Are the doses physiologic? Does the effect reflect a truly physiologic event? The principal brain peptides that have been postulated to have a function in feeding behavior are reviewed here.

Cholecystokinin. As a candidate for an endogenous peptide satiety signal, cholecystokinin (CCK) has received the most attention. The first work by Smith, Gibbs and their coworkers[108,109] on the appetite-suppressing effects of peripherally administered CCK was performed before recognition that the peptide was also present in brain. Their studies demonstrated that peripheral administration of small quantities was capable of suppressing food intake in several species, work since confirmed by other investigators. Whether peripherally administered CCK reaches the brain remains uncertain, but the demonstration that its effects are largely prevented by vagotomy has led to the suggestion by Smith that it acts upon vagal afferents in the gut. McHugh[79] has shown that the rate of emptying of the stomach is regulated by CCK acting on a CCK-responsive circular muscle sphincter in the pylorus. He proposes, therefore, that the vagal signal is stomach distention. There is also evidence suggesting a direct effect of CCK on the hypothalamus. Cholecystokinin is present in brain, CCK receptors are also present, and intracranial injections of CCK induce satiety. Moreover, acute CCK injection in the sheep inhibits eating, and antibodies to CCK given into the CSF stimulate eating.[31] However, many negative studies have also been reported.[105] The mode of action of brain CCK, if it does in fact elicit satiety, remains unclear. The highest concentrations of CCK are found in cortex, not hypothalamus, and anatomic studies of its localizations do not strongly support a major function in the hypothalamic or limbic systems involved in feeding behavior. Although changes in CCK receptor occur in relation to feeding, the claim that CCK levels are altered by feeding has not been confirmed.[100] In conclusion, despite conflicting results and many interspecies variations, there is good pharmacologic evidence to indicate that CCK may act both peripherally and centrally to modify feeding behavior, acting in both sites to induce satiety. However, these experiments do not prove that CCK has a physiologic function in appetite regulation.

Insulin. Discovery of insulin in brain at concentrations greater than those present in plasma led to the suggestion that insulin might be synthesized within the CNS. Insulin receptors are found in the hypothalamus, and the possibility that either endogenous or pancreatic-derived insulin might regulate food ingestion was proposed. Hyperinsulinemia is a constant finding in virtually all forms of human and animal obesity. It was suggested by Woods and Porte[125] that high plasma insulin concentrations might slowly enter the CSF, causing an elevation of CSF insulin levels. Such an increase might be a signal to relevant centers in the brain to regulate insulin secretion over long periods of time. Indeed, insulin can be detected in the CSF of experimental animals after intravenous injection of large supraphysiologic doses. Elevated levels of CSF insulin have been reported in obese patients.[92] Evidence that blood-borne insulin can reach selected sites in brain was provided by *in vivo* radioautographic studies.[118,119] Insulin appeared in the endothelium of microvessels distributed in the brain and in certain of the circumventricular organs that lack an effective blood-brain barrier. Locally applied insulin can alter hypothalamic electrical activity, affect peripheral glucose metabolism, and interfere with norepinephrine turnover. In summary, it is evident that insulin and its receptors present in brain might function to mediate food ingestion. The origin of CNS insulin remains unresolved awaiting demonstration of messenger ribonucleic acid (RNA) levels. It is possible that plasma insulin constitutes one of the afferent components of the short- or long-term nutritional control systems.

Endogenous Opiates. Morphine administration stimulates eating in experimental animals,[105] and naloxone, an endogenous opiate antagonist, decreases food intake in rats with congenital forms of obesity such as the Zucker fat rat.[76] Stress-induced eating is also blocked by naloxone.[19,76,84] These observations and others give strong indication that endogenous opioids are involved in appetite regulation. The most specific evidence that opioids act centrally is the demonstration that intraventricular injection of either β-endorphin[51,80,104] or dynorphin[85] stimulate eating in food-sated rats, and central administration of systemically ineffective doses of naloxone stimulates food intake.[67]

That these findings may be relevant to food intake in the human being is the report that naloxone administration inhibits food intake in patients with Prader-Willi syndrome, a disorder of excessive food intake, and that morphine-addicted individuals tend to be chronically undernourished.

Bombesin. Central administration of bombesin reduces feeding behavior in rats and inhibits stress-induced feeding, elicited in rodents by pinching the tail. The satiety-inducing effects of bombesin are not abolished by vagotomy, indicating that its action is independent of the effects of CCK. Cholecystokinin and bombesin given together have additive effects. Bombesin receptors are found in the CNS, highest concentrations being in the hypothalamus. Intraventricular administration reduces feeding in rats, sheep, and pigs. Intraventricular administration of bombesin also decreases water intake. In contrast, direct intrahypothalamic injection of bombesin causes satiety, appropriate postprandial behavior, and normal water intake.

Thyrotropin-releasing Hormone and Other Anorexigenic Peptides

The administration of TRH and of its metabolite cyclo-His-Pro reduce food and water intake.[90,101,122]

Anorexigenic Peptide. Trygsted and colleagues[117] isolated a tripeptide, pGLU-His-Gly-OH, from the urine of patients with anorexia nervosa and claimed that injections of this material inhibited food intake. However, subsequent studies in other laboratories have not confirmed this claim.[12,105]

These pharmacologic studies provide evidence that several brain peptides can alter feeding behavior either directly or by interacting with monoamines or other neurotransmitter systems. It is likely that further research will disclose other peptides with effects on feeding. It is evident that more refined methods of study are required to determine their physiologic roles. Whether any will be demonstrated to contribute to pathologic conditions such as anorexia nervosa or tumor-induced cachexia is unknown.

TUMOR ANOREXIA

The clinical observation has frequently been made that patients with certain kinds of cancer suffer from profound anorexia, a finding interpreted to mean that tumors may secrete anorexigenic factors. One such factor, isolated from a Leydig-cell tumor in experimental rats, was shown to be estrogen,[132] but other factors are probably present. Tumor neurosis factor (also called cachexin) has been purified from tumor tissue.[133-135] It induces profound anorexia and weight loss when injected into experimental animals. The possibility that secretion from tumors may cause cachexia in human beings is currently under investigation.

EXTRAHYPOTHALAMIC REGULATION

It would be gross oversimplification to imply that the hypothalamus is the only region of the brain with an important influence on food intake. The studies of Chi and Flynn[25] showed that experimental animals with hypothalamic islands that separate the hypothalamus from the rest of the brain do not develop aphagia, as would be expected if the only region for this drive were located in or restricted to the hypothalamus. Other areas also must be capable of initiating this form of behavior. It should not be surprising that such highly integrated activity as seeking, discriminating, and ingesting appropriate quantities of food must involve extensive areas of the limbic brain. Klüver and Bucy[71] described aberrations in discrimination of food following temporal lobe lesions in the monkey, and frontal lobotomy was also sometimes followed by hyperphagia and obesity. Similar syndromes have been described in humans.[75] Bilateral lesions of the amygdala are reported in several species to produce varying syndromes of adipsia and aphagia, and disorders of perception, recognition, and behavior in respect to food intake have been described in the human which have features akin to the Klüver-Bucy syndrome. Extensive neurophysiologic data relating the limbic system to hypothalamic food regulation have been accumulated by Morgane.[82]

HYPOTHALAMIC FACTORS IN HUMAN OBESITY

Although it is generally agreed that obesity may arise from hypothalamic lesions, it is equally likely that in most cases of obesity no significant hypothalamic abnormalities are involved. Nevertheless, a number of writers have emphasized the physiologic similarities between VMN-lesioned rats and obese humans. As summarized by Girvin,[47] both VMN-lesioned rats and obese humans (1) eat more of a good-tasting food, (2) eat less of a bad-tasting food, (3) eat only a slight excess of food during each day, (4) eat fewer meals each day, (5) eat more at each meal, (6) eat more quickly, (7) react more emotionally, (8) are less active, (9) eat more when food is easily accessible, (10) eat less when food is difficult to obtain, and (11) fail to regulate food consumption when the food consumed is preloaded with solids but regulate normally when preloaded with liquids. External controls (tastes, psychic factors, and the social milieu) rather than internal food signals appear to take over regulation of food intake in both obese individuals and VMN-lesioned rats. These superficial similarities may be a clue to the pathophysiology of human hyperphagia. Compulsive eating may occur with rather nonspecific brain lesions. Green and Pau[52] have reported a series of 10 such patients, 9 of whom had abnormal electroencephalograms and were successfully treated with anticonvulsants. Bulimia, a disorder of excessive food intake, often associated with vomiting, is discussed in chapter 21. Patients with hypothalamic hyperphagia show stress- and depression-activated eating, as do obese patients without hypothalamic disease (Reichlin, unpublished).

LATERAL HYPOTHALAMIC LESIONS: THE LATERAL HYPOTHALAMIC SYNDROME IN THE HUMAN BEING

In marked contrast to the VMN syndrome are the effects of lesions in the lateral hypothalamus immediately adjacent to the VMN: These result in aphagia, which can lead to cachexia and death.

Anorexia secondary to a hypothalamic lesion is rare. In a case reported by White and Hain,[123] a 62-year-old woman died weighing 67 pounds after progressive emaciation. On postmortem examination, a small discrete cystic lesion in the wall of the third ventricle was noted that had resulted in a decrease in hypothalamic tissue. The primary lesion was in the hypothalamus. More recently, Lewin and coworkers[73] reported the case of a young woman who suffered from severe anorexia nervosa. She was found at autopsy to have an astrocytoma involving the inferior surface of the hypothalamus. A direct correlation between the lateral hypothalamic lesions described in experimental animals and the presence of an anorexia syndrome in the human being does not appear to have been reported. Anorexia nervosa, generally assumed to be a psychiatric disorder,[9] is discussed in chapter 21.

DIENCEPHALIC SYNDROME

A rare disorder of infancy is the diencephalic syndrome caused most commonly by a glioma arising in the anterior hypothalamic area.[21,36] No counterpart has been described in experimental animals. The infant, usually a boy, follows a stereotyped course. After normal birth and early development, the infant begins to lose weight, usually between the third and twelfth months of life, and emaciation becomes progressive despite normal food intake (Fig. 9). In most cases, the infant is described as being unusually cheerful and alert, despite the apparent cachexia. Emaciation is unrelenting, and death occurs before the second year. The lesions in these infants have been remarkably consistent, usually being low-grade astrocytomas of the anterior hypothalamus or optic nerve[21] (Tables 6, 7) The pathophysiology of the disturbance is unexplained. It is apparent that this is not due to aphagia produced by lateral hypothalamic lesions, inasmuch as food intake

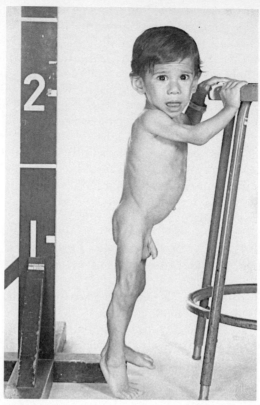

FIGURE 9. This photograph shows a two-year-old child with diencephalic syndrome due to astrocytoma of anterior hypothalamus. There is loss of subcutaneous fat and growth failure. (Courtesy of H. Guyda).

may be increased. Hypothalamic lesions in this age group appear to result consistently in this wasting syndrome rather than in the more typical picture of later childhood and adolescence in which similar lesions result in obesity, somnolence, rage, and precocious puberty (Table 8). The remarkable lack of subcutaneous fat in these cases is so striking as to be of diagnostic assistance on plain roentgenograms of the extremities. Several reports have noted elevated GH levels in cases of diencephalic syndrome owing conceivably to loss of the anterior hypothalamic GH-inhibiting pathways. Paradoxical rises in GH after glucose are reported similar to the response in acromegaly.

Treatment by surgical removal or radiation has been effective in a few cases.[1,21]

DISORDERS OF CONSCIOUSNESS ASSOCIATED WITH HYPOTHALAMIC DISEASE

A disturbance of consciousness attributable to hypothalamic lesions was first described by Gayet in 1875 in a patient with severe somnolence whose autopsy examination disclosed necrotic periventricular lesions of the third ventricle.[121] This was probably the first description of what was to become known as Wernicke's encephalopathy, the pathology of which was de-

TABLE 6. Clinical Features of Diencephalic Syndrome (Pooled Data of 67 Anatomically Defined Tumors)

Clinical Features	%
Emaciation	100
Alert appearance	87
Increased vigor and/or hyperkinesis	72
Vomiting	68
Euphoria	59
Pallor	55
Nystagmus	55
Irritability	32
Hydrocephalus*	33
Optic atrophy	24
Tremor	23
Sweating	15
Large hands/feet	5
Large genitals	5
Polyuria	5
Papilledema	5
Positive pneumoencephalogram	98
Endocrine anomalies	90
CSF protein	64
CSF abnormal cells	23

*Hydrocephalus includes clinical plus pneumoencephalographic findings. Positive in 9 of 10 with adequately recorded investigation. (Occasionally, patients had electrolyte and blood pressure anomalies and eosinophilia.)

From Burr, IM, et al,[21] with permission.

scribed by him in 1881. This condition commonly is associated, in the acute stage, with somnolence and confusion. In 1890, Mauthner described several cases of encephalitis in which somnolence was predominant and lesions demonstrated in the basal diencephalon.[121] Probably these cases were early examples of epidemic encephalitis, later described in detail by

TABLE 7. Histology of Tumors Producing Diencephalic Syndrome

Tumors	No. of Patients
Gliomas	56
Astrocytoma	37
Not subclassified	10
Spongioblastoma	5
Astroblastoma	1
Oligodendroglioma	1
Mixed astrocytoma/spongioblastoma	1
Mixed astrocytoma/oligodendroglioma	1
Ependymoma	2
Ganglioglioma	1
Dysgerminoma	1
No histology	10

From Burr, IM, et al,[21] with permission.

TABLE 8. Etiology of Hypothalamic Disease by Age

1. Premature infants and neonates
   Intraventricular hemorrhage
   Meningitis: bacterial
   Tumors: glioma, hemangioma
   Trauma
   Hydrocephalus, kernicterus
2. 1 month to 2 years
   Tumors
      Glioma, especially optic glioma
      Histocytosis X
      Hemangiomas
      Hydrocephalus, meningitis
      "Familial" disorders: Laurence-Moon-Biedl, Prader-Labhart-Willi
3. 2 to 10 years
   Tumors
      Craniopharyngioma
      Glioma, dysgerminoma, hamartoma, histiocytosis X, leukemia
      Ganglioneuroma, ependymoma, medulloblastoma
   Meningitis
      Bacterial
      Tuberculous
   Encephalitis
      Viral and demyelinating
      Various viral encephalides and exanthematous demyelinating encephalides
      Disseminated encephalomyelitis
      "Familial" disorders: diabetes insipidus, etc.
4. 10 to 25 years
   Tumors
      Craniopharyngioma
      Glioma, hamartoma, dysgerminoma
      Histiocytosis X, leukemia
      Dermoid, lipoma, neuroblastoma
   Trauma
      Subarachnoid hemorrhage, vascular aneurysm, arteriovenous malformation
      Inflammatory diseases, meningitis, encephalitis, sarcoid, tuberculosis
      Associated with midline brain defects; agenesis of corpus callosum
      Chronic hydrocephalus or increased intracranial pressure
5. 25 to 50 years
   Nutritional: Wernicke's disease
   Tumors
      Sarcoma, glioblastoma, lymphoma
      Meningioma, colloid cysts, ependymoma, pituitary tumors
   Vascular
      Infarct, subarachnoid hemorrhage
      Pituitary apoplexy
   Inflammation: Encephalitis, sarcoid, meningitis

From Plum, F, AND Van Uitert, R,[97] with permission.

Von Economo. His descriptions were the first to indicate an association of somnolence with lesions in the posterior hypothalamus. This conclusion has been confirmed by both experimental and clinical observations.

Aberrations in the level of consciousness ranging from increased periods of sleeping, from which arousal is easily obtained, to frank coma have been attributed to hypothalamic lesions.[43,107] The site responsible for these disturbances of alertness and responsiveness, perhaps more than any other aspect of hypothalamic function, has been difficult to define anatomically. By the time the patient dies, lesions are frequently extensive and the secondary effects of increased intracranial pressure have supervened. The opposite condition, insomnia, occasionally has been associated with specific hypothalamic lesions. For example, the reports of Von Economo indicated that anterior hypothalamic-preoptic lesions in encephalitis were associated with hyperactivity and decreased sleeping periods.

Despite difficulties in precise localization, tentative conclusions with respect to hypothalamic function in the regulation of consciousness which agree closely with the experimental literature can be formulated. Clearly, the hypothalamus is neither the sole site of, nor need be implicated at all with, lesions that cause a disorder in consciousness.

Regions of the brain, destruction of which result in altered alertness, awareness,and consciousness, range from bilateral anterior mesial cortical lesions (involving the cingulate gyri) to lesions in the rostral pons. This subject is critically reviewed by Plum and Posner.[96] The effect of a given lesion depends to a major degree on the acuteness of onset. A very large lesion in the basal hypothalamus, developing slowly — as can occur with an expanding craniopharyngioma, pituitary adenoma, or meningioma — may not be associated with any alteration of consciousness. On the other hand, the abrupt occurrence of a small posterior hypothalamic or rostral mesencephalic lesion often produces profound coma. The survival time following an acute lesion may affect the manifestations of that lesion. Remarkable recovery of function following extensive lesions of the upper midbrain and posterior hypothalamus has been reported in patients who have survived for weeks or months after the initial episode. Animal studies closely parallel this finding.

Lesions along the neural axis described above can produce similar effects on alertness and responsiveness.[29] A syndrome of disinterest, slowed responsivity, and lack of spontaneity and attention (sometimes called *abulia*) can occur with bilateral lesions of the cingulate gyrus (sometimes even with unilateral dominant lesions), the hypothalamus, and the midbrain reticular formation. In the case reported by Nielsen and Jacobs,[88] a 46-year-old woman developed a peculiar, abrupt-onset stupor during which she stood immobile with eyes open and a vacant stare and did not appear to respond to auditory or visual stimuli. She survived several days during which she remained mute and unresponsive yet frequently appeared to be awake. She was incontinent and made no effort to eat. At autopsy, bilateral lesions were found in the distribution of the anterior cerebral arteries, which had resulted in necrosis of the anterior portions of both cingulate gyri. The corpus callosum was not involved. The authors pointed out the similarities between this case and those of Marchiafava-Bignami disease, in which lesions of the corpus callosum are found.

The description of this case is not unlike that of so-called *akinetic mutism*, a term coined by Cairns in 1941[22,23] to describe the clinical findings in a 14-year-old girl with a craniopharyngioma extending deeply into the tuberal region of the hypothalamus. The patient had a history of progressive somnolence from which she could not be aroused. At the time of admission, although appearing awake, the patient showed no response to questions and appeared to be in a trance. Her eyes moved to follow an object, and she would fixate upon the examiner as if about to speak but nothing was forthcoming. She was mute and showed virtually no spontaneous movement (hence the term akinetic mutism). In addition, she showed minimal responses to painful stimuli with absence of any observable signs of emotional expression. She was able to swallow food and liquid when it was placed in her mouth but made no signs of desiring either. She was incontinent of both feces and urine.

The remarkable feature of this case was that following operative drainage of tumor under local anesthesia, the patient immediately began to respond and to speak. She had no recollection of the period of coma. This unusual clinical picture also has been referred to as "coma vigil."[22,24,27]

Fulton and Bailey[43] described a similar case in a 28-year-old woman with a lesion in the same region. She had suffered for many years from amenorrhea, polyuria, and polydipsia. About five years before death, episodes of drowsiness began to occur, during which the patient would suddenly drop asleep in the midst of an animated conversation or in the middle of routine duties. She could always be aroused from such episodes, and they appeared to be normal periods of sleeping rather than seizures. Prior to death, extreme somnolence occurred, progressing to coma. At autopsy, a sarcoma of the tuberal region was found. There was no associated hydrocephalus, and the pituitary gland appeared normal. It is apparent in such cases that the anatomic localization of the defect is not precise. Nor is it always possible to exclude pressure effects on the posterior hypothalamic region or upper midbrain.

A lesion in the posterior-basal hypothalamus was considered to be the cause of somnolence and hypothermia in the case of glioblastoma reported by Davison and Demuth.[30] The tumor in this instance involved the medial posterior hypothalamus and extended from the posterior region of the infundibulum through the mammillary region but did not extend into the midbrain.

Lesions of the upper mesencephalic reticular formation initially produce profound coma and are usually irreversible. Occasionally, with prolonged survival, recovery to a stage similar to akinetic mutism may occur (vegetative state).[113] It is important with lesions in the pons to make certain that coma is actually present. Such lesions, which interrupt corticospinal, corticobulbar, and corticopontine fibers, can result in total paralysis with preservation only of eye or lid movement. The patient may appear superficially to have akinetic mutism. However, consciousness may be entirely preserved and the electroencephalogram (EEG) may show a normal alpha pattern. Recognition of this fact is of upmost importance in the management of the patient. This paralytic form with preserved awareness is called the "locked-in syndrome."

These cases illustrate that no precise anatomic area controls consciousness. The maintenance of normal sleep—waking sequences appear to depend on brainstem influences as well as on those of certain areas of the limbic system. Disturbances at a number of levels may produce profound disorders of attention and responsiveness. Having made this generalization, it is still accurate to say that the areas most likely to result in the greatest disturbance of consciousness are the midbrain reticular formation and the posterior hypothalamus.[106,113,114]

Experiments in animals confirm this view.

Ranson[99] demonstrated in primates that lateral hypothalamic lesions in the regions adjacent to the mammillary bodies produced a syndrome of akinesia, hypothermia, tameness, lethargy, and temporary aphagia. Acute lesions in the mesencephalic tegmentum caused a more severe disorder of consciousness.

Studies in cats indicate that the degree and persistence of somnolence produced by hypothalamic lesions are proportional to the extent of involvement of pathways from the ventromedial nucleus and posterior hypothalamus to ventral mesencephalic nuclei. Swett[96] described in the cat a distinguishing feature of posterior hypothalamic lesions, depending on whether they are medial or lateral. Medial posterior hypothalamic lesions resulted in minimal disturbance of consciousness, feeding, or grooming, whereas lateral posterior hypothalamic lesions induced drowsiness, cataplexy, and absence of feeding. It was concluded (as Ransom had earlier suggested) that lateral pathways in or close to the medial forebrain bundle are of great importance in the maintenance of normal alertness.

MEMORY AND THE HYPOTHALAMUS

For many years it was considered likely that lesions of the mammillary bodies which occur in Wernicke's encephalopathy were responsible for deficit in memory (Korsakoff's psychosis). The extensive studies of Victor and associates[121] cast doubt on this hypothesis. The lesions that they found to be most consistently associated with memory deficits in patients with Wernicke-Korsakoff disease were located in the medial dorsal nucleus of the thalamus. Several other descriptions of patients with memory disorders and lesions in this area owing to other causes have been reported confirming this anatomic localization. Presumably, medial dorsal thalamic lesions cause a deficit in memory by interrupting connections between the thalamus and medial frontal and temporal lobe areas.

A number of case reports have emphasized an association between hypothalamic tumors and defects in memory that mimic the amnestic syndrome of the Wernicke-Korsakoff syndrome. Some have had infarcts in the dominant thalamus.[50] Not all have extended to include the thalamus, although secondary effects owing to compression cannot be excluded. One is left with the conclusion that hypothalamic lesions in isolation can alter the processes of acquisition of new memories. But the precise anatomic sites affected remain undefined. In the case of Reeves and Plum described above, memory disturbance was prominent, and the lesion was restricted to the VMN-infundibular region of the hypothalamus.

PERIODIC HYPOTHALAMIC DISEASE

KLEINE-LEVIN SYNDROME

The Kleine-Levin syndrome is characterized by the appearance, usually in adolescent boys, of recurrent episodes of somnolence, hyperphagia, and sexual hyperactivity.[11,37,46] Individual attacks appear at intervals of three to six months and may last for one to three weeks. During the attack the patient sleeps for extended periods of time, often 18 to 20 hours daily. Episodes of arousal may be associated with gorging of food, masturbation, and overt sexual advances. The attack is self-limited and there is afterward complete or partial amnesia for the episode.

No demonstrable neurologic abnormality can be demonstrated during an attack, and endocrine studies are unrevealing. In one report, diurnal variations in steroids were absent during the attack. No structural lesions have been described; occasionally, a patient with an encephalitis-like illness may present a similar pattern. One patient was said to have had a recent toxoplasmosis infection.

In the interval between attacks, the patient demonstrates no abnormalities. In general, the disorder is self-limited and disappears by late adolescence or early adult life.

The term Kleine-Levin syndrome was given to this disorder by Critchley in 1942.[28] He described two cases of his own and found another 16 in the early literature, the first reports being separate cases reported by Kleine and by Levin.

In recent years, cases of similar periodic disorders have been observed in girls and in adult patients. Because of the characteristic symptoms, the disorder is thought to reflect deranged hypothalamic function, although proof of this is lacking.

PERIODIC SYNDROME OF WOLFF

In 1964, Wolff and associates[124] described a case of periodic hyperthermia, vomiting, weight loss, and hypercortisolemia that he attributed to cyclic hypothalamic discharge. The attacks occurred with remarkable regularity every three weeks. Treatment with chlorpromazine was effective in controlling the episodes. The relationship of this case to diencephalic epilepsy is not clear at this time. As noted above, this disorder has been present for more than 22 years with no evidence of specific neurologic disease.

DIENCEPHALIC EPILEPSY

Episodes of autonomic dysfunction characterized by tachycardia, flushing, hypertension, salivation, sweating, and deviations in temperature regulation have been called diencephalic epilepsy.[95,112] The EEG was abnormal in many of the cases reported in early series, and about half of the patients have responded favorably to anticonvulsants. In the majority of cases that have been examined at autopsy, a space-occupying lesion has been found in the region of the third ventricle. Cholesteatoma, colloid cyst of the third ventricle, and gliomas have been reported. Paroxysmal attacks of autonomic activation appear, therefore, to be caused by direct pressure effects of obvious anatomic lesions on the hypothalamus. Although rare, when suspected, such cases require complete investigation in an attempt to discover a lesion. Most are not due to a seizure disorder per se but rather to compressive effects that intermittently disturb hypothalamic function. Instances of *episodic hypercortisolemia* also have been reported. A few of these have associated seizure disorders, and others seem to be an early stage in the development of Cushing's disease (see chapter 8).

MISCELLANEOUS HYPOTHALAMIC SYNDROMES

The association of obesity, hypogonadism, and mental retardation has been described in several disorders that are thought to be due to hypothalamic dysfunction.

Prader-Willi Syndrome

A disorder characterized by mental retardation, short stature, hypogonadism (and cryptorchidism), obesity, and neonatal hypotonia was described by Prader, Labhart, and Willi in 1956 and 1963.[127] Over 100 cases that fulfill these criteria now have been reported, and it probably occurs with some frequency but is not diagnosed properly. A few cases are associated with a defect on chromosome 15.[139-142] The condition occurs sporadically, and it is not certain that the syndrome is a single nosologic entity. The disorder is recognized at birth by severe hypotonia and inactivity. The infant is motionless, sleepy, difficult to arouse, and areflexic. Temperature regulation may be abnormal. Tube-feeding is frequently required for several weeks.

Feeding difficulties are replaced by hyperphagia between ages 6 months and 2 years. The child eats continuously and seems to lack normal satiety mechanisms. Gross obesity may result. Diabetes mellitus is frequently associated. Moderate to severe mental retardation are present and make management difficult.

The constellation of abnormalities in these patients suggests hypothalamic dysfunction. However, clinical investigations fail to reveal lesions, and autopsied cases have not shown definite abnormalities. Endocrinologic studies rarely have been performed in the postpubertal age group. In the report of Hamilton and coworkers,[55] three patients between the ages of 19 and 23 were studied. Each had evidence of hypogonadotropic hypogonadism, and one patient responded to clomiphene with a rise in testosterone that persisted after discontinuation of the drug. Thyroid-stimulating hormone, adrenocorticotropic hormone, and growth hormone responses were normal.

Bray and coworkers[143] studied 40 patients with the syndrome. Subjects had normal glucose tolerance, and rise in GH after insulin hypoglycemia and arginine. TRH testing was normal, but GnRH responses were absent in all subjects tested.

It is likely that the disorder is the result of an undefined organic lesion of the hypothalamus that interferes with normal regulation of gonadotropins. The possibility exists that perinatal insult owing to an as yet unspecified cause may result in the rather selective hypothalamic abnormality. The best established treatment of this disorder is behavior modification in a specialized institutional setting. Trials of naloxone have been promising.[129] The families of patients with Prader-Willi syndrome need good family counseling.

Laurence-Moon-Biedl Syndrome

An autosomal recessive hereditary condition characterized by hypogonadism, obesity, retinitis pigmentosa, mental deficiency, and polydactyly has been called the Laurence-Moon-Biedl syndrome. Diabetes mellitus is rare, but diabetes insipidus is common. Other manifestations reported in certain families include nerve deafness and hyperlipemia. Chromosome studies are normal.

Autopsy studies generally have demonstrated normal pituitary architecture, and it is assumed that the hypogonadism is secondary to hypothalamic dysfunction. Hypothalamic lesions have not been described. The endocrine manifestations of the syndrome are variable; affected members of a family may show normal gonadal function, and pregnancy has been reported to occur.

SUMMARY

Hypothalamic disturbances in the human being are rare. When they occur, they show remarkably close agreement with descriptions found in experimental lesions of the hypothalamus. It is possible to localize tentatively certain disorders of function to hypothalamic regions. Preoptic lesions are associated with autonomic disturbances such as cardiac arrhythmia, bladder incontinence, and pulmonary edema. Hyperthermia is common with acute lesions of the anterior hypothalamic-preoptic region. Lesions of the anterior hypothalamus may produce disturbances in food intake, and in infancy can result in cachexia despite normal food intake. Lesions in the lateral regions of the anterior hypothalamus are associated with loss of thirst drive or with alterations in food intake.

Lesions of the ventromedial hypothalamic area in the human being produce hyperphagia, obesity,and abnormal emotional states. Lesions in this region that extend into the median eminence also commonly produce endocrine disorders, including diabetes insipidus, hypogonadism, and abnormalities of secretion of adrenocorticotropin hormone, growth hormone, and prolactin. Mid-lateral-hypothalamic lesions have been infrequently documented in man but may cause anorexia and weight loss. Caudal hypothalamic lesions result in disorders in consciousness, somnolence, hypokinesia, and hypothermia or poikilothermia.

REFERENCES

1. ALLEN, JC, HELSON, L, JEREB, B: *Preradiation chemotherapy for newly diagnosed childhood brain tumors. A modified Phase II trial.* Cancer 51:2001–2006, 1983.
2. ANAND, BK, AND BROBECK, JR: *Hypothalamic control of food intake in rats and cats.* Yale J Biol Med 24:123, 1951.
3. ANDERSSON, B: *The central control of water and salt balance.* In MOGENSON, GJ, AND CALARESU, FR (EDS): *Neural Integration of Physiological Mechanisms and Behavior.* University of Toronto Press, Toronto, 1975, p 213.
4. ARONSOHN, E, AND SACHS, J: *Die Beziehungen des Gehirns zur Komperwarme und zum Fieber; Experimentelle untersuch Engen.* Arch Ges Physiol 37:232, 1885.
5. BAILE, CA, DELLA-FERA, MA, MCLAUGHLIN, CL: *Hormones and feed intake.* Proc Nutr Soc 42:113–127, 1983.
6. BALDESSARINI, RJ: *Chemotherapy in Psychiatry.* Harvard University Press, Cambridge, MA, 1985.
7. BANDLER, RJ, CHI, CC, FLYNN, JP: *Biting attack elicited by stimulation of the ventral midbrain tegmentum of cats.* Science 177:364, 1972.
8. BARRETT, R, MERRIT, HH, WOLF, A: *Depression of consciousness as a result of cerebral lesions.* In *Sleep and Altered States of Consciousness.* Assoc Res Nerv Ment Dis 45:241, 1967.
9. BATES, GW, AND WHITWORTH, NS: *Effects of body weight on female reproductive function.* In GIVENS, JR (ED): *The Hypothalamus.* Year Book Medical Publishers, Chicago, IL, 1984, pp 97–115.
10. BAUER, HG: *Endocrine and other clinical manifestations of hypothalamic disease: A survey of 60 cases, with autopsies.* J Clin Endocrinol Metab 14:13–31, 1954.
11. BILLIARD, M, GUILLEMINAULT, C, DEMENT, WC: *A menstruation-linked periodic hypersomnia. Kleine-Levin syndrome or new clinical entity?* Neurology 25:436, 1975.

12. BLAVET, N, DeFEUDIS, FV, CLOSTRE, F: *Lack of effect of the peptide pvro-Glu-His-Gly-OH on food consumption in mice and rats.* Gen Pharmacol 13:173–176, 1982.
13. BLESSING, WW, SVED, AF, REIS, DJ: *Destruction of noradrenergic neurons in rabbit brainstem elevates plasma vasopressin, causing hypertension.* Science 217:661–663, 1982.
14. BLIGH, J: *Neuronal models of hypothalamic temperature regulation.* In LEDERIS, K, AND COOPER, KE (EDS): *Recent Studies of Hypothalamic Function,* S Karger, Basel, 1973, pp 315–330.
15. BLUM, B, ISREALI, J, DUJOVYN, M, ET AL: *Angina-like cardiac disturbances of hypothalamic etiology in cat, monkey, and man.* Isr J Med Sci 18:127–139, 1982.
16. BRAY, GA, AND GALLAGHER, TF, JR: *Manifestations of hypothalamic obesity in man: A comprehensive investigation of eight patients and a review of the literature.* Medicine 54:301–333, 1975.
17. BRAY, GA, AND YORK, DA: *Hypothalamic and genetic obesity in experimental animals: An autonomic and endocrine hypothesis.* Physiol Rev 59:719–809, 1979.
18. BROWN, DR, AND HOLTZMAN, SG: *Suppression of deprivation-induced food and water intake in rats and mice by naloxone.* Pharmacol Biochem Behav 11:567–573, 1979.
19. BROWN, MR: *Thermoregulation.* In KRIEGER, DT, BROWNSTEIN, MJ, AND MARTIN, JB (EDS): *Brain Peptides.* John Wiley & Sons, New York, 1983, pp 301–314.
20. BROWN, M, AND TACHE, Y: *Hypothalamic peptides: Central nervous system control of visceral functions.* Fed Proc 40:2565–2569, 1981.
21. BURR, IM, SLONIM, AE, DANISH, RK, ET AL: *Diencephalic syndrome revisited.* J Pediatr 88:429–436, 1976.
22. CAIRNS, H, OLDFIELD, RC, PENNYBACKER, JB, WHATTERIDGE, D: *Akinetic mutism with an epidermoid cyst of the third ventricle (with a report on the associated disturbance of brain potentials).* Brain 64:273–290, 1941.
23. CAIRNS, H: *Disturbances of consciousness with lesions of brain-stem and diencephalon.* Victor Horsley Memorial Lecture. Brain 75:109–139, 1952.
24. CAROFF, S, ROSENBERG, H, GERBER, JC: *Neuroleptic malignant syndrome and malignant hyperthermia.* Lancet 1:244–249, 1983.
25. CHI, CC, AND FLYNN, JP: *Neural pathways associated with hypothalamically elicited attack behavior in cats.* Science 171:703–706, 1971.
26. CLARK, WG: *Influence of opioids on central thermoregulatory mechanisms.* Pharm Biochem Behav 10:609–613, 1979.
27. CRAVIOTO, H, SILBERMAN, J, FEIGIN, I: *A clinical and pathologic study of akinetic mutism.* Neurology 10:10–21, 1960.
28. CRITCHLEY, M: *Periodic hypersomnia and megaphagia in adolescent males.* Brain 85:627–656, 1962.
29. DANIEL, PM, AND TREIP, CS: *The pathology of the hypothalamus.* Clin Endocrinol Metab 6:3–19, 1977.
30. DAVISON, C, AND DEMUTH, EL: *Disturbances in sleep mechanism: Clinicopathological study: lesions at diencephalic level (hypothalamus).* Arch Neurol Psychiat 55:111, 1946.
31. DELLA-FERA, MA, BAILE, CA, SCHNEIDER, BS: *Cholecystokinin antibody injected in cerebral ventricles stimulates feeding in sheep.* Science 212:687–689, 1981.
32. DINARELLO, CA: *An update on human interleukin-1 from molecular biology to clinical relevance.* J Clin Immunol 5:287–297, 1985.
33. DINARELLO, CA, AND WOLFF, SM: *Molecular basis of fever in humans.* Am J Med 72:799, 1982.
34. DIZ, DI, AND JACOBOWITZ, DM: *Cardiovascular effects produced by injections of thyrotropin-releasing hormone in specified preoptic and hypothalamic nuclei in the rat.* Peptides 5:801–808, 1984.
35. DOBA, N, AND REIS, DJ: *Acute fulminating neurogenic hypertension produced by brainstem lesions in rat.* Circ Res 32:584–593, 1973.
36. DROP, SL, GUYDA, HJ, COLLE, E. *Inappropriate growth hormone release in the diencephalic syndrome of childhood: Case report and 4 year endocrinological follow-up.* Clin Endocrinol (Oxf) 13:181–187, 1980.
37. DUFFY, JP, AND DAVISON, K: *A female case of the Kleine-Levin syndrome.* Br J Psychiat 114:77–82, 1968.
38. EVANS, DE, AND GILLIA, RA: *Reflux mechanisms involved in cardiac arrhythmias induced by hypothalamic stimulation.* Am J Physiol 234:199–209, 1978.
39. FELDBERG, W, AND MYERS, RD: *Effects on temperature of amines injected into the cerebral ventricles. A new concept of temperature regulation.* J Physiol (London) 173:226–245, 1964.
40. FOX, RH, WILKINS, DC, BELL, JA, ET AL: *Spontaneous periodic hypothermia: Diencephalic epilepsy.* Br Med J 2:693–695, 1973.
41. FROHLICH, A: *Ein Fall von Tumor dert Hypophysis Cerebri ohne Akromegalie.* Wien Klin Runcsch 15:883–886, 1901.
42. FROHMAN, LA: *Glucoregulation.* In KRIEGER, DT, BROWNSTEIN, MJ, MARTIN, JB. (EDS): *Brain Peptides.* John Wiley & Sons, New York, 1983, pp 281–300.

43. FULTON, JF, AND BAILEY, P: *Tumors in the region of the third ventricle: Their diagnosis and relation to pathological sleep.* J Nerv Ment Dis 69:1–32, 1929.
44. GALE, CC: *Neuroendocrine aspects of thermoregulation.* Ann Rev Physiol 35:391–432, 1973.
45. GIBBS, J, AND SMITH, GP: *The neuroendocrinology of postprandial satiety.* In MARTINI, L, AND GANONG, WF (EDS): *Frontiers in Neuroendocrinology,* vol 8. Oxford University Press, London, 1984, pp 223–246.
46. GILLIGAN, BS: *Periodic megaphagia and hypersomnia—an example of the Kleine-Levin syndrome in an adolescent girl.* Proc Aust Assoc Neurol 9:67–72, 1973.
47. GIRVIN, JP: *Clinical correlates of hypothalamic and limbic system function.* In MOGENSON, GJ, AND CALARESU, FR (EDS): *Neural Integration of Physiological Mechanisms and Behavior.* University of Toronto Press, Toronto, 1975, pp 412–422.
48. GOLDSTEIN, M: *Brain research and violent behavior (a summary and evaluation of the status of biomedical research on brain and aggressive violent behavior).* Arch Neurol 30:1–21, 1974.
49. GOWERS, WR: *Epilepsy and Other Chronic Convulsive Diseases: Their Causes, Symptoms and Treatment.* Dover Publications, New York, 1885.
50. GRAFF-RADFORD, NR, ESLINGER, PJ, DAMASIO, AR, ET AL:*Nonhemorrhagic infarction of the thalamus: Behavioral, anatomic, and physiologic correlates.* Neurology 34:14–23, 1984.
51. GRANDISON, AND GUIDOTT, A: Neuropharmacology, 161:553–536, 1977.
52. GREEN, S, AND PAU, RH: *Treatment of compulsive eating disturbances with anticonvulsant medication.* Am J Psychiatry 131:428–437, 1974.
53. GROSSMAN, SP: *Direct adrenergic and cholinergic stimulation of hypothalamic mechanisms.* Am J Physiol 202:872–883, 1962.
54. GUIHARD, J, ET AL: *Hypothermie spontanee recidivante avec agenesie du corps calleux. Syndrome de shapiro nouvelle observation.* Ann Pediatr 18:645–649, 1971.
55. HAMILTON, CR, SCULLY, RE, KLIMAN, B: *Hypogonadotropinism in Prader-Willi syndrome. Induction of puberty and spermatogenesis by clomiphene citrate.* Am J Med 52:322–325, 1972.
56. HARDY, JD: *Control of body temperature.* In MOGENSON, GJ, AND CALARESU, FR (EDS): *Neural Integration of Physiological Mechanisms and Behavior.* University of Toronto Press, Toronto 1975, pp 294–321.
57. HENSEL, H: *Neural processes in thermoregulation.* Physiol Rev 53:948–982, 1973.
58. HERSCH, C: *Electrocardiographic changes in subarachnoid haemorrhage, meningitis, and intracranial space-occupying lesions.* Br Heart J 26:785–793, 1964.
59. HESS, WR: *The functional organization of the diencephalon.* In HUGHES, JR (ED): p 275, Grune & Stratton, New York, 1957.
60. HETHERINGTON, AW, RANSON, JW: *Hypothalamic lesions and adiposity in the rat.* Anat Rec 78:149–161, 1940.
61. HILTON, SM: *The role of the hypothalamus in the organization of patterns of cardiovascular response.* In LEDERIS, K, AND COOPER, KE (EDS): *Recent Studies of Hypothalamic Function.* S Karger, Basel, 1973, pp 306–322.
62. HUANG, YH, AND MOGENSON, GJ: *Neural pathways mediating drinking and feeding in rats.* Exp Neurol 37:306–318, 1972.
63. ISENSCHMID, R, AND KREHL, L: *Uber den Einfluss des Gehirms auf die Warmerregulation.* Arch Exp Path Pharmakol 70:109–115, 1912.
64. ISHIZUKA, B, QUIGLEY, ME, YEN, SSC: *Pituitary hormone release in response to food ingestion: Evidence for neuroendocrine signals from gut to brain.* J Clin Endocrin Metab 57(6):1111–1116, 1983.
65. JOHNSON, RH, AND PARK, DM: *Intermittent hypothermia.* J Neurol Neurosurg Psych 36:411, 1973.
66. JOHNSON, RH, AND SPALDING, JM: *Disorders of the Autonomic Nervous System.* FA Davis, Philadelphia, 1975.
67. JONES, JF, AND RICHTER, JA: Life Sci 28:2055–2064, 1981.
68. KASTIN, NW, AND MARTIN, JB: *Push-pull perfusion technique in the median eminence: A model system for evaluating releasing factor dynamics.* Methods Enzymol 103:176–187, 1983.
69. KENNEDY, GC: *Some aspects of the relation between appetite and endocrine development in the growing animal.* In MOGENSON, GH, AND CALARESU, FR (EDS): *Neural Integration of Physiological Mechanisms and Behavior.* University of Toronto Press, Toronto, 1975, pp 326–341.
70. KENNEDY, GC: *The regulation of food intake.* Discussion Adv Psychosom Med 7:91–92, 1972.
71. KLUVER, H, AND BUCY, PC: *Preliminary analysis of functions of temporal lobes in monkeys.* Arch Neurol Psychiat 42:979–991, 1939.
72. KASTING, NW, VEALE, WL, COOPER, KE, LEDERIS, K: *Effect of hemorrhage on fever: The putative role of vasopressin.* Can J Physiol Pharmacol 59:324–328, 1981.
73. LEWIN, K, MATTINGLY, D, MILLS, RR: *Anorexia nervosa associated with hypothalamic tumour.* Br Med J 2:629–636, 1972.
74. LEWITT, PA, NEWMAN, RP, GREENBERG, HS, ET AL: *Episodic hyperhidrosis, hypothermia and agenesis of corpus callosum.* Neurology 33:1122–1129, 1983.
75. LILLY, R, CUMMINGS, JL, BENSON, F, FRANKEL, M: *The Human Klüver-Bucy Syndrome.* Neurology 33:1141–5, 1983.

76. MARGULES, DL, MOISSET, B, LEWIS, MJ, SHIBUYA, H, PERT, CB: *Beta-endorphin is associated with overeating in genetically obese mice (ob/ob) and rats (fa/fa)*. Science 202:988–991, 1978.

77. MARTIN, JB, AND REICHLIN, S: *Neural regulation of the pituitary-thyroid axis*. In KENNY, AD, AND ANDERSON, RR (EDS): *Proceedings of the Sixth Midwest Thyroid Conference*. University of Missouri Press, Columbia, MO 1970, pp 1–36.

78. MAYER, J: *Some aspects of the problem of regulation of food intake and obesity*. N Engl J Med, 274:610–615, 1966.

79. McHUGH, PR: *The control of gastric emptying*. J Autonom Nerv Syst, 9:221–231, 1983.

80. McKAY, LD, KENNEY, NJ, EDENS, NK, WILLIAMS, RH, WOODS, SC: Life Sci 29:1429–1434, 1981.

81. MOGENSON, GJ: *Changing views of the role of the hypothalamus in the control of ingestive behaviors*. In LEDERIS, K, AND COOPER, KE (EDS): *Recent Studies of Hypothalamic Function*. S Karger, Basel, 1974, pp 268–284.

82. MORGANE, PJ: *Anatomical and neurobiochemical bases of the central nervous control of physiological regulations and behaviour*. In MOGENSON, GJ, AND CALARESU, FR (EDS): *Neural Integration of Physiological Mechanisms and Behavior*. University of Toronto Press, Toronto, 1975, pp 24–45.

83. MORGANE, PJ: *The function of the limbic and rhinic forebrain-limbic midbrain systems and reticular formation in the regulation of food and water intake*. Ann NY Acad Sci 157:806, 1969.

84. MORLEY, JE, AND LEVINE, AS: *Stress-induced eating is mediated through endogenous opiates*. Science 209:1259–1261, 1980.

85. MORLEY, JE, AND LEVINE, AS: *Dynorphin (1–13) induces spontaneous feeding in rats*. Life Sci 29:1901–1903, 1981.

86. MORRISON, SD, AND MAYER, J: *Adipsia and aphagia in rats after lateral subthalamic lesions*. Am J Physiol 191:248–269, 1957.

87. MYERS, RD: *Ionic concepts of the setpoint for body temperature*. In LEDERIS, K, AND COOPER, KE (EDS): *Recent Studies of Hypothalamic Function*. S Karger, Basel, 1973, pp 371–382.

88. NIELSEN, JM, AND JACOBS, LL: *Bilateral lesions of the anterior cingulate gyri*. Bull Los Angeles Neurol Soc 16:231–235, 1951.

89. NELSON, TE, AND FLEWELLEN, EH: *The malignant hyperthermia syndrome*. N Engl J Med 309:416–421, 1983.

90. NANCE, DM, COY, DH, KASTON, AJ: *Experiments with a reported anorexigenic tripeptide: Pyro-Glu-His-Gly-OH*. Pharmacol, Biochem Behav 11:733–735, 1979.

91. NOEL, P, HUBERT, JP, ECTORS, M, ET AL: *Agenesis of the corpus callosum associated with relapsing hypothermia: A clinicopathological report*. Brain 96:359–368, 1973.

92. OWIN, OE, REICHARD, GA, JR, BODEN, G: *Comparative measurements of glucose beta-hydroxy-butyrate, acetoacetate, and insulin in blood and cerebrospinal fluid during starvation*. Metabolism 23:7–14, 1974.

93. OOMURA, Y: *Contribution of electrophysiological techniques to the understanding of central control systems*. In MOGENSON, GJ, AND CALARESU, FR (EDS): *Neural Integration of Physiological Mechanisms and Behavior*. University of Toronto Press, Toronto, 1975, p 375.

94. PANSKEPP, J: *On the nature of feeding patterns—primarily in rats*. In NOVIN, D, WYRWICKA, W, BORAY, GA (EDS): *Hunger: Basic Mechanisms and Clinical Implications*, Raven Press, New York, 1976, pp 369–382.

95. PENFIELD, W: *Diencephalic autonomic epilepsy*. Arch Neurol Psychiat 22:358–369, 1929.

96. PLUM, F, AND POSNER, J: *The Diagnosis of Stupor and Coma*, ed 3. FA Davis, Philadelphia, 1980.

97. PLUM, F, AND VAN UITERT, R: *Nonendocrine diseases and disorders of the hypothalamus*. In REICHLIN, S, AND BALDESSARINI, RJ (EDS): *The Hypothalamus*, vol 56: Raven Press, New York, 1978, pp 415–473.

98. RABIN, BM: *Ventromedial hypothalamic control of food intake and satiety: A reappraisal*. Brain Res 43:317–336, 1972.

99. RANSON, SW: *Somnolence caused by hypothalamic lesions in the monkey*. Arch Neurol Psychiat 41:1–29, 1939.

100. REEVES, AG AND PLUM, F: *Hyperphagia, rage and dementia accompanying a ventromedial hypothalamic neoplasm*. Arch Neurol 20:616–624, 1969.

101. REICHELT, KL, FOSS, I, TRYGSTAD, O, EDMINSON, PD, JOHANSEN, JH, BOLER, JB: *Humoral control of appetite-II, purification and characterization of an anorexogenic peptide from human urine*. Neuroscience 3:1207–1211, 1978.

102. ROTHBALLER, AB: *Some endocrine manifestations of central nervous system disease. An approach to clinical neuroendocrinology*. Bull NY Acad Med 42:257–269, 1966.

103. RUSSEK, M: *Current hypotheses in the control of feeding behavior*. In MOGENSON, GH, AND CALARESU, FR (Eds): *Neural Integration of Physiological Mechanisms and Behavior*. University of Toronto Press, Toronto, 1975, pp 128–141.

104. SANGER, DJ, AND McCARTHY, PS: *Increased food and water intake produced in rats by opiate receptor agonists*. Psychopharmacology 74:217–220, 1981.

MANIFESTATIONS OF HYPOTHALAMIC DISEASE

105. SCHNEIDER, BS, FRIEDMAN, JM, HIRSCH, J: *Feeding behavior.* In KRIEGER, DT, BROWNSTEIN, MJ, MARTIN, JB (EDS): *Brain Peptides.* John Wiley & Sons, New York, 1983, pp 251–268.

106. SHAPIRO, WR, EILLIAMS, GH, PLUM, F: *Spontaneous recurrent hypothermia accompanying agenesis of the corpus callosum.* Brain 92:423–436, 1969.

107. SKULTETY, FM: *Clinical and experimental aspects of akinetic mutism. Report of a case.* Arch Neurol 19:1–5, 1968.

108. SMITH, GP, AND GIBBS, J:*Cholecystokin and satiety: Theoretic and therapeutic implications.* In NORVIN, D, WYRWICKA, W, BORAY, GA (EDS): *Hunger: Basic Mechanisms and Clinical Implications.* Raven Press, New York, 1976, pp 349–361.

109. SMITH, GP, JEROME, C, CUSHIN, B, ET AL: Science 213:1036–1037, 1981.

110. SMITH, GT, MORAN,TH, COYLE, JT, KUHAR, MJ, O'DONAHUE, TL, MCHUGH, PR: *Anatomic localization of cholecystokinine receptors to the pyloric sphincter.* Am J Physiol 246:R127–R130, 1984.

111. SMITH, OA, AND DEVITO, JL: *Central neural integration for the control of autonomic responses associated with emotion.* Ann Rev of Neurosci 7:43–66, 1984.

112. SMITH, OA, STEPHENSON, RB, RANDALL, DC: *Range of control of cardiovascular variables by the hypothalamus.* In LEDERIS, K, AND COOPER, KE (EDS): *Recent Studies of Hypothalamic Function,* S Karger, Basel, 1973, pp 294–310.

113. SOLOMON, GE: *Diencephalic autonomic epilepsy caused by a neoplasm.* J Pediatr 83:277–282, 1973.

114. SPRAGUE, JM: *Chronic brainstem lesions.* In *Sleep and altered states of consciousness.* Res Pub Assoc Res Nerv Ment Dis 45:157–201, 1965.

115. SWETT, CP, AND HOBSON, JA: *The effects of posterior hypothalamic lesions on behavioral and electrographic manifestations of sleep and waking in cats.* Arch Ital Biol 106:283–296, 1968.

116. TALMAN, WT: *Cardiovascular regulation and lesions of the central nervous system.* Ann Neurol 18:1–12, 1985.

117. TRYGSTAD, O, FOSS, I, EDMINSON, PD, JOHANSEN, JH , REICHELT, KL: Acta Endocrinol 89:196–208, 1978.

118. VAN HOUTEN, M, AND POSNER, BI: *Insulin binds to brain blood vessels in vivo.* Nature 282:623–625, 1979.

119. VAN HOUTEN, M, POSNER, BI, KOPRIWA, BM, BRAWER, JR: *Insulin-binding sites in the rat brain: In vivo localization to the circumventricular organs by quantitative radioautography.* Endocrinology 105:666–673, 1979.

120. VEALE, WL, AND COOPER, KE: *Evidence for the involvement of prostaglandins in fever.* In LEDERIS, K, AND COOPER, KE (EDS): *Recent Studies in Hypothalamic Function.* S Karger, Basel, 1973, pp 359–368.

121. VICTOR, M, ADAMS, RD, COLLINS, GH: *Wernicke-Korsakoff Syndrome.* FA Davis, Philadelphia, 1971.

122. VIJAYAN, E, AND MCCANN, SM: *Suppression of feeding and drinking activity in rats following intraventricular infection of thyrotropin releasing hormone (TRH).* Endocrinology 100:1727–1730, 1977.

123. WHITE, LE, AND HAIN, RF: *Anorexia in association with a destructive lesion of the hypothalamus.* Arch Pathol 68:275–279, 1959.

124. WOLFF, SM, ADLER, RC, ET AL: *A syndrome of periodic hypothalamic discharge.* Am J Med, 36:956–967, 1964.

125. WOODS, SC, AND PORTE, D, JR: *Regulation of food intake and body weight in insulin.* Diabetologia, 20:274–280, 1981.

126. WYLLIE, E, LUDERS, H, MACMILLAN, JP, ET AL: *Serum prolactin levels after epileptic seizures.* Neurology 34:1601–1604, 1984.

127. ZELLWEGER, H, AND SCHNEIDER, HJ: *Syndrome of hypotonia-hypomentia-hypogonadism-obesity (HHHO) or Prader-Willi syndrome.* Am J Dis Child 115:588–592, 1968.

128. SILVA, JE: *Brown adipose tissue: An extrathyroidal source of triiodothyronine.* News Physiol Sci 1:119–122, 1986.

129. MASCHERPA, G, COGLIATI, F, MAURI, R, RESENTINI, M: *The probable anorexigenic effect of naloxone in the Prader-Labhart-Willi syndrome (letter).* Minerva Pediatr 34:675, 1982.

130. REICHLIN, S: *Actual and potential diagnostic and therapeutic uses of hypophysiotropic hormones in pituitary and neurological diseases: An overview.* In MÜLLER, EE, MACLEOD, RM (EDS): *Neuroendocrine Perspectives* vol 5. Elsevier, Amsterdam, 1986, pp 121–136.

131. ERDHEIM, J: *Veber Hypophysengangsgeschwülste und hirn Cholesteatome.* Sitzungsb. D.K. Akad. d. Wissensch. Math.-Natur W. Cl., Wien 113:537–726, 1904.

132. MORDES, JP, LONGCOPE, C, FLATT, JP, ET AL: *The rat LTW(m) Leydig cell tumor: Cancer anorexia due to estrogen.* Endocrinology 115:167–173, 1984.

133. BEUTLER, B, AND CERAMI, A: *Cachectin and tumor necrosis factor as two sides of the same biological coin.* Nature 320:584–588, 1986.

134. BEUTLER, B: Nature 316:552–554, 1985.

135. PENNICA, D: Nature 312:724–729, 1984.

136. Dinarello, CA, Cannon, JG, Mier, JW, Bernheim, HA, LoPrester, G, Lynn, DL, Love, RN, Webb, AC, Auron, DE, Reuben, RC, et al: *Multiple biological activities of human recombinant interleukin 1.* J Clin Invest 77:1734–1739, 1986.

137. Perlmutter, DH, Goldberger, G, Dinavello, CA, Mizel, SB, Colten, HR: *Regulation of class III major histocompatability complex gene products by interleukin-1.* Science 232:850–852, 1986.

138. Auron, PE, Webb, AC, Rosenwasser, LJ, Mucci, SF, Rich, A, Wolff, SM, Dinarello, CA: *Nucleotide sequence of human monocyte interleukin 1 precursor cDNA.* Proc Natl Acad Sci USA 81:7907–7911, 1984.

139. Hood, OJ, Rouse, BM, Lockhart, LH, Bodensteiner, JB: *Proximal duplications of chromosome 15: Clinical dilemmas.* Clin Genet 29:234–240, 1986.

140. Witkowski, R, Ullrich, E, Pietsch, P, et al: *Infant hypotonia, obesity, hypogenitalism and oligophrenia—new viewpoints on the etiology and symptoms of Prader-Willi syndrome.* Psychiatr Neurol Med Psychol (Leipz) 37:255–261, 1985.

141. Pauli, RM, Meisner, LF, Szmanda, RJ: *"Expanded" Prader-Willi syndrome in a boy with an unusual 15q chromosome deletion.* Am J Dis Child 137:1087–1089, 1983.

142. Wisniewski, L, Hassold, T, Heffelfinger, J, Higgins, JV: *Cytogenetic and clinical studies in five cases of inv dup(15).* Hum Genet 50:259–270, 1979.

143. Bray, GA, Dahms, WT, Swerdloff, RS, et al: *The Prader-Willi syndrome: A study of 40 patients and a review of the literature.* Medicine 62:59–80, 1983.

Chapter 12

PITUITARY ADENOMAS: PATHOLOGY AND PATHOGENESIS

Pituitary adenomas are common benign tumors that arise in the pars distalis and occasionally in the pars intermedia. This chapter considers their pathology, pathogenesis, and management.

CELL TYPES IN THE NORMAL PITUITARY GLAND

Pathologic changes in pituitary adenoma correlate with the types and distribution of cells in the normal pituitary gland. The relative proportion of cell types and their morphology are modified by endocrine status, such as target gland disease and pregnancy. At least five types are distinguishable by immunohistochemical staining of their secretions:[40-49,88] somatotropes (GH), lactotropes (PRL), corticotropes (ACTH, POMC), thyrotropes (TSH), and gonadotropes (LH, FSH). At least one group of cells has no detectable secretions, but some of these have been shown by *in situ* hybridization to express specific hormonal mRNA. Somatotropes (50 percent) are located principally in the lateral portions of the gland. Lactotropes (10 to 25 percent) occur randomly and uniformly throughout the pars distalis. Corticotropes (10 to 20 percent) are found chiefly in the central portion (median wedge) and within the rudimentary pars intermedia as lining cells of the cystic cavities. Thyrotropes (less than 10 percent) are located mainly in the anteriormedial portion. Gonadotropes (10 percent) are randomly distributed in the gland, intermingled with other cells. There appear to be at least three populations of gonadotropes: those that secrete only LH, those that secrete only FSH, and those that secrete both. Although immunohistochemical staining suggests that the majority of cells secrete only one gonadotropin, mRNA hybridization suggests that most gonadotropes contain both LH and FSH.

PATHOGENESIS OF PITUITARY ADENOMAS

Pituitary microadenomas (usually 1 to 3 mm in diameter) are found in 8 to 27 percent of routine autopsies in which serial sections of the adenohypophysis are performed,[9,14,62] but they emerge as clinical problems far less frequently. The different percentages reported may reflect different criteria used by pathologists, some of whom refer to focal hyperplasia as an adenoma.[68] Even true adenomas lack a defined capsule. The factors that deter-

cally as enhancement of GH release to various stimuli and increasing pituitary responses to releasing factors.

TUMORS ARISING FROM LOSS OF NEGATIVE-FEEDBACK CONTROL

In rodents, pituitary TSH-secreting tumors can develop after thyroidectomy. Such tumors initially can be transplanted only into thyroidectomized rats (thyroxine-deficiency dependent), but after serial passage the tumors gain variable degrees of autonomy and increased resistance to feedback inhibition by thyroxine.[23,67] Although enlargement of the pituitary gland occurs quite commonly in chronic hypothyroidism in the human, tumors rarely develop[72] (see chapter 5). Even more rare are gonadotropin-secreting tumors arising after gonad deficiency.

Pituitary adrenotrope adenomas in patients with Cushing's disease may grow aggressively after adrenalectomy (Nelson's syndrome), presumably due to loss of feedback inhibition, but in these cases an adenoma had already been present.

Although target gland deficiency can cause pituitary adenomas in rodents, similar mechanisms do not seem important in the great majority of human adenomas. The defect causing most PRL, GH and ACTH secreting tumors appears to be intrinsic to the pituitary or secondary to altered hypothalamic control.

ROLE OF THE HYPOTHALAMUS IN PATHOGENESIS OF PITUITARY ADENOMAS

The discovery of the hypothalamic regulatory factors and recognition that virtually all anterior pituitary functions depend on the hypothalamus has led to the hypothesis that hypothalamic hyperfunction could give rise to adenomas.[50,51] Conclusive evidence supporting this view has not been obtained to date, however.

The main approaches to this problem have been (1) to identify abnormalities of hypothalamic-pituitary regulation in patients with adenoma, (2) to compare the extent to which pituitary secretory responses in adenoma cases resemble normal physiologic responses before and after tumor removal, and (3) to attempt to identify the presence of abnormal amounts of hypophysiotropic hormones in body fluids of patients with pituitary hypersecretion.

GH-Secreting Adenomas

Residual Normal Regulation. Many patients with acromegaly retain some residual of normal physiologic responsivity.[15,16] For example, some show spontaneous surges in plasma GH level, partial suppression with glucose loading, and responses to hypoglycemia and arginine infusion.[67]

Regulatory Abnormalities. In acromegaly, GH control mechanisms are qualitatively and quantitatively abnormal.[68] Approximately 60 percent of patients show "paradoxical" responses to glucose loading (that is, an in-

426   HYPOTHALAMIC-PITUITARY DISEASE

crease, instead of a decrease, in blood GH levels). Although spontaneous fluctuations in GH levels are common, sleep does not induce GH release as it does in normal persons. In contrast to normal individuals, in whom GH levels increase following the administration of dopamine agonists like L-dopa or bromocriptine, acromegalic persons almost without exception show a decrease in GH levels following such treatment.[7,31,58] In some cases, the response to bromocriptine is sufficiently great to be useful therapeutically.[7,10] Because the inhibitory effect of L-dopa on GH secretion is blocked by carbidopa, an inhibitor of peripheral conversion of L-dopa to dopamine, the tumor-cell membranes can be assumed to have dopamine receptors that are inhibitory to GH secretion. It is postulated that under normal conditions, dopamine acts on the hypothalamus to stimulate release of growth hormone releasing hormone (GHRH) and that this effect predominates, so that direct inhibitory effects of dopamine are not manifested. The majority of patients with acromegaly also show an increase in plasma GH following the injection of TRH, a response that does not occur in normal individuals.[61,81] This paradoxical effect has been attributed to the appearance of TRH receptors on the abnormal adenoma. However, the appearance of paradoxical responses to glucose administration, TRH, and dopamine can no longer be taken as evidence of intrinsic pituitary abnormality because of recent studies in patients with acromegaly owing to ectopic GHRH secretion. In three of five such patients, similar paradoxical responses of GH to these stimuli occurred,[81] and when studied, these reverted to normal following removal of the source of ectopic GHRH. Hence it appears that GHRH can induce these abnormalities in normal pituitary glands.

Few cases of acromegaly have been studied in detail prior to and after apparent complete removal of a microadenoma. One case, reported by Hoyte and Martin,[37] showed return of normal responsiveness and loss of the paradoxical GH response to TRH and L-dopa. These findings indicate that hypothalamic abnormalities had not preceded the tumor. The extent to which this finding is typical of the disease is not known.

Efforts to identify excess secretion of GHRH or decreased secretion of somatostatin in acromegaly have been made. From a theoretic point of view, excessive amounts of hypothalamic GHRH could bring about pituitary GH hypersecretion by a mechanism similar to that occurring with ectopic GHRH secreting tumors. To date, more than 15 such cases have been reported, including instances of remission of the GH hypersecretion after removal of the tumor.[21,22,63,78] In the cases of ectopic GHRH secretion in which pituitary pathology has been examined, some show hyperplasia (as was the case in Thorner's patient whose pancreatic tumor yielded GHRH) and others adenomas. Thus the possibility exists that prolonged stimulation of somatotropes by endogenous GHRH, whether of tumor or hypothalamic origin, may induce adenoma formation. Six cases are reported by Asa and associates[2] of hypothalamic gangliocytomas that caused acromegaly. Immunocytochemical studies revealed that the tumors contained GHRH, presumably the cause of the GH overstimulation (Fig. 1).

Proof that GHRH is secreted in excess in acromegaly of the usual variety has been claimed by Hagen and colleagues,[30] who reported that GH release from monkey pituitary gland *in vitro* was stimulated following

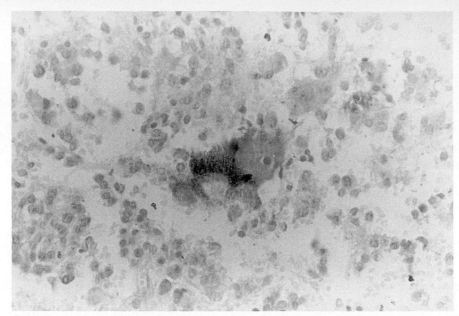

FIGURE 1. Intrasellar gangliocytoma associated with pituitary somatotropic adenoma and acromegaly. A large neuron contains immunoreactive hpGRF-40; small round cells of the adenoma are negative. Avidin-biotin-peroxidase complex technique with hematoxylin counterstain (× 128). (Courtesy Dr. K. Kovacs, St. Michael's Hospital, Toronto.)

exposure to acromegalic plasma. Recent studies in which measurement of circulating GHRH by radioimmunoassay has been accomplished show that less than 1 percent of acromegalies have increased levels of the stimulating peptide in the peripheral blood; but the critical studies, not as yet available, would be the measurement of GHRH levels in hypophysial-portal blood.

As to the possibility that acromegaly is due to somatostatin deficiency, measurements of cerebrospinal fluid (CSF) in acromegalics show normal levels, but CSF concentration cannot be taken as a reflection of hypothalamic somatostatin secretion rate.[64] Somatostatin deficiency has not been excluded as a cause in some cases of acromegaly.

The critical problem in all studies of the role of the hypothalamus in the pathogenesis of acromegaly (as is true for the other pituitary hypersecretory disorders) is that definitive proof will require unambiguous methods for measurement of hypothalamic hormone secretion rate, preferably to include direct measurement of hypophysial-portal blood concentrations.

The findings that some cases of acromegaly persist despite removal of all gland in contact with the base of the hypothalamus suggest a high degree of autonomy for the GH secreting adenoma. In brief, a definitive answer cannot be given as to the role of hypothalamic hypersecretion in the pathogenesis of acromegaly. Furthermore, there may be considerable heterogeneity in this disorder, a few cases being due to well-localized adenomas (entirely due to intrinsic pituitary disease), and a smaller number may have mainly diffuse hyperplasia. It is this group that conceivably could be of hypothalamic origin. The various etiologies of hypersomatotropism are listed in Table 2.

HYPOTHALAMIC-PITUITARY DISEASE

TABLE 2. Etiology of Hypersomatotropism

I. Pituitary
  1. Densely granulated GH cell adenoma
  2. Sparsely granulated GH cell adenoma
  3. Mixed GH cell and PRL cell adenoma
  4. Acidophil stem cell adenoma
  5. Mammosomatotroph cell adenoma
  6. Plurihormonal adenoma (unclassified)
  7. GH cell carcinoma
  8. GH cell hyperplasia
II. Extrapituitary
  1. Eutopic GH cell adenoma
    a. Sphenoid sinus
    b. Parapharyngeal
  2. Ectopic GH-producing tumors
    a. Lung; ovary; breast
  3. Excess GH-releasing factor secretion
    a. Eutopic
      (1) Hypothalamic hamartoma or choristoma
    b. Ectopic
      (1) Pancreatic islet cell tumors
      (2) Bronchial and intestinal carcinoid tumors

ACTH-secreting Adenomas

Excessive secretion of glucocorticoids is most commonly secondary to ACTH hypersecretion, accounting for approximately 70 percent or more of cases of spontaneous Cushing's syndrome (chapter 6). This group, characterized by bilateral hyperplasia of the adrenal cortex and an inappropriate elevation of ACTH (Cushing's disease), has been shown in various series to be accompanied by either radiologic or histologic evidence of adenoma of the pituitary gland in between 40 and 64 percent[8,66] (see chapter 6). Recent series that have utilized arteriography and recent generation of computerized axial tomography (CAT) scan techniques indicate an incidence of abnormality of 82 percent in Cushing's disease.[71] Exploration of the pituitary gland even in the absence of radiologic abnormalities revealed in the series of Tyrrell and others[82] 15 microadenomas in 20 patients, and in these and one other, removal of "suspicious" tissue resulted in a cure. In Hardy's series,[33] all of 10 patients with Cushing's disease were cured by microadenonectomy. Thus, the majority of cases of this disorder appear to be due to ACTH-secreting adenomas;[70] a few may be due to rather more diffuse hyperplasia of the adrenotrope cell or to minute tumors. Besser and colleagues have proposed that an unsuspectedly high proportion of patients with Cushing's disease have occult ACTH secreting tumors. Following adrenalectomy, previously unrecognized tumors may become evident, and established tumors may become even larger (Nelson's syndrome). It is considered likely that such patients have had adenomas all along, but that onset of tumor growth is due to loss of normal feedback inhibition. Transient resistance to the feedback action of cortisol also has been observed in patients with primary Addison's disease.[12]

    In attempts to determine whether the central nervous system (CNS) may be involved in the pathogenesis of Cushing's disease, many studies have been carried out on the response of such patients to physiologic stimuli; these have become the basis of sophisticated and specific tests of the pituitary-adrenal axis, but of themselves they have not as yet established whether the disease is due to excessive secretion of a hypothalamic factor or whether the retention of some normal responses is due to residual CNS functions of the adenomatous tissue.[6]

One hallmark of Cushing's disease is that the setpoint for feedback control of secretion of ACTH is established at a higher level. Much recent work reviewed by Jones[38] indicates that feedback effects of cortisol may be directed at the pituitary gland as well at the level of the hypothalamus or other CNS structures. Higher setpoint, therefore, cannot be taken as evidence for or against a pituitary abnormality as compared with brain hypersecretion of corticotropin-releasing hormone (CRH).

More specific evidence of an intrinsic defect in the pituitary gland in Cushing's disease is the demonstration that some patients with this disorder show ACTH discharge following the administration of TRH, a response never seen in normal persons;[53] in a few, the administration of dopamine agonists such as bromocriptine suppresses ACTH secretion, again a response not seen in the normal person.[56] The latter observations (as in the analogous case of GH-secreting adenomas) are interpreted to indicate that the tumor cells express TRH and dopamine receptors either through unmasking or other enhancement of receptors that have been there all along or through dedifferentiation. A direct effect of bromocriptine in experimental ACTH-secreting tumors *in vitro* has been demonstrated by MacLeod and Krieger.[60]

Cushing's disease patients characteristically lose normal circadian rhythms early in the disease, which could be attributed to either pituitary or central nervous system abnormality. The finding that normal GH circadian rhythms also are lost in Cushing's disease and that this defect persists after clinical cure led Krieger[50] to propose that there is an intrinsic neural abnormality in such patients. However, it has been shown more recently that the abnormality gradually clears if sufficient time elapses.[55] In view of the finding that cortisol can produce a number of changes in brain function in the human (including cerebral atrophy), it is equally likely that the changes are secondary to steroid effects on the brain.

The use of neurotransmitter antagonists has been proposed by Krieger as a means of identifying a neural basis of Cushing's disease. The most interesting results have been obtained using the serotonin antagonist cyproheptadine, which was assumed to act on the serotonergic hypothalamic system regulating CRH secretion.[52,54] Approximately 60 percent of cases are reported to respond, partially or completely, to this therapy, although it may take very high doses (up to 32 mg) or prolonged treatment (4 to 5 months) to see an effect. Cyproheptadine also restores circadian periodicity and reverses paradoxical ACTH response to TRH and lowers ACTH in some cases of Nelson's syndrome. Krieger suggests that "the existence of a subgroup of patients who do not respond to cyproheptadine raises the question that there may be at least two types of Cushing's disease, one dependent upon abnormal central nervous system drive (perhaps by a serotonergic mechanism), the other of primary pituitary origin, the latter perhaps representing those patients who respond to microadenomectomy.''[50] However, the demonstration that cyproheptadine can inhibit ACTH by a direct action on adenomas (*in vitro*) weakens the argument for a central defect in CRH secretion.

Excessive hypothalamic CRH secretion can cause Cushing's disease. A single case of hypothalamic CRH secreting gangliocytoma has been described (Fig. 2), as have several cases of ectopic CRF secretion.[5]

Tests using synthetic CRH in Cushing's disease have given some new insights into the pathogenesis of this disease. Most cases show exaggerated ACTH-cortisol responses, whereas responses in ectopic ACTH syndrome and in primary adrenal adenomas are blunted or abolished (see chapter 15). Following removal of the adenoma, basal ACTH secretion in most patients with Cushing's disease falls to extremely low levels and the pituitary gland becomes unresponsive to CRH. Recovery of normal function may take months. These observations suggest that the nontumorous portion of the gland has been suppressed by the adenoma. An additional observation to suggest that CRH hypersecretion is not the cause of most cases of Cushing's disease is that CRH-induced ACTH responses are blunted in patients with pituitary-adrenal hypersecretion associated with psychotic depression. Because the likelihood is great that pituitary-adrenal secretion in depression is due to chronic neural activation, Gold and colleagues have proposed that depression leads to CRF hypersecretion, which in turn causes mild hypersecretion of ACTH and cortisol, which in turn inhibits adrenocorticotrope secretory response to CRH (see chapter 15).

The most convincing evidence that adenomas are not due to hypothalamic dysfunction is the study of ACTH regulatory responses in patients

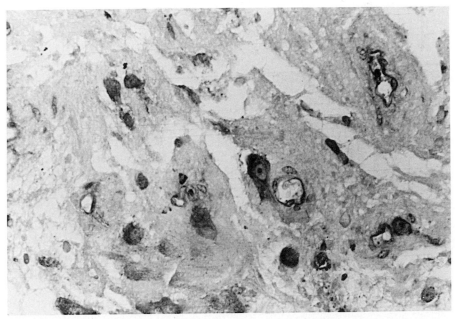

FIGURE 2. Corticotropin-releasing factor immunopositivity is localized within cell bodies and axonal processes of neurons in a sellar gangliocytoma associated with pituitary corticotropic hyperplasia and Cushing's disease. Avidin-biotin-peroxidase complex technique with hematoxylin counterstain (× 80). (Courtesy of Dr. SL Asa, St. Michael's Hospital, Toronto.)

cured by microadenomectomy. Several series have been published.[6,55,71,73] In general, these show a return to normal feedback regulatory control and hence suggest that CRH abnormalities were not the cause of the disease. As noted above, preoperative and postoperative testing with CRH indicates a return of feedback regulatory control to normal, but this recovery is preceded by a transient period of hypoadrenalism. Most patients show a return to normal responsiveness to feedback inhibition by the "low-dose" dexamethasone test and normal responses to metyrapone. In the patient of Lagerquist and associates,[55] circadian rhythms returned, as was true for the case of Bigos et al.[92] These authors provide a complete summary of the literature and also point out the association of galactorrhea, slight PRL excess secretion in Cushing's disease, and remission after surgery. Similar findings were reported by Schnall and colleagues.[73]

Although these findings may not be uniform in all patients with Cushing's disease, the high incidence of microadenoma in this disease and complete cure following pituitary microadenomectomy are strong evidence that intrinsic pituitary disease underlies most instances of this disorder.

In our opinion, the role of the brain in the pathogenesis of Cushing's disease has not been established. We believe that all the observations that have been made can be explained by the view that adenomas develop in the presence of a normal neural and steroid milieu. Abnormalities are intrinsic to the tumor. We believe it likely that the abnormality is due to loss of cortisol feedback by a group of cells which then hypersecrete ACTH, which leads to excessive cortisol, which in turn suppresses the remaining normal gland.

Prolactin-secreting Tumors

Of all cases of hyperprolactinemia, about one third can be shown to be due to adenomas (see chapter 7). The precise frequency with which adenomas are present is still uncertain, and the role of the hypothalamus in the pathogenesis or maintenance of the disorder is still a subject of speculation.

Although no unique pattern characterizes PRL regulatory responses in patients with adenomas, it can be stated in general that such cases lose characteristic circadian rhythms and become less responsive to the stimulating effects of TRH, and dopamine antagonists, such as chlorpromazine and metoclopramide, but retain partial or complete responsivity to the inhibitory effects of dopamine agonists (see chapter 7).[3] The impaired responsiveness of the adenoma to secretagogues is not due to the fact that such patients already have high PRL levels, because pregnant women, with similarly elevated PRL levels, show exuberant responses to TRH and to metoclopramide.[3] The abnormality in the adenoma cases thus indicates either a defect in receptor mechanism or the presence of small, rapidly turning over pools of PRL.

Crucial to the question of whether there is an underlying nervous system abnormality is the extent to which normal PRL secretory responses return after removal of the microadenoma. This question has been addressed by Barbarino and coworkers,[3] who studied seven women with PRL-secreting tumors before and after microadenomectomy. Prior to surgery, all had blunted or absent responses to metoclopramide and to TRH. After surgical cure (as indicated by return to menses and of PRL level to normal), responses to these physiologic tests returned to normal in six of seven cases. In a series of 20 cases studied by Molitch and colleagues,[68,90] 12 were cured, and their secretory responses returned to normal.[27] In the remainder, blood PRL levels remained elevated, and physiologic responses were persistently abnormal. It is not clear whether these patients have an abnormality of CNS function or whether there is residual adenoma, despite the surgeon's perception that all tumor has been removed.

In the series from our clinic, a study has been made of the presurgical and postsurgical results of testing with L-dopa-carbidopa pretreatment. This approach, utilized by Fine and Frohman[19] and also studied by Camanni and colleagues[10] in patients with acromegaly, is based on the fact that L-dopa is converted to dopamine in both the brain and the pituitary gland (and hence could theoretically act in either place) but that carbidopa (which blocks the enzymatic conversion step) acts only in regions outside the blood-brain barrier. Fine and collaborators[19] showed that L-dopa inhibition of PRL release in normal subjects is not blocked by carbidopa, but it is in tumors. The conclusion was drawn that in normal persons, the principal effect of L-dopa is at the level of the hypothalamus, but in adenoma patients, it is at the pituitary level. In seven patients cured by microadenomectomy,[27] all had abnormal responses to L-dopa-carbidopa, and all reverted to normal after microadenomectomy. We conclude that the microadenoma is an intrinsic abnormality in most patients.

Although a defect in hypothalamic catecholamine secretion has been proposed in the pathogenesis of prolactinoma,[18,84] we think the evidence to date is unconvincing.

These observations suggest at most a permissive role for the nervous system in the pathogenesis of prolactinoma. However, a finding that suggests a hypothalamic abnormality in prolactinoma is the demonstration by Garthwaite and Hagen[26] of PRL-releasing activity in the plasma of patients with galactorrhea-amenorrhea, 8 of 13 of whom had demonstrable tumors. The forcefulness of this observation in providing convincing evidence of hypothalamic dysfunction in this disorder is conditioned by uncertainty as to the chemical nature of prolactin-releasing factor, of its site of secretion, and of the effect of microadenomectomy on its concentration. This interesting work will require further study.

Recently Weiner and colleagues[89] have proposed that differences in regional perfusion lead to local regions of low dopamine concentration. These could lead to local foci of lactotrope hyperplasia.

PATHOLOGY OF PITUITARY TUMORS

The elegant studies of Kovacs and coworkers[34,35,40-49] have clarified the varieties of pituitary tumors that occur. Their classification (see Table 1) will be used in this discussion. From a clinical perspective, tumors have also been graded according to size and to degree of invasiveness. Microadenomas are defined as tumors less then 10 mm in diameter (grade I). Macroadenomas, defined as greater than 10 mm, may be enclosed (grade II) with or without suprasellar extension or be invasive, either localized (grade III) or diffuse (grade IV). Illustrative of the utility of this grading system is the

PROLACTINOMAS
(355 cases)

SELLA TURCICA RADIOLOGICAL CLASSIFICATION			WOMEN NO. CASES	WOMEN %	MEN NO.	MEN %
A D E N O M A S (ENCLOSED)	GR. 0	NORMAL	17	6	0	0
	GR. I <10mm	MICRO-ADENOMA	178	59	8	15
	GR. II >10mm	NO SSE	69	29	21	70
		SSE	18		18	
A D E N O M A S (INVASIVE)	GR. III LOCALIZED	NO SSE	9	3	0	0
		SSE	0		0	
	GR. IV DIFFUSE	NO SSE	3	3	3	15
		SSE	6		5	
TOTAL			300	100	55	100

FIGURE 3. Radiologic classification of the sella turcica and grading of the tumor in 355 cases of PRL adenomas. SSE: Suprasellar expansion. (From Hardy, J.[32] with permission.)

breakdown of 355 cases of prolactinoma operated on by Jules Hardy[32] (Fig. 3). Of these cases, 17 in women had no radiologic evidence of tumor (grade 0); 178 were grade I; 87, grade II; 9, grade III; and 9, grade IV. It is evident in all the surgical reports that prognosis of treatment by adenomectomy corresponds closely to tumor size. Thus, microadenomas are successfully removed by experienced surgeons in 70 to 90 percent of cases, whereas invasive macroadenomas are virtually never cured by surgery alone.

GH Cell Adenomas

Growth hormone cell adenomas can be divided morphologically into densely and sparsely granulated tumors[1,2] (see Table 1) (Figs. 4 and 5). Although this distinction has no endocrinologic significance with respect to levels of hormone secreted or clinical symptoms, their separation has been important from a treatment standpoint. Sparsely-granulated tumors are more aggressive and have a faster growth rate.

Densely granulated GH cell adenomas appear to be acidophilic by conventional stains and show a diffuse cytoplasmic positivity for GH by the immunoperoxidase technique. Sparsely granulated GH cell adenomas appear as chromophobic adenomas histologically. By using anti-GH as the primary antibody, the immunoperoxidase technique reveals brown cytoplasmic deposits in the forms of streaks, cres-

HYPOTHALAMIC-PITUITARY DISEASE

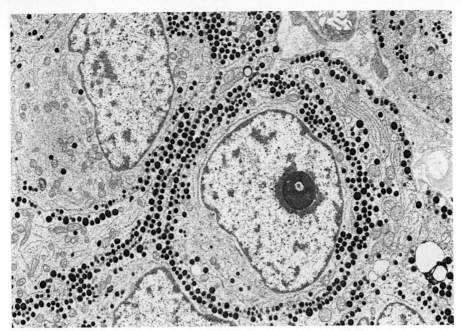

FIGURE 4. Electron micrograph of a densely granulated growth hormone cell adenoma of the pituitary gland with well-developed cytoplasm containing numerous secretory granules (×7500). (Courtesy Dr. K. Kovacs, St. Michael's Hospital, Toronto.)

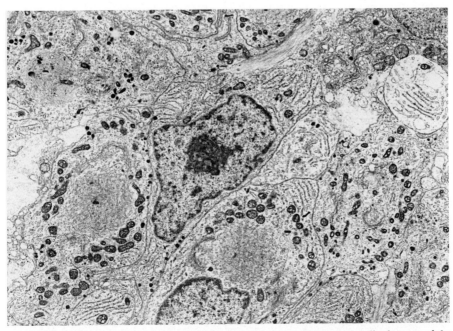

FIGURE 5. Electron micrograph of a sparsely granulated growth hormone cell adenoma of the pituitary gland with fibrous bodies. The cytoplasm of adenoma cells contains fibrous bodies and a few secretory granules (×7500). (Courtesy Dr. K. Kovacs, St. Michael's Hospital, Toronto.)

cents, or ring-like structures corresponding to the Golgi apparatus. In a few cells, GH immunopositivity is more diffuse and stronger. In most of the cells, it is not as prominent as in densely granulated GH cell adenomas. At the electron microscopic level, the immunoprecipitate is found over the secretory granules.[2]

Prolactin Cell Adenomas

In women, PRL secreting adenomas are commonly recognized when they are small due to their endocrine effects. In men, on the other hand, symptoms of tumor mass itself (headache and visual disturbance) more often bring the tumor to attention. Despite these differences in timing of presentation, representing in all probability a longer duration of tumor presence in men, there are no pathologic features that distinguish the tumors in the two sexes.

Adenomas composed of PRL cells can be densely or sparsely granulated (Figs. 6 and 7). The former type corresponds to the acidophilic adenoma and occurs infrequently. The latter is chromophobic and is the most common type of pituitary adenoma.

By using anti-PRL as the primary antibody, densely granulated PRL cell adenomas show diffuse immunopositivity in the form of brown deposits over the entire cytoplasm. In sparsely granulated adenomatous PRL cells, the immunopositivity has a streak or crescent shape or forms a ring-like structure representing the conspicuous Golgi complex. By electron microscopy, immunostaining is localized over the secretory granules, and the immunoreactive material of Golgi sacculi is lost.

Mixed GH-PRL Adenomas

These tumors are true mixed-cell adenomas that contain two separate populations of cells, one secreting PRL, the other GH.[13,29,40,44] According to the Kovacs classification, they are *bihormonal, bimorphous* tumors. Clinical signs and biochemical documentation of elevated serum levels of both GH and PRL are found. Pathologically, various combinations of sparsely or densely granulated cells may be present.

Acidophil Stem Cell Adenomas

These are rapidly growing, invasive tumors containing a *bihormonal, monomorphous* cell type, usually with prominent PRL immunoreactivity and sparse GH immunoreactivity contained within the same cells.[35] The tumors usually present clinically with the symptoms of hyperprolactinemia and tumor mass (headache and visual disturbance). Growth hormone secretion documented by elevated GH levels is rare, but the tumor cells clearly contain both PRL and GH. It is speculated that the tumor arises from an acidophil stem cell, the presumed common precursor of GH and PRL cells.

Mammosomatotrope Cell Adenomas

These are bihormonal, monomorphous tumors consisting of one cell type, the mammosomatotrope, which secretes GH and PRL.[40,44] They give rise usually to clinical manifestations of acromegaly. The cells are acidophilic, and immunoperoxidase staining reveals both PRL and GH. Less than 50

HYPOTHALAMIC-PITUITARY DISEASE

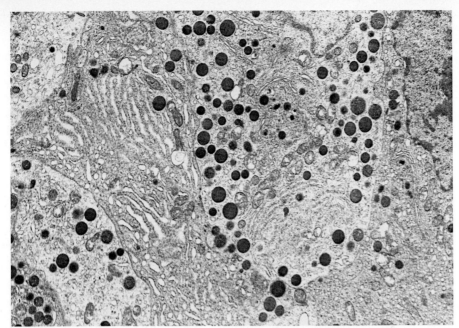

FIGURE 6. Electron micrograph of a densely granulated prolactin cell adenoma of the pituitary gland. The adenoma cells possess many large, spherical, and evenly distributed electron dense secretory granules (×8800). (Courtesy Dr. K. Kovacs, St. Michael's Hospital, Toronto.)

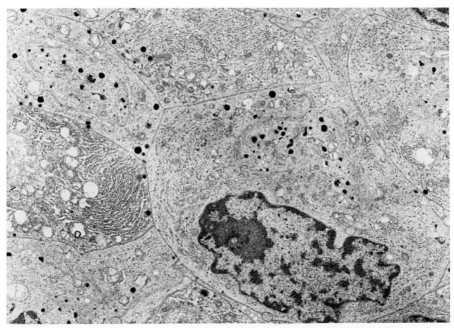

FIGURE 7. Electron micrograph of a sparsely granulated prolactin cell adenoma of the pituitary gland showing well-developed cytoplasm, prominent RER membranes, and Golgi apparatus, as well as a few irregular secretory granules (×7500). (Courtesy Dr. K. Kovacs, St. Michael's Hospital, Toronto.)

PITUITARY ADENOMAS: PATHOLOGY AND PATHOGENESIS 437

percent secrete PRL in amounts sufficient to result in hyperprolactinemia. The tumors grow slowly.

Corticotrope Cell Adenomas

Corticotrope cell adenomas are found in patients with Cushing's disease or Nelson's syndrome.[25,46] So-called silent corticotrope cell adenomas contain immunoreactive ACTH-related peptides but are unassociated with clinical and biochemical evidence of increased ACTH secretion.

> Corticotrope cell adenomas with increased ACTH secretion are usually densely granulated, basophilic, and strongly periodic acid-Schiff stain (PAS) positive. Occasionally they are chromophobic and sparsely granulated. The immunoperoxidase technique demonstrates the presence of ACTH and related peptides such as β-lipotropin and endorphins in the cytoplasm of adenoma cells. The immunopositivity is usually intense, located over the secretory granules, and often concentrated along the cell membrane where secretory granules line up in large numbers.

Silent corticotrope cell adenomas are chromophobic or basophilic by conventional stains. Despite the clinical absence of hormone secretion, these tumors show positive immunostaining for ACTH and related peptides.[34,45] The immunopositivity obtained with antibodies directed against various parts of the proopiomelanocortin molecule shows considerable variations from case to case and even within the same tumor. It appears that silent corticotrope cell adenomas represent heterogeneous tumors which can be divided into various subtypes based on their electron microscopic appearance.

Thyrotrope Cell Adenomas

Thyrotrope cell adenomas are rare, usually accompanied by elevated blood TSH levels (see chapter 5).[1,59,80] They develop in patients with long-standing primary hypothyroidism or are seen in association with hyperthyroidism secondary to excessive TSH secretion by the tumor. Certain thyrotrope cell adenomas occur in euthyroid patients; apparently these tumors are silent and do not secrete excessive amounts of biologically active TSH.

> Thyroid-stimulating hormone cell adenomas are chromophobic and show positive immunostaining for TSH. In a few tumors, regarded as TSH cell adenomas by electron microscopy, no TSH immunopositivity is evident, suggesting that they do not store immunologically reactive TSH in sufficient amounts to be demonstrable by the immunoperoxidase technique. As an alternative explanation, these tumors may produce an abnormal TSH which does not react with the TSH antibody.

Gonadotrope Cell Adenomas

Gonadotrope cell adenomas are uncommon, occurring either in patients with long-standing primary hypogonadism or unassociated with apparent gonadal abnormality.[47,49,76] Clinically, local symptoms prevail, such as visual disturbances and headache.

Gonadotrope cell adenomas are chromophobic by conventional staining and contain FSH[87] and/or LH, which may be documented by the immunoperoxidase technique.

The immunoprecipitate almost always is located over the secretory granules, which may be small and sparse, rendering the demonstration of FSH/LH by the immunoperoxidase technique uncertain. This difficulty can be successfully overcome by the application of the avidin-biotin technique or pronase digestion prior to immunoperoxidase staining. In some adenomas, only FSH or LH is noted.

Pituitary tumors comprised of thyrotropes or gonadotropes, although appearing to be hormonally silent, may in fact secrete only one of the two subunits making up the glycoproteins.[69]

The two subunits, termed α and β, are encoded by separate messenger RNA species, derived from distinct genes on separate chromosomes. According to Ridgway, "discordant and excessive alpha subunit production has been considered a characteristic feature of the tumors in some but not all circumstances." Although initially considered to be rare, the frequency of glycoprotein hormone or subunit production by pituitary tumors may reach 5 to 20 percent of all cases. Thus, many so-called nonfunctioning chromophobe adenomas, when studied carefully for glycoprotein hormone production, are found to be associated with FSH and/or α-subunit production.

Null Cell Adenomas

According to Kovacs, "null cell adenomas lack biochemical, clinical, and morphologic markers; they are unaccompanied by clinical and biochemical evidence of hormone secretion."[40,48] These tumors are common in older patients; they are PAS-negative and chromophobic. By electron microscopy (EM), cells invariably contain cytoplasmic secretory granules and possess all the cell constituents required for hormonal secretion. Based on EM studies, they have been divided into two types: *oncocytic*, characterized by an abundance of mitochondria;[42,57] and *nononcocytic*, without abnormal numbers of mitochondria. The significance of this pathologic difference is unknown.

In some cases, null cell adenomas contain scattered cells which show positive immunostaining for various adenohypophysial hormones, such as TSH, FSH, LH, α-subunit, ACTH, or PRL. The interpretation of this focal immunopositivity is difficult. It is possible that the immunopositivity is due to cellular differentiation; certain adenoma cells from the precursor state may differentiate into cells that become capable of synthesizing and storing immunocytologically demonstrable hormonal compounds.

Plurihormonal Adenomas

Plurihormal adenomas may be monomorphous (one cell secreting two or more hormones) or plurimorphous (multiple cell types). Various combinations of hormone secretion may occur, such as GH and TSH; GH, PRL, and TSH; GH, PRL, and ACTH; GH, PRL and α-subunit. Although rare, such tumors likely will be highly informative of the origins and embryologic development of pituitary secretory cells.

Parasellar Tumors

Aside from adenomas, a variety of other pituitary and parapituitary masses can occur (Table 3). Of particular importance to the clinician are cranio-

TABLE 3. Tumors and Tumor-like Conditions in the Sella Turcica and Parasellar Regions

Abscess	Glioma (optic nerve, infundibulum, posterior lobe, hypothalamus)
Adenoma (pituitary)	
Aneurysm	Granular cell tumor (posterior lobe, stalk)
Angioma	Hamartoma (hypothalamus)
Carcinoma (pituitary)	Histiocytosis X
Carcinoma (sphenoid sinus, nasopharynx)	Hypophysitis (chronic, lymphocytic)
Chordoma	Leukemia
Choristoma	Lymphoma
Craniopharyngioma	Melanoma
Cryptococcosis	Meningioma
Cysts (various types)	Metastasis (carcinoma, sarcoma)
Fibroma	Osteosarcoma
Fibrosarcoma	Paraganglioma
Gangliocytoma	Plasmacytoma
Ganglioneuroma	Sarcoidosis
Germinoma (ectopic pinealoma)	Syphilis
Giant cell granuloma	Tertoma
	Tuberculosis

pharyngioma and metastatic tumor. Craniopharyngiomas may occur as pituitary tumors, particularly in children or young adults. They are assumed to arise from the remnants of Rathke's pouch and they produce no hormones. Because craniopharyngiomas contain keratin, immunostaining using antikeratin antibody is a valuable approach confirming the diagnosis.

Metastatic carcinomas to the pituitary gland may destroy large areas of the normal parenchyma. Except for those causing the ectopic ACTH syndrome, they contain no pituitary hormones. The application of the immunoperoxidase technique can be useful in the differential diagnosis to exclude pituitary tumor.

Primary carcinomas arising from adenohypophysial cells are extremely rare and can be diagnosed morphologically only when distant metastases are present.[74,75] They may produce GH, PRL, or ACTH or may be unassociated with hormone excess. The immunoperoxidase technique can reveal the presence of hormone in the cell cytoplasm.

The immunocytologic approach also may be valuable in exploring the cellular composition of metastatic tumors whose primary site is unknown and when pituitary origin is suspected. The presence of GH or PRL indicates adenohypophysial derivation of the tumor. In cases of ACTH-producing tumors, clarification of the primary site is more complicated, because ACTH may be produced by nonpituitary neoplasms as a part of the ectopic ACTH syndrome.

REFERENCES

1. Afrasiabi, A, Valenta, L, Gwinup, G: *A TSH-secreting pituitary tumour causing hyperthyroidism: Presentation of a case and review of the literature.* Acta Endocrinol (Copenh) 72:448–460, 1979.
2. Asa, SL, Scheithauer, BW, Bilboa, JM, Horvath, E, Ryan N, Kovacs, K, Randall, RV, Law, ER, Jr, Singer, W, Linfoot, JA, Thorner, MO, Vale, W: *A case for hypothalamic acromegaly: A clinicopathological study of six patients with hypothalamic gangliocytomas producing growth hormone-releasing factor.* J Clin Endocrin Metab 58:796–803, 1984.
3. Barbarino, A, deMarinis, L, Maira, G, Menini, E, Anile, C: *Serum prolactin response to*

thyrotropin-releasing hormone and metoclopramide in patients with prolactin-secreting tumors before and after transsphenoidal surgery. J Clin Endocrinol Metab 47:1148–1155, 1978.

4. BAYLIN, SB: *The multiple endocrine neoplasia syndromes: Implications for the study of inherited tumors.* Semin Oncol 5:35–45, 1978.

5. BELSKY, JL, CUELLO, B, SWANSON, LW, SIMMONS, DM, JARRETT, RM, BRAZA, F: *Cushing's syndrome due to ectopic production of corticotropin-releasing factor.* J Clin Endocinol Metab 60:496–500, 1985.

6. BERLINGER, FG, RUDER, HL, WILBER, JF: *Cushing's syndrome associated with galactorrhea, amenorrhea and hypothyroidism: A primary hypothalamic disorder.* J Clin Endocrinol Metab 45:1205–1210, 1977.

7. BESSER, GM, WASS, JAH, THORNER, MO: *Acromegaly—Results of long term treatment with bromocriptine.* Acta Endocrinol (Suppl) (Copenh) 88:187–198, 1978.

8. BURKE, CW, AND BEARDWELL, CG: *Cushing's syndrome. An evaluation of the clinical usefulness of urinary free cortisol and other urinary steroid measurements in diagnosis.* Q J Med 42:175–204, 1973.

9. BURROW, GN, WORTZMAN, G, REWCASTLE, NB, HOLGATE, PC, KOVACS, K: *Microadenomas of the pituitary and abnormal sellar tomograms in an unselected autopsy series.* N Engl J Med 304:156–158, 1981.

10. CAMANNI, F, PICCOTTI, GB, MASSERA, F, MOLINATTI, G, MANTEGAZZA, P, MÜLLER, EE: *Carbidopa inhibits the growth hormone and prolactin suppressive effects of L-dopa in acromegalic patients.* J Clin Endocrinol Metab 47:647–653, 1978.

11. CARLSON, HE, LEVINE, GA, GOLDBERG, NJ, HERSHMAN, JM: *Hyperprolactinemia in multiple endocrine adenomatosis. Type I.* Arch Intern Med 138:1807–1808, 1978.

12. CLAYTON, R, BURDEN, AC, SCHRIEVER, V, ROSENTHAL, RD: *Secondary pituitary hyperplasia in Addison's disease.* Lancet Nov 5, pp. 954–956, 1977.

13. CORENBLUM, B, SIREK, AMT, HORVATH, ET, KOVACS, K, EZRIN, C: *Human mixed somatotrophic and lactotrophic pituitary adenomas.* J Clin Endocrinol Metab 42:857–865, 1976.

14. COSTELLO, RT: *Subclinical adenomas of the pituitary gland.* Am J Pathol 12:205–216, 1936.

15. DAUGHADAY, W, AND CRYER, PE: *Growth hormone hypersecretion and acromegaly.* Hosp Pract 13:75–80, 1978

16. DAUGHADAY, W, CRYER, PE, JACOBS, LS: *The role of the hypothalamus in the pathogenesis for pituitary tumors.* In KOHLER, PO, AND ROSS, GT, (EDS): *Diagnosis and treatment of pituitary tumors.* Excerpta Medica, New York, 1973, pp 26–34.

17. DELELLIS, RA, AND WOLFE, HJ: *Multiple endocrine adenomatosis syndromes: Origins and interrelationships.* In HOLLAND, J, AND FREI, E (EDS): *Cancer Medicine,* ed 2. Lea & Febiger, Philadelphia, 1979.

18. FAGLIA, G, SPADA A, MORIONDO, P, ET AL: *What is the role of dopamine in the pathogenesis of prolactinomas.* In CAMANNI E, AND MÜLLER, EE, (EDS): *Pituitary Hyperfunction.* Raven Press, New York, 1984, pp 279–288.

19. FINE, SA, AND FROHMAN, LA: *Loss of central nervous system component of dopaminergic inhibition of prolactin secretion in patients with prolactin secreting pituitary tumors.* J Clin Invest 61:973–980, 1978.

20. FRIEND, JN, JUDGE, DM, SHERMAN, BM, SANTEN, J: *FSH-secreting pituitary adenomas: Stimulation and suppression studies in two patients.* J Clin Endocrinol Metab 43:650–657, 1976.

21. FROHMAN, LA: *Ectopic hormone production by tumors: Growth hormone releasing factor.* In MÜLLER, EE, AND MACLEOD, RM (EDS): *Neuroendocrine Perspectives.* Elsevier, Amsterdam, 1984, pp 201–224.

22. FROHMAN, LA, THOMINET, JL, SZABO, M: *Ectopic growth hormone-releasing factor syndromes.* In RAITI, S, AND TOLAMN, RA (EDS): *Human Growth Hormone.* Plenum, New York, 1986, pp 347–360.

23. FURTH, J, AND CLIFTON, KH: *Experimental pituitary tumors.* In HARRIS, GW, AND DONOVAN, BT, (EDS): *The Pituitary Gland.* Buttersworth, London, 1966, pp 460–497.

24. GAGEL, RF, MELVIN, KEW, TASHJIAN, AH, JR, MILLER, HH, FELDMAN, ZT, WOLFE, HJ, DELELLIS, RA, CERVI-SKINNER, S, REICHLIN, S: *Natural history of the familial medullary thyroid carcinoma-pheochromocytoma syndrome and the identification of preneoplastic stages by screening studies: A five year report.* Trans Assoc Am Phys 88:177–191, 1975.

25. GARCIA, JH, KALIMO, H, GIVENS, JR: *Human adenohypophysis in Nelson syndrome: Ultrastructural and clinical study.* Arch Pathol Lab Med 100:253–268, 1976.

26. GARTHWAITE, TL, AND HAGEN, TC: *Plasma prolactin-releasing factor-like activity in the amenorrhea-galactorrhea syndrome.* J Clin Endocrinol Metab 47:885–891, 1978.

27. GOODMAN, R, BILLER, B, MOSSES, AC, MOLITCH, M, FELDMAN, S, POST, K: *Restoration of normal prolactin secretory dynamics after surgical cure of prolactinoma is evidence against underlying hypothalamic dysregulation. Program of the 61st Annual Meeting of the Endocrine Society,* Anaheim, California, June 1979.

28. GRAZE, K, SPILER, IJ, TASHJIAN, AH, JR, MELVIN, KEW, CERVI-SKINNER, S, GAGEL, RF, MILLER, HH, WOLFE, HJ, DELELLIS, RA, LEAPE, L, FELDMAN, ZT, REICHLIN, S: *Natural history of familial*

medullary thyroid carcinoma: Effect of a program for early diagnosis. N Engl J Med 299:980–985, 1978.

29. GUYDA, H, ROBERT, F, COLLE, E, ET AL: *Histologic, ultrastructural, and hormonal characterization of a pituitary tumor secreting both hGH and prolactin.* J Clin Endocrinol Metab 36:531–538, 1973.

30. HAGEN, TC, LAWRENCE, AM, KIRSTEINS, L: *In vivo release of monkey pituitary growth hormone by acromegalic plasma.* J Clin Endocrinol 33:448–454, 1978.

31. HANEW, K, AIDA, M, TANO, T, YOSHINAGA, K: *Abnormal growth hormone responses to L-dopa and thyrotropin releasing hormone in patients with acromegaly.* Tohoku J Exp Med 121:197–206, 1977.

32. HARDY, J: *Transsphenoidal microsurgery of prolactinomas.* In BLACK, PM, ZERVAS, NT, RIDGEWAY, EC, MARTIN, JB (EDS): *Secretory Tumors of the Pituitary Gland.* Raven Press, New York, 1984, pp 73–82.

33. HARDY, J: *Transsphenoidal surgery for hypersecreting adenomas.* In KOHLER, PO, AND ROSS, GT (Eds): *Diagnosis and treatment of pituitary tumors.* Elsevier, New York, 1973, pp 179–198.

34. HORVATH, E, KOVACS, K, KILLINGER, DW, ET AL: *Silent corticotropic adenomas of the human pituitary gland: A histologic, immunocytologic and ultrastructural study.* Am J Pathol 98:617–627, 1980.

35. HORVATH, E, KOVACS, K, SINGER, W, ET AL: *Acidophil stem cell adenoma of the human pituitary: Clinico-pathological analysis of 15 cases.* Cancer 47:761–771, 1981.

36. HORVATH, E, KOVACS, K, SINGER, W, ET AL: *Acidophil stem cell adenoma of the human pituitary.* Arch Pathol Lab Med 101:594–599, 1977.

37. HOYTE, KM, AND MARTIN, JB: *Recovery from paradoxical growth hormone responses in acromegaly after transsphenoidal selective adenomectomy.* J Clin Endocrinol Metab 41:656–659, 1975.

38. JONES, MT: *Control of corticotrophin (ACTH) secretion.* In JEFFCOATE, SL, AND HUTCHINSON, JSM (Eds): *The Endocrine Hypothalamus.* Academic Press, London, 1978, pp 386–419.

39. KATZ, MS, GREGERMAN, RI, HORVATH, E, ET AL: *Thyrotroph cell adenoma of the human pituitary gland associated with primary hypothyroidism: Clinical and morphological features.* Acta Endocrinol (Copenh) 95:41–49, 1980.

40. KOVACS, K: *Light and electron microscopic pathology of pituitary tumors: Immunohistochemistry.* In BLACK, PM, ZERVAS, NT, RIDGWAY, EC, MARTIN, JB: *Tumors of the Pituitary Gland.* Raven Press, New York, 1984, pp 365–376.

41. KOVACS, K, BILBAO, JM, ASA, SL: *The pathology of parasellar and hypothalamic lesions.* In GIVENS, JR (ED): *The Hypothalamus.* Yearbook Medical Publishers, Chicago, 1984, pp 17–38.

42. KOVACS, K, AND HORVATH, E: *Pituitary "chromophobe" adenoma composed of oncocytes: A light and electron microscopic study.* Arch Pathol 95:235–242, 1973.

43. KOVACS, K, AND HORVATH, E: *Pituitary tumors: Pathologic Aspects.* In TOLIS, G, LABRIE, F, MARTIN, JB, NAFTOLIN, F (EDS): *Clinical Neuroendocrinology: A Pathophysiological Approach.* Raven Press, New York, 1979, pp 367–384.

44. KOVACS, K, AND HORVATH, E: *Pathology of pituitary adenomas.* In GIVENS, JR (ED): *Hormone Secreting Pituitary Tumors.* Yearbook Medical Publishers, Chicago, 1982, pp 97–119.

45. KOVACS, K, HORVATH, E, BAYLEY, TA, ET AL: *Silent corticotroph cell adenoma with lysosomal accumulation and crinophagy: A distinct clinicopathologic entity.* Am J Med 64:492–499, 1978.

46. KOVACS, K, HORVATH, E, KERENYI, NA, ET AL: *Light and electron microscopic features of a pituitary adenoma in Nelson's syndrome.* Am J Clin Pathol 65:337–342, 1976.

47. KOVACS, K, HORVATH, E, REWCASTLE, NB, ET AL: *Gonadotroph cell adenoma of the pituitary in a woman with long-standing hypogonadism.* Arch Gynecol 229:57–65, 1980.

48. KOVACS, K, HORVATH, E, RYAN, N, ET AL: *Null cell adenoma of the human pituitary.* Virchows Arch (Pathol Anat) 387:165–176, 1980.

49. KOVACS, K, HORVATH, E, VAN LOON, GR, ET AL: *Pituitary adenomas associated with elevated blood follicle-stimulating hormone levels: A histologic, immunocytologic and electron microscopic study of two cases.* Fertil Steril 29:622–638, 1978.

50. KRIEGER, DT: *The central nervous system and Cushing's disease.* Med Clin North Am 62:268–285, 1978.

51. KRIEGER, DT: *The hypothalamus and neuroendocrine pathology.* In KRIEGER, DT, HUGHES, JC, (EDS): *Neuroendocrinology.* Sinauer Associates, Sunderland, MA, 1980, pp 13–22.

52. KRIEGER, DT, AMOROSA, L, LINICK, F: *Cyproheptadine-induced remission of Cushing's disease.* N Engl J Med 293:893–902, 1975.

53. KRIEGER, DT, AND CONDON, EM: *Cyproheptadine treatment of Nelson's syndrome: Restoration of plasma ACTH circadian periodicity and reversal of response to TRF.* J Clin Endocrinol Metab 46:349–352, 1978.

54. KRIEGER, DT, AND LURIA, M: *Effectiveness of cyproheptadine in decreasing ACTH concentration in Nelson's syndrome.* J Clin Endocrinol Metab 43:1179–1182, 1976.

55. LAGERQUIST, LG, MEIKLE, AW, WEST, CD, TYLER, FH: *Cushing's disease with cure by resection of*

pituitary adenoma: Evidence against a primary hypothalamic defect. Am J Med 57:826–836, 1974.

56. LAMBERTS, SWJ, AND BIRKENHAGER, JC: *Effect of bromocriptine in pituitary-dependent Cushing's syndrome.* J Endocrinol 70:315–316, 1976.

57. LANDOLT, AM, AND OSWALD, UW: *Histology and ultrastructure of an oncocytic adenoma of the human pituitary.* Cancer 31:1099–1110, 1973.

58. LAWRENCE, AM, GOLDFINE, ID, KIRSTEINS, L: *Growth hormone dynamics in acromegaly.* J Clin Endocrinol Metab 31:239–247, 1970.

59. LEONG, ASY, CHAWLA, JC, TEH, EC: *Pituitary thyrotropic tumour secondary to long-standing primary hypothyroidism.* Pathol Eur 11:49–56, 1976.

60. MACLEOD, RM, AND KRIEGER, DT: *Differential effect of ergotamine on ACTH and prolactin secretion.* Program of the 58th Annual Meeting of the Endocrine Society, San Francisco, 1976 (Abstract 317).

61. MAEDA, K: *Critical review: Effects of thyrotropin releasing hormone on growth hormone release in normal subjects and in patients with depression, anorexia nervosa and acromegaly.* Kobe J Med Sci 22:263–270, 1976.

62. MCCORMICK, WF, AND HALMI, NS: *Absence of chromophobe adenomas from a large series of pituitary tumors.* Arch Pathol 92:231–238, 1971.

63. MELMED, S, BRAUNSTEIN, GD, HORVATH, E, EZRIN, C, KOVACS, K: *Pathophysiology of acromegaly.* Endocrine Rev 4:271–286, 1983.

64. PATEL, Y, RAO, K, REICHLIN, S: *Somatostatin in human cerebrospinal fluid.* N Engl J Med 296:529–533, 1977.

65. PEARSE, AGE, AND TAKOR TAKOR, T: *Neuroendocrine embryology and the APUD concept.* Clin Endocrinol 5 (Suppl):229, 1976.

66. PLOTZ, CM, KNOWLTON, AI, RAGAN, C: *Natural history of Cushing's syndrome.* Am J Med 13:597–614, 1952.

67. REICHLIN, S: *Etiology of Pituitary Adenomas.* In POST, KD, JACKSON, IMD, REICHLIN, S, (EDS): *The Pituitary Adenoma.* Plenum, New York, 1980, pp 29–45.

68. REICHLIN, S, AND MOLITCH, ME: *Neuroendocrine aspects of pituitary adenoma.* In CAMANNI, F, AND MÜLLER, EE, (EDS): *Pituitary Hyperfunction.* Raven Press, New York, 1984, pp 47–70.

69. RIDGWAY, EC: *Gycoprotein hormone production by pituitary tumors.* In BLACK, PM, ZERVAS, NT, RIDGWAY, EC, MARTIN, JB, (EDS): *Secretory tumors of the pituitary gland.* Raven Press, New York, 1984, pp 343–364.

70. ROBERT, F, PELLETIER, G, HARDY, J: *Pituitary adenomas in Cushing's disease.* Arch Pathol Lab Med 102:448–460, 1978.

71. SALASSA, RM, LAWS, ER, JR, CARPENTER, PC, NORTHCUTT, RC: *Transsphenoidal removal of pituitary microadenoma in Cushing's disease.* Mayo Clin Proc 53:24–28, 1978.

72. SAMAAN, NA, OSBORNE, BM, MACKAY, B, LEAVENS, ME, DUELLO, TM, HALMI, NS: *Endocrine and morphologic studies of pituitary adenomas secondary to primary hypothyroidism.* J Clin Endocrinol Metab 45:903–911, 1977.

73. SCHNALL, AM, BRODKEY, JS, KAUFMAN, B, PEARSON, OH: *Pituitary function after removal of pituitary microadenomas in Cushing's disease.* J Clin Endocrinol Metab 47:410–418, 1978.

74. SCHOLZ, DA, GASTINEAU, CF, HARRISON, EG: *Cushing's syndrome with malignant chromophobe tumor of the pituitary and extracranial metastases: Report of a case.* Proc Staff Meet Mayo Clin 37:31–35, 1962.

75. SHELDON, WH, GOLDEN, A, BONDY, PK: *Cushing's syndrome produced by a pituitary basophil carcinoma with hepatic metastases.* Am J Med 17:134–141, 1954.

76. SNYDER, PJ, AND STERLING, FH: *Hypersecretion of LH and FSH by a pituitary adenoma.* J Clin Endocrinol Metab 42:544–553, 1976.

77. TAKOR TAKOR, T, AND PEARSE, AGE: *Cytochemical identification of human and murine pituitary corticotrophs and somatotrophs as APUD cells.* Histochemie 37:207–214, 1973.

78. THORNER, MO, PERRYMAN, RL, CRONIN, MJ, ET AL: *Somatotroph hyperplasia: Successful treatment of acromegaly by removal of a pancreatic islet tumor secreting a growth hormone releasing factor.* J Clin Invest 70:965–977, 1982.

79. TINDALL, GT, AND TINDALL, SC: *Transsphenoidal surgery for acromegaly: Long term results in 50 patients.* In BLACK, PM, ZERVAS, NT, RIDGWAY, EC, MARTIN, JB, (EDS): *Secretory Tumors of the Pituitary Gland.* Raven Press, New York, 1984, pp 175–178.

80. TOLIS, G, BIRD, C, BERTRAND, G, ET AL: *Pituitary hyperthyroidism: Case report and review of the literature.* Am J Med 64:177–183, 1978.

81. TOLIS, G, KOUTSILIERIS, M, BERTRAND, G: *Endocrine diagnosis of growth hormone secreting pituitary tumors.* In BLACK, PM, ZERVAS, NT, RIDGWAY, EC, MARTIN, JB: *Secretory tumors of the pituitary gland.* Raven Press, New York, 1984, pp 145–154.

82. TYRRELL, JB, BROOKS, RM, FITZGERALD, PA, COFOID, P, FORSHAM, PH, WILSON, CB: *Cushing's disease: Selective transsphenoidal resection of pituitary microadenomas.* N Engl J Med 298:753–758, 1978.

83. VANDEWEGHE, M, BRAXEL, K, SCHUTYSER, J, VERMUELEN, A: *A case of multiple endocrine adenomatosis with primary amenorrhea.* Postgrad Med J 54:618–622, 1978.
84. VAN LOON, GR: *A defect in catecholamine neurons in patients with prolactin-secreting pituitary adenoma.* Lancet 2:868–871, 1978.
85. VELDHUIS, JD, GREEN, JE, III, KOVACS, E, WORGUL, TJ, MURRAY, FT, HAMMOND, JM: *Prolactin-secreting pituitary adenomas. Association with multiple endocrine neoplasia. Type I.* Am J Med 67:830–837, 1979.
86. WOLFE, HJ, MELVIN, KEW, CERVI-SKINNER, SJ, ALSAADI, AA, JULIAR, JF, JACKSON, CE, TASHJIAN, AH: *C-cell hyperplasia preceding medullary thyroid carcinoma.* N Engl J Med 289:437–441, 1973.
87. WOOLF, PD, AND SCHENK, EA: *An FSH-producing pituitary tumor in a patient with hypogonadism.* J Clin Endocrinol Metab 38:561–570, 1974.
88. ZIMMERMAN, EA, DEFENDINI, R, FRANTZ, AG: *Prolactin and growth hormone in patients with pituitary adenomas. A correlative study of hormone in tumor and plasma by immunoperoxidase technique and radioimmunoassay.* J Clin Endcorinol Metab 38:577–585, 1974.
89. ELIAS, KA, WEINER, RI: *Direct arterial vascularization of estrogen-induced prolactin-secreting anterior pituitary tumors.* Proc Natl Acad Sci USA 81(14):4549–4553, 1984.
90. MOLITCH, ME: *Growth hormone hypersecretory states.* In RAITI, S, AND TOLAMN, RA (EDS): *Human Growth Hormone.* Plenum, New York, 1986.
91. MOLITCH, ME, AND REICHLIN, S: *Hypothalamic hyperprolactinemia.* In MACLEOD, RM, SCAPAGNINI, U, THORNER, MO (EDS): *Prolactin.* Springer-Verlag, New York, 1985, pp 709–720.
92. BIGOS, ST, SOMMA, M, RASIO, E, ET AL: *Cushing's disease: management by transsphenoidal pituitary microsurgery.* J Clin Endocrinol Metab 50(2):348–354, 1980.

Chapter 13

HYPOTHALAMIC-PITUITARY DISORDERS: NEUROLOGIC AND OPHTHALMOLOGIC ASSESSMENT

NEUROLOGIC ASPECTS

In the evaluation of patients with suspected disturbance of the hypothalamus or pituitary, it is necessary to assess: (1) the local effects of compression, distortion, or destruction of neural structures; (2) the extent of hormonal disturbance; and (3) alterations in nonendocrine visceral and behavioral functions (see chapter 11). As in all clinical medicine, the major clues to the nature of the disorder come from a complete history, general physical examination, and neurologic examination, including evaluation of mental status. It is particularly important to interview knowledgeable members of the patient's family or friends, because behavioral disturbances (including sexual dysfunction) are common manifestations of both pituitary and hypothalamic diseases, and the patient may not be aware of these abnormalities or, if aware, unwilling to discuss them. General physical examination is also important because a number of neuroendocrine diseases are manifestations of systemic disorders such as granuloma, or malignancy.

Pituitary tumors can cause symptoms and signs by several mechanisms. The majority are first recognized by the clinical manifestations of excess prolactin (PRL) (see chapter 7), growth hormone (GH) (see chapter 8), or adrenocorticotropic hormone (ACTH) (see chapter 6) secretion. The small percentage of tumors that secrete thyroid-stimulating hormone (TSH), luteinizing hormone (LH), follicle-stimulating hormone (FSH), or inactive hormones (α or β subunit) usually present as tumor masses. The same is true for the 20 to 30 percent of pituitary tumors that secrete no known hormone, that is, are nonfunctional by current criteria. These latter tumors present usually with neurologic symptoms of headache and visual disturbance. Or they may cause hypothalamic symptoms or give rise to pituitary insufficiency owing to compression of surrounding pituitary tissue.

SPECIAL ASPECTS OF MEDICAL HISTORY

HEADACHE

Headache due to pituitary tumor is usually bitemporal or bifrontal; it may be felt as a deep discomfort behind the eyes. Headache is thought to result from pressure effects on an intact diaphragma sellae; evidence in support of this is the finding that in some patients headaches become less severe when the tumor grows into the suprasellar region. Pituitary tumors may be asymmetric, and the headaches associated with local pressure may be ipsilateral. Nausea and vomiting, occurring together with papilledema, suggest increased intracranial pressure. Direct pressure on the optic chiasm or tract may cause visual hallucinatory effects associated with "whiteness," "visual glow," "spots," or "a film of water."[12,19] These symptoms may be confused with the aura, scotomata, pulsating headache, and nausea of classic migraine, which does not occur, except by coincidence, in pituitary-tumor patients. It should be recalled that migraine may be activated or accentuated by hormone therapy in a hypopituitary patient, or by administration of oral contraceptives to susceptible individuals. A colloid cyst of the third ventricle may cause repeated sudden attacks of bitemporal headaches, which are often positional and associated with drop attacks.

Libido

Disturbances of libido frequently occur in patients with tumors of the pituitary gland. Suppression of libido usually results from gonadotropin deficiency secondary to pituitary or hypothalamic disease. Elevation of prolactin is often associated with decreased sexual activity in both men and women and in men may be accompanied by impotence. Whether this is due to the associated gonadal hormone deficiency or to direct effects of prolactin on the brain is unknown, but treatment with bromocriptine commonly restores libido to normal even when testosterone levels are not restored (see chapter 7).

Hypersexuality also has been reported in association with hypothalamic lesions. Boys with precocious puberty may show precocious sexual interest and drive, but this is much less common than might be anticipated. Increased sexuality with aggressive sex drive also has been seen in the Kleine-Levin syndrome, an episodic disorder (see chapter 11).

Sleep

Alternations in sleep which may occur with pituitary or hypothalamic disease include hypersomnia, inability to sleep, and reversal of day-night rhythms (see chapter 11). Somnolence is a common presenting complaint in hypothalamic tumors. Headaches or diabetes insipidus also may interfere with sleep. Aberrations of circadian rhythms are known to occur (see chapter 10).

Vision and Visual Field Evaluation

Anatomic Considerations

The boundaries of the sella turcica are continuous with a number of neural structures whose functions must be assessed in suspected disorders of the hypothalamus and pituitary gland.[5,21] Because the ventral hypothalamus and pituitary gland are so close to the optic nerves, optic chiasm, and optic

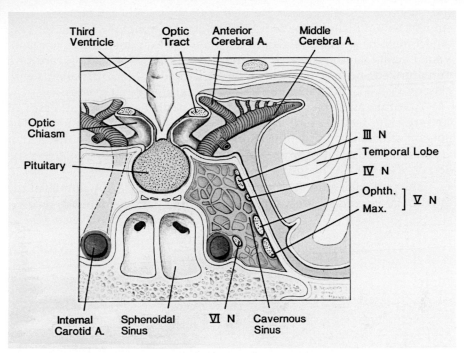

FIGURE 1. This is a diagrammatic representation of the anatomic relations of the pituitary fossa and cavernous sinus. The lateral wall of the sella turcica is formed by the cavernous sinus. The sinus contains the carotid artery, two branches of the fifth cranial nerve (ophthalmic and maxillary), the III nerve (oculomotor), IV nerve (trochlear), and VI nerve (abducens). The optic chiasm and optic tract are located superior and lateral, respectively, to the pituitary gland. (Drawing by B Newberg, modified from AK Maxwell in *Gray's Anatomy*, ed 35. WB Saunders, Philadelphia, 1973.)

tracts, careful testing of visual acuity and visual fields is an essential part of the clinical evaluation. Serial measurements help to follow progress of the clinical disturbance and of the effects of therapy. The state of visual function is also often crucial in determining the type and urgency of the therapy to be used. Lateral extension of pituitary tumors may compromise the function of the third, fourth, or sixth cranial nerves within the cavernous sinus, resulting in diplopia (Fig. 1).[25] The ophthalmic division of the fifth cranial nerve also may be affected in the cavernous sinus, causing a reduced corneal reflex or decreased facial sensation on the same side. Involvement of the cranial nerves is much less frequent than is involvement of the visual system.

Visual Field Examination

Initial assessment of visual fields by confrontation is relatively reliable, provided certain precautions are followed.[8] The use of finger movements is not adequate. A small, round object such as the white head of a pin, measuring 2 to 3 mm in diameter, is a satisfactory test object. The periphery of the visual fields can be compared with that of the examiner; a red or blue-green object provides a more senitive index of loss of vision within a portion of a field than does a white object and can be used to search for scotomata or a vertical field cut by asking the patient to note desaturation of the color (particularly of red). The size of the blind spot can be assessed by confrontation. It should be remembered in confrontation testing that the object must be placed equidistant between the examiner and the patient. Visual acuity can be assessed by the use of a Jaegher reading card or a miniaturized Snellen chart held at the prescribed distance. In patients with glasses, visual acuity should be tested with and without glasses.

Accurate assessment of visual fields, particularly in early cases of compression, requires evaluation by tangent screen and perimetry. The tangent screen permits identification of focal scotomata within the field of vision near the point of fixation. Perimetry is essential to document the details of defects in the visual fields.

The particular pattern of visual symptoms produced by tumors of the hypothalamus and pituitary gland in an individual case depends on ana-

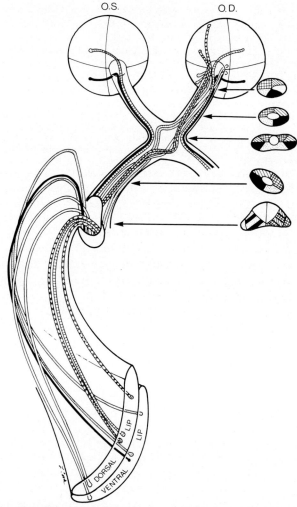

FIGURE 2. The nerve fiber anatomy of the visual pathways from retina to occipital cortex. Cross-sections on right show location of fibers at various levels in the pathway. (Courtesy of DD Donaldson. From Wray, SH: *Neuro-ophthalmology: Visual fields, optic nerve, and pupil.* In Pavan-Langston, D (ed): *Manual of Ocular Diagnosis and Therapy.* Little, Brown & Co., Boston, 1980.)

HYPOTHALAMIC-PITUITARY DISEASE

tomic features, such as the position of the chiasm in relation to the pituitary fossa, the configuration of the diaphragma sellae, and the size and rate of growth of the tumor.[2,4] The decussating fibers in the optic chiasma are arranged in well-defined laminae (Fig. 2). Nasal retina fibers, which constitute approximately 50 to 60 percent of the total retinal fibers from one eye, cross over to join the temporal fibers of the opposite eye to form the optic tract. These fibers subserve vision in the temporal visual field. The ventral fibers, which subserve the upper temporal fields, are located in the anterior, inferior part of the chiasm; they form a short loop that extends into the optic nerve of the opposite side before passing backward to form the optic tract. The dorsal fibers, which subserve the lower temporal visual field, loop into the ipsilateral optic tract before crossing in the posterosuperior chiasm to form a portion of the contralateral optic tract. Fibers from the macular region of the retina occupy the posterior part of the chiasm.

The positions of the retinal axons in the optic nerves, optic chiasm, and optic tracts explain patterns of abnormality following lesions in the visual pathways. In the studies of Hoyt[14] in the macaque monkey, lesions of retina were made and the pattern of fiber degeneration in the visual pathway examined. These studies showed that macular fibers contributed to all parts of the chiasm except for narrow zones of the anterior and posterior inferior chiasm. This no doubt explains the early involvement of central fields and acuity in chiasmal compression. These studies also showed that fibers from the lower nasal retina project forward into the contralateral optic knee (the knee of von Willebrand). A lesion in the posterior optic nerve or anterior chiasm affecting these fibers produces a hemianopic scotoma in the ipsilateral eye and a superior temporal defect in the opposite eye.

The visual disturbance produced by a lesion in the parasellar region depends on the part of the chiasm compressed.[8,10] Midline pressure on the optic chiasm from below first affects the fibers subserving vision in the upper temporal fields, leading to a characteristic *bitemporal superior quadrantanopsia or hemianopsia* (Fig. 3).[9,13,16,18,27,28] However, because of the complex pattern of fiber crossovers, visual defects are commonly asymmetric. With further chiasm compression, visual loss in the temporal field progresses circularly from the upper temporal to the lower temporal regions. Complete bitemporal hemianopsia occurs with functional transection of the chiasm. Visual acuity is normal in bitemporal hemianopsia unless there is also involvement of the uncrossed fibers from the macular region of the same eye. Commonly, visual field loss is greater in one eye, owing to a predominantly lateral involvement of the chiasm as the tumor mass extends upward asymmetrically. The compromise of vision from compression of the chiasm probably arises in part from vascular impairment.[3,6] The vessels that supply the chiasm arise from the arteries of the circle of Willis, most of which enter the chiasm from its ventral side.

Lesions impinging on the posterior chiasm may result in *bitemporal hemianopic* scotomas owing to macular-fiber involvement. Visual acuity remains normal in such cases unless the adjacent optic nerve is also affected, resulting in disturbance of nasal macular fibers. Occasionally, monocular visual deficits occur with compression of the chiasm or optic nerves.[17] Most often they occur as a superior temporal defect.

Chiasm lesions occasionally produce a *central unilateral scotoma* that may be confused with that caused by papillitis or retrobulbar neuritis (Fig.

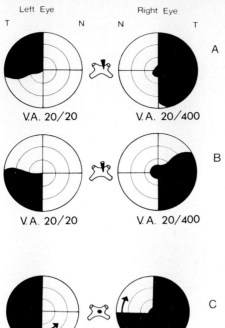

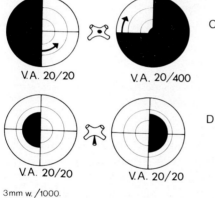

FIGURE 3. Types of bitemporal field defects are illustrated here. (A) Central visual fields of a lesion anterior and inferior to chiasm with compression of the optic nerve. (B) Lesion located anterior and superior to the chiasm, affecting predominantly the right side. (C) Progressive lesion inferior to the chiasm. (D) Lesion posterior to the chiasm, causing bitemporal hemianopic scotomas. (Adapted from Vaughn, D, Cook, R, Asbury, T: *General Ophthalmology*. Lange Medical Publications, Los Altos, CA, 1974.)

4).[1,11,22] An arcuate defect, common in glaucoma, also may occur.[15] Papilledema rarely occurs and develops only when the tumor extends into the third ventricle and causes obstructive hydrocephalus and increased intracranial pressure.[2,23,24] A large tumor that compresses one optic nerve and also causes increased intracranial pressure may result in pallor of the ipsilateral optic nerve associated with papilledema in the opposite eye (Foster-Kennedy syndrome). A *binasal field* loss rarely may occur as a result of lateral chiasmal compression.

The location of the chiasm in relation to the sella may be important in some cases in determining the extent of visual symptoms. In the majority of cases (approximately 75 percent), the chiasm lies directly over the dorsum sella; in 15 to 20 percent the chiasm lies more anteriorly over the tuberculum sellae (prefixed chiasm); and in a small number (less than 5 percent), it is situated behind the dorsum sellae (postfixed).[4] The position of the chiasm also is important in the transfrontal surgical approach to the sellar region, because a prefixed chiasm limits visualization of the sellar region. The pituitary stalk is always posterior to the chiasm.

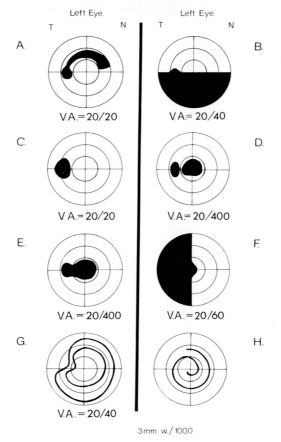

Left Eye   Left Eye

A.   V.A.=20/20

B.   V.A=20/40

C.   V.A.=20/20

D.   V.A.=20/400

E.   V.A.=20/400

F.   V.A.=20/60

G.   V.A.=20/40

H.

3mm w./1000

FIGURE 4. Types of monocular visual field loss in left eye are illustrated here. (A) Superior arcuate scotoma (inferior nerve fiber bundle defect). (B) Inferior altitudinal field defect respecting the horizontal meridian (superior nerve fiber bundle defect). (C) Enlargement of the blind spot in the left eye. (D) Central scotoma, normal blind spot. (E) Centrocecal scotoma. (F) Temporal hemianopsia respecting the vertical meridian but with involvement of central vision. (G) Generalized construction of the visual field to two isopters. (H) Nonorganic "corkscrew" field defect (hysteria, malingering) to one isopter. (Wray, SH: *Neuro-ophthalmology: Visual fields, optic nerve, and pupil.* In Pavan-Langston D (ed): *Manual of Ocular Diagnosis and Therapy.* Boston, Little, Brown & Co. 1980.)

Tumors arising above the stalk lead initially to loss of acuity in the outer, lower quadrants of the visual field. Either suprasellar or infrasellar lesions may cause a combination of total blindness in one eye and an opposite temporal hemianopsia.

In a series of 1000 cases of pituitary adenomas reported by Hollenhorst and Younge[12] from the Mayo Clinic, 421 presented with visual complaints (Tables 1 and 2).

> These were by far the most common neurologic symptoms associated with pituitary tumor. Diplopia was rare (7 cases) and other central nervous system (CNS) signs and symptoms (seizures, dizziness, confusion, subarachnoid hemorrhage) occurred in 24. Diabetes insipidus was a symptom in 10 cases, and cerebrospinal fluid (CSF) rhinorrhea in 5. Headache and complaints referrable to acromegaly were less frequent than visual complaints.

separately, the patient being asked to close his or her eyes and to sniff two or three times, trying to identify the substance. If initial testing suggests a deficit, more careful testing is required using stronger scents, such as oil of wintergreen, cloves, or strawberry extract. Irritative compounds such as ammonia and alcohol are to be avoided because they may stimulate receptors of the fifth cranial nerve to give a false-positive test. Henkin has described more precise methods for testing olfaction; these are important in quantitation of abnormalities of smell such as occur in patients with thyroid or adrenal dysfunction or in hyposmia as occurs in some patients with Kallmann's syndrome.

PINEAL TUMORS

Tumors of the pineal gland or other structures in the posterior region of the third ventricle can result in distinctive clinical manifestations. Pressure on the posterior commissure and superior colliculi causes paralysis of conjugate upward gaze (Parinaud's syndrome), which may be associated with pupillary asymmetry and, rarely, with nystagmus retractoruis, a condition in which the eyes move rhythmically inward and outward on convergence. Pupillary abnormalities with epithalamic lesions result from interruption of pretectal and posterior commissure connections to the oculomotor-nerve nucleus. These pathways subserve the light reflex (pupillary vasostriction). Argyll Robertson pupils (nonreactive to light but reactive to accommodation) may be present. Defects in downward gaze are rare and are associated with lesions of the midbrain tegmentum below the aqueduct, superior and medial to the red neclus.

Compression of the aqueduct of Sylvius results in obstructive hydrocephalus, headaches, vomiting, and papilledema. Pressure on the upper brainstem in advanced cases can result in cerebellar ataxia, pyramidal tract signs (weakness, spasticity, and extensor plantar responses), and coma.

OTHER NEUROLOGIC MANIFESTATIONS

Lateral extension of pituitary tumors into the medial part of the temporal lobe may result in seizures, often with gustatory or olfactory auras. Lateral extension into the internal capsule may cause hemiplegia. Hypothalamic lesions rarely occur with disorders of temperature regulation, abnormal emotionality, altered thirst, and appetite, or changes in the level of consciousness (for detailed discussion see chapters 4 and 11).

VISUAL EVOKED RESPONSES

Visual evoked responses (VER's) are measured by presenting patterned visual stimuli at various frequencies and, with the use of computer averaging, determining the responses arising from the visual cortex.[7] Intrinsic lesions of the optic nerves due to demyelination are detected easily. Abnormal VER's also may occur after compression of the optic pathways, but the changes are less reliable and less often abnormal. Compression tends to produce distortion of the VER waveforms with loss of amplitude but minimal or no changes in latency. Rapid reappearance of an absent VER can occur after surgical relief of a compressive lesion.

REFERENCES

1. ASBURY, T: *Unilateral scotoma as the presenting sign of pituitary tumor.* Am J Ophthalmol 59:510, 1965.
2. BATZDORF, U, AND STERN, WE: *Clinical manifestations of pituitary adenomas: A pilot study using computer analysis.* In KOHLER, PO, AND ROSS, GT (EDS): *Diagnosis and Treatment of Pituitary Tumors.* Excerpta Medica, Amsterdam, 1973, pp 17–35.
3. BERGLAND, R, AND RAY, BS: *The arterial supply of the human optic chiasm.* J Neurosurg 31:327, 1969.
4. BERGLAND, RM, RAY, BS, TORACK, RM: *Anatomical variations in the pituitary gland and adjacent structures in 225 human autopsy cases.* J Neurosurg 28:93, 1968.
5. BLOCH, HJ, AND JOPLIN, GF: *Some aspects of the radiological anatomy of the pituitary gland and its relationship to surrounding structures.* Br J Radiol 32:527, 1959.
6. BOGHEN, DR, AND GLASER, JS: *Ischemic optic neuropathy—the clinical profile and natural history.* Brain 98:689, 1975.
7. CHIAPPA, K: *Pattern-shift visual evoked potentials: Interpretation.* In *Evoked Potentials in Clinical Medicine.* Raven, New York, 1983 p. 80–81.
8. COGAN, DG: *Neurology of the visual system.* Charles C Thomas, Springfield, IL, 1966.
9. CUSHING, H: *The chiasmal syndrome of primary optic atrophy and bitemporal field defects in adults with a normal sella turcica.* Arch Ophthalmol 3:505–551, 704–735, 1930.
10. GITTINGER, JW: *Ophthalmological evaluation of pituitary adenomas.* In POST, KD, JACKSON, IMD, REICHLIN, S, (EDS): *The Pituitary Adenoma.* Plenum, New York, 1980, pp 259–283.
11. HOLLENHORST, RW, SVIEN, HJ, BENOIT, CF: *Unilateral blindness occurring during anesthesia for neurosurgical operation.* Arch Ophthalmol 52:819, 1954.
12. HOLLENHORST, RW, AND YOUNGE, BR: *Ocular manifestations produced by adenomas of the pituitary gland: Analysis of 1000 cases.* In KOHLER, PO, AND ROSS GT (EDS): *Diagnosis and Treatment of Pituitary Tumors.* Excerpta Medica, Amsterdam, 1973, p 53.
13. HOLMES SELLORS, PJ: *Visual abnormalities in pituitary tumors.* In JENKINS, JS (ED): *Pituitary Tumors.* Butterworth, Boston, 1972, p 106.
14. HOYT, WF: *Correlative anatomy of the optic chiasm—1969.* Clin Neurosurg 17:189, 1970.
15. KEARNS, TP, AND RUCKER, CW: *Arcuate defects in the visual fields due to chromophobe adenomas of the pituitary gland.* Am J Ophthalmol 45:505, 1958.
16. KIRKHAM, TH: *The ocular symptomatology of pituitary tumors.* Proc R Soc Med 65:517, 1972.
17. KNIGHT, CL, HOYT, WF, WILSON, CB: *Syndrome of incipient prechiasmal optic nerve compression.* Arch Ophthalmol 81:1, 1972.
18. LYLE, TK AND CLOVER, P: *Ocular symptoms and signs in pituitary tumors.* Proc R Soc Med 54:611, 1961.
19. NEETENS, A, AND SELOSSE, P: *Oculomotor anomalies in sellar and parasellar pathology.* Ophthalmologica 175:80, 1977.
20. ROBERT, CM, JR, FEIGENBAUM, JA, STERN, WE: *Ocular palsy occurring with pituitary tumors.* J Neurosurg 38:17, 1973.
21. SCHAEFFER, JP: *Some points in the regional anatomy of the optic pathway, with especial reference to tumors of the hypophysis cerebri and resulting ocular changes.* Anat Rec 28:243, 1924.
22. SUGITA, K, SATO, O, HIROTA, T, TSUGANE, R, KAGEYAMA, N: *Scotomatous defects in the central visual fields in pituitary adenomas.* Neurochirurgica 18:155, 1975.
23. TSO, MOM, AND FINE, BS: *Electron microscopic study of papilledema in man.* Am J Ophthalmol 82:424, 1976.
24. TSO, MOM, AND HAYREH, SS: *Optic disc edema in raised intracranial pressure. III. A pathologic study of experimental papilledema.* Arch Ophthalmol 95:1448, 1977.
25. WEINBERGER, LM, ADEN, FH, GRANT, FC: *Primary pituitary adenoma and the syndrome of the cavernous sinus: A clinical and anatomic study.* Arch Ophthalmol 24:1197, 1940.
26. WELCH, K, AND STEARS, JC: *Chiasmapexy for the correction of traction on the optic nerves and chiasm associated with their descent into an empty sella turcia—case report.* J Neurosurg 35:760, 1971.
27. WRAY, SH: *Neuro-ophthalmologic manifestations of pituitary and parasellar lesions.* Clin Neurosurg 24:86, 1977.
28. WRAY, SH: *The neuro-ophthalmic and neurologic manifestations of pinealomas.* In SCHMIDEK, H (ED): *Pineal Tumors.* Masson, New York, 1977, p 21.
29. WRAY, SH: *Neuro-ophthalmologic diseases.* In ROSENBERG, R (ED): *The Clinical Neurosciences,* vol 3. Churchill, New York, 1984.

Chapter 14

HYPOTHALAMIC-PITUITARY DISORDERS: RADIOLOGIC ASSESSMENT

Major advances have occurred in the radiologic evaluation of lesions in sellar and parasellar locations. High resolution computerized axial tomography (CAT) scans, which are now widely available, combined with multiplanar, thin-slice techniques make possible, after administration of contrast material, the detailed visualization of the median eminence, pituitary stalk, and the superior margin of the pituitary gland.[63,64] The optic chiasm, optic nerves, and optic tracts are usually seen. The introduction of metrizamide into the cerebrospinal fluid (CSF) pathway permits more precise delineation of anatomic structures in the suprasellar region. More recently the application of nuclear magnetic resonance imaging (MRI), in which bone contrast disappears, has provided an additional sensitive radiologic imaging technique for visualization of the hypothalamic-pituitary region.

RADIOLOGIC ASSESSMENT

Radiologic assessment of the skull formerly was considered important in all patients with suspected hypothalamic-pituitary disorders, unexplained visual disturbance, optic atrophy, or diplopia.[50] Anteroposterior and lateral views of the skull were screened for evidence of calcification, increased intracranial pressure, and focal erosions in the region of the sella turcica. Views of the optic canal were important if glioma of the optic nerve was considered. Complete examination of the sella turcica, particularly in suspected cases of microadenomas of the pituitary gland, now requires CAT scans, which have largely replaced plain radiographs of the skull for assessment of most intracranial lesions. A consideration of the standard radiologic features of the sella turcica is important for historical purposes and because the assessment remains an appropriate one if fourth generation CAT scans are not available.

Sella Turcica

The outline and landmarks of the sella turcica are illustrated in Figure 1. The normal sella turcica, as seen on lateral projection, consists of the posterior part of the planum sphenoidale, the tuberculum sellae, the anterior clinoid processes, the floor, and the dorsum sellae; the latter includes the

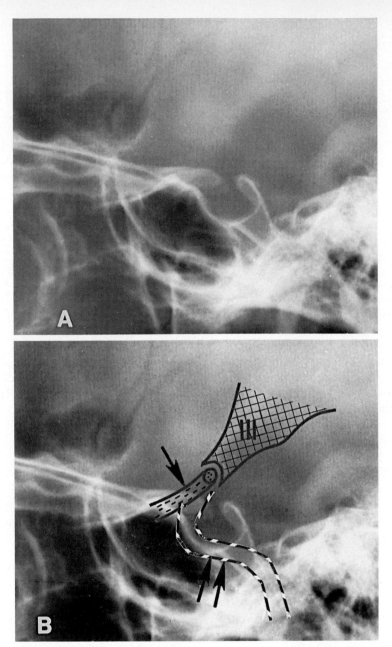

FIGURE 1. *(A)* Radiologic view of the normal sella in lateral projection. *(B)* Lateral view of the sella turcica indicating carotid artery *(double arrows)*, optic nerve *(single arrow)*, and anterior third ventricle *(III)*.

posterior clinoid processes and the adjacent part of the sphenoid and occipital bone that form the clivus (Fig. 2).

Size

The profile of the sella may be oval, round, or flat. A small sella turcica usually has no clinical significance, although long-standing pituitary insufficiency occasionally may result in a small fossa. Enlargement of the sella is an important finding and requires careful delineation of the cause.[36,37] The anteroposterior diameter of the sella, determined by measuring the maximum distance from the anterior concavity of the sella to the anterior rim of the dorsum sellae, varies from 5 to 16 mm, with an average of 10.5 mm. The depth of the pituitary fossa is measured as the greatest distance from the floor to a perpendicular line drawn between the tuberculum sellae and the top of the dorsum sellae. The upper limit is usually stated as 13 mm. The width of the sella is determined in films taken in an anteroposterior projection by calculating the distance across the floor of the sella, which can be seen as a thin, horizontal plate of bone approximately 1 cm below the anterior clinoid processes. The normal width varies from 10 to 15 mm. In a series of 100 normal sellae, Mahomoud[32] calculated the area of the sella by planimetry as visualized on lateral projection. The range was 22 to 130 mm.[3] In 45 of 49 patients with pituitary tumors, the area was 130 to 823 mm; four patients had sellae measurements slightly below 130 mm.[3]

The volume of the sella can be calculated using a formula derived by Di Chiro and coworkers.[13,14] Anteroposterior, depth, and width measurements are multiplied and then divided by two. The volume of the sella was considered to be abnormal when it exceeded 1092 mm; the mean volume was 594 mm. In practice there is considerable variation, and one cannot always decide with certainty whether a particular sella is enlarged or not.[3] In general, changes in contour or asymmetry, demineralization, and local erosions or resorption are more reliable indicators of intrasellar disease.

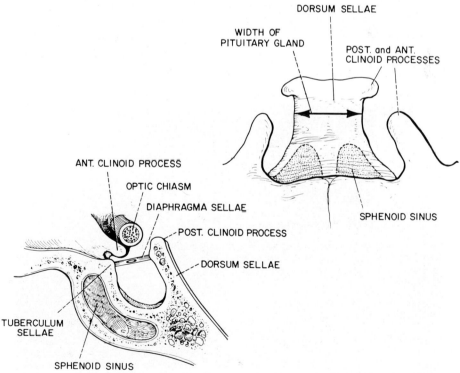

FIGURE 2. Radiologic landmarks of the sella turcica projected in lateral *(left)* and anteroposterior planes *(right)*.

RADIOLOGIC ASSESSMENT 459

Calcification

Calcification of sellar or extrasellar contents may occur normally, particularly in an elderly subject. A curved arch of calcification evident in the sella on lateral view often is due to calcification in the internal carotid artery (Fig. 3). A line of calcification extending posteriolaterally from the dorsum sella is a normal finding, the consequence of calcification in the petroclinoid ligaments. Occasionally, one may see bridging of the anterior and posterior clinoid processes by a linear line of calcification along the intraclinoid ligaments. Craniopharyngiomas (60 to 70 percent) and meningiomas (30 percent) are commonly calcified; pituitary adenomas are rarely calcified, but both chromophobe and prolactin-secreting tumors have been reported to show calcification.

Causes of Enlargement

The sella may be enlarged secondary to increased pituitary size, increased intracranial pressure, defective diaphragm (empty sella), or erosion caused by extrasellar structures.[37,38] Long-standing hypothyroidism also can cause enlargement of the pituitary fossa owing to secondary pituitary enlargement. Common intrasellar lesions are pituitary adenomas, craniopharyngiomas, and pituitary cysts. Rarely, tumors of the nasopharynx extend superiorly into the sella. Parasellar lesions may mimic intrasellar tumors and therefore must be considered in the differential diagnosis. Aneurysms of the internal carotid artery arising in the cavernous sinus or at the origin of the anterior cerebral artery may cause lateral erosion and enlargement of the sella turcica.[5,7] Radiologic findings in this condition may resemble in every respect an enlarging asymmetric pituitary tumor and can be distinguished only by CAT scan with contrast or carotid angiography.

Chronic increased intracranial pressure rarely may lead to sellar en-

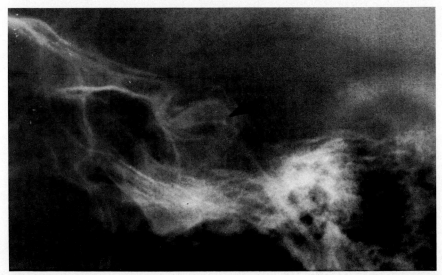

FIGURE 3. Calcification of an intracavernous portion of the internal carotid artery *(arrow)*. The artery is tortuous and displaced upward.

TABLE 1. Common Tumors of the Sellar Region

Intrasellar tumors	Anterior suprasellar tumors
Adenomas	Meningiomas
Craniopharyngiomas	Optic gliomas
Meningioma	Posterior suprasellar tumors
Pituitary cyst	Adenoma
Glioma	Meningioma
Suprasellar tumors	Craniopharyngioma
Adenomas	Chordmas
Craniopharyngioma	Epidermoid cysts
Ependymoma	Intraventricular tumors
Hamartoma-infundibuloma	Colloid cyst
Glioma	Arachnoid cyst
Teratoma-germinoma, ectopic pinealoma	Papilloma
Meningioma	Astrocytoma
Arachnoid cysts	Craniopharyngioma

largement. More commonly enlargement occurs without increased intracranial pressure, as a result of extension of the subarachnoid space through a defective diaphragma sellae (primary empty-sella syndrome). It is believed that continued pulsations within the subarachnoid space transmit hydraulic forces which remodel the bone and eventually enlarge the sella. Although the pituitary gland is compressed into a rim of tissue around the wall of the sella, function usually remains surprisingly normal (see chapter 17). By conventional roentgenography, one cannot distinguish an enlarged sella turcica caused by an intrasellar lesion from an empty-sella syndrome. This differentiation often can be made definitively with a CAT scan or an MRI study. In many cases, the CAT scan is diagnostic, especially if the infundibulum can be traced to the floor of the sella (infundibular sign), but we have seen a case in which the CAT scan failed to detect the empty sella, and a pituitary cyst was erroneously labeled an empty sella. Empty sella occurs in association with benign intracranial hypertension (pseudotumor cerebri) in about 15 percent of cases (see chapter 17). Rarely, intrasellar extension of a suprasellar or tuberculum sellae meningioma may give the appearance of an enlarged pituitary fossa. Common tumors of the sella and parasellar region are summarized in Table 1.

    Intrasellar tumors typically produce an asymmetric ballooning of the sella, with undercutting of the clinoid processes either anteriorly or posteriorly.[28,32] Microadenomas may cause asymmetric focal erosion of the floor of the sella, which may be evident only on lateral or anteroposterior tomography. With experience gained from transsphenoidal surgery, it is now evident that microadenomas as small as 3 to 5 mm in diameter can cause erosion of the floor. Although this sign is of particular importance in the diagnosis of prolactin- or ACTH-secreting microadenomas, many instances are reported of *false-positives*, that is, an erosion present that does not correspond to the site of the microadenoma at surgery or *false-negatives*, normal tomography with adenomas found at surgery.

Radiologic Signs of Increased Intracranial Pressure

The earliest detectable radiologic sign of increased intracranial pressure is erosion of the anterior aspect of the dorsum sellae; the cortical bone on the inside of the fossa becomes thin and indistinct. This is followed by atrophy of the superior margins of the posterior clinoid processes. Long-standing increases in intracranial pressure result in complete loss of the tips of the posterior clinoids. By this time, changes are usually evident in the floor of the fossa, with thinning of the cortical bone; this is often followed by enlargement of the pituitary fossa. Eventually, atrophic changes can occur also in the anterior clinoid processes.

COMPUTERIZED AXIAL TOMOGRAPHY SCANS OF THE HYPOTHALAMIC-PITUITARY REGION

The advent of sellar tomography combined with pluridirectional CAT scanning has revolutionized the identification, followup, and management of pituitary adenomas and of other lesions of the hypothalamic-pituitary axis. Pneumoencephalography is now rarely undertaken.[63,64] Instillation of a water-soluble contrast agent like metrizamide into the lumbar CSF can be maneuvered into the suprasellar cistern. Computerized axial tomography scans in combination with metrizamide allow precise anatomic study of the optic chiasm, medial basal hypothalamus, infundibular stem, and the superior aspect of the pituitary gland.

The CAT scan after administration of intravenous contrast material provides visualization of the normal pituitary gland, suprasellar region, third ventricle, and retrochiasmatic region.[23] The contrast-enhanced infundibular stalk often can be identified in the coronal or horizontal plane. Microadenoma greater than 5 mm in diameter may be identified as either

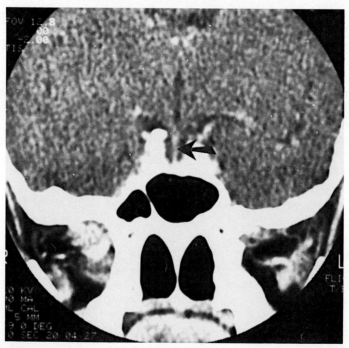

FIGURE 4. This is a contrast-enhanced coronal CAT scan showing partially empty sella. The normal enhancement of the infundibulum and pituitary stalk is evident (arrow). The third ventricle is seen above the infundibulum.

HYPOTHALAMIC-PITUITARY DISEASE

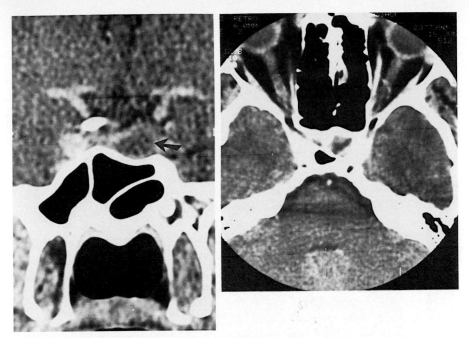

FIGURE 5. This is a pituitary macroadenoma demonstrating nonenhancement after administration of intravenous contrast material. *(Left)* Coronal CAT showing asymmetry of sellar floor, and round mass indicative of adenoma *(arrow)*. *(Right)* Horizontal CAT scan showing position of tumor.

contrast-enhanced or low-density defects in the pituitary gland (see below). Sellar enlargement, an empty (CSF-containing) sella (Fig. 4), a suprasellar extension of tumor (Fig. 5), and cavernous sinus invasion are commonly readily visible on coronal or horizontal thin sections (Fig. 6).

A few investigators have examined pituitary adenomas 3 to 4 hours after contrast administration. Lesions that initially are low density may become enhanced. It remains uncertain whether this technique will improve the identification of small adenomas.

Recently Wolpert[64] reviewed the radiologic characteristics of pituitary adenomas. The following description of the utility of high-resolution coronal CAT scanning is a summary of his observations.

RADIOLOGIC ANATOMY OF CORONAL CAT SCANS

Vascular Structures

The internal carotid arteries, the proximal anterior cerebral arteries, the basilar artery, the pituitary gland, the infundibulum, and the cavernous sinuses can be seen. Pituitary lesions may show less than normal enhancement or none at all.[59]

Gland Density

The density of the normal pituitary gland usually appears similar to the cavernous sinuses. The gland is more or less homogeneous in density; care

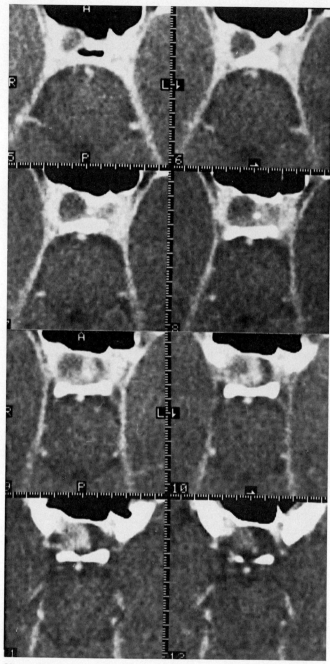

FIGURE 6. Shown here is a contrast-enhanced pituitary prolactinoma. These eight consecutive 1 mm CAT sections in horizontal plane demonstrate macroadenoma.

must be taken not to mistake image noise caused by CAT artifact for heterogeneity or cystic change in the pituitary.

Low-Density Areas (Simulation of Microadenoma)

Originally, the hallmark of a pituitary microadenoma (a tumor 10 mm or less in diameter) was thought to be a low-density cystic area within the gland.[58] However, neuroepithelial, Rathke cleft, adenomatous, and arachnoid cysts may mimic a tumor.[56,58] In one autopsy series, pituitary cysts measuring 1 to 6 mm in diameter were seen in 18 of 205 (8.7 percent) specimens.[40] In another autopsy series of 100 cases, 14 had microadenoma; 6, pars intermedia cysts; 4, metastases; and 3, pituitary infarcts.[9] A review of the past history available in 80 of these 100 patients revealed no clinical signs or symptoms of pituitary disease.

Wolpert notes the importance of silent microadenomas. "That a microadenoma may exist silently in the general population has been known for a number of years. The incidence of such microadenomas varies between 8.5 percent and 27 percent.[8,10,30,35,43] with 40 to 50 percent of the tumors being prolactinoma as determined by immunohistochemical techniques.[8,30] The majority of these tumors occur in the sixth and seventh decades, without sex predominance."

These observations point to the fact that there are many potential causes for a low-density area within the pituitary gland, including microadenoma. In Wolpert's own series of 107 women ages 18 to 65 who were referred for suspected intracranial lesions other than pituitary tumor, a low-density area measuring 3 mm or more in diameter was seen in 7 patients.[62] In another series of 50 pituitary scans performed for orbital symptoms, there were 10 low-density areas 3 mm in diameter or larger.[9] Thus the specific diagnosis of a tumor can be very difficult.

A low-density area also may be due to an empty sella.[51] These are usually readily diagnosable if the infundibulum extends to the floor of the sellar.[24] Adenomas have been reported to coexist with an empty sella.[15,39,55]

High-Density Areas

High-density areas also may occur within the normal sella. Tortuous intracavernous carotid arteries and transsellar communicating channels between the carotid arteries may exist. Indentation of the lateral aspect of the pituitary gland by a carotid artery was found in 14 of 50 cadaver specimens.[48] Intrasellar venous communications between the cavernous sinuses are common. The density of the pituitary gland also may vary on different examinations, so that comparison studies are difficult to evaluate.

Gland Height

Wolpert emphasizes the importance of assessing the height of the pituitary gland. "Because the border between the pituitary gland and the cavernous sinus is poorly defined, increase in size is best determined by assessing the height of the gland. . . . Ideally the height of the gland should be measured at right angles to the diaphragma sellae, but this may require an unobtainable degree of neck hyperextension.

"The height of the normal gland, as measured by CT in 20 normal patients in one series, was reported as not exceeding 7 mm in females and 6 mm in males.[58] A mean height of 5.3 ± 1.7 mm was found in 50 normal patients in another series.[9] According to Cusick et al,[11] a gland height in excess of 9 mm is abnormal, an opinion also close to that of Swartz et al,[57] who found the height of the gland in 50 normal females age 18-35 to range between 5.4 and 9.7 mm."

In Wolpert's own studies of 107 asymptomatic women, ages 18 to 65, with no signs or symptoms of pituitary disease, two patients had a gland height of 9 mm, and eight had a gland height of 8 mm, as measured by direct coronal CAT.[62] Both patients with 9 mm gland height (ages 21 and 65) had a normal serum prolactin level. The possibility of an asymptomatic tumor being present in these two patients could not be excluded. The gland height varied with age, being larger in younger patients. The normal height reported in cadavers varies from 5 to 9 mm.[9,38]

The normal pituitary gland varies in weight between 450 and 900 mg in women and between 350 and 800 mg in men.[46] Weight increases progressively during pregnancy and with multiparity. The superior surface of the gland is usually flat or concave but may be convex.[9,40] The superior surface bulged upward in 19 of Wolpert's 107 asymptomatic female patients,[62] more frequently with the larger glands. The superior surface may be dented if the carotid siphons are relatively close together.[46,47,48] A small bulge is often present at the point of insertion of the infundibulum on the pituitary.

Infundibulum

The infundibulum should be seen in almost all normal patients (see Figure 4) extending between the pituitary gland and the infundibular recess of the third ventricle. It is best seen on the more posterior scans because it most often lies immediately anterior to the dorsum sellae. The infundibulum is usually midline, but it may be slightly off center in some normal cases.

Cavernous Sinus

The cranial nerves can be seen as filling defects in the lateral wall of the enhanced cavernous sinus. The anatomic relations of this region are shown in Figure 2 and in Figure 1, chapter 13. The III and IV cranial nerves are seen lying superolaterally between the two folds of dura that form the lateral walls of the cavernous signs. The first and second divisions of the V nerve are positioned slightly inferiorly in the same dural plane. The third division of nerve V does not lie within the cavernous sinus; it extends forward from Meckel's cave below the sinus. Nerve VI is rarely seen within the cavernous sinus. Because the lateral wall of the cavernous sinus is usually straight, a lateral bulge suggests a pituitary mass[29] or lesion within the cavernous sinus.

HYPOTHALAMIC-PITUITARY DISEASE

Suprasellar Structures

The chiasmatic cistern is seen as a low-density area immediately above the sella. The optic chiasm is visible on coronal scans but can be better defined on axial scans using thicker sections (4 or 5 mm), or after metrizamide instillation. The anteroinferior third ventricle is seen above the optic chiasm. The interpeduncular cistern is seen behind and above the dorsum, extending superiorly to the hypothalamus. The apex of the basilar artery also can be defined.

Sellar Floor and Subsellar Structures

With direct coronal CAT scanning, details of both the pituitary gland and the bony floor of the sella are visualized on the same cut. An abnormality of the sellar floor adjacent to a pituitary adenoma is helpful in making a tumor diagnosis. However, false-positive results may occur; a pituitary adenoma may lie at some distance from an area of cortical thinning or a depressed sellar floor.[8,40,60]

The sphenoid sinus and its septa are seen inferiorly. Knowledge of the anatomy of the septa is important prior to transsphenoidal adenomectomy.

Axial CAT Scanning

If the patient cannot tolerate the hyperextended head position, axial scanning may be necessary. Sagittal reconstruction of axial images can also provide excellent detail of the suprasellar structures.

Metrizamide Suprasellar CAT Cisternography

Intracisternal metrizamide in conjunction with axial or direct coronal CAT scans provides an excellent visualization of the optic chiasm and adjacent vascular structures (Fig. 7).[16,53] Only 3.5 to 5 ml of dilute metrizamide (170 mg iodine per ml) is necessary.[21]

Magnetic Resonance Imaging (MRI)

The application of MRI to defining pituitary and juxtapituitary tumors has evolved rapidly (Figs. 8, 9).[25] The normal pituitary gland is contrasted against the bright bone marrow and air within the basisphenoid. The multiplanar facility of MRI shows sagittal, coronal, and axial images of tumors without the need for the neck hyperextension required for CAT. Another attractive feature of MRI is its ability to demonstrate parasellar aneurysm when blood-flow-dependent MRI sequences are used. It is likely that thinner high-resolution MRI sections will provide data to rival and to surpass those of CAT scans.

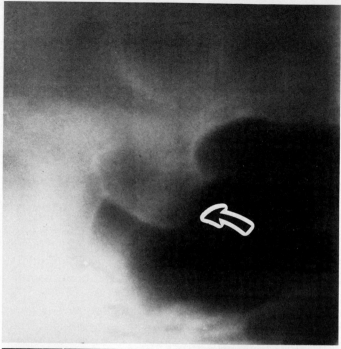

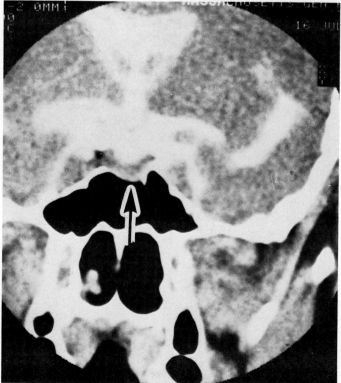

FIGURE 7. Metrizamide cisternography demonstrating partial filling of pituitary fossa in a patient with acromegaly. *(Top)* Lateral skull x-ray showing ballooning of pituitary fossa with thinning of sellar floor *(arrow)*. Metrizamide fills suprasellar cistern. *(Bottom)* Coronal CAT showing metrizamide within suprasellar cistern and within upper pituitary fossa. Thinning of sellar floor is also evident *(arrow)*.

HYPOTHALAMIC-PITUITARY DISEASE

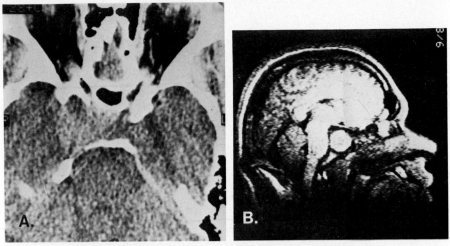

FIGURE 8. CAT scan and MRI of pituitary adenoma. *(A)* CAT scan without contrast showing R pituitary mass extending into cavernous sinus. Erosion of sellar bony landmarks is apparent. *(B)* MRI of massive prolactinoma in 51-year-old man complaining of decreased libido.

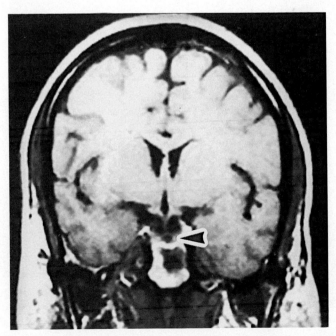

FIGURE 9. This is a high-resolution MRI showing details of third ventricle, median eminence, and pituitary stalk. A low-density microadenoma is visualized in the inferior region of the sella *(arrow)*.

RADIOLOGIC ASSESSMENT

469

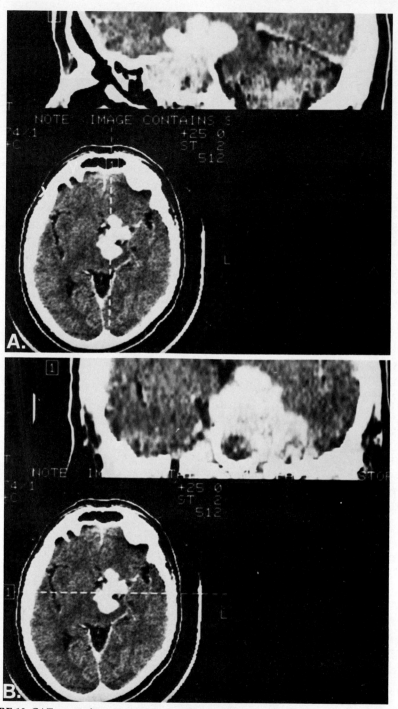

FIGURE 10. CAT scans after contrast administration in patient with invasive macroadenoma. *(A)* Combined horizontal *(lower)* and sagittal *(upper)* projections to show extent of left lateral and suprasellar extension of tumor. *(B)* Combined horizontal *(lower)* and coronal *(upper)* projections of same tumor. Extensive invasion of left cavernous sinus is evident.

HYPOTHALAMIC-PITUITARY DISEASE

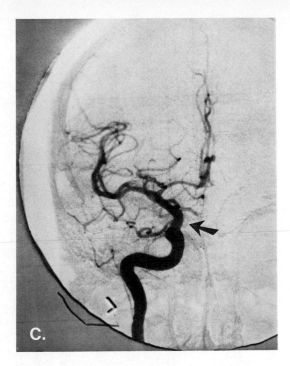

FIGURE 10 *(continued). (C)* Left carotid angiogram showing lateral displacement *(arrow)* of intracavernous portion of internal carotid artery.

RADIOLOGY OF SECRETORY ADENOMAS

PROLACTINOMA

Wolpert's experience with pituitary tumors is extensive. "Most prolactinomas appear as a low density or even cystic lesions (see Figure 5).[6,11,26,59] Since pituitary gland enhancement parallels the blood iodine level, it is advisable to scan patients as the iodine-containing contrast medium is being administered in order to 'highlight' the prolactinoma. The infundibulum is often displaced by the tumor but this is not a reliable sign, since it may normally be off the midline. It is important to view the scans with both soft tissue and bone techniques. Thinning and depression of the sellar floor are strong confirmatory indications of a pituitary adenoma if the bony changes are contiguous with the soft tissue tumor.[59]

"Not all prolactinomas are of a low density, however. Gardeur et al[20] described focal hypodensity in 12 and focal hyperdensity in 15 of 63 prolactinomas. Unfortunately, surgical proof was not available in all their patients. Sakoda et al[52] found that 25 surgically proven adenomas showed enhancement, and that small zones of decreased attenuation found in 4 of them represented cystic degeneration or necrosis within tumor." Certain signs appear to be reliable in determining the presence of a tumor in a patient with hyperprolactinomia. A gland height of 10 mm or more is highly suggestive. If the gland height is under 10 mm, the combination of a low-density focal area at least 3 mm in diameter, asymmetrically situated in the gland, and associated with an asymmetrical bulge in the superior margin of the gland is also reliable.

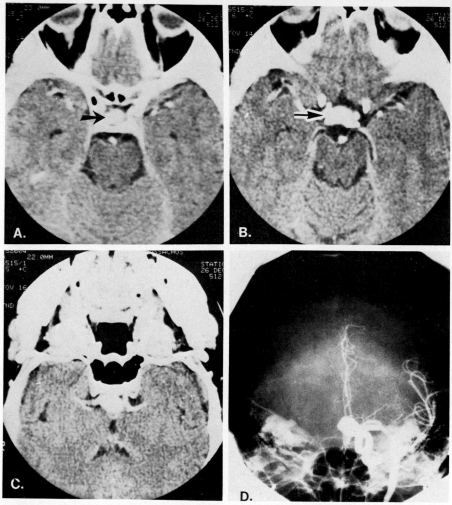

FIGURE 11. These are radiologic studies of a carotid aneurysm that mimics intrasellar tumor. *(A, B)* Contrast-enhanced intrasellar mass *(arrow)*. *(C)* Coronal view of densely enhanced intrasellar mass. *(D)* Anterior view of aneurysm after right carotid angiogram.

ACTH-producing Tumors

There is little information in the literature about the enhancement pattern of ACTH tumors. Both hyperdense and hypodense ACTH-secreting adenomas were reported in one study.[61] These tumors were usually but not invariably hypodense in another series.[26] Suprasellar extension may occur.

Acromegaly

Because patients with GH-secreting tumors present clinically with acromegaly, plain skull radiographs often establish the diagnosis. Excessive growth of the skeletal tissue is manifested by thickening of the skull vault, increased bone density, and enlargement of the paranasal sinuses and mastoid air cells. If sellar enlargement and prognathism accompany these

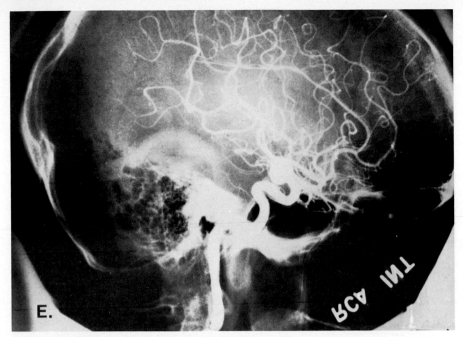

FIGURE 11 *(continued). (E)* Lateral view of aneurysm.

skull changes, the diagnosis is established. No consistent enhancement pattern has been described with GH-secreting tumors.

Acromegalic patients often present when the disease is well advanced and sellar enlargement and erosion are prominent (see Figure 7).

PITUITARY APOPLEXY

Several lesions may be seen. A sellar or suprasellar mass containing a high-density area indicates hemorrhage. An area of mottled, mixed density is commonly seen within a tumor.[17,44] Occasionally a fluid-blood density level is visualized in the suprasellar mass.[19]

NONSECRETORY ADENOMAS

Patients with nonsecretory adenomas often first present with a large tumor that has grown out of the sella or into the cavernous sinus (Fig. 10). The tumor usually is homogeneous after contrast enhancement, although, occasionally, ring enhancement may be seen.[31]

CALCIFICATION

Calcification may be detected in either nonsecreting or secreting adenomas. In one series[49] it was seen histologically in 4 and radiologically in 2 of 132 tumors (about 5 percent). When calcification is present within a nonsecreting adenoma, distinction from a craniopharyngioma, hypothalamic glioma, and meningioma may be very difficult.[2] If the calcification is curvilinear, an aneurysm should be suspected.

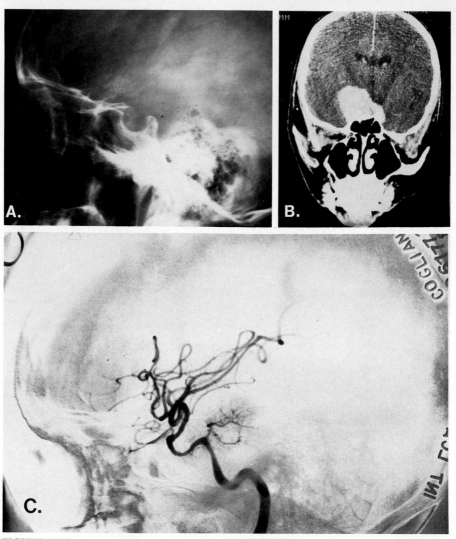

FIGURE 12. These are radiologic findings in a patient with parasellar meningioma. *(A)* Lateral skull x-ray examination showing "moth-eaten" appearance of dorsum sellae and floor of sella. *(B)* Contrast-enhanced coronal CAT scan showing large asymmetric mass in sellar and parasellar region. *(C, D, E)* Sequences of tumor enhancement during left carotid angiogram. *(C)* Early filling.

According to Wolpert, "microscopic calcifications were seen in 51 of a surgical series of 755 pituitary adenomas (6.7 percent) and by plain radiographs and conventional tomography in 13 of these patients (1.7 percent).[49] The majority of the tumors were prolactinomas. There is nothing specific about pituitary calcification, since it can also be physiological[42] ('pituitary stones')." Craniopharyngioma should be the first consideration in a patient with an intrasellar calcification.

DIFFERENTIAL DIAGNOSIS OF PITUITARY ADENOMAS

Parasellar lesions, both neoplastic and nonneoplastic, may mimic adenoma radiologically. Pituitary lesions are best studied by direct coronal scans; and suprasellar lesions, by axial scans 4 to 5 mm thick, with and without

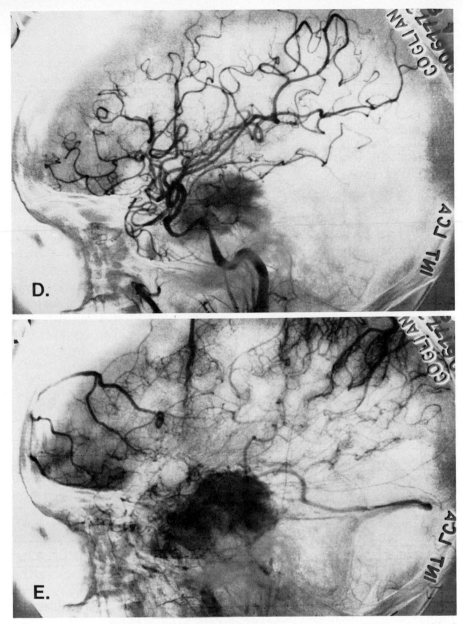

FIGURE 12 *(continued)*. *(D)* Tumor blush during arterial phase of angiogram. *(E)* Dense tumor blush during early venous phase.

enhancement. In the diagnosis of unilateral visual loss, orbital scans parallel to the plane of the optic nerve and canal as well as high bone resolution images utilizing a thin section collimator are indicated.[64]

ANEURYSM

Mistaking an aneurysm in the suprasellar or parasellar area for pituitary adenoma may result in aneurysm rupture during surgery for an anticipated adenoma (see chapter 17)[61] (Fig. 11). Bone destruction together with abnormal calcification, usually curvilinear in configuration, should alert the radiologist to the possibility of an aneurysm. Dynamic CAT can demonstrate the entire aneurysm, including the lumen and clot, during the rapid injection of the contrast medium. The aneurysm may originate from the cavernous portion of the carotid or the circle of Willis. Unfortunately, an aneurysm may coexist with a pituitary adenoma and lead to diagnostic confusion.[27] Acromegalic patients may show ectasia of the cranial vessels and have increased incidence of cerebral artery aneurysms.

TUBERCULUM SELLAE MENINGIOMA

Meningiomas frequently occur in the region of the sella, particularly at the dural attachments (Fig. 12). This tumor may arise from the tuberculum sellae, the diaphragma sellae, the cerebellopontine angle cistern, the cavernous sinus, or the medial sphenoidal ridge and spread as a parasellar mass.[64] An important clue to the diagnosis is the presence of hyperostosis or erosion of the adjacent bone which can be seen in 50 percent of cases by plain films.[13] Calcium may be seen in the lesion on the nonenhanced scan. After contrast administration, meningiomas which are highly vascular enhance in a mottled or homogeneous manner (see Figure 12). The diagnosis can be made preoperatively by angiography using selective internal carotid studies and subtraction, which shows in about a third of the cases a characteristic blush and/or feeding arteries.[64]

CRANIOPHARYNGIOMA

This tumor accounts for about 5 to 10 percent of brain tumors in children (see chapter 17). About 70 percent arise within the sella, and the remainder arise above it.[33] The tumor usually presents as a calcified sellar or suprasellar mass with or without sellar erosion (Figs. 13 and 14). It occurs mostly in the young, but a second peak in incidence occurs in middle age. Calcification is seen more frequently in younger patients (80 percent) than in older ones (50 percent).

Computerized axial tomography scanning is very useful for diagnosis because flocculent or curvilinear calcification is such a frequent finding. Calcification, if seen in conjunction with a low-density cystic midline tumor in a child, is almost pathognomonic of a craniopharyngioma. Enhancement was rare in one series[41] but was seen in 6 of 8 children in another.[18]

HYPOTHALAMIC GLIOMA

Wolpert[64] points out that "hypothalamic glioma and optic nerve glioma should be considered together, because both pathologically and radiologically they may appear almost identical. The hypothalamic glioma often presents clinically in children with the diencephalic syndrome, since it arises in the anterior hypothalamus in the floor of the third ventricle. Because the tumor occurs in the suprasellar area, the suprasellar cistern should be examined with axial or direct coronal scanning. The lesion indents the suprasellar cistern from above and the third ventricle from below.

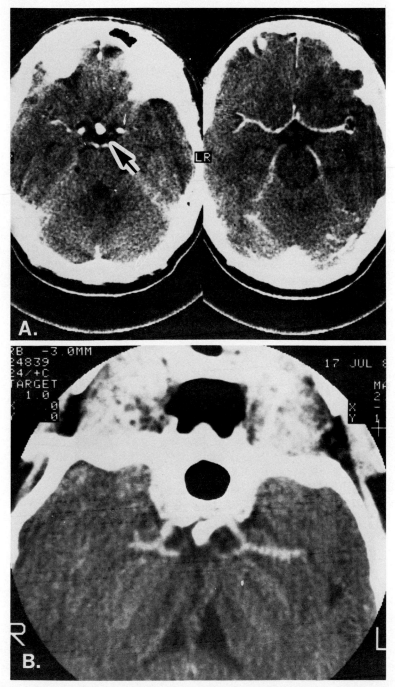

FIGURE 13. Shown here is a calcified intrasellar mass proven at surgery to be craniopharyngioma. *(A)* Horizontal contrast-enhanced CAT scan showing intrasellar dense mass *(arrow)*. *(B)* Coronal projection.

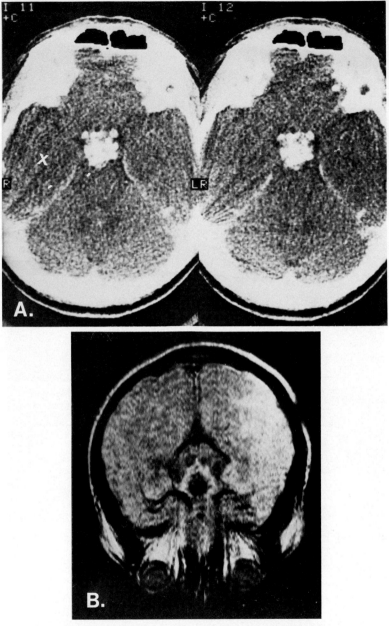

FIGURE 14. These are CAT and MRI scans of a craniopharyngioma. *(A)* Contrast-enhanced CAT scan showing suprasellar cystic, irregular mass. *(B)* Coronal MRI showing cystic suprasellar mass.

It may enhance slightly. Since it may be very small at the time of clinical presentation, metrizamide CAT cisternography may be necessary to make the diagnosis.''

The optic nerve glioma is situated immediately anterior to the hypothalamus and presents with visual loss.[45] Because this is a tumor of childhood and visual loss may not be appreciated in the very young, the lesion may not become evident until it has grown posteriorly to involve the hypothalamus. The association of optic nerve glioma and neurofibromatosis is well known. Skull films may show enlargement of the optic foramen, and this is readily confirmed by thin section high-detail CAT scans of the optic canals. Usually the sella is normal, but there may be undercutting of the anterior clinoid process with deepening of the chiasmatic groove. The tumor is usually isodense on the nonenhanced scan and shows moderate enhancement. Metrizamide cisternography may be of considerable help in the diagnosis.

METASTASIS

Metastases to the pituitary gland may originate from carcinoma of the breast, bronchus, kidney, or colon.[45] In an autopsy series, clinically silent pituitary metastases were seen in 3.6 percent of 500 patients dying from cancer. In the same group, a silent pituitary adenoma was found in 1.8 percent.[34] Radiographically, the sella is enlarged or destroyed, and the lesion generally appears as an enhancing mass. It may be difficult to differentiate metastasis from other causes of sellar enlargement. The diagnosis is usually considered only when the patient presents with a sellar lesion and a known primary tumor.

MISCELLANEOUS

A collection of unrelated lesions, including arachnoid cyst, Rathke cleft cyst, chordoma, atypical teratoma, dermoid, epidermoid, hamartoma, sarcoid granuloma, eosinophilic granuloma, and sphenoid sinus mucocele may cause abnormalities on CAT scan. Cystic lesions such as arachnoid, dermoid, and epidermoid cysts appear as a low-density suprasellar lesion and mimic craniopharyngioma. Chordoma is a destructive lesion of the clivus that usually contains calcium, and sphenoid sinus mucocele is an expanding lesion of the sphenoid sinus with destruction of the floor of the sella. Sarcoid and eosinophilic granulomas may show as nonspecific suprasellar masses and contrast enhancement may occur.

BRAIN SCAN

The radioisotope brain scan now has limited value in the assessment of suprasellar or hypothalamic lesions.[12] Only tumors extending well above the sella can be detected reliably. Radioactive[99m] technetium is the isotope most commonly used, at the recommended dose of approximately 8 to 10 mCi. The half-life of the isotope is 6 hours; as a result, the total dose of body radioactivity is very small (less than 0.13 rad per 10 mCi intravenous dose). Suprasellar chromophobe adenomas, craniopharyngiomas, meningiomas, and teratomas often can be visualized on brain scan. It is commonly positive with tumors in the pineal region. Although the radioisotope brain scan provides a simple, safe, noninvasive preliminary screening test, it is rarely indicated or used. Computerized axial tomography scans have replaced brain scans almost entirely.

CEREBRAL ANGIOGRAPHY

Cerebral angiography of the internal carotid and its branches and of the vertebrobasilar system is accomplished by selective catheterization by the femoral-aortic route. Angiography carries a 1 to 2 percent risk of morbidity associated with transient or permanent neurologic deficit or vascular occlusion. This hazard is substantially increased in elderly patients, in severe atherosclerosis, in diabetes, and in hypertension. Although increasing use of CAT scans has greatly reduced the need for angiography, its use is still advocated to exclude a parasellar or suprasellar aneurysm as a cause of radiographic changes in the sella or parasellar region (see Figure 11); to outline cerebral vessels, in particular the internal carotid and its branches that form the anterior circle of Willis in cases where surgery is envisioned; and to demonstrate lateral displacements of the carotid within the cavernous sinus, inasmuch as this region cannot be visualized adequately by the CAT scan.[1,4] Because of the risk of hemorrhage from an unsuspected aneurysm, angiography is considered by most neurosurgeons to be mandatory when direct surgical intervention is planned by the transfrontal route. Angiography is usually not necessary prior to surgical removal of microadenomas via the transsphenoidal route. Digital subtraction angiography with intravenous dye administration rapidly is replacing direct arterial injections for identifying aneurysms.

REFERENCES

1. BAKER, HL, JR.: *The angiographic delineation of sellar and parasellar masses.* Radiology 104:67, 1972.
2. BANNA, M, BAKER, HL, HOUSER, OW: *Pituitary and parapituitary tumours on computed tomography.* Br J Radiol 53:1123, 1980.
3. BATZDORF, U, AND STERN, WE: *Clinical manifestations of pituitary adenomas: A pilot study using computer analysis.* In KOHLER, PO, AND ROSS, GT (EDS): *Diagnosis and Treatment of Pituitary Tumors.* Elsevier, New York, 1973, p 17.
4. BENTSON, JR: *Relative merits of pneumographic and angiographic procedures in the management of pituitary tumors.* In KOHLER, PO, AND ROSS, GT (EDS): *Diagnosis and Treatment of Pituitary Tumors.* Elsevier, New York, 1973, p 86.
5. BLOCH, HJ, AND JOPLIN, GF: *Some aspects of the radiological anatomy of the pituitary gland and its relationship to surrounding structures.* Br J Radiol 32:527, 1959.
6. BONAFE, A, SOBEL, D, MANELFE, C: *Relative value of computed tomography and hypocycloidal tomography in the diagnosis of pituitary microadenoma. A radio-surgical correlative study.* Neuroradiol 22:133, 1981.
7. BULL, JWD, AND SCHUNK, H: *The significance of displacement of the cavernous portion of the internal carotid artery.* Br J Radiol 35:801, 1962.
8. BURROW, GN, WORTZMAN, G, REWCASTLE, NB, ET AL: *Microadenomas of the pituitary and abnormal sellar tomograms in an unselected autopsy series.* N Engl J Med 304:156, 1981.
9. CHAMBERS, EF, TURSKI, PA, LAMASTERS, D, ET AL: *Regions of low density in the contrast-enhanced pituitary gland: Normal and pathologic processes.* Radiology 144:109, 1982.
10. COSTELLO, RT: *Subclinical adenoma of the pituitary gland.* Am J Pathol 12:205, 1936.
11. CUSICK, JF, HAUGHTON, VM, HAGEN, TC: *Radiological assessment of intrasellar prolactin-secreting tumors.* Neurosurgery 6:376, 1980.
12. DECK, MDF: *Radiographic and radioisotopic techniques in diagnosis of pituitary tumors.* In KOHLER, PO, AND ROSS GT (EDS): *Diagnosis and Treatment of Pituitary Tumors.* Excerpta Medica, Amsterdam 1973, p 71.
13. DICHIRO, G, AND LINDGREN, E: *Bone changes in cases of suprasellar meningiomas.* Acta Radiol 38:133, 1952.
14. DICHIRO, G, AND NELSON, KB: *The volume of the sella turcica.* Am J Roentgenol 87:989, 1962.
15. DOMINGUE, JN, WING, SD, WILSON, CB: *Coexisting pituitary adenomas and partially empty sellas.* J Neurosurg 48:23, 1978.

16. DRAYER, BP, ROSENBAUM, AE, KENNERDELL, JS, ET AL: *Computed tomographic diagnosis of suprasellar masses by intrathecal enhancement.* Radiology 123:339, 1977.

17. EBERSOLD, MJ, LAW, ER, SCHEIHAUER, BW, ET AL: *Pituitary apoplexy treated by transsphenoidal surgery. A clinicopathological and immunocytochemical study.* J Neurosurg 58:315, 1983.

18. FITZ, CR, WORTZMAN, G, HARWOOD-NASH, DC, ET AL: *Computed tomography in craniopharyngiomas,* Radiology 127:687, 1978.

19. FUJIMOTO, M, YOSHINO, E, VEGUCHI, T, ET AL: *Fluid blood density level demonstrated by computerized tomography in pituitary apoplexy. Report of two cases.* J Neurosurg 55:143, 1981.

20. GARDEUR, D, NAIDICH, TP, METZGER, J: *CT analysis of intrasellar pituitary adenomas with emphasis on patterns of contrast enhancement.* Neuroradiology 20:241, 1981.

21. GHOSHHAJRA, K: *High-resolution metrizamide CT cisternography in sellar and suprasellar abnormalities.* J Neurosurg 54:232, 1981.

22. GYLDENSTED, C, AND KARLE, A: *Computed tomography of intra- and juxtasellar lesions.* Neuroradiology 14:5, 1977.

23. HATAM, A, BERGSTROM, M, GREITZ, T: *Diagnosis of sellar and parasellar lesions by computed tomography.* Neuroradiology 18:249, 1979.

24. HAUGHTON, VM, ROSENBAUM, AE, WILLIAMS, AL, ET AL: *Recognizing the empty sella by CT: The infundibulum sign.* AJNR 1:527, 1980.

25. HAWKES, RC, HOLLAND, GN, MOORE, WS, ET AL: *The applications of NMR imaging to the evaluation of pituitary and juxasellar tumors.* AJNR, 1983.

26. HEMMINGHYTT, S, KALKHOFF, RK, DANIELS, DL, ET AL: *Computed tomographic study of hormone-secreting microadenomas.* Radiology 146:65, 1983.

27. JAKUBOWSKI, J, AND KENDALL, B: *Coincidental aneurysms with tumours of pituitary origin.* J Neurol Neurosurg Psychiatr 41:972, 1978.

28. KAUFMAN, B, ET AL: *Radiographic features of intrasellar masses and progressive asymmetrical nontumorous enlargement of the sella turcica, the "empty" sella.* In KOHLER, PO, AND ROSS, GT (EDS): *Diagnosis and Treatment of Pituitary Tumors.* Elsevier, New York, 1973, p 100.

29. KLINE, LB, ACKER, JD, POST, MJD, ET AL: *The cavernous sinus: A computed tomographic study.* AJNR 2:299, 1981.

30. KOVACS, K, RYAN, N, HORVATH, E, ET AL: *Pituitary adenomas in old age.* J Gerontol 35:16, 1980.

31. KUULIALA, I: *Computed axial tomography of pituitary adenomas.* Clin Radiol 1:32, 1981.

32. MAHOMOUD, MS: *The sella in health and disease: Value of the radiographic study of the sella turcica in morbid anatomical and topographic diagnosis of intracranial tumors.* Br J Radiol (Suppl)8:1, 1958.

33. MATSON, D: *Neurosurgery of Infancy and Childhood,* ed 2. Charles C Thomas, Springfield, IL, 1969.

34. MAX, MB, DECK, MDG, ROTTENBERG, DA: *Pituitary metastasis: Incidence in cancer patients and clinical differentiation from pituitary adenoma.* Neurology 31:998, 1981.

35. MCCORMICK, WF, AND HALMI, NS: *Absence of chromophobe adenomas from a large series of pituitary tumors.* Arch Pathol 92:231, 1971.

36. MCLACHLAN, MSF, ET AL: *Estimation of pituitary gland dimensions from radiographs of the sella turcica: a post-mortem study.* Br J Radiol 41:323, 1968.

37. MCLACHLAN, MSF, ET AL: *Applied anatomy of the pituitary gland and fossa: a radiological and histopathological study based on 50 necropsies.* Br J Radiol 41:782, 1968.

38. MCLACHLAN, MSF, WILLIAMS, ED, FORTT, RW, ET AL: *Estimation of pituitary gland dimensions from radiographs of the sella turcica. A post-mortem study.* Br J Radiol 41:323, 1968.

39. MOLITCH, ME, HIESHIMA, GB, MARCOVITZ, S, ET AL: *Coexisting primary empty sella syndrome and acromegaly.* Clin Endocrinol (Oxf) 7:261, 1977.

40. MUHR, C, BERGSTROM, K, GRIMELIUS, L, ET AL: *A parallel study of the roentgen anatomy of the sella turcica and the histopathology of the pituitary gland in 205 autopsy specimens.* Neuroradiology 21:55, 1981.

41. NAIDICH, TP, PINTO, RS, KUSHNER, MJ, ET AL: *Evaluation of sellar and parasellar masses by computed tomography.* Radiology 120:91, 1976.

42. OZANOFF, MB: *Intracranial calcification.* in NEWTON, TH, AND POTTS, DG (EDS): *Radiology of the Skull and Brain,* vol I, book 2, ed 1. CV Mosby, St. Louis, 1971, p 823.

43. PARENT, AD, BEBIN, J, SMITH, RR: *Incidental pituitary adenomas.* J Neurosurg 54:228, 1981.

44. POST, KD: *General considerations in the surgical treatment of pituitary tumors.* In POST, KD, JACKSON, IMD, REICHLIN, S (EDS): *The Pituitary Adenoma.* Plenum, New York, 1980, p 341.

45. POST, KD, AND KASDON, DL: *Sellar and parasellar lesions mimicking adenomas.* In POST, KD, JACKSON, IMD, REICHLIN, S (EDS): *The Pituitary Adenoma.* Plenum, New York, 1980, p 159.

46. RASMUSSEN, AT, cited by BERGLAND, RM, RAY, BS, TORACK, RM: *Anatomical variations in the pituitary gland and adjacent structures in 225 human autopsy cases.* J Neurosurg 28:93, 1968.

47. RENN, WH, AND RHOTON, AL: *Microsurgical anatomy of the sellar region.* J Neurosurg 43:228, 1975.

48. RHOTAN, AL, HARRIS, FS, RENN, WH: *Microsurgical anatomy of the sellar region and cavernous sinus.* Clin Neurosurg 24:54, 1977.

RADIOLOGIC ASSESSMENT   481

TABLE 1. Recommended Routine Endocrine Studies for Evaluation of Endocrine Disturbances in Hypothalamic-Pituitary Disease

I. Acromegaly or Gigantism
  1. Plasma GH levels at rest in fasting state on two or three occasions.
  2. Three-hour glucose suppression test with samples for glucose and GH taken at 0, 15, 30, 60, and 120 minutes.
  3. TRH stimulation test.
  4. Bromocriptine suppression test (2.5 mg single dose sampled at 0, 60, and 120 minutes).
  5. Evaluation of other pituitary hormones.
     a. ACTH-adrenal function
        1. Diurnal cortisol rhythm (8 AM, 4 PM)
        2. ACTH reserve (either insulin tolerance or oral metyrapone test).
     b. Pituitary-thyroid
        1. Plasma TSH, thyroxine (T_4) and triiodothyronine (T_3).
     c. Prolactin
        1. Random serum sample at rest in fasting state, response to TRH
     d. Gonadotropins
        1. Plasma testosterone or estradiol.
        2. LH and FSH.
     e. ADH
        1. If urine volume less than 2000 ml/day and urine gravity of 1.012 or more in overnight specimen, no further tests are indicated. If not, overnight or 12 hr dehydration test (see below).
  6. Serum somatomedin C levels.
II. Galactorrhea or Hyperprolactinemia
  1. Prolactin
     a. Three random samples at rest in fasting state.
     b. If prolactin values over 100 ng/ml, bromocriptine 1.25 or 2.5 mg single dose administration. Plasma samples removed for prolactin determination at 0, 60, and 120 minutes.
  2. Growth hormone
     a. One random sample at rest in fasting state
     b. GH secretory reserve (usually hypoglycemia, or L-dopa, see below).
  3. ACTH-adrenal
     a. Diurnal cortisol rhythm.
     b. ACTH reserve.
  4. Pituitary-thyroid
     a. Plasma TSH, T_4, and T_3.
  5. Gonadotropins
     a. Plasma testosterone or estradiol.
     b. LH and FSH
     c. LHRH Test (rarely helpful).
  6. ADH
     a. If urine volume less than 2000 ml/day, or first AM urine specimen with specific gravity 1.012 or more, no further test indicated.
     NOTE: If CAT scan shows either a microadenoma or no abnormality, it is not usually necessary to test pituitary functions other than GH, estradiol, and testosterone. Macroadenoma or suspected suprasellar lesion requires a full workup.
III. Cushing's Disease
  1. Plasma cortisol, 8 AM and 10 PM.
  2. Twenty-four hour urinary 17-OH corticosteroids or free cortisol (abnormal if greater than 25 mg or 120 μg, respectively).
  3. Plasma ACTH (abnormal if greater than 90 ng/ml.).
  4. a. Low single dose dexamethasone suppression test (1 mg at 11:00 PM; suppression of 8:00 AM cortisol to less than 50% or 5 μg/dl).
     b. Low multiple dose dexamethasone suppression test (0.5 mg q 6 h for two days).
     c. High single dose (8 mg) overnight dexamethasone suppression test to exclude Cushing's syndrome.
     d. High multiple dose (dexamethasone suppression test 2.0 mg q 6 h for two days). Positive suppression excludes most cases of Cushing's disease.
  5. Other pituitary hormones
     a. Basal GH, PRL, TSH, T_4, T_3, testosterone, and estradiol. If normal, no further tests.

TABLE 1. *Continued*

IV. Panhypopituitarism
  1. Growth hormone
    a. Insulin tolerance test (0.05 U/kg b w). Blood sugar must be reduced to 40 mg/dl. or 50% of initial blood sugar or less. Blood samples taken for GH and glucose at 0, 20, 40, and 60 minutes. Test terminated with IV glucose, 10 gm. Test contraindicated in older individuals, those with heart disease or long-standing hypothyroidism or potential for seizures. Patient must be observed to avoid serious problems. If IV insulin test is not feasible, recommend L-dopa test or clonidine test:
    b. L-dopa test, 500 mg p o. Blood samples taken for GH assay at 0, 15, 30, and 60 minutes.
  2. Prolactin
    a. AM sample in resting state.
    b. TRH, 500 μg IV. Blood samples taken at 0, 15, 30, 60, and 90 minutes. Samples at 0 and 30 minutes are usually sufficient.
  3. ACTH-adrenal
    a. Diurnal cortisol rhythm.
    b. ACTH reserve test with either IV insulin or metyrapone.
  4. Pituitary-thyroid
    a. Plasma TSH, T_4, and T_3.
    b. TRH test, 500 μg IV. Blood samples at 0, 15, 30, 60, and 90 minutes. A sample at 0 and 30 minutes is usually sufficient, but in differentiating hypothalamic and pituitary abnormality may require more samples.
  5. Gonadotropins
    a. Plasma testosterone or estradiol.
    b. Serum LH and FSH.
  6. Overnight dehydration test plus vasopressin, if abnormal.

tion of the pituitary gland), and men over the age of 40 have rather meager responses, so that increments of 2 μU/ml, a relatively modest response and one that is barely in the range of most immunoassays, may be seen in normal persons of this age group.

Criteria for abnormality must therefore be adjusted for age and sex. Although the dose of 500 μg given intravenously as a bolus over 30 seconds has been used widely for testing in the United States and Canada, it is likely that a smaller dose given over a somewhat longer time would be equally effective and would have the advantage of producing fewer side effects.

TABLE 2. Normal TSH Responses to TRH

Sex	Dose (μg. IV)	Δ Response (μU/ml)	Investigator
Women	500	>6	Snyder et al[43]
Men			
age <30	500	>6	Snyder et al[43]
age 40–79	500	>2	
Men and women	500	Mean 15(8.5–27.0)*	Fleischer et al[11]
Men and women	25 to 200	>5.9	Sakoda et al[35]
Men	200	3.5 to 15.6	Ormston et al[54,55]
Women	200	6.5 to 20.5	Ormston et al[54,55]
Men	200	3.5 to 15.0	Faglia et al[10]
Women	200	6.0 to 30.0	Faglia et al[10]
Men	200 (60-min infusion)	mean 10.4(6.8–23.3)*	Lundberg and Wide[55]
Women	200 (60-min infusion)	mean 15.7(10.8–23.7)*	Lundberg and Wide[55]
Children (1-10/12 14-3/12)	500	23.3±3.3 SEM	Kaplan et al[67]

*Range of responses

Proper clinical trials in large numbers of patients have not been carried out using this more conservative regimen, and for this reason diagnostic standards do not exist for doses lower than 200 μg. The effects of estrogen priming have not been standardized for clinical testing.

The important side effects of TRH administration are a rise in blood pressure and sense of urinary urgency in about half of the patients.[25] Rare idiosyncratic responses have been observed, including a brief period of unconsciousness in two individuals, with documented absent pulse in one, lasting for only a few moments.[2] There also was one case of pituitary apoplexy following administration of the triple test[1] (see below), which includes GnRH, TRH, and insulin-induced hypoglycemia. (Side effects of TRH are also discussed in chapter 5.)

The TRH test is of greatest value in the differential diagnosis of hyperthyroidism, in patients with high normal or elevated thyroid hormone levels.[43] Suppressed response (increment less than 5 μU/ml in women and men under the age of 40, and increment less than 2 μU/ml in older men) in the absence of pituitary disease is virtually diagnostic of thyrotoxicosis; and if responses exceed these values, thyrotoxicosis can be excluded with a certainty of about 95 percent. Fasting can inhibit the response to TRH.[3]

The use of the TRH test in the differential diagnosis of hypothalamic disease from pituitary disease is somewhat disappointing because hypothyroid patients with intrinsic pituitary disease may have normal responses, and patients with intrinsic hypothalamic disease may have blunted TSH responses to TRH (Tables 3 and 4). These problems came to light early in the study of the usefulness of TRH as a diagnostic agent. In the large series of Snyder and coworkers,[43] 24 of 26 cases with pituitary lesions giving rise to hypothyroidism had blunted responses; but in Faglia and colleagues' series,[10] half had normal responses. In the Abbott Laboratories combined experience with 76 hypothyroid pituitary cases, 60 percent had TSH responses that were less than 2 μU/ml, and an additional 23 percent had responses between 2 and 6 μU/ml. In this series, 17 percent fell within the normal range of responses.

In addition to age and sex differences, the state of GH secretion also may modify responses to TRH. High GH levels inhibit TSH responsiveness, and low GH levels potentiate them. Early in the course of efforts to characterize "hypothalamic hypothyroidism," it was noted that in patients

TABLE 3. TRH Responses in Pituitary-Hypothalamic Disease in Children

	Mean Peak TSH (μml./ml.)	Peak Prolactin (ng./ml.)
Normal Children (Age 1-10/12 to 14-3/12)	23.3±3.3 (SEM)	25.9±1.8 (SEM)
Isolated GH Deficiency (Age 5 to 25)	20.7±2.8	30.7±4.1
Multiple Hypopituitarism (Age 5-1/2 to 24-10/12)	27.7±4.4	25.9±1.8

(Adapted from Kaplan, S. L., et al.: *Thyrotropin-releasing factor (TRF) effect on secretion of human pituitary prolactin and thyrotropin in children and in idiopathic hypopituitary dwarfism: Further evidence for hypophysiotropic hormone deficiencies.* Endocrinol Metab 35:825–834, 1972.)

HYPOTHALAMIC-PITUITARY DISEASE

TABLE 4. TRH Responses in Pituitary-Hypothalamic Disease in Adults

Diagnosis	No of Cases	Response	Author
Acromegaly	16 Euthyroid	43% Impaired	Snyder et al[43]
	10 Hypothyroid	7 Normal	Faglia et al[10]
		0 Absent	
		2 Impaired	
		1 Exaggerated	
Nonfunctioning pituitary tumor with hypothyroidism	12	7 Absent or impaired	Snyder et al[43]
	8	2 Absent, 2 impaired	Faglia et al[10]
	6	6 Absent	Fleischer et al[11]
Hypothalamic disease	4 Hypothyroid	2 Normal	Snyder et al[43]
	2 Euthyroid	1 Impaired	Snyder et al[43]
Craniopharyngioma	3 Hypothyroid (includes above)	2 Reduced	Snyder et al[43]

with hypothalamic disease, TSH responses tended to be prolonged with a late peak. This is not a useful differential point in diagnosis because some patients with pituitary disorder show the same kind of response.

An important aspect of TRH testing of patients with hypothalamic-pituitary disease is that responsiveness may be abnormal even in patients who are not clinically hypothyroid. For example, in Snyder and associates' series,[43] 9 of 13 women had impaired responses, but only 5 were hypothyroid. In men, 10 of 11 without hypothyroidism had impaired responses. Therefore, the TRH test can be used in a few patients to demonstrate hypothalamic-pituitary disease even in the absence of demonstrable TSH deficiency. As noted in chapter 8, TRH induces GH release in more than 50 percent of acromegalic patients, and hence it is useful in bringing out the abnormality in borderline cases and in following postoperative status.

Thyrotropin-releasing hormone is a useful gauge of prolactin (PRL) secretory reserve. Prolactin responses follow the same dose–response characteristics as those of TSH responses. A normal PRL response to TRH (defined as >100 percent rise over baseline) is indicative of normal PRL secretory cell reserve, but responses are blunted in virtually all cases of hyperprolactinemia regardless of cause. Blunting of PRL in this situation has been attributed to the existence, in most cases of hyperprolactinemia, of a small pituitary pool that is turning over rapidly.[26] This is true for the bulk of prolactinomas which are sparsely granulated, and for the pituitary isolation syndrome which is associated with deficient prolactin-inhibiting factor (PIF). Thyroid-stimulating hormone responses are also blunted in about 30 percent of depressed individuals (see chapter 21).

GONADOTROPIN HORMONE RELEASING HORMONE (GNRH) TEST

Gonadotropin hormone releasing hormone (GnRH) is usually administered for diagnostic test purposes in doses ranging from 25 to 100 μg

TABLE 7. Serum LH and FSH Response to GnRH in 155 Patients with Hypothalamic-Pituitary-Gonadal Dysfunction

Condition	Total	LH				FSH			
		Normal	Absent	Impaired	Exaggerated	Normal	Absent	Impaired	Exaggerated
Hypothalamic disease									
Isolated gonadotrophin deficiency	15	4	3	8		9	3	3	
Craniopharyngioma	10	4	5	1		2	5	3	
Isolated TRH deficiency	1			1				1	
Tumors	2		1	1		1		1	
Pituitary disease									
Nonfunctioning pituitary tumors	31	11	1	19		28		3	
Acromegaly	27	6		21		11		16	
Cushing's disease	3	1		1	1	2		1	
Sheehan's syndrome	2			2		2			
Idiopathic hypopituitarism	6	1	4	1		4	2		
Amenorrhea syndromes									
Delayed puberty — primary amenorrhea	4	1		2	1	2		2	
Anorexia nervosa	13	6		2	5	8		2	3
Secondary amenorrhea and galactorrhea	15	7			8	14			1
Polycystic ovary syndrome	3	2			1	2		1	
Turner's syndrome	2				2				2
Male syndromes									
Delayed puberty	3	3				2		1	
Precocious puberty	1	1				1			
Testicular feminization	1				1				1
Primary gonadal failure	7	2			5	1			6
Anorexia nervosa	1			1				1	
Galactorrhea	3	2	1			2		1	
Gynecomastia	2	2				2			
Miscellaneous									
Internal hydrocephaly	2	1	1			2			
Werner's syndrome	1				1				1
Total	155	54 (35%)	16 (10%)	60 (39%)	25 (16%)	95 (61%)	10 (7%)	36 (23%)	14 (9%)

(Adapted from Mortimer, C H, et al.[27])

The loss of sensitivity of GnRH is restored by giving repeated injections of GnRH. Responses initially absent may thus be restored to normal. Because this may occur in some patients with intrinsic pituitary disease (as well as in patients with hypothalamic disease), it is likely that GnRH can stimulate the function (or hyperplasia) of remnant gonadotropic cells. Although gonadotropic failure is one of the earliest manifestations of hypothalamic or pituitary disease in many patients, GnRH responsiveness is often retained even when adrenocorticotropin hormone (ACTH), TSH, or GH deficiency is present.

The foregoing discussion indicates that the GnRH test alone given as a single bolus injection is of no value in differentiating between hypothalamic disease and pituitary disease. Failure to respond to repeated doses would be diagnostic of intrinsic pituitary disease. However, in states of primary gonadal insufficiency, GnRH-induced LH and FSH responses usually are exaggerated, suggesting that the hyperfunctional state in some way is a hyperresponsive state. This is also true in postmenopausal women.

In prepubertal children, responses to GnRH are absent or minimal. This may be due to the low gonadal hormone levels or, more likely, to the fact that endogenous GnRH is not being secreted. It is probable that endogenous GnRH, released as puberty unfolds, accounts for pubertal development of the pituitary gland and of its sensitization.

It can be anticipated that the GnRH test will be refined for diagnostic purposes by means of various steroid priming regimens (see Seyler and coworkers[40]) and by the use of more precisely determined doses, but data of this sort have not yet been accumulated in sufficient amount.

The superagonists of GnRH have been used successfully in differentiating true precocious puberty (due to central nervous system disease) from other forms. In normal sexually mature individuals, or in those with true precocious puberty,[5,23,53] high doses of GnRH suppress gonadotropin secretion, presumably owing to "down regulation" of GnRH receptors. In individuals with primary hypersecretion of the gonads (for example, ovaries in polyostotic fibrous dysplasia[5,18] or testes in familial testotoxicosis[6,17]—see chapter 9), GnRH agonists do not suppress gonadal secretion. These agents have not yet been approved for general use, but doses used have been approximately 4 μg/kg per day for 8 to 12 weeks of the agonist D-Trp^6-Pro^9-Ne^t-GnRH.[18]

CORTICOTROPIN-RELEASING HORMONE (CRH) TEST

Ovine CRH is administered for test purposes as a bolus intravenous injection of either 1 μg/kg body weight or a standard dose of 100 μg. The agent has not been approved for general clinical use in the United States, and a standard method has not as yet been determined. In normal individuals (Fig. 1), a rise in ACTH is detected as early as 5 minutes, with peak values between 30 and 60 minutes. Plasma cortisol is significantly elevated by 15 minutes and reaches peak values between 30 and 90 minutes.[7,22,30,38,39,47] Neither cortisol nor ACTH return to baseline levels by 180 minutes, a reflection of the long half-life of the CRH peptide (see chapter 6). The duration of elevation is a function of the dose.[7] The side effects noted have

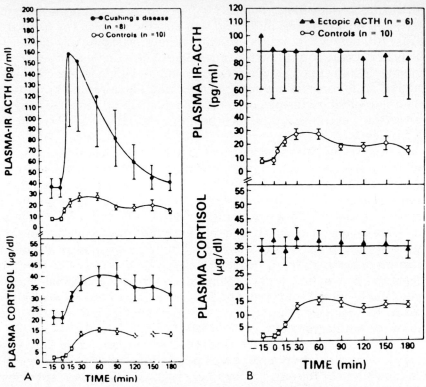

FIGURE 1. Plasma ACTH and cortisol responses to CRH in patients with Cushing's disease *(A)* and hypercortisolism due to ectopic ACTH secretion *(B)* are shown here. Patients with Cushing's disease show hyperresponsiveness to CRH; those with ectopic secretion show unchanged plasma ACTH. These data demonstrate the suppressive effect of ACTH-cortisol excess on pituitary responsiveness. Similar results are obtained in patients with adrenal adenoma. (From Chrousos, GP, et al.[4] Reprinted by permission of The New England Journal of Medicine.)

been facial flushing lasting up to 120 minutes in about 30 percent of cases. No changes in supine blood pressure or heart rate were noted.[22]

One variable conceivably affecting the response to CRH is the time of day that the test is given. Gold and colleagues,[15] for example, suggest that the best time for the test is in the evening (2000 hours), when basal function is at its lowest, but most other workers use a more convenient time in the morning (about 0800 hours). This question was specifically addressed by Tsukada and coworkers,[46] who report that the increment in ACTH and cortisol are the same at either time, although basal levels are higher in the morning. Not all workers agree with this conclusion. Several series of cases have been reported in which various forms of pituitary-adrenal disorders were studied (Table 8).

The studies available thus far indicate that Cushing's disease is characterized by hyperresponsiveness, most reported cases showing responses at or above the upper limit of normal.[15,22,28,29,32,64] However, in the more recent studies of Müller and others,[64] 1 out of 21 patients with ACTH-dependent Cushing's disease failed to respond to CRH. In contrast, ectopic ACTH production is associated with suppression of response inferred either from ACTH or cortisol measurements. Exceptions have been re-

TABLE 8. Summary of CRH Provocative Tests

Group / Dose	No	Mean Increment ACTH (pg/ml)	Mean Increment Cortisol (µg/dl)	Time	Reference
Normal					
1 µg/kg	10	19.1	13.0	PM	Chrousos et al[4]
1 µg/kg	30	20.0*	12.0*	PM	Gold et al[15]
200 µg	5	46.0	6.2	AM	Pieters et al[32,33]
100	20	—	7.3±1	AM	Lytras et al[22]
Cushing's disease					
1 µg/kg	7	135.0	28.0	PM	Chrousos et al[4]
200 µg	5	172.0	15.2	AM	Pieters et al[32,33]
1 µg/kg	2	120.0*	12.0*	AM	Orth et al[29]
100 µg	7			AM	Muller et al[28]
Ectopic ACTH secretion					
1 µg/kg	6	6	0.2	PM	Chrousos et al[4]
100 µg	1			AM	Muller et al[28]
Adrenal adenoma					
1 µg/kg	2	0		AM	Lytras et al[22]
Dexamethasone RX					
100 µg	6		0	AM	Chrousos et al[4]
Depression					
1 µg/kg	19	9*	10*	PM	Gold et al[15]
Hypopituitarism with ACTH deficiency					
100 µg	4†		7.5	AM	Lytras et al[22]
100 µg	2			AM	Tsukada et al[46]
1 µg/kg				PM	Schulte et al[39]
Hypopituitarism with normal ACTH					
100 µg	9		7.6	AM	Lytras et al[22]
Hypothalamic disease with ACTH deficiency					
100 µg	4			AM	Tsukada et al[46]
1 µg/kg				PM	Schulte et al[39]
Primary adrenal insufficiency					
1 µg/kg	3			PM	Schulte et al[39]

*Estimated from published graph   †Not certain whether pituitary or hypothalamic disease

TABLE 9. Summary of GRH Test Results in Selected Series of Normals and GH Disorders

Group	Dose	Maximum Increment (ng/ml)	Reference
Normal young adult males			
GRH 1–40	0.1 µg/kg	11.4	Vance et al[48]
	0.33 µg/kg	14.6	
	1.0	17.0	
	3.3	14.5	
	10.0	15.6	
GRH 1–44	1 µg/Kg	34±28 SD	Gelato et al[13,14]
GRH 1–44	75 µg	21.4	Sassolas et al[36]
	150	27.8	
	300	20.8	
	600	23.0	
Normal women, premenopausal			
GRH 1–40	3.3	29.5	Evans et al[9]
GRH 1–44	1.0	53±10 SD	Gelato et al[13,14]
Normal women, postmenopausal			
GRH 1–40	1 µg/kg	15.3±3.1	Dawson-Hughes et al[51]
GH Deficiency			
Idiopathic	7/19 cases, abnormal*		Schriock et al[37]
	5/10 cases, abnormal*		Rogol et al[34]
Optoseptal Dysplasia	3 cases	8.7, 2.3, 15.5 ng/ml	Schriock et al[37]
Craniopharyngioma	3 cases	2.3, 0.7, 1.9 ng/ml	Schriock et al[37]
	4 cases	2.0, 1.0, 2.0, 6.0, 2.0, 8.0 ng/ml	Rogol et al[34]
Intrauterine Growth failure	5 cases	19.4 (5–51) ng/ml	Rogol et al[34]
Familial short stature	18 cases	17.6 (5–33) ng/ml	Rogol et al[34]
GH excess			
Acromegaly, untreated			
GRH 1–40	1 µg/kg	39.7, ±36.8 (8.0–110.5)	Gelato et al[13,14]
GRH 1–44	100 µg	70.0 (2–1088, n = 35) ng/ml	Shibasaki et al[41]
GRH 1–44	100 µg		Chiodini et al[52]
Acromegaly, treated			
GRH 1–40	1 µg/kg	7.5±6.9 (1.0–23.5)	Gelato et al[13,14]

*Unresponsive (less than 5 ng/ml)

(nor may there ever be) adequate clinicopathologic correlation. The possibility exists that long-standing GHRH deficiency could lead to impaired initial GH responses, as is typical for the GnRH response in patients with hypothalamic hypogonadotropinism. That this interpretation may be valid comes from an examination of responses in patients with unequivocal hypothalamic disease. In the series of patients reported by Schriock[37] of three cases with optic-septal hypoplasia, there were two normal responses and one impaired response (increment 2.3 ng/ml). In patients with craniopharyngioma, 3 of 3 cases reported by Schriock[37] had subnormal responses, and 4 of 6 in Rogol's series[34] had subnormal responses (increment less than 5 ng/ml), including one case that had never had any therapy. Single injections may not prove to be of crucial value in differential diagnosis between hypothalamic disease and pituitary disease. In patients with either intrauterine growth failure (5 cases) or familial short stature (18 cases), all had normal responses (more than 5 ng/ml). Hence, failure to release GH means that there is a defect in either hypothalamus or pituitary gland, but a normal response is compatible with idiopathic GH deficiency.

Two relatively large series of acromegalic patients have been reported. In Shibasaki and coworkers' series[41] of 10 cases, about one third had subnormal responses, and the majority had normal responses. In Gelato and associates'[13] series of 6 untreated cases, all were either in the normal range or slightly greater than normal (mean increment 39.7±36.8 ng/ml). However, in a large series of treated cases, the mean increment was 7.5±6.9, including 6 of 15 who had responses below 5 ng/ml. Bromocriptine inhibits responsiveness to GHRH (Goldman, Motch, Reichlin, unpublished). These findings indicate that active acromegaly may be associated with subnormal, normal, or supranormal responses, and hence the test is not an indicator of the state of metabolic activity of the disease. There are no qualitative differences in active acromegalic cases either. It appears, therefore, that the TRH test, which causes paradoxical GH release in about 60 percent of active acromegalic patients, is a more revealing provocative test.

The use of GHRH may help define the type of neuroendocrine dysfunction in patients with so-called neurosecretory dysfunction.[58,59] These patients show growth failure and diminished spontaneous GH secretion, with partial or complete preservation of pharmacologic responses to dopaminergic or α-adrenergic stimulation. From the therapeutic point of view, it is worth pointing out that GHRH 1-40 is effective by intranasal injection, but its potency is only 1/30 that of the intravenous route.[8]

Growth hormone releasing hormone also has been given by constant infusion over periods as long as 6 hours. Initial studies found that blood GH levels were transiently elevated and then gradually fell in the face of continued elevated GHRH levels.[16] However, more recent studies have shown enhancement of pulsatile secretion with continuous infusion of 2.5 or 1.5 ng/kg per minute of GHRH.[60]

REFERENCES

1. GARD, TG, BERNSTEIN, B, LARSEN, PR: *Studies on the mechanism of 3,5,3'-triiodothyronine-induced suppression of secretogogue-induced thyrotropin release in vitro.* Endocrinology 108:2046–2053, 1981.

responses to intravenous injection of corticotropin-releasing factor in the morning and evening. J Clin Endocrinol Metab 57:869–871, 1983.

47. TSUKADA, T, NAKAI, Y, KOH, T, TSUJII, S, INADA, M, NISHIKAWA, M, SHINODA, H, KAWAI, I, TAKEZAWA, N, IMURA, H: *Plasma adrenocorticotropin and cortisol responses to ovine corticotropin-releasing factor in patients with adrenocortical insufficiency due to hypothalamic and pituitary disorders.* J Clin Endocrinol Metab 58:758–760, 1984.

48. VANCE, ML, BORGES, JLC, KAISER, DL, EVANS, WS, FURLANETTO, R, THOMINET, JL, FROHMAN, LA, ROGOL, AD, MACLEOD, RM, BLOOM, S, RIVIER, J, VALE, W, THORNER, MO: *Human pancreatic tumor growth hormone-releasing factor: Dose-response relationships in normal man.* J Clin Endocrinol Metab 58:838–844, 1984.

49. VON WERDER, K, MULLER, OA, HARTL, R, LOSA, M, STALLA, GK: *Growth hormone releasing factor (hpGRF)-stimulation test in normal controls and acromegalic patients.* J Endocrinol Invest 7:185–191, 1984.

50. WILLIAMS, T, BERELOWITZ, M, JOFFE, SN, THORNER, MO, RIVIER, J, VALE, W, FROHMAN, LA: *Impaired growth hormone responses to growth hormone-releasing factor in obesity.* N Engl J Med 311:1403–1407, 1984.

51. DAWSON-HUGHES, B, STERN, D, GOLDMAN, J, REICHLIN, S: *Regulation of growth hormone and somatomedin-C secretion in postmenopausal women: Effect of physiological estrogen replacement.* J Clin Endocrinol Metab 63:424–432, 1986.

52. CHIODINI, PG, LIUZZI, K, DALLABONZANA, D, ET AL: *Changes in growth hormone (GH) secretion induced by human pancreatic GH-releasing hormone-44 in acromegaly: A comparison with thyrotropin-releasing hormone and bromocriptine.* J Clin Endocrinol Metab 60:48–52, 1985.

53. BOEPPLE, PA, MANSFIELD, MJ, WIERMAN, ME, ET AL: *Use of a potent, long acting agonist of gonadotropin-releasing hormone in the treatment of precocious puberty.* Endocr Rev 7:24–33, 1986.

54. ORMSTON, BJ, ALEXANDER, L, EVEFED, DC, ET AL: *Thyrotrophin response to thyrotrophin-releasing hormone in ophthalmic Grave's disease: Correlation with other aspects of thyroid function, thyroid suppressibility and activity of eye signs.* Clin Endocrinol (Oxf) 2:369–376, 1973.

55. LUNDBERG, PO, AND WIDE, L: *The response of TRH, metyrapone and vasopressin in patients with hypothalamo-pituitary disorders.* Eur J Clin Invest 3:49–56, 1973.

56. HALL, R, BESSER, GM, ORMSTON, BJ, ET AL: *Response to thyrotrophin-releasing hormone.* Lancet 2:213, 1971.

57. LIPPE, BM, VAN-WERLE, AJ, LAFRANCHI, SH, ET AL: *Reversible hypothyroidism in growth hormone-deficient children treated with human growth hormone.* J Clin Endocrinol Metab 40:612–618, 1975.

58. BERCU, BB, SHULMAN, DI, ROOT, AW, ET AL: *Growth hormone (GH) provocative testing frequently does not reflect endogenous GH secretion.* J Clin Endocrinol Metab 63:709–716, 1986.

59. BERCU, BB, ROOT, AW, SHULMAN, DI: *Preservation of dopaminergic and α-adrenergic function in children with growth hormone neurosecretory dysfunction.* J Clin Endocrinol Metab 63:968–973, 1986.

60. SASSOLAS, G, GARRY, J, COHEN, R, ET AL: *Nocturnal continuous infusion of growth hormone (GH)-releasing hormone results in a dose-dependent accentuation of episodic GH secretion in normal men.* J Clin Endocrinol Metab 63:1016–1022, 1986.

61. LEMARCHAND-BERAUD, T, ZUFFEREY, M, REYMOND, M, ET AL: *Pituitary responsiveness to LHRH and TRH in adolescent girls.* Bull Schwiez Akad Med Wiss 34:241–254, 1978.

62. MOSS, AM, MILLER, M: *Diabetes insipidus.* Curr Diagn 3:705–710, 1971.

63. MOSES, AM, STREETEN, DHP: *Disorders of the hypothalamic-neurohypophyseal system.* In KOHLER, PO, (ED): *Clinical Endocrinology.* John Wiley & Sons, New York, 1986, pp 53–72.

64. MÜLLER, E: *Growth enhancement by clonidine treatment in children with growth disorders.* In MÜLLER, EE, MACLEOD, RM (EDS): *Neuroendocrine Perspectives,* vol 5. Elsevier, Amsterdam, 1986, pp 309–314.

65. SNYDER, PJ, RUDENSTEIN, RS, GARDNER, DF, ROTHMAN, JG: *Repetitive infusion of gonadotropin-releasing hormone distinguishes hypothalamic from pituitary hypogonadism.* J Clin Endocrin Metab 48:864–868. 1979.

66. LARON, Z, TOPPER, E, GIL-AD, I: *Oral clonidine—A simple, safe, and effective test for growth hormone secretion.* In *Evaluation of Growth Hormone Secretion.* S Karger, Basel, 1982, pp 103–115.

67. KAPLAN, SL, ET AL: *Thyrotropin-releasing factor (TRF) effect on secretion of human pituitary prolactin and thyrotropin in children and in idiopathic hypopituitary dwarfism: Further evidence for hypophysiotropic hormone deficiencies.* Endocrinol Metab 35:825, 1972.

68. PIMSTONE, BL, BECKER, DJ, KRONHEIM, S: *FSH and LH response to LH releasing hormone in normal and malnourished infants.* In LUFT, R, AND YALOW, RS (EDS): *Radioimmunoassay: Methodology and Applications in Physiology and in Clinical Studies, Hormone and Metabolic Research.* Supplement Series, vol. 5, Georg Thieme, Stuttgart, 1974, p 179.

HYPOTHALAMIC-PITUITARY DISEASE

APPENDIX

Glucose – Growth Hormone Suppression Test

Substance	Oral glucose, as used in the glucose tolerance test, is used.
Dose	75 to 100 g glucose p o.
Principle	Glucose, acting via the hypothalamus, suppresses GH release. Acromegalic patients usually fail to suppress GH after glucose or may show a paradoxical response.
Method	The patient should be fasted and on bed rest after midnight. Oral glucose is administered and blood samples for GH and glucose are taken at 0, 30, 60, 90, 120, and 180 minutes.
Possible adverse effects	None, although an occasional subject is nauseated owing to gastric irritation.
Interpretation	Normal subjects almost invariably show suppression in GH to less than 5 ng/ml by 90 to 180 minutes. Patients with acromegaly, starvation, anorexia nervosa, and certain other conditions may fail to suppress or may show a paradoxical rise.

Insulin Hypoglycemia Test for GA, PRL, and ACTH-Adrenal Reserve

Substance	Crystalline zinc insulin administered intravenously.
Dose	0.1 U/kg (normal patient); 0.05 U/kg (suspected hypopituitary patient), 0.15 or 0.2 U/kg if usual doses fail to induce response, usually in obese (i.e. insulin-resistant patients).
Principle	Insulin given IV causes hypoglycemia which is monitored by CNS glucoreceptors. Stimulation of GH, ACTH-cortisol, and PRL release occurs in 30 to 60 minutes, provided significantly hypoglycemia (usually less than 50 percent of pretest levels) is induced.
Method	The patient should be fasted and on bed rest after midnight. Any symptoms or signs of hypoglycemia should be recorded. Blood samples for glucose, GH, and cortisol are taken at 0, 30, 60, 90, and 120 minutes.
Possible adverse effects	Symptomatic hypoglycemia is necessary for adequate stimulation of GH secretion, but in the event of marked CNS signs or symptoms, glucose should be given intravenously. Care should be taken with suspected hypopituitary patients who may have insufficiency of both GH and adrenal functions and who may show exaggerated responses to hypoglycemia. Elderly

proven to be more reliable and effective than L-dopa for assessing GH reserve. Apomorphine also causes prolactin suppresion in patients with prolactin-secreting tumors.

Thyrotropin-releasing Hormone (TRH) Test

Substance	TRH is a synthetic tripeptide.
Dose	The usual test dose is 500 μg. IV.
Principle	TRH acts directly on pituitary cells to cause release of both TSH and prolactin. TSH induces the release of T_3, and hence this test also is useful in evaluating thyroid disease. T_4 usually does not change appreciably.
Method	TRH is administered IV over a 30-second period after an initial baseline blood sample has been taken. Subsequent samples are taken at 15, 30, 60, and 90 minutes. For simplicity and economy, samples taken prior to injection and at 15 and 30 minutes are usually sufficient. If the test is being done to distinguish between pituitary disease and hypothalamic disease, several authors have suggested that the full five-sample procedure be carried out, because "hypothalamic" hypothyroid cases are more likely to have a delayed peak response. However, patients with pituitary disease occasionally show this same response.
	Because some patients show slight hypertension (less than 20 percent) or occasionally hypotension, patients should be kept prone for 15 minutes after injection.
Possible adverse effects	Symptoms in about 50 percent of subjects include flushing, sweating, palpitations, nausea, sensation of urinary urgency, mild hypertension, or mild hypotension. No serious complications have been reported. Probably a somewhat slower administration (2 to 3 minutes instead of a single bolus injection) is equally effective without causing side effects, but tests done this way have not been standardized.
Interpretation	A TSH response to TRH greater than 5 μU/ml is seen in more than 90 percent of normal individuals. In men over the age of 40, normal responses may be as low as 2 μU/ml. Ninety-eight percent of hyperthyroid patients fail to show a response. In hypothyroidism, about 70 percent of patients have a greater response than normal, and also prolonged. However, the overlap between normal and hypothyroid patients makes

this test valuable only in the group of hyperresponders.

Gonadotropin Hormone Releasing Hormone (GnRH) Test

Substance	GnRH, a synthetic decapeptide.
Dose	100 μg. IV
Principle	GnRH directly stimulates the pituitary to release LH and FSH.
Method	With the patient at rest during the test, blood samples are taken at 0, 30, 45, 60, and 90 minutes after administration. Serum determinations of LH are usually sufficient for diagnostic purposes, but FSH also should be measured if possible.
Interpretation	An increase in plasma LH of 10 to 20 mIU/ml is considered normal. Follicle-stimulating hormone usually shows a lesser response, and the peak is delayed. In some patients with hyperprolactinemia, the FSH response is exaggerated, and in prepubertal children FSH response is greater than LH response. Responses within the normal range indicate that the pituitary is intrinsically normal, but many cases with gonadotropin failure due to intrinsic pituitary disease may respond nevertheless. However, failure to respond does not always indicate that the pituitary gland is abnormal. As in male patients with hypogonadotropic hypogonadism, long-standing GnRH deficiency can cause secondary unresponsiveness to exogenous GnRH, and normal responsivity can be restored by prolonged stimulation. Proper criteria for the longer-term diagnostic stimulation of LH and FSH have not been developed. An example of this problem is anorexia nervosa, in which a single injection of GnRH is often ineffective in stimulating the pituitary gland until the patient has regained some body weight.

GRH Test

Substance	GRH, a synthetic peptide. Three forms have been utilized: GRH 1-29, GRH 1-40, and GRH 1-44-OH. All forms give similar results.
Dose	1 μg/kg or 100 μg, IV bolus
Principle	GRH directly stimulates the pituitary to release GH.
Method	With the patient supine after an overnight fast, blood samples are taken at 0, 30, 60, 90, and 120 minutes for determination of serum GH. For practical purposes, values at 0, 30, and 60 min-

| Interpretation | aborted if more than 3 percent of body weight is lost. |

If patient probably has DI, the dehydration test can be begun at either midnight or 4 PM. Initial serum osmolality in excess of 295 mOsm/kg in a patient with access to water who is not hyperglycemic is strongly suggestive of a urinary concentrating deficit. Maximally concentrated urine should reach a level of 800 mOsm/kg or more except in cases of debility, malnutrition, and anorexia nervosa, in whom maximum concentration may be as low as 450 mOsm/kg.

In severe DI, urine osmolality remains below serum osmolality even after prolonged water deprivation. Pitressin (or desmopressin)-induced increase in urine Osm by 50% or more is good evidence of vasopressin deficiency. Normals show less than 9 percent increase in urine osmolality (after plateau dehydration), patients with partial ADH deficiency more than 9% and less than 50%. For further details, including differentiation from compulsive water drinking, see Moses, and others.[62,63]

HYPOTHALAMIC-PITUITARY DISEASE

Chapter 16

TREATMENT OF HYPOTHALAMIC-PITUITARY DISORDERS

PITUITARY ADENOMAS

Pituitary adenomas account for 5 to 10 percent of all symptomatic intracranial tumors. Routine autopsy studies show that they are far more common than these statistics indicate; 10 to 25 percent of pituitary glands contain small discrete adenomas, most asymptomatic.[4,19] Although more than 75 percent of pituitary adenomas in adults are classified as chromophobes on the basis of classic histologic stains and light microscopy, studies by electron microscopy show that the cells of most, if not all, chromophobe adenomas contain secretory granules (see chapter 12). After the development of prolactin radioimmunoassays and immunohistochemical methods, it became apparent that 20 to 50 percent of so-called chromophobe tumors secrete prolactin, with similar incidences in men and women. That many of these tumors were originally thought to be nonfunctional can be attributed to the fact that hyperprolactinemia may not produce recognizable symptoms, particularly in men. Pituitary adenomas are rare in childhood, and when they occur, they are most often associated with growth hormone (GH) secretory excess (i.e, gigantism) or Cushing's disease. This chapter discusses the available forms of treatment of functional (secretory) and nonfunctional adenomas. Specific details about management of secretory tumors also are given in chapters on individual tropic hormones, and they should be read in conjunction with this chapter. Several recent reviews also address this topic.[2,16,35-37]

SURGERY

The earliest treatment used for pituitary adenomas was surgical. As early as 1906, Horsley approached the pituitary gland by way of the middle cranial fossa, and Schloffer in 1907 operated by the extracranial, transsphenoidal route. According to MacCarty and colleagues,[25] the first successful endonasal, transsphenoidal approach was that of Hirsch, who in 1910 removed two tumors. Cushing initially favored the extracranial approach, but later he developed the transfrontal procedure, which became the most widely used technique. More recently, the development of microsurgical methods,[13,14] the availability of antibiotics, and improved roentgenologic techniques[33] have repopularized the transsphenoidal approach, which is

hormone secreted and the certainty that the endocrine hypersecretory state is due to pituitary disease rather than depending on radiologic diagnosis. For example, most clinical endocrinologists now advocate transsphenoidal surgery for patients with Cushing's disease, whether or not investigations reveal a pituitary adenoma (see chapter 6). On the other hand, prolactin microadenomas, which only five years ago were treated widely by surgery, are now nearly universally treated with bromocriptine (see chapter 7). Growth hormone secreting tumors usually are evident on CAT scan (see chapter 8), and most endocrinologists advocate surgical removal (see chapter 8).

Grade I tumors by the Hardy classification (see chapter 12) are those less than 10 mm in diameter which show minor radiologic evidence of erosion; the success of their surgical treatment is not different than grade 0. A survey of the results of treatment of microadenomas by surgery was compiled recently by Zervas.[34] Information was obtained by a questionnaire obtained from 22 neurosurgical centers. A total of 2606 cases of surgery for secreting microadenomas was collected. Remission, assessed by strict endocrine criteria during the first year of life, was 77 percent for all microadenomas. The results by tumor type showed remission in 74 percent of prolactinomas, 78 percent of GH-secreting tumors, and 81 percent of adrenocorticotropin hormone (ACTH)-secreting tumors. Grade II tumors are defined as macroadenomas and fall into two groups: those confined to the sella, and those with suprasellar extension but without bony invasion. Grade III and grade IV are invasive tumors that erode and destroy bone. The success of surgery, in terms of cure, is much lower with macroadenomas. In the series reviewed by Zervas,[34] remission rates were 30 percent for patients with prolactinomas, 33 percent for those with acromegaly, and 61 percent for those with Cushing's disease (Table 1).

Risk of Transsphenoidal Surgery

The mortality for transsphenoidal surgery in skilled hands is less than 1.0 percent. Zervas[34] reported 23 deaths in 2677 operations for macroadenomas (0.9 percent). The combined figure includes patients with Cushing's disease and acromegaly who are undoubtedly greater risks than those with prolactinoma. Of these fatalities, 10 were secondary to hypothalamic injury, and 5 to meningitis (Table 2). The most frequent serious complications of surgery for macroadenomas were visual loss (39 cases), cerebrospinal fluid rhinorrhea (88 cases), permanent diabetes insipidus (28 cases), and

TABLE 1. Remission Rates for Macroadenomas

Disorder	No of Cases	No of Remissions	Rate (%)
Prolactinomas	1022	310	30
Acromegaly	440	146	33
Cushing's disease	70	43	61

(From Zervas, NT,[34] with permission.)

TABLE 2. Mortality and Morbidity in Macroadenomas*

Risk	No
Death (N = 23)	
Pulmonary embolism	1
Hypothalamic injury	10
Vascular damage	3
Cardiac	3
Meningitis	5
Pneumocephalus	1
Complications (N = 371)	
Visual loss	33†
Oculomotor palsy	16†
CSF rhinorrhea	88
Meningitis	13
Abscess	1
Vascular damage	7
Pulmonary embolism	3
Permanent DI	28†
Transient DI	163
Hematoma	8
Hemiparesis	1†
GI bleed	1
Encephalopathy	1†
Epistaxis	2

*N = 2677
†Permanent injury
(From Zervas, NT,[34] with permission.)

oculomotor palsy (16 cases) (see Table 2). The mortality in patients operated for microadenoma was 0.27 percent (7 of 2606 patients). The morbidity for transsphenoidal surgery of microadenomas is less than 0.05 percent. In the survey of Zervas,[34] 10 serious complications occurred in 2606 patients. Although all these data were obtained by a retrospective questionnaire and are therefore subject to considerable potential error, they do indicate that this surgical approach to treatment has little risk in experienced hands.

Long-term followups of patients considered cured by surgery, exceeding 5 years in some series and approaching 10 to 15 years in others, are now being reported. These results to date show considerable variation. Serri et al[27] reported recurrence in 12 of 24 patients with prolactin adenomas after 4 years. In our experience, recurrence is about 2 to 3 percent per year in patients treated for prolactin microadenomas. The recurrence in Cushing's disease is reported to be less than 1 percent per year, if remission after surgery is sustained more than 6 months. The results in acromegaly are similar.

Surgical Management of Recurrent or Persistent Adenoma

A surgical attempt to manage recurrent or persistent pituitary adenoma is often considered. Detailed analysis of the outcome of transsphenoidal surgery in 127 such cases was presented by Laws and colleagues.[38] Their cases included mainly second surgical procedures, but also individuals with failed radiation and medical therapy.

In roentgenographically visualized prolactinomas, 12 of 41 (29 percent) were successful; in acromegaly, 5 of 12 (42 percent); in Cushing's disease, 1 of 4 (25 percent); and in Nelson's syndrome, 5 of 24 (21 percent). In patients operated upon only for persistent hyperfunction, success was obtained in acromegaly in 5 of 9 (56 percent); in prolactin excess, in 12 of 35 (34 percent); in Cushing's disease, 5 of 19 (26 percent).

Complications were most frequent in patients with prior craniotomy; these authors state that "irradiation alone does not produce consistent changes in the nature of tumor tissue and does not usually make removal of the tumor significantly more difficult or hazardous."

Taking secondary transsphenoidal surgery as a whole for all forms of sellar and parasellar disease, in a group of 158 cases, new complications occurred in a substantial proportion. Nine patients developed CSF leaks, 11 developed permanent diabetes insipidus, and 13 developed new hypopituitarism. It is clear that the odds for success are greatest in therapy of acromegaly (56 percent benefitted) and poorest in recurrent Nelson's syndrome (21 percent benefitted), but that the risks of additional hypophysial function deficits and local surgical complications are considerable. The risk of death is quite low (4 of 158) and was seen only in patients with marked and severe intracranial disease.

RADIATION THERAPY

Roentgenotherapy (conventional or supervoltage) is still widely used in the treatment of pituitary adenomas, either alone or in addition to surgical therapy.[2,3,5,20,28,29] Proton-beam or heavy particle irradiation[10,17,18,21,22,24] has been used in the management of hyperfunctioning adenomas in two centers in the United States. Other ablative approaches such as direct implanation of radioactive substances (yttrium or gold) are rarely used in the United States.[8,9]

Conventional Radiation

The often quoted series of Sheline[2,28] is representative of radiation treatment regimens used for adenomas. Bilateral opposed fields using a 4 or 6 MeV linear accelerator with total dose to the pituitary gland of 4000 to 5000 rads are given in 20 to 25 fractions over a period of 5 to 6 weeks. Most centers now administer doses of 4500 rads. Doses above 5000 rads do not further improve the success of treatment and do increase the frequency of complications. Lower doses appear to be less effective. A total of 140 patients with chromophobe adenomas was included in the study reported by Sheline and colleagues[29] of tumors treated from 1940 to 1970 (Table 3). How many of these patients had prolactinomas and how many had nonfunctioning pituitary adenomas is unknown. All were macroadenomas, judged in retrospect to correspond to grade III or IV adenoma according to the Hardy-Vezina classification system. Visual field defects were present in 92 percent. The sella was markedly enlarged in 96 percent. Hypopituitarism was diagnosed in 53 percent. Twenty-three received radiation therapy (RT) alone, 37 had surgical decompression, and 80 had a combination of surgery and RT; the surgery performed was via a craniotomy in 115 pa-

TABLE 3. Chromophobe Adenomas, University of California, San Francisco

Pretreatment finding	Treatment (%)			Patients (N = 140)	
	RT (N = 23)	Surgery (N = 37*)	Surgery + RT (N = 80)	N	%
Visual field deficit(s)	78	97	94	129	92
Grossly enlarged sella	100	95	96	135	96
CNS invasion	4	19	8	14	10

*Including eight surgical deaths.
(From Sheline, et al,[29] with permission.)

tients. Immediate improvement during the first 1 to 2 years was similar in all three groups, but recurrence was much more frequent in the surgically treated group who did not receive radiation therapy. The addition of surgery to RT was no better than RT alone at either 5 or 10 years after treatment. Because the recurrence rate after surgery alone was much greater, Sheline[29] recommended RT of all surgically treated macroadenomas, particularly if invasive. No complications were attributed definitely to radiation treatment.

The surgical mortality in this early series was high (8 of 80), and complications were frequent; the latter included increase in visual deficit, cerebrospinal fluid rhinorrhea, and postoperative epilepsy. Postradiation and postoperative followup for tumor recurrence focused primarily on visual field assessment. In this series when visual deficit involved one quarter or less of a visual field, 65 to 67 percent of visual field abnormalities reverted to normal after either surgery or RT. For more serious visual field deficits, involving up to one half of a visual field loss, surgery was superior to RT. The 5-year recurrence-free survival rate was 93 percent for RT alone, 25 percent for surgery alone, and 90 percent for surgery plus RT. At 10 years these had declined to 71, 9, and 70 percent, respectively.

A recent review of those patients who had survived more than 10 years after treatment revealed that none of the RT only treated group had shown a recurrence; the longer the period of followup, the greater was the difference in favor of nonrecurrence for the RT-treated group over those treated with surgery alone. From these data Sheline[28,29] concludes that with modern methods of RT, at doses of 4500 to 5000 rads, the cure rate should be about 95 percent for macroadenomas. The results of more recent studies of the efficacy and safety of radiotherapy indicate that it continues to have an important role in the treatment of pituitary macroadenomas. This impression is supported by data from the University of California, San Francisco, series obtained during the years 1970 to 1979 (Table 4).[29] Of 15 patients treated with RT alone and 61 with surgery plus RT, none have had recurrences after followup intervals of 6.5 and 4.5 years, respectively. Other series suggest similar results. Henderson[16] reported 5-year recurrence-free rates of 33 percent for surgery alone (performed transsphenoidally) and 65 percent for surgery followed by RT. Transfrontal resection increased these rates to 58 and 87 percent, respectively. Emmanuel[6] reported a 93 percent

TABLE 4. Nonfunctional Prolactinomas 1970–1979, University of California, San Francisco

Parameter	RT	Surgery + RT
No. of patients	15	61
Known prolactinomas	4	14
Followup (years)	1–10 (6.5)*	1–9 (4.5)
Field defects/invasion	10	51
Sphenoid sinus involved	5	10
Dead, intercurrent disease	2	2
Recurrence	0	0
Suprasellar cyst formation	0	2

*parentheses show mean values.

4-year recurrence-free survival rate for combined surgery and RT, compared with 30 percent for resection alone.

The main disadvantage of conventional radiation is the long delay in reducing pituitary hypersecretion. Other disadvantages are that a significant proportion of patients are not brought under control (as many as 25 percent at 5 years); the treatment requires daily visits to the hospital for five to six weeks and thus may not be feasible for many patients; epilation of the temporal area is extremely common, but almost always transient.

Prolactinoma

It can be concluded that postoperative RT improves the long-term recurrence-free rate for mass effects of large pituitary tumors of the chromophobe/prolactinoma type. We recommend that large tumors be resected by the transsphenoidal route, whenever possible, and that postoperative radiation in divided doses (4 to 5 doses weekly of 180 rads) be given for 5 weeks to a total dose of 4500 to 5000 rads. Prolactin levels can be used in most cases of prolactinoma to determine whether residual tumor is present postsurgery, but the levels of prolactin do not indicate reliably the amount of residual tumor. Bromocriptine is used after radiation to maintain maximum reduction in prolactin levels in patients with persistent hyperprolactinoma. In almost all cases bromocriptine is effective in preventing further increase in tumor size.

Microadenomas

Few series have examined the efficacy of RT in microadenomas. Grossman and associates[12] studied 36 women (ages 18 to 48 years) who had amenorrhea-galactorrhea. Prolactin levels ranged from 75 to 5600 ng/ml. Radiation therapy was given in a regimen as described above, that is, 180 rads daily $\times 5 \times 5 = 4500$ to 5000 rads, and patients were placed on dopamine antagonists (bromocriptine, lisuride, or pergolide). After a period of 2 to 10 years (mean 4.2 years), serum prolactin levels were normal (<18 ng/ml) in 8 of 28 patients evaluated after medication was withdrawn. Postradiation hypopituitarism evidenced by GH deficiency was found in 21 patients.

We do not advocate RT for small prolactinomas. Medical treatment alone suffices for most patients (see chapter 7).

Acromegaly and Cushing's Disease

Conventional RT has been used for decades in the treatment of acromegaly. Bloom and Kramer[3] reviewed the results of 40 patients treated between 1957 and 1982. Three quarters of the patients are alive and well after RT treatment (7 patients also had surgery; 3 by craniotomy, 4 by the transsphenoidal approach). Recurrence occurred in 4 patients (10 percent). Acromegalic patients seem more susceptible to visual nerve damage after RT than patients with chromophobe adenomas. Thus, five patients in the Bloom and Kramer series had visual complications (four patients were blind in one eye, one patient was totally blind). In contrast, the results of RT of prolactinomas showed that not a single patient of 140 treated with RT had visual compromise.[29] Nor was visual damage experienced in 43 patients with craniopharygioma treated with the same doses. This damaging effect of RT on the visual pathway may be secondary to the small vessel disease that is common in acromegaly. Readjustment of their treatment course to 180 rads daily and maximum total of 4600 rads has eliminated this complication.

Postradiation hypopituitarism was a common complication in the series of acromegalic patients reported by Eastman and colleagues.[5] Twenty-five to 50 percent of patients showed evidence of pituitary insufficiency 5 to 10 years after RT.

We recommend transsphenoidal surgery as initial therapy for all acromegalic patients with pituitary adenomas, with conventional irradiation treatment given if hormonal hypersecretion persists. The rare occurrence of the ectopic GHRH syndrome presenting with acromegaly necessitates careful clinical assessment of all patients prior to surgery (see chapter 8).

Cushing's disease also can be treated effectively with RT. This has also been advocated by a few for children. We recommend that pituitary exploration be undertaken in adult patients and in most children. Failure to identify a microadenoma (10 to 15 percent of cases) requires secondary forms of treatment (see chapter 6).

Complications of Radiation Therapy

The only acute complication of RT is local hair loss, usually restricted to the temporal areas of the scalp. Late complications include hypopituitarism, carcinogenesis, and injury to the visual system or nervous system. The true incidence of individual hormonal failure is unknown. Growth hormone is particularly susceptible. Carcinogenesis and central nervous system injury are rare; seven cases of fibrosarcomas or osteosarcomas are reported in patients treated with less than 5000 rads. Central nervous system injury has been reported in only two patients who received this dose. The possibility of subtle brain damage, known to be important in children, has been considered also in adults, but has not been established by specific study.

Heavy Particle Therapy

Two alternative forms of external radiation therapy are available. Both utilize cyclotron-activated heavy particles administered through a carefully collimated beam whose pathway is defined by preliminary radiologic study of the pituitary gland and surrounding structures. In one technique, pioneered by Lawrence, Linfoot, and Tobias and their colleagues at the Donner Laboratory, University of California, Berkeley, α (helium) particles are utilized.[21,22,24] In the other technique developed by Kjellberg and Kliman[17,18] at the Massachusetts General Hospital in Boston, protons are utilized. Protons are generated from hydrogen atoms by removing the orbital electrons. A particle beam with a flux of more than 2 billion protons per second is emitted. The protons induce ionization at the end of range of the beam, generating a Bragg peak within the sella turcica. A total of 12 portal entry sites, six on each side of the head, provide a central dose of up to 12,000 rads. Because the energy release of protons is highly localized (as compared with electrons or x-rays), it is possible to deliver as much as 12,000 to 15,000 rads to the pituitary gland without damaging skin or skull. The intensity of this form of energy necessitates extremely careful control to avoid damage to the optic nerves, cranial nerves, temporal lobe, and hypothalamus. The method is appropriate only in patients whose lesions are confined to the pituitary fossa, are regular in outline, and are unaccompanied by local signs of hypothalamic or optic-chiasm compression. The procedure also requires preliminary CAT scans and cavernous sinograms to outline the tumor adequately.

The experience with proton beam irradiation has been reviewed recently by Kliman and Kjellberg.[18] Over the past 20 years, more than 500 patients with acromegaly, 145 patients with Cushing's disease, and 29 patients with Nelson's syndrome have been treated. Although precise endocrinologic data are lacking in many of these patients, it is evident that the treatment is relatively effective, convenient for the patient (a single exposure), and relatively safe.

In the Kjellberg and Kliman series,[18] 435 of 510 patients with acromegaly treated with proton beam were available to followup over the 20-year period. Fifty-one (11.7 percent) had died, most of cerebrovascular or cardiovascular disease. Only three were considered to have died of a cause related to the pituitary tumor or its treatment. Two of these had invasive pituitary tumors; one developed a fibrosarcoma.

Median GH levels in groups of patients fall after treatment, but data in individual patients are lacking. They conclude that normalization of plasma GH levels to less than 5 ng/ml occurred in 75 percent at 10 years, and 92.5 percent at 20 years. Only one patient was said to have relapsed after treatment.

Eight of 435 cases (1.8 percent) available for analysis had visual field defects.[17,18] Transient oculomotor defects occurred in 6 other patients, with permanent defects in 2. The incidence of partial or total hypopituitarism is considerable after proton beam therapy. Forty-two of 510 patients (9.7 percent) had thyroid deficiency attributed to the therapy, 39 (9.0 percent) had adrenal deficiency, and 29 (6.7 percent) had gonadal deficiency. Similar results are reported by this group in Cushing's disease.

Proton beam radiation has the following advantages: It produces maximum effects within 2 years (in contrast to 3 years or longer with conventional therapy), requires only a 2- to 4-day hospitalization instead of a 6-week course of daily treatments, and is usually unaccompanied by epilation. The incidence of side effects, however, is somewhat greater after proton beam radiation than after conventional radiation. In the compilation of Kjellberg and Kliman[18] of their second 100 cases (in which most of the technical problems of radiation, dosimetry, and localization had been resolved), the following complications were observed: temporary disturbance in extraocular movements, 12 percent; visual impairment, 2 percent; partial hypopituitarism, 3 percent; total hypopituitarism, 6 percent; transient diabetes insipidus, 3 percent; seizures, 2 percent. Other complications, observed in a small number of cases, were minor temporal-lobe disturbance (episodes of sensory or olfactory aura) requiring anticonvulsants, and disturbed mentation.

Proton beam radiation has the disadvantages of requiring high technology available only in one center in the United States, being applicable only when the tumor is confined to the sella, and not being fully effective in an appreciable number of cases.

Alpha particle pituitary irradiation has been carried out by Linfoot and Lawrence[22,24] in 314 cases, and data are available on 299. Treatment is by plateau or by use of Bragg peak, depending upon the anatomy of the tumor. Results reported have not been broken down by modality used. By 1 year, median fasting GH had fallen to approximately 9.5 from an initial median of 23 ng/ml, and by 4 years to a median of 5 ng/ml. Levels continued to fall over the ensuing 18 years of followup. Growth hormone levels fell to 5 ng/ml in 30 percent of patients within 2 years, 68 percent within 6 years, and 95 percent within 8 years. Relapses were usually the result of some degree of extrasellar extension: suprasellar, intrasphenoidal, posterior inferior into region of the clivus, lateral extension. Because many of the cases in the series were treated prior to the use of CAT scans, there is an appreciable incidence of these abnormalities.

Approximately 34 percent of the patients developed ACTH deficiency, and TSH deficiency, and 25 percent developed gonadotropic insufficiency, but these values are not certain because gonadotropin deficiency was not treated in older individuals. Neurologic complications include partial field cuts in 29 percent (asymptomatic). Three patients developed unilateral extraocular motor nerve lesions, usually affecting the third nerve. These usually cleared and were relatively asymptomatic. Three developed temporal lobe epilepsy (all in cases treated previously). Overall CNS complication rate in 298 cases was 4 percent.

Because of the high incidence of optic-nerve and cranial-nerve damage and brain necrosis in patients treated with more than 5000 rads by conventional methods or 15,000 rads by proton beam, it is widely recommended that patients not be given a second course of radiation therapy if they have already received one full course. Also the incidence of sarcoma of the pituitary gland is increased in patients given more than one course of treatment.

The medical treatment of secretory tumors is discussed in chapters 6 (adrenocorticotropin hormone), 7 (prolactin), and 8 (growth hormone).

MANAGEMENT OF HYPOPITUITARISM

Chronic Replacement

ACTH Deficiency

In the evaluation of patients with pituitary insufficiency, the identification of ACTH deficiency is of paramount importance; the consequent adrenal insufficiency can be life-threatening, particularly in stress.[30] Most patients are well controlled on 25 mg of cortisone or the equivalent (20 mg hydrocortisone or 5 mg prednisone) per day, given in two, equal, divided doses. There are patients who feel perfectly well on a single daily dose. A few patients require a larger dose for regular maintenance, for example, 37.5 mg of cortisone per day (30 mg hydrocortisone or 7.5 mg prednisone given as 5 mg in the morning and 2.5 mg at night). We noted that several hypopituitary patients given the higher dose of cortisone or prednisone as a standard dose develop mild signs of steroid overdosage.

The benefit from the use of hydrocortisone or cortisone is no greater than from prednisone; the much lower cost of the latter and the longer duration of action (owing to slower degradation), in fact, make prednisone superior. Because ACTH deficiency does not lead to complete mineralocorticoid (aldosterone) deficiency, hypopituitary patients, unlike addisonian patients, rarely require supplemental treatment with synthetic mineralocorticoids such as desoxycorticosterone acetate (DOCA) or fludrocortisone acetate. During stress, patients must increase the dosage twofold or threefold, and they must also be instructed to contact a physician if they are unable to take medications by mouth. It is imperative to instruct and repeatedly to remind the patient of the necessity for close medical supervision, particularly if under stress. It is also imperative that the patients carry identification (wallet card, necklace, or bracelet) indicating that they are "cortisone dependent." If medical attention will not be available in an emergency, as, for example, when traveling in an underdeveloped country or in a wilderness area, we insist that our patients be accompanied by a companion and carry a vial or two of a soluble preparation of steroid. Monitoring the adequacy of adrenal steroid replacement includes evaluation of appetite, weight, sense of well-being, and measurements of plasma sodium concentration and appropriate postural blood pressure changes. There is no completely objective measure of adequacy of corticoid replacement independent of careful and experienced clinical judgment.

Thyroid Deficiency

Most TSH-deficient patients are well treated with 100 to 200 μg per day of synthetic L-thyroxine given as a single dose. Monitoring the adequacy of replacement involves clinical evaluation, but measurements of plasma T_4 and T_3 are a good guide to therapy because they accurately reflect circulating hormone; values should fall within the usual normal range. Because of the danger of precipitating angina, coronary insufficiency, and arrhythmia in patients with long-standing pituitary disease, thyroid hormone replacement is usually initiated stepwise: in a older person, 25 μg T_4 for 2 weeks, 50

μg for the next 2 weeks, and then 100 μg per day for 2 weeks. Additional increments of 50 μg per day are then given at 2-week intervals until full replacement is achieved.

Gonadotropin Deficiency

Unless the patient wants to have children, gonadotropin deficiency is satisfactorily managed with gonadal steroid replacement therapy alone. *In the adult male,* most workers recommend testosterone dosage equivalent to 12 to 15 mg per day, given intramuscularly in a long-acting preparation every 2 to 3 weeks.[26] This form of treatment is the least expensive. Thus, testosterone enanthate or testosterone proprionate can be given in a dose of 200 to 300 mg every two or three weeks. The patient is usually instructed in self-administration. Testosterone also can be administered by mouth in the form of fluoxymesterone tablets, the only commercially available derivative of testosterone that is absorbed readily by the gut. Absorption of this form is somewhat irregular, and all orally taken testosterone preparations have the potential to cause cholangitis with the appearance of obstructive jaundice. Parenteral preparations are free of this problem. Preparations for use by inunction are under investigation. They have the advantage that they avoid "first pass" metabolism by the liver. The criteria for adequate replacement include maintenance of beard growth, libido, and potency. Excess dosage may result in edema formation, gynecomastia, disturbing sexual drive, nightmares, and acne. Because hypogonadal men do not express genetically determined baldness, normal replacement doses may bring about baldness in those who are susceptible, which in a sense can be regarded as a side effect of therapy. It is important to inform the patient of this possibility. Long-standing gonadal insufficiency may require many months of therapy before adequate sexual drive and performance can be restored. The longer the deficiency has been present, the longer it takes to achieve the desired response, and if the patients have been untreated for many years, particularly throughout the teens and early twenties, full restoration of normal male development may never occur. This lack of sex drive may lead to the peculiar situation in which the patient is not motivated to maintain adequate sex hormone replacement therapy. Another point of practical importance is that a surprisingly large number of individuals may have been hypogonadal for many years prior to its recognition and have therefore adopted a lifestyle appropriate to hypogonadism. This can include the choice of marital partner or of vocation. Replacement therapy may create difficulties in such patients, inasmuch as it may threaten a harmonious marriage or cause sex drive that cannot be fulfilled. The physician must exercise sound judgment in the institution of gonad replacement therapy.

In *women,* adequate sex hormone replacement therapy is given with one of several estrogenic preparations (ethinyl estradiol 10 to 15 μg per day, conjugated estrogens 0.65 to 1.25 mg per day). Diethylstilbestrol, the least costly of the estrogens, has been declared by the FDA to have carcinogenic potential and is no longer used for replacement treatment. Therapy is given for 25 days of each month, and a menstrual period is induced by the administration, on days 21 to 25 inclusive, of an orally effective progestin such as medroxyprogesterone, 5 to 10 mg per day. Other acceptable regimens include one of the birth control pills in daily doses not to exceed the equivalent of 20 μg per day of estradiol; doses in the range of 10 μg per day are probably adequate. Estrogen inunctions by skin patches are now available. By avoiding "first pass" exposure to the liver, stimulation of angiotensinogen (a peptide that causes hypertension in some cases) and of low-density lipoproteins (a factor thought to increase risk of atherosclerosis) is reduced or prevented altogether. Recent evidence indicates that the administration of estrogenic hormones increases the frequency of endometrial carcinoma twofold to fivefold. For this reason we now insist that patients given hormone replacement take regular progestin treatment to induce menses (because of the finding that progesterone reverses endometrial hyperplasia) and have gynecologic evaluations at yearly intervals. The smallest dose that is effective is the one that should be used. In young women, the advantage of taking estrogen replacement includes the maintenance of secondary sex characteristics, reduced risk of cardiac disease, sense of well-being, increased breast size, vaginal and vulvar tissue turgor, and reduced risk of osteoporosis. Whether these advantages persist after the mid-forties is still a matter of controversy. The physician and the patient together should discuss the pros and cons of therapy and decide, in the individual case, how replacement therapy will be managed. We advise sex-hormone replacement in young hypopituitary women who may have greater need and desire for restoration and maintenance of normal physiologic function. Cervical exfoliative cytology (Pap test) and breast examinations should be evaluated at six-month intervals in women on estrogen replacement therapy.

Estrogenic hormones alone do not usually restore normal libido to the panhypopituitary woman. The addition of small amounts of an androgenic hormone is required to make up for the loss of adrenal androgen secretion. This can be accomplished by the administration of a long-acting testosterone preparation such as testosterone enanthate or testosterone proprionate in oil, 25 mg every 4 to 6 weeks. Excessive dosage is indicated by the development of hirsutism. Clinicians usually fail to ask their women hypopituitary patients about abnormalities in libido, and many patients are unaware that anything can be done about their loss of sex drive.

Infertility

It is in the management of infertility that the greatest advances have been made recently in the therapy of hypopituitarism.

Women. The etiology of gonadotropin failure is the major determinant of the choice of therapy of pituitary failure in women. In women with functional amenorrhea, the first line of treatment is with the drug clomiphene (Clomid). This agent acts as an estrogen antagonist at both the pituitary and possibly the hypothalamic levels. It is administered in 5-day courses beginning at the dose of 50 mg per day by mouth. If the patient fails to menstruate after two courses of therapy given at monthly intervals, the dose is increased to 100 mg per day for 5 days, and then to 150 mg per day. Two hundred mg per day is the highest dose that should be administered.

Clomiphene is also used to induce ovulation in women who are having anovulatory cycles, including those with polycystic ovaries. When anovulatory menses are occurring, the clomiphene is timed to be given 5 days after the first day of the menstrual cycle; ovulation usually takes place 5 to 12 days following the last day of therapy. A number of side effects are caused by clomiphene, but most important and potentially dangerous is the occurrence of hyperstimulation of the ovaries, which is most likely to occur in patients with polycystic ovary syndrome. The physician caring for such patients must monitor ovarian size during therapy. There is an appreciable risk of multiple pregnancies in patients in whom ovulation has been induced by clomiphene.

In patients who fail to respond to clomiphene, two alternative therapies are available to induce ovulation: pulsatile gonadotropin-releasing hormone (GnRH) infusion, or injections of menopausal gonadotropin followed by human chorionic gonadotropins (HCG). In individuals with functional or structural hypothalamic disease, GnRH treatment is much superior to the gonadotropin therapies, but in those with complete gonadotropin deficiency owing to intrinsic disease (for example, Sheehan's syndrome), it may be necessary to administer the gonadotropins.

Pulsatile GnRH is administered by a special pump which provides an injection every 90 minutes day and night. The pump is worn on a belt, and the infusion is delivered either subcutaneously or intravenously. The rate of success in several series is shown in Table 5. Therapy may extend through 1 to 3 cycles. Because the negative-feedback of ovarian secretion is preserved in this mode of therapy, multiple pregnancies are rare in contrast to the situation with clomiphene and HMG therapy.

If clomiphene and pulsatile GnRH are ineffective, or if the latter is unavailable, ovulation can be produced by administering a course of human menopausal gonadotropin (rich in follicle-stimulating-hormone (FSH)-like gonadotropins) for 2 weeks followed for 5 days by daily injections of (HCG) (which has luteinizing-hormone (LH)-like effects). References on gynecologic endocrinology should be consulted for details of dosage, precautions, and side effects of these therapies. It is reasonable to tell patients whose infertility is due to hypothalamic or pituitary disorder that approximately 80 percent fertility rate can be achieved by one or other of the methods available. Of course, complete evaluation of the reproduc-

TABLE 5. Results of Ovulation and Pregnancy in the Use of Different Doses, Frequency, and Routes of GnRH Pulses

Source	μg/pulse	Interval	Route	No. cycles	No. ovulations	No. pregnancies
Leyendecker et al.	2.5–5–10–15–20	89	IV*	26	26	6
Schoemaker et al.	10–20	90–120	IV†	24	21	6
Miller et al.	1–5	96–120	IV‡	23	20	7

*Zyklomat pump.
†Direct intravenous administration.
‡Autosyringe pump.
(From Yen, SSC: *Clinical applications of gonadotropin-releasing hormone and gonadotropin-releasing hormone analogs.* Fertil Steril 39:257–266, 1983, with permission.)

tive status of both partners should be carried out before initiating such therapies to exclude structural abnormalities of the reproductive tract.

Men. *Infertility in men* owing to hypothalamic-pituitary insufficiency is best treated with pulsatile GnRH injections. Infertility in men is much more difficult to treat than in females. This is due in part to the very long time required to nurture the developing sperm. In contrast to the ripening of the ovum, which takes only 2 weeks, 70 days are required for the full cycle of sperm maturation and growth. Therapy must thus be given over a much longer period of time. If the pituitary gland is destroyed, GnRH likely will not work, and a course of human menopausal gonadotropin and HCG is indicated. However, the success rate is not much over 30 percent with this approach. Androgen replacement is not needed while GnRH or gonadotropins are being administered because the endocrine secretions of the testes also are stimulated by GnRH and HCG.

We advise fertile men who are to undergo ablative surgery in the pituitary-hypothalamic area to consider the advisability of placing sperm in a sperm bank, even if they are not married and do not contemplate having children in the near future. Sperm can be kept in a viable state for seven years or more in such banks.

Growth Hormone Deficiency

The shortage of human growth hormone (hGH), and the failure to define a clear-cut syndrome of GH deficiency in the adult are the main factors that have limited the use of this agent in adults. However, with the present availability of biosynthetic hGH, we anticipate that some experience with GH therapy will soon accumulate. Until these data have been obtained, GH substitution therapy will be directed toward children (see also chapter 8). The occurrence of four cases of Creutzfeldt-Jakob disease in recipients of hGH from cadaver sources has stopped effectively the use of natural hormone for new cases (see chapter 8), because it will take many years to carry out the necessary infectivity studies, even if new methods are developed to rid the hormone preparations of infective particles. However, several companies currently are planning to introduce biosynthetic hGH. The preparation now available in North America has the disadvantage of possessing a methionyl terminal amino acid which has induced antibody formation in about one third of cases. However, the need for hGH for treatment of hypopituitary dwarfs is pressing and has led to Food and Drug Administration approval of this compound. Several manufacturers have prepared methionine-free hGH, and these will undoubtedly be introduced in the near future.

The correct dose to be used has not been fully established because current regimens utilizing the native hormone have tended to undertreat, that is, to use the minimum dose of hormone. One suggested regimen is to administer 2 mg three times a week after an initial trial of 1 mg three times a week. Secondary failure occurs frequently, and GH therapy may bring about hypothyroidism that requires therapy. We anticipate that the availability of virtually unlimited quantities of hGH and the use of new regimens of pulsatile administration may lead to important improvements in therapy.

In addition to biosynthetic GH, clinical trials now underway suggest that in 60 percent or more of children with idiopathic GH deficiency administration of growth hormone releasing hormone (GHRH) may prove equally beneficial in stimulating growth (see chapter 8). It has not yet been shown that secondary growth occurs when this approach is taken. Clonidine also has been reported to stimulate growth in children with intact hypothalamic-pituitary function, but it is too early to know whether this will prove to be a useful therapy.

Prolactin Deficiency

There is no currently available source of human prolactin (hPRL) other than cadaver pituitaries; distribution of the limited amount of hPRL that has been isolated by the National Hormone Distribution Program of the National Institute of Health has been stopped because of the suspicion that these preparations may be contaminated with Creutzfeldt-Jakob virus.

ADH Deficiency

The treatment of diabetes insipidus (DI) is discussed in chapter 4. The treatment of choice now for partial DI is an oral agent such as chlorpropamide, which potentiates endogenous vasopressin. The treatment of choice for severe DI is nasal insufflation with desmopressin (see chapter 4).

TREATMENT OF ACUTE SEVERE HYPOPITUITARISM

Particularly in stressed individuals, it may be necessary to give treatment on an emergency or semiemergency basis. Adrenocorticotropin hormone deficiency is best treated with a glucocorticoid preparation. Treatment can be initiated with intravenous injection of a soluble solution of cortisol or hydrocortisone in doses of 100 to 300 mg per day, which are from three to ten times the normal replacement doses. Cortisone can be given as an intramuscular injection in a similar dose. In this form, it is absorbed somewhat more slowly but also somewhat less dependably. Oral absorption is equal to or better than absorption following intramuscular injection, and for this reason the latter route should not be used as the sole method in a critically sick patient. Patients with long-standing hypopituitarism given usual or large replacement doses of corticoids may develop euphoria abruptly, or even acute psychotic reactions; for this reason, it is generally better to avoid large doses unless the clinical situation is urgent.

In the treatment of pituitary coma or precoma, both corticoid and thyroid hormone replacement urgently is indicated. However, excessively rapid thyroid hormone replacement can result (in susceptible patients) in the precipitation of coronary insufficiency, myocardial infarction, angina, or arrhythmias. The clinician often must steer the difficult course between life-threatening myxedema coma and potential cardiac disturbance. Given a patient with severe TSH-thyroid deficiency requiring urgent treatment, most clinicians now administer the usual normal daily requirement of thyroid hormone for 2 or 3 days by mouth, if possible, or otherwise by vein (50 μg per day of T_3, or 150 μg per day of T_4). The dose is decreased after 3 to 4 days of treatment to 50 to 100 μg of thyroxine per day, and a week to 10 days later, after the urgent situation is past, therapy is increased in the usual way (see above).

The management of other disorders affecting the hypothalamic-pituitary region is discussed in chapter 21.

REFERENCES

1. ATKINSON, RL, ET AL: *Acromegaly. Treatment by trans-sphenoidal microsurgery.* JAMA 233:1279, 1975.
2. BLACK, PM, ZERVAS, NT, RIDGWAY, EC, MARTIN, JB (EDS): *Secretory Tumors of the Pituitary Gland.* Raven Press, New York, 1984.
3. BLOOM, B, AND KRAMER, S: *Conventional radiation therapy in the management of acromegaly.* In BLACK, PM, ZERVAS, NT, RIDGWAY, EC, MARTIN, JB (EDS): *Secretory Tumors of the Pituitary Gland.* Raven Press, New York, 1984, pp 73.
4. BURROW, GN, WORTZMAN, G, REWCASTLE, NB, ET AL: *Microadenomas of the pituitary and abnormal sellar tomograms in an unselected autopsy series.* N Engl J Med 304:156, 1981.
5. EASTMAN, RC, CORDEN, P, ROTH, J: *Conventional supervoltage is an effective treatment for acromegaly.* J Clin Endocrinol Metab 48:931, 1979.
6. EMMANUEL, IG: *Symposium on pituitary tumors: Three historical aspects of radiotherapy, present treatment, techniques, and results.* Clin Radiol 17:154, 1966.
7. FAGER, CA, ET AL: *Indications for and results of surgical treatment of pituitary tumors by the intracranial approach.* In KOHLER, PO, AND ROSS, GT (EDS): *Diagnosis and Treatment of Pituitary tumors.* Elsevier, New York, 1973, p 146.
8. FRASER, R, ET AL: *The assessment of the endocrine effects and the effectiveness of ablative pituitary treatment by Y and Au implantation.* In KOHLER, PO, AND ROSS, GT (EDS): *Diagnosis and Treatment of Pituitary Tumors.* Elsevier, New York, 1973, p 35.
9. FRASER, R, ET AL: *Needle implantation of ytrium seeds for pituitary ablation in cases of secondary carcinoma.* Lancet 1:382, 1959.
10. GARCIA, JF, ET AL: *Treatment of pituitary tumors with heavy particles.* In KOHLER, PO, AND ROSS, GT (EDS): *Diagnosis and Treatment of Pituitary Tumors.* Elsevier, New York, 1973, p 253.
11. GORDEN, P, AND ROTH, J: *The treatment of acromegaly by conventional pituitary irradiation.* In KOHLER, PO, AND ROSS, GT (EDS): *Diagnosis and Treatment of Pituitary Tumors.* Elsevier, New York, 1973, p 230.
12. GROSSMAN, A, COHEN, B, PLOWMAN, N, REES, LH, JONES, AE, BESSER, GM: *The circulating prolactin response to radiotherapy in patients with prolactinomas.* (In preparation.)
13. GUIOT, G: *Transsphenoidal approach in surgical treatment of pituitary adenomas: General principles and indications in non-functioning adenomas.* In KOHLER, PO, AND ROSS, GT (EDS): *Diagnosis and Treatment of Pituitary Tumors.* Elsevier, New York, 1973, p 159.
14. HARDY, J: *Transsphenoidal surgery of hypersecreting pituitary tumors.* In KOHLER, PO, AND ROSS, GT (EDS): *Diagnosis and Treatment of Pituitary Tumors.* Elsevier, New York, 1973, p 179.
15. HARDY, J: *Transsphenoidal microsurgery of prolactinomas.* In BLACK, PM, ZERVAS, NT, RIDGWAY, EC, MARTIN, JB (EDS): *Secretory Tumors of Pituitary Gland.* Raven Press, New York, 1984, p 73.
16. FAHLBUSCH, R, WERDER, K, VON (EDS): *Clinical aspects of the hypothalamus.* Acta Neurochirurgica 75:1–152, 1985.
17. KJELLBERG, RN, KLIMAN, B, SWISHER, B, BUTLER, W: *Proton beam therapy of Cushing's disease and Nelson's syndrome.* In BLACK, PM, ZERVAS, NT, RIDGWAY, EC, MARTIN, JB (EDS): *Secretory Tumors of the Pituitary Gland.* Raven Press, New York, 1984, p 295.
18. KLIMAN, B, KJELLBERG, RN, SWISHER, B, BUTLER, W: *Proton beam therapy of acromegaly.* In BLACK, PM, ZERVAS, NT, RIDGWAY, EC, MARTIN, JB (EDS): *Secretory Tumors of the Pituitary Gland.* Raven Press, New York, 1984, p 191.
19. KOVACS, K: *Light and electron microscopic pathology of pituitary tumors: Immunohistochemistry.* In BLACK, PM, ZERVAS, NT, RIDGWAY, EC, MARTIN, JB (EDS): *Secretory Tumors of the Pituitary Gland.* Raven Press, New York, 1984.
20. KRAMER, S: *Indications for, and results of, treatment of pituitary tumors by external radiation.* In KOHLER, PO, AND ROSS, GT (EDS): *Diagnosis and Treatment of Pituitary Tumors.* Elsevier, New York, 1973, p 217.

HYPOTHALAMIC-PITUITARY DISEASE

21. LAWRENCE, JH, ET AL: *Heavy particle therapy in acromegaly and Cushing's disease.* JAMA 235:2307, 1976.

22. LAWRENCE, JH: *Heavy particle irradiation of intracranial lesions.* In WILKINS, RH, AND RENGACHARY, SS (EDS): *Neurosurgery.* McGraw Hill, New York.

23. LAWS, ER, JR: *The neurosurgical management of acromegaly.* In BLACK, PM, ZERVAS, NT, RIDGWAY, EC, MARTIN, JB (EDS): *Secretory Tumors of the Pituitary Gland.* Raven Press, New York, 1984, p 169.

24. LINFOOT, JA: *Heavy ion therapy: Alpha particle therapy of pituitary tumors.* In LINFOOT, JA (ED): *Recent Advances in the Diagnosis and Treatment of Pituitary Tumors.* Raven Press, New York, 1979, p 245.

25. MACCARTY, CS, ET AL: *Indications for and results of surgical treatment of pituitary tumors by the transfrontal approach.* In KOHLER, PO, AND ROSS, GT (EDS): *Diagnosis and Treatment of Pituitary Tumors.* Elsevier, New York, 1973, p 139.

26. MARTIN, JB, AND COPELAND, PM: *Hypothalamic hypopituitarism.* In KRIEGER, DT, AND BARDIN, CW (EDS): *Current Therapy in Endocrinology and Metabolism.* BC Decker, Philadelphia, 1985, p 11.

27. SERRI, O, RASIO, E, BEAUREGARD, H, HARDY, J, SOMMA, M: *Recurrence of hyperprolactinemia after selective transsphenoidal adenomectomy in women with prolactinoma.* N Engl J Med 309:280, 1983.

28. SHELINE, GE: *Treatment of chromophobe adenomas of the pituitary gland and acromegaly.* In KOHLER, PO, AND ROSS, GT (EDS): *Diagnosis and Treatment of Pituitary Tumors.* Elsevier, New York, 1973, p 201.

29. SHELINE, GE, GROSSMAN, A, JONES, AE, BESSER, GM: *Radiation therapy for prolactinomas.* In BLACK, PM, ZERVAS, NT, RIDGWAY, EC, MARTIN, JB (EDS): *Secretory Tumors of the Pituitary Gland.* Raven Press, New York, 1984, p 93.

30. VELDHUIS, JD: *Hypopituitarism.* In KRIEGER, DT, AND BARDIN, CW (EDS): *Current Therapy in Endocrinology and Metabolism.* BC Decker, Philadelphia, 1985, p 16.

31. WILLIAMS, RA, ET AL: *The treatment of acromegaly with special reference to transsphenoidal hypophysectomy.* Q J Med 64:79, 1975.

32. WILSON, CB: *The long term results following pituitary surgery for Cushing's disease and Nelson's syndrome.* In BLACK, PM, ZERVAS, NT, RIDGWAY, EC, MARTIN, JB (EDS): *Secretory Tumors of the Pituitary Gland.* Raven Press, New York, 1984, p 287.

33. WOLPERT, SM: *The radiology of pituitary adenomas.* Sem Roentgenol 19:53, 1984.

34. ZERVAS, NT: *Surgical results for pituitary adenomas: Results of an international survey.* In BLACK, PM, ZERVAS, NT, RIDGWAY, EC, MARTIN, JB (EDS): *Secretory Tumors of the Pituitary Gland.* Raven Press, 1984, p 377.

35. FAHLBUSCH, R, SCHRELL, U: *Surgical therapy of lesions within the hypothalamic region.* Acta Neurochirugica 75:125–135, 1985.

36. WERDER, K, VON, MULLER, OA: *Medical therapy of hypothalamic diseases.* Acta Neurochirurgica 75:147–152, 1985.

37. BELCHETZ, PE (ED): *Management of Pituitary Disease.* Chapman & Hall, London, 1984.

38. LAWS, ER, JR, FODE, NC, REDMOND, NJ: *Transsphenoidal surgery following unsuccessful prior therapy.* J Neurosurg 63:823–829, 1985.

Chapter 17

SPECIAL TOPICS IN HYPOTHALAMIC-PITUITARY DISEASE

The clinical manifestations of hypothalamic-pituitary disease usually can be predicted on the basis of anatomic and physiologic principles. However, the natural history of an individual case depends on the special etiology of the underlying disease. This is also true in considering diagnostic and therapeutic approaches. In this chapter, a number of specific causes of hypothalamic-pituitary dysfunction are considered.

NONPITUITARY TUMORS OF THE THIRD-VENTRICLE REGION

The midline region around the third ventricle is a common site of involvement of a variety of tumors, particularly those arising from cell rests, germ cells, or developmental abnormalities (Table 1).[11,29,115] The effects of such tumors depend on location, its rate of growth, and the occasional production of ectopic hormones by tumor cells. Tumors in the region of the anteromedial basal hypothalamus or inferior part of the third ventricle produce disorders of neuroendocrine regulation and of visual and olfactory functions. Tumors of the anterior-superior portion of the third ventricle may give rise to hydrocephalus by obstructing the foramina of Monro. Papilledema, visual loss, headaches, and vomiting may supervene. Dementia and memory disorders may occur as a result of interruption of connections between the dorsomedial thalamic nucleus and the frontal lobe. Mass lesions in the epithalamic or pineal region of the third ventricle cause Parinaud's syndrome (paralysis of conjugate vertical gaze), pupillary abnormalities, nystagmus, and brainstem signs. Obstruction of the aqueduct of Sylvius results in increased intracranial pressure. Posteroinferior involvement commonly causes hydrocephalus, ocular palsies, cerebellar ataxia, and corticospinal tract symptoms and signs.

PITUITARY CYSTS AND CRANIOPHARYNGIOMA

Rathke's Cleft Cysts

Cysts of Rathke's pouch occur in vestigial remnants of the craniopharyngeal anlage that gives rise to the anterior pituitary, the intermediate lobe,

dysfunction occurs. Diabetes insipidus rarely occurs with pituitary adenoma, but it is common with craniopharyngioma and with granulomatous, inflammatory, or infiltrative lesions at the base of the brain.

Treatment. The treatment of craniopharyngioma, usually surgical, is difficult at best. The choice of radical versus partial removal of the cyst is still debated. In the pediatric series reported by Matson and Crigler,[63] 57 of 74 children underwent radical excision. Remarkably, in the 40 that had not been previously operated on, there were no deaths. Of the total series, 40 cases were judged by long-term followup to represent a good result. Recurrences were rare. In adults, such radical removal is more difficult and accompanied by much higher mortality, up to 30 to 40 percent in some series and much greater morbidity in the survivors. Recently, there has been increasing evidence that radiation may help arrest growth of the remaining tumor. In the long-term followup of 23 patients treated with radiation as primary therapy, 18 of 23 were functioning normally, whereas only 3 of 14 cases treated by aggressive surgical attempts to remove the entire tumor were functioning normally.[30] Baskin and Wilson[119] reported on the surgical management of 74 cases. Forty were male patients and 34 were female patients. Twenty-eight patients were less than 18 years of age. The authors reported remission in 91 percent of patients (followed for a mean period of 4 years) after subtotal radical resection followed by irradiation. Operative morbidity was 12 percent, and mortality 3 percent. In another series of 125 patients, those who underwent x-ray therapy had a 76 percent 10-year survival compared with 21 percent for the group that had not received x-ray therapy.[122] Total excision is not the treatment of choice; aspiration of the cyst or partial excision combined with postoperative radiation may provide better management. This controversial issue is discussed in detail by Tindall and Barrow.[121] The complications of radiation, including GH deficiency, indicate that radiation therapy should be delayed as long as possible.[30]

Epidermoid Tumors (Cholesteatomas)

Epidermoid tumors are benign and arise from epithelial cell rests. According to Russell and Rubinstein,[80] epidermoid tumors cannot be clearly differentiated from craniopharyngiomas, because both commonly contain histologic features of squamous epithelium and contain cholesterol crystals. The relationship of craniopharyngioma and epidermoid cyst to Rathke's pouch and its derivatives has never been firmly established. Multiple sectioning of craniopharyngioma tissue almost invariably results in some sections that resemble in every respect the classic picture of the epidermoid cyst. It would thus appear that separation of the two tumor types is artificial.

HAMARTOMAS, INFUNDIBULOMAS, AND PITUICYTOMAS

Hamartomas are defined by Blackwood and coworkers[11] as a "congenital malformation with a potentiality for growth which does not exceed that of the normal tissue in which they are situated." In most instances, such

HYPOTHALAMIC-PITUITARY DISEASE

tumors represent ectopias, or abnormal localization or organization of neural tissue in the developing brain. Hamartomas may arise spontaneously and singly or they may occur in multiple sites in combination with hereditary disorders such as tuberous sclerosis, Lindau's syndrome, von Recklinghausen's neurofibromatosis, and perhaps Sturge-Weber disease.

Hamartomas occur rather commonly in the tuberal region of the hypothalamus, both as isolated tumors as reported in the case of Reeves and Plum (see chapter 11) and in combination with the syndromes described above. They may produce a variety of hypothalamic hormones; cases of hamartomas are reported that contain gonadotropin hormone releasing hormone (GnRH), growth hormone releasing hormone (GHRH), (see chapter 8) and corticotropin releasing hormone (CRH). They may be associated with precocious puberty, acromegaly, or Cushing's disease.

Other symptoms associated with hamartomas are due to local pressure that disturbs endocrine and autonomic functions of the hypothalamus. Tuberous sclerosis has been reported to cause growth failure, hypogonadism, or precocious puberty. Neurofibromatosis may result in diabetes insipidus and anterior pituitary deficiency. A curious, unexplained clinical observation is the association of neurofibromatosis with excessive somatic growth and of cerebral gigantism (see chapter 11). These patients do not secrete growth hormone (GH) excessively, and the mechanism of the growth acceleration is unknown.

The term infundibuloma was originally applied to tumors of the infundibular region that were thought to arise from pituicytes. The true histologic nature of these tumors is in some doubt, and Russell and Rubinstein[80] argue that they are likely astrocytomas. Tumors may arise in the neurohypophysis itself and have been called pituicytomas. They are exceedingly rare. Gangliocytomas consisting of primitive-appearing nerve cells also may occur in the basal hypothalamus. They may secrete hypothalamic hormones. The most common primary tumor of the posterior pituitary is the granular cell tumor, but metastatic tumor to the neurohypophysis is even more common (see chapter 4).

ARACHNOID CYSTS

Fluid-filled cysts arising from arachnoid membrane may occur in the suprasellar subarachnoid space and in the third ventricle.[81,82] The latter are believed to develop from entrapments of arachnoid that occur during development.

Arachnoid cysts occur predominantly in childhood and may give rise to rather specific neurologic signs. Russman and coworkers[82] reviewed the neurologic and endocrinologic abnormalities in four cases reported in the literature and included three of their own. The cysts, most commonly intraventricular, resulted in macrocephaly (hydrocephalus) and head and trunk tremor. The head tremor was characterized in most cases by a rhythmic bobbing. The ventricle was dilated. Endocrinologic abnormalities included precocious puberty, diabetes insipidus, obesity, hypothyroidism, and adrenal insufficiency. Arachnoid cysts of the suprasellar area may give rise to visual-field defects and blindness. It is important to recognize this syndrome in children, because the cysts are benign and can be removed

Few studies have been done to characterize endocrine function in these patients. In early reports it was suggested that panhypopituitarism might occur, and enlargement of the sella turcica has been described. In a report of three cases of congenital stenosis of the aqueduct, Fielder and Krieger[28] conducted detailed endocrine assessments and reviewed the endocrine status of five other cases from the literature. The clinical presentations varied in these cases, and endocrine disturbances were mild; hypogonadism and abnormalities in dynamic GH and ACTH secretion were the commonest disorders. Improvement in endocrine status was observed in some cases after surgical placement of a shunt.

VASCULAR LESIONS OF THE HYPOTHALAMIC-PITUITARY REGION

Aneurysms are uncommon causes of pituitary destruction. Cushing was the first to point out that an aneurysm can simulate an adenoma, although he never encountered such a lesion; but the first case was reported much earlier, by Silas Weir Mitchell in 1888.[21]

In a dramatic account, White[111] records the difficulty in distinguishing between an expanding intrasellar aneurysm and a hypophysial tumor by roentgenographic means. He illustrated his paper with a series of roentgenograms reproduced in a standard textbook to show progressive sellar destruction by a pituitary adenoma. "Unfortunately, the lesions turned out to be an aneurysm and the error in diagnosis caused this patient her life." In this case, a large aneurysm arising from the infraclinoid portion of the right internal carotid artery had compressed the optic nerves, eroded into the pituitary fossa, and destroyed the pituitary by pressure. In White's review of the literature and collection of unpublished cases, he was able to discuss 36 examples in which "the differential diagnosis between hypophysial tumor and intrasellar aneurysm without routine angiography would have been difficult or impossible." Less than 1.9 percent of all intracranial aneurysms manifest this abnormality. The average age was 46.5 years, the oldest 67, and the youngest 16. An aneurysm presenting as diabetes insipidus was seen in a 6-month-old boy by Shucart and Wolpert.[97] There seems to be no sex difference in aneurysm distribution. Most aneurysms arise from the internal carotid, and in this group the infraclinoid portion is the most frequent site of origin. Rarely is the anterior cerebral, posterior communicating, or basilar artery the site of the lesion. Progressive loss of anterior pituitary function and optic nerve compression are the most common manifestations. Cranial nerve compression giving rise to ocular palsies is reported in less than 15 percent of the cases. Headaches occur, but they are not common. Because the aneurysm may become thrombosed, even bilateral arteriography may not reveal the lesion in every case.

It is important to know that ectasia of the carotid arteries is extremely common in acromegaly (6 of 13 cases reported by Hatam and Greitz[41]), and in the series of Jakubowski and Kendall,[44] 11 incidental silent aneurysms were found in 183 patients with adenomas and craniopharyngioma.

Hypothalamic Damage Following Rupture of a Berry Aneurysm

Following the rupture of an anterior communicating aneurysm, insufficiency of pituitary function[24] or the syndrome of inappropriate secretion of antidiuretic hormone (ADH)[48] may appear. In an extensive pathologic study of the hypothalamus, Crompton[21] observed hypothalamic lesions in 61 percent of cases. Anterior and posterior communicating aneurysms were most frequently the cause. Ischemic lesions, varying from minute foci of necrosis to large areas 5 mm in diameter or more, were found in a few cases. Small or large hemorrhagic lesions were also observed. Massive hemorrhages in the path of rupture of an aneurysm into the lateral ventricles occurred in a few. Microhemorrhages consisting of subarachnoid blood forced up perivascular sheaths of perforating arteries, greatly distending the sheaths and then rupturing into the cerebral parenchyma through the wall of the sheath to form ball hemorrhages, were found along the course of the vessel. Microhemorrhages were often localized in the paraventricular and supraoptic nuclei, which were completely destroyed if the hemorrhage became confluent. Extensive endocrine testing has not been carried out in such patients,[70] but in one series, Jenkins and collaborators[45] showed a high frequency of impaired responses to metyrapone, and loss of the diurnal cortisol rhythm.

Pituitary Apoplexy

Acute hemorrhage into the pituitary gland was first reported in 1905 by Bleibtau, and at the time of Rovit and Fein's 1972 review[78] approximately 180 cases had been reported in addition to their own personally observed series of nine cases. Hemorrhage almost always occurs in a previously abnormal gland, most commonly a functioning adenoma.[24,59,102] Precipitating causes include anticoagulant therapy, head trauma, radiation therapy, estrogen therapy, and upper respiratory infection.[104] Spontaneous hemorrhage unrelated to any antecedent event occurs most frequently.

Rovit and Fein[78] proposed the following course of events in the pathogenesis of this disorder, a description that has not since been improved upon.

> An epithelial tumor, probably a chromophobe adenoma, gradually enlarges, expanding the pituitary fossa and compressing the remnants of functioning contiguous pituitary tissue. As the tumor continues to enlarge, it gains additional room for expansion by stretching the diaphragma sella. Further expansion superiorly may be accomplished if the attenuated diaphragm splits or if the diaphragmatic notch itself is unusually voluminous. Otherwise the neoplasm must squeeze itself through a narrow channel between the firm fibrous peripheral limbs of the diaphragma sella and the hypophysial stalk centrally. It is precisely at this juncture where we believe the chain of events leading to pituitary apoplexy occurs. . . .
>
> Virtually all the afferent blood supply destined for the pars distalis and the tumor itself is contained in a fine complex of vessels lying within and adjacent to the now compressed and distorted hypophysial stalk. Impairment of the infundibular circulation by impaction of tumor at the diaphragmatic notch may accordingly render virtually the entire anterior lobe ischemic, necrotic and hemorrhagic, as well

with which this condition follows pregnancy. The hyperplastic, highly vascular pituitary gland of the pregnant woman is especially sensitive to ischemic insult. It has been reported that the average sella size in such patients is smaller than normal. The crowding of tissue may contribute to its vulnerability to loss of blood flow. The bulk of new cells are lactotropes arising under stimulation of placental estrogens. It is most likely that Sheehan's syndrome arises when this highly vascular gland, with its high rate of metabolism, is suddenly deprived of blood flow because of shock. The roles of local spasm and of circulating vasoconstrictor substances have not been evaluated fully. Rarely, postpartum necrosis may occur in the absence of any evidence of hemorrhage.

The observed frequency of Sheehan's syndrome is to some extent a function of the adequacy of obstetric care. In 1963, Sheehan estimated, on the basis of the occurrence in routine autopsies and on the mean survival (22 years) of his patients, that in Liverpool 55 patients per million had severe hypopituitarism, and a similar number moderate hypopituitarism.[91] The estimated maximum was between 240 and 350 live patients per million. Sheehan stated that if a woman dies in the puerperium, there is a 38 percent chance that a massive or large pituitary necrosis will be found at autopsy. It is likely that many patients suffer from unrecognized mild pituitary failure following childbirth. The contemporary incidence of this disorder is not known.

Pituitary Necrosis of Diabetes Mellitus

Although the histologic findings and course in pituitary necrosis of diabetes resemble those of postpartum pituitary necrosis, there is no convincing explanation for the occurrence of this disorder in the diabetic patient. Stalk vessels occasionally appear to be sclerotic in diabetes, but in most cases the blood supply is not abnormal. Infarctions have been reported in young diabetic patients under the age of 20.

Clinical Manifestations

Ischemic necrosis causes no local symptoms or signs; rather, the manifestations are due to partial or complete loss of anterior pituitary secretions. Rarely, the onset of hypopituitarism may be abrupt, leading to severe ACTH-adrenal insufficiency, and thus complicating the clinical management of shock. Usually, hypopituitarism appears more gradually. Commonly, milk is not produced postpartum, owing to prolactin deficiency; normal menses are not resumed, owing to gonadotropin deficiency; weakness, loss of body hair, and loss of libido ensue, owing to gonadotropin and ACTH insufficiency; varying degrees of hypothyroidism may be noted. Because so many women are given estrogens at the time of delivery to prevent lactation, and birth control pills to prevent subsequent pregnancy, the usual hallmarks of Sheehan's syndrome may be missed for months or years. Hypopituitarism may develop after a few apparently normal periods. Although it is usual for amenorrhea to occur in such cases, there have been reports of patients with normal menstrual periods in whom deficiencies of the other pituitary hormones occurred. Pregnancies occur in a few such patients. Several patients have had hypogonadism and hypothyroidism. Thyroid replacement has restored normal gonadotropin secretion in a few cases.

The occurrence of ischemic infarction in a diabetic patient is heralded by the sudden amelioration of the severity of the carbohydrate disturbance, including a marked decrease in insulin requirement. In fact, a sudden decrease in insulin requirement in a diabetic patient suggests pituitary infarction. This occurrence is the clinical analog of the "Houssay phenomenon" in the dog: the amelioration of postpancreatectomy diabetes following hypophysectomy. Infarction may beneficially affect the course of the disease. In the classic case of Poulsen,[72] pituitary infarction led to a reversal of the changes of diabetic retinopathy. This observation, in fact, was one of the important findings that led to the widespread use of hypophysectomy and stalk section in the human being for the management of vascular disease in diabetes.

RADIATION-INDUCED HYPOTHALAMIC-PITUITARY DYSFUNCTION

Although the normal pituitary gland resists radiation damage, a number of patients have developed pituitary insufficiency after radiation of the head for various malignant conditions, including carcinoma of the nasopharynx, carcinoma of the maxillary sinus, intracranial medulloblastoma, glioma, ependymomas, and angiomas.[17,21,22,33,125,126] The dose of radiation responsible for this effect is variable.

The most frequent manifestation of pituitary insufficiency is growth failure following radiation in children.[40,86] Growth hormone secretory reserve is diminished in these cases — 11 of 16, for example, in the series of Shalet and coworkers,[86] studied a year or more after treatment. The importance of GH deficiency in growth failure was demonstrated by showing adequate growth after replacement therapy. Secondary amenorrhea owing to gonadotropin failure also has been reported. Growth disturbance occurs so frequently that it should be evaluated routinely in all children receiving radiation therapy to the head. In adults, deficiency of all anterior pituitary functions has been demonstrated in some patients after head or nasopharyngeal radiation. In one study, 15 of 1200 patients gave evidence of hypothalamic-pituitary dysfunction after whole-brain irradiation.[120] The commonest finding was hyperprolactinemia. In several cases, the use of the thyrotropic-hormone-releasing-hormone (TRH) test has shown that pituitary responses are normal,[55] as are responses to GHRH.[125] From this it has been inferred that the disorder is caused by radiation-induced hypothalamic lesions.

In common with other neural tissues, the hypothalamus is relatively sensitive to the damaging effects of ionizing radiation, and as shown by Arnold and collaborators[1] in the monkey, it is more sensitive than is the pituitary gland.[14] Gross necrosis of the hypothalamus and other parts of the brain in the human being has been produced by repeated courses of radiation to resistant acromegalic patients (doses recorded by Peck and McGovern[68] were 9775, 8150, and 10,126 rads). The late clinical manifestations of postradiation necrosis can include the appearance of localizing neurologic signs, papilledema, and dementia. Sarcomas and gliomas in the brain also have been reported following ionizing radiation.[35,36] Fortunately, the routine use of prophylactic cerebral radiation of children being treated for acute leukemia has not been followed by demonstrable impairment of intelligence. In a study of 34 children by Soni and collaborators[101] treated prospectively with 2400 rads from ^{60}Co, there was no disturbance in neurologic or psychologic function 18 months later. Eleven other patients studied four years after radiation also were indistinguishable from a control group. However, this is a significant incidence of GH failure after whole brain radiation.

Several authors have given estimates of the maximum dose that can be tolerated by brain tissue. Boden[14] estimated that the largest dose the brainstem can tolerate is 4500 rads in 17 days (250 KV) for small- and medium-size fields, and 3500 rads in 17 days for large fields over 100 cm^3. Arnold and collaborators[1] suggest that doses should not exceed 4500 rads in 30 days for centrally located tumors. According to Peck and McGovern,[68] "the degree of radionecrosis is proportional to the total size of the dose and time factors in its administration." It becomes more pronounced as the time interval from radiation is lengthened. Lindgren[56] calculated time-dose relationship curves for human brains on the basis of 13 cases adequately described in the literature, plus four of his own drawn from previously radiated autopsied gliomas. He stated that the minimal dose that produced necrosis on delivery of the rays through medium-size fields was between 4500 and 5000 rads in 30 days. Peck and McGovern recommended "a mid-plane tissue dose of 4000 r through stationary fields in 28 days using 4 × 4 cm portals at the surface. . . . There is little excuse for repeated courses of therapy."

Peck and McGovern[68] note that "the relative radiosensitivity of the brain varies from one region to another. The cortex and immediate subcortical medullary region are less sensitive than the deep-seated white matter. The sensitivity of the latter also appears to vary from region to region." There are two phases to the radiation injury. Initially, there is an acute inflammatory vasculitis, meningitis and choroid plexitis, with leukocytic infiltration.[6,84] The nuclei of the granular cells of the cerebellum show contraction and pyknosis. These early changes are established within 2 hours of irradiation, increased over 8 to 24 hours, and regress by 4 days. The delayed response, weeks and months later, includes damage to glia, astrocytosis, vascular endothelial proliferation, hyalinization of basement membranes, and necrosis.[37,105] The neuron damage may be due in part to the ischemic change.

There is no known treatment for radiation-induced brain damage. Only preventive measures can be used, that is, restricting doses to maximum recommended levels of 4000 rads to central brain structures. Radiation-induced hypothalamic injury should be considered in the differential diagnosis of hypothalamic-pituitary insufficiency in patients who have received head or upper-neck radiation.

HISTIOCYTOSIS X, EOSINOPHILIC GRANULOMA

Histiocytosis X is a granulomatous disease of unknown etiology and highly variable course, characterized by solitary or multiple lesions that can in-

HYPOTHALAMIC-PITUITARY DISEASE

volve virtually any tissue in the body and, although most common in early childhood, can occur at any age.[4,5,106] It is important to the clinical neuroendocrinologist as a cause of lesions of the hypothalamus. The term histiocytosis X includes several clinical varieties of disease, now believed by most pathologists to be different manifestations of a single underlying pathogenetic defect. The most common variety is termed *Hand-Schuller-Christian disease*, so named because of classic descriptions of cases, the first reported by Hand in 1893. This patient had the so-called classic triad: polyuria, exophthalmos, and skull defects. Much less common is the type termed *Letterer-Siwe disease*, seen in infants in a rapidly progressive form with widespread parenchymal involvement. The term eosinophilic granuloma was originally applied to solitary bone lesions. Because similar cytologic findings can be demonstrated in each of the forms of histiocytosis X, this term has come into common use.

Diabetes insipidus is the most frequent endocrine manifestation of histiocytosis and occurs in somewhat less than half of the cases of the chronic disseminated type (Hand-Schuller-Christian disease).[52,67] It is often seen in partial form and can present as the earliest sign of the disease in the absence of any other manifestation. Other endocrine abnormalities include impaired growth,[15] hypogonadism, and partial and complete hypopituitarism.[26,100] The growth failure is caused by GH deficiency. Other, less common, neurologic findings include those caused by mass lesions in the basal third ventricle and hypothalamus, indistinguishable from those caused by any type of localized hypothalamic disease. The lesion in the basal hypothalamus usually consists of a localized infiltrating granulomatous lesion, sometimes well circumscribed in nodular form. Histiocytes and eosinophils are seen on microscopic study.[4,5,9] The nodules may involve the dura also and distort the adjacent pituitary. Localized tumor-like infiltrations have been observed also in the hypothalamus.[52] It is uncommon for the tumor to replace the pituitary; evidently hypopituitarism in these cases generally is caused by damage to the hypothalamus or stalk.

DIAGNOSIS AND COURSE

The diagnosis of histiocytosis X should be the first consideration in differential diagnosis of diabetes insipidus in infants or young children. In fully established cases, 90 percent show skeletal lesions in some part of the body, especially in membranous bone of the skull. Lesions of the hypothalamus rarely give rise to roentgenographic changes in the sella; cases have been observed showing sellar lesions without hypopituitarism. Exophthalmos, usually unilateral but occasionally bilateral, is caused by retrobulbar infiltration of granulomatous tissue. Early in the illness, and sometimes even after the illness is well established, diabetes insipidus may be the only neuroendocrine abnormality present. Computerized axial tomography scan is often positive, revealing an enhancing infiltrating lesion. Some presentations are difficult to diagnose; the first clue to the nature of the illness may come from biopsy of the intracranial lesion.

The course of histiocytosis X is highly variable. Patients with single skeletal lesions (common in the jaw or mastoid) may be managed with local treatment, such as radiation treatment or curettage, and have no further manifestations. Others may follow a smoldering course, with new lesions occurring from time to time over many years, and a few who present with parenchymal infiltration may show a rapid and explosive course. Most cases fit the second category, and the prognosis for the disease as a whole is generally good, with a mortality of less than 15 percent of all cases.

TREATMENT

The variable and indolent nature of the disease has made it difficult to evaluate therapy.[23] There is no evidence that therapy directed at the CNS can reverse damage already inflicted, but it may arrest further progress of disease. In contrast, skeletal lesions can heal completely. Among the modalities that have been used for bone are local excision and curettage of accessible lesions and radiation therapy for well-circumscribed or inaccessible lesions. High-dosage corticosteroid therapy has been useful in treating the systemic manifestations, such as pulmonary involvement, which can be immediately life-threatening. Some patients have been reported to go into remission for 12 to 30 months after this treatment, and others require continued low-dose treatment for active peripheral manifestations such as infiltration of lung and skin.

The most significant advance in the treatment of disseminated histiocytosis has been the introduction of chemotherapy. Vogel and Vogel[106] summarize the results of therapy with alkylating agents, such as nitrogen mustard, cyclophosphamide, leukoblastine, and methotrexate, and show an 80 to 90 percent remission rate. There is remarkably little data on the course of hypothalamic lesions treated with either chemotherapy or x-ray treatment.

Whether one gives a single course of therapy or an initial course followed by low-dose maintenance therapy depends upon one's concept of therapy. Experts in cancer chemotherapy tend to try for a cure by giving high doses and repeated courses in order to decrease tumor cell mass and to destroy resistant cells. Because the etiology of histiocytosis X (neoplasm versus infection) has not been established, no dogmatic position can be followed on this question. It is obvious that a proper approach to patients with histiocytosis requires collaboration with experienced chemotherapists and radiation therapists.

SARCOIDOSIS OF THE HYPOTHALAMIC-PITUITARY UNIT

Sarcoidosis is a granulomatous illness of unknown etiology that can involve any part of the body. First described by Boeck in 1899 as a skin lesion, the systemic form of the disease was recognized by Schaumann in 1914, and diabetes insipidus owing to sarcoid was first described by Tillgren[103] in 1935. The course can be relatively benign and self-limiting or progressive. Evidence of systemic infection is often completely absent. Central nervous system involvement is relatively uncommon, but by 1948, Colover[20] could report 118 cases, including 3 of his own. The brain can be involved very early in the course of the illness, so that the common systemic manifestations are inapparent or can appear late.[3] The hypothalamic-pituitary axis is particularly liable to damage by sarcoidosis, as evidenced by the finding that 35 percent of the reported cases with neurologic findings presented symptoms of diabetes insipidus at some time during the course of their illness.[12,69,73,128] The special vulnerability of the stalk probably is a reflection of its superficial location in relation to a basilar meningitis: an infiltrative basilar meningitis extends upward into the hypothalamus along the perivascular cuffs.[34,71,85] Infiltrative nodules also may appear in the hypothalamus and pituitary gland and may present as a parasellar tumor[127] (Fig. 1). All degrees of pituitary insufficiency have been reported, ranging from panhypopituitarism to partial deficiencies.[85,87,103] Other evidence of hypothalamic involvement, such as somnolence and hyperphagia, also has been reported.[3] Optic atrophy and bitemporal or homonymous hemianopsia may result from local pressure on the visual system. Extension of granulomatous tissue along the base of the brain is common and results in unilateral or bilateral cranial nerve palsies.

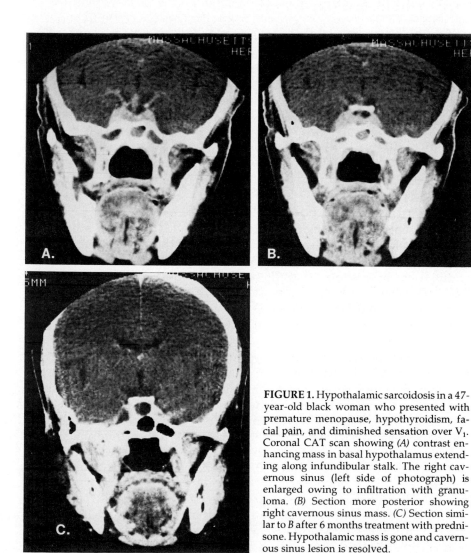

FIGURE 1. Hypothalamic sarcoidosis in a 47-year-old black woman who presented with premature menopause, hypothyroidism, facial pain, and diminished sensation over V_1. Coronal CAT scan showing (A) contrast enhancing mass in basal hypothalamus extending along infundibular stalk. The right cavernous sinus (left side of photograph) is enlarged owing to infiltration with granuloma. (B) Section more posterior showing right cavernous sinus mass. (C) Section similar to B after 6 months treatment with prednisone. Hypothalamic mass is gone and cavernous sinus lesion is resolved.

Patients with cerebral sarcoidosis usually have abnormal CSF findings; protein concentration is slightly or markedly elevated, a modest pleocytosis is present, and in many patients low CSF sugar is reported. One case studied by Pennell[69] had values as low as 10 mg/100 ml. Thus, the appearance of tuberculosis is mimicked. Computerizied axial tomography scans with contrast enhancement frequently demonstrate a lesion in the medial basal hypothalamus or pituitary stalk. It is obvious that sarcoidosis should be considered in the differential diagnosis of any patient with localized hypothalamic or pituitary disorder, particularly in young adult blacks, in whom the disease is most common in North America. The only known treatment of sarcoidosis is the use of corticosteroids in anti-inflammatory doses. Some patients have prolonged remissions of diabetes insipidus after such treatment, and a few even remain in remission despite the progress of other systemic manifestations of the disease.

EMPTY-SELLA SYNDROME

The term empty-sella syndrome refers to enlargement of the sella turcica secondary to extension of the subarachnoid space through a partially defective diaphragma sella.[41,44,49,50] Although the pituitary gland becomes compressed to the rim of the fossa, hypothalamic-pituitary connections usually are preserved, and endocrine disturbances, if any, are minimal.[8] On plain x-ray examinations, the enlarged pituitary fossa cannot be readily distinguished from that owing to an expanding intrasellar tumor.[110] However, CAT scans readily demonstrate low density in the sella compatible with CSF.

ETIOLOGY

The term empty-sella syndrome was first applied to this condition by Busch[16] in 1951. Early descriptions emphasized the development of the disorder after operative or x-ray ablation of pituitary tumors. More recently, it has been shown that the condition frequently occurs spontaneously in patients with no history of pituitary disease.[49] The abnormality commonly is noted first on routine skull roentgenograms taken in patients who present with headaches. Such cases are referred to as the *primary* empty-sella syndrome.

Several theories have been proposed with respect to the etiology of primary empty-sella syndrome.[49,50] Kaufman has emphasized that the condition develops because of a congenitally defective diaphragma sella. The condition is more common in women, particularly in the obese, and may occur with associated conditions such as benign intracranial hypertension,[109] pickwickian syndrome,[110] extrasellar tumor, hydrocephalus, and congestive heart failure. However, the majority of cases occur in the absence of these conditions and without evidence of increased intracranial pressure.

The diaphragma sellae was partially incomplete in 58 percent of cases.[16] Of these only 5.5 percent were associated with remodelling of the pituitary fossa. As this indicates, the condition is not uncommon, and several cases are seen each year on any major endocrine service.

CLINICAL MANIFESTATIONS

Neurologic

In the series of 31 cases reported by Neelon and coworkers,[66] 87 percent were women, and 93 percent were obese. Headache was the presenting symptom in 71 percent, and 29 percent had hypertension. The ages of onset centered in the fifth decade but ranged from the third to the eighth. Nontraumatic CSF rhinorrhea or visual field disturbances occur rarely. The occurrence of visual field disturbance is attributed to herniation of the optic chiasm into the sella turcica, with vascular or compressive neuropathy.

Four patients in this series had papilledema owing to benign intracranial hypertension. The sella turcica was enlarged by measurements in 26 of the 31 patients, but the configuration remained normal in 15. The result was a "symmetrically ballooned sella," without evidence of bone erosion.

Endocrine

In the patients reported by Neelon and coworkers,[66] the endocrine status was normal in 63 percent of cases, panhypopituitarism existed in four cases, and acromegaly was diagnosed in four cases. Testing of pituitary-hormone reserve indicated partial hypopituitarism in 11 patients, the most common abnormality being a decreased response of plasma GH to insulin-induced hypoglycemia. Reduced levels of LH were present in five cases but FSH was normal. Diabetes insipidus and disturbance of other hypothalamic functions were extremely rare. Secondary amenorrhea and hyperprolactinemia with galactorrhea have been reported in primary empty-sella syndrome.[7,64,103]

MANAGEMENT

The primary management problem with empty-sella syndrome is to distinguish it from an enlarging intrasellar pituitary tumor. This differentiation can be made definitely by high resolution CAT scans in most cases. Confirmation on CAT scan requires demonstration of the "infundibular sign," that is, an image of the stalk extending to the floor of the sella (see chapter 14). The presence of low-density fluid does not completely exclude the diagnosis of pituitary cyst or of infarct of the pituitary gland. Occasionally metrizamide cisternography is required to define the sellar contents. Normal pituitary tissue lining the rim of the sella is often visible, but there is no correlation between this observation and the likelihood of pituitary insufficiency.

The rare association of the condition with other causes of increased intracranial pressure should lead to the search for the possibility of benign intracranial hypertension,[109] abnormalities of cardiac or pulmonary function,[110] and, rarely, of extrasellar brain tumor. Except for the recognized association with benign intracranial hypertension, these conditions are fortunately uncommon.

A difficult clinical problem is the question of whether headaches are caused by the empty sella. A few case reports have appeared in which surgical repair by muscle grafting of the defective diaphragma sellae has resulted in remission of headache. However, no clear presenting feature of the headache permits separation from the much more common tension or muscle-spasm headache, and it is often very difficult to decide, in a given case, whether the headache is in fact related to the presence of the empty sella.

Occasionally, surgery is required in empty-sella syndrome (whether primary or secondary) because of visual field disturbances. In a recent case in our practice, the presence of optic atrophy and visual field abnormality were shown at surgery to be associated with entrapment of the optic chiasm into the superior portion of the sella turcica by arachnoid tissue adhesions. The excision of these tissues was followed by complete recovery of visual function. Usually, however, once the diagnosis of empty-sella syndrome is established, further investigations are not required, and the principal therapy is reassurance.

BENIGN INTRACRANIAL HYPERTENSION

Benign intracranial hypertension (pseudotumor cerebri) (BIH) presents clinically as a combination of headache, papilledema, and raised intracranial pressure in the absence of a space-occupying lesion of the brain or of obstructive hydrocephalus.[13,46,47,116] The majority of patients are obese females in the third to fifth decades of life. The CSF pressure is invariably increased, but its protein and sugar concentrations are normal, and diagnostic studies including electroencephalogram (EEG), CAT scan, and cerebral angiography are normal. Computerized axial tomography or magnetic resonance imaging (MRI) scans usually show normal or small cerebral ventricles; in a small number of cases the ventricles are slightly enlarged. If these criteria are strictly applied, over 95 percent of cases are self-limiting, and followup fails to reveal underlying disturbance. The other 5 percent have recurrent bouts of the disorder.

The presenting symptoms are usually headache and/or disturbance of vision. Headache is often relatively mild and may be aggravated by coughing or straining. Visual complaints include blurring, and more seriously, transient, sudden episodes of dimming or complete loss of vision (visual obscurations), which may occur many times during the day. Although visual loss may be minimal despite severe chronic papilledema, these episodes of fleeting visual loss are ominous warnings of optic ischemia, secondary to the increased intracranial pressure. They must be attended to promptly because permanent visual loss may follow. Diplopia owing to sixth cranial nerve involvement may also occur as a result of the increased pressure.

ETIOLOGY

A small percentage of cases have been shown to occur following dural venous sinus occlusion, toxic agents, antibiotics, and excessive vitamin A therapy, and a causative relationship with these factors is suggested (Table 2). The majority of cases are idiopathic and occurred most frequently in obese women.[46,47,107,108] An association with minor menstrual irregular-

TABLE 2. Differential Diagnosis of Syndrome of Benign Intracranial Hypertension (Papilledema, Headache, and Increased Intracranial Pressure)

I. Endocrine
   Steroid administration and withdrawal
   Contraceptive medication
   Addison's disease
   Obesity
   Pregnancy and postpartum
   Empty sella syndrome
II. Metabolic diseases
   Uremia
   Hypocalcemia-hypoparathyroidism
   Diabetic ketoacidosis
   Eclampsia
III. Toxic agents and drugs
   Heavy metal poisoning
   Hypervitaminosis A
   Tetracycline
   Nalidixic acid
   Chlordane
IV. High cerebrospinal fluid proteins
   Guillain-Barre syndrome
V. Circulatory diseases
   Congestive heart failure
   Chronic pulmonary hypoventilation
   Mediastinal obstruction
   Hypertensive encephalopathy
VI. Vascular or infectious diseases
   Disseminated lupus erythematosus
   Bacterial endocarditis
   Lateral-sinus and superior sagittal sinus thrombosis
   Meningitis or encephalitis
VII. Hematologic diseases
   Iron deficiency anemia
   Infectious mononucleosis
   Idiopathic thrombocytopenia purpura
   Polycythemia
VIII. Intracranial hypertension due to structural disease, without focal neurologic abnormalities
   Mass lesions
   Obstructive hydrocephalus
   Chronic meningitis.
IX. Idiopathic BIH

ities, contraceptive medication, or pregnancy has been noted by several investigators, but the frequency of these conditions in the general population makes definite correlation impossible.[77] It is possible that estrogens and progesterone have a direct effect on the transport function of glial cells. This hypothesis is suggested by the finding that meningiomas (tumors arising from arachnoid cells of brain and spinal cord) display a high incidence of receptors for both estradiol and progesterone,[129] and that the growth of these tumors is stimulated by estradiol and progesterone.[130] Glucocorticoid therapy with subsequent withdrawal of adrenal corticoids has been one of the more common events believed to play a role in the development of the condition.[13,18] Benign intracranial hypertension can occur following cure of Cushing's disease.

Pathophysiology

The evidence pertaining to the pathophysiology of the disorder has been summarized by Fishman.[31] The signs and symptoms are related directly to increased intracranial pressure, which commonly ranges from 300 to 600 mm CSF. Studies of patients have sought evidence for (1) alterations in intracranial venous or arterial pressure and (2) alterations in cerebral blood, CSF, and brain volumes.

Increased intracranial venous pressure is the likely cause of those cases of pseudotumor cerebri that follow thrombosis of the superior sagittal or lateral sinuses. These cases are rare, however. The association of the condition with obesity has suggested the possibility that local venous obstruction in the neck might contribute to the process. However, there is no direct evidence to support this hypothesis.

Arterial hypertension does not cause increased intracranial pressure, except in hypertensive encephalopathy, in which abnormalities in vascular integrity of small vessels secondary to the hypertensive disease result in microscopic infarcts and vasogenic edema.

The limited data available on changes in the *cerebral circulation* in idiopathic benign intracranial hypertension point to a significant increase in cerebral blood flow and increase in cerebral blood volume.[62] More recently, Raichle and others[74] reported a minor decrease in cerebral blood flow accompanied by a small but significant increase in cerebral blood volume.

Abnormalities of CSF absorption have been reported by several investigators using spinal infusion tests.[17,61] These observations suggest a defect in CSF absorption analogous to the occurrence of papilledema and intracranial hypertension in association with the Guillain-Barré syndrome.[76]

The finding of small ventricles in many patients points to the likelihood that *brain volume* may be increased in these patients. Fishman concludes:

> Thus, clinical and experimental evidence supports the hypothesis that BIH is associated with an increase in brain volume due to an increase in water content and is therefore a form of brain edema. What kind of brain edema does this represent? There is no evidence for vasogenic edema, that is, there is no evidence of increased capillary permeability assessed by isotope encephalography or by contrast-enhanced computed tomography. Similarly, the CSF protein is not increased — further evidence against the presence of vasogenic edema. There is also no evidence of cellular (cytotoxic) edema, in that neurological function is not affected and the EEG is normal in BIH. Thus, assuming that the increase in brain volume and brain water associated with BIH represent edema, then the findings would be best explained as a form of interstitial (hydrocephalic) edema. Such a mechanism is supported by the evidence, noted earlier, for the association of BIH with impaired CSF absorption.
>
> The fact that ventricular dilatation does not develop is quite consistent with the proposed mechanism. Patients with spinal cord tumors or polyneuritis associated with intracranial hypertension do not necessarily develop hydrocephalus. . . . the presence of free communication between the ventricular system and the cortical subarachnoid spaces in BIH would protect the periventricular white matter from the pressure atrophy that characterizes hydrocephalus.
>
> In summary, the evidence favors the occurrence of increased extracellular fluid volume characteristic of interstitial brain edema in both obstructive hydrocephalus and BIH. The fundamental defect may be a block to CSF absorption. Such a mechanism appears to underlie the development of BIH, whether due to occlusive venous

HYPOTHALAMIC-PITUITARY DISEASE

disease or associated with the other multiple factors, although the precise pathophysiology is obscure.

In view of the variety of factors associated with the syndrome, probably no single abnormality can account for all instances of the disorder. In the case of adrenal corticoid deficiency or steroid withdrawal, it is likely that the syndrome results from effects of corticoids on the permeability of cerebral capillaries. The relative steroid deficiency may result in alteration of transport of fluid across the blood-brain barrier, resulting in increased brain water.

The frequent occurrence of BIH in women, and its occurrence after contraceptive use and during pregnancy, has resulted in the listing of "endocrinopathy" as an etiologic factor. Estrogens are known to cause relaxation of vascular smooth muscle and to decrease the elasticity within blood vessels, factors that are thought to contribute to venous stasis and phlebothrombosis in the leg veins. There are, however, no data to confirm or to deny a specific effect of estrogens on brain vessels.

TREATMENT

The majority of patients with BIH require no treatment. Exclusion of mass lesions may require close followup with repeated CAT or MRI scans. Modification of factors that may contribute is important in a few cases. But most of the patients fall into the idiopathic group. A systematic approach to the management of these patients is given by Wall and Weinberg.[107]

The major threat to the patients with idiopathic BIH is visual failure. Daily lumbar punctures are effective in some patients, removing 15 to 30 ml of CSF. Acetazolamide (Diamox) (2 – 4 g per day) is the initial drug of choice and is moderately effective. Furosemide may be added, if needed. Both act by independent mechanisms to reduce CSF formation. If BIH persists after these drugs have been given for 2 to 3 weeks, a trial of high-dose corticosteroids is indicated. We prefer dexamethasone. Intermittent or progressive visual compromise may require a lumboperitoneal shunt or an optic nerve sheath fenestration.[107] Weight reduction is effective in most patients in terminating the progression of the disorder in those patients (less than 5 percent) who have difficulties that persist for 1 or more years.

REFERENCES

1. ARNOLD, A, BAILEY, P, HARVEY, RA: *Intolerance of the primate brainstem and hypothalamus to conventional and high energy radiations.* Neurology 4:575, 1954.
2. ARRAS, MJ, JR, AND SAUNDERS, AM: *Renal cortical necrosis with pituitary infarction in a nonpregnant woman.* Arch Pathol 85:262, 1968.
3. ASZKANAZY, CL: *Sarcoidosis of the central nervous system.* J Neuropath Exp Neurol 11:392, 1952.
4. AVERY, ME, MCAFEE, JG, GUILD, HG: *The course and prognosis of reticuloedotheliosis (eosinophilic granuloma, Schuller-Christian disease and Letterer-Siwe disease).* Am J Med 22:636, 1957.
5. AVIOLI, LV, LASERSOHN, JT, LOPRESTI, JM: *Histiocytosis X (Christian disease): A clinicopathological survey, review of ten patients and the results of prednisone therapy.* Medicine 42:119, 1963.
6. BAILEY, OT: *Basic problems in the histopathology of radiation of the central nervous system.* In HALEY, TJ, AND SNIDER, RS (EDS): *Response of the Nervous System to Ionizing Radiation.* Academic Press, New York, 1962, p 783.

7. Bar, RS, Massaferri, EL, Malarkey, WB: *Primary empty sella, galactorrhea, hyperprolactinemia, and renal tubular acidosis.* Am J Med 59:863, 1975.

8. Berke, JP, Buxton, LF, Kokmen, E: *The "empty" sella.* Neurology 25:1137, 1975.

9. Bernard, JD, and Agilar, MJ: *Localized hypothalamic histiocytosis X.* Arch Neurol 20:368, 1969.

10. Berry, RG, and Schlezinger, NS: *Rathe-cleft cysts.* Arch Neurol 1:648, 1959.

11. Blackwood, W, et al: *Neuropathology.* Williams & Wilkins, Baltimore, 1973.

12. Bleisch, UR, and Robbins, SS: *Sarcoid-like granuloma of the pituitary gland.* Arch Int Med 89:877, 1952.

13. Boddie, HG, Banna, M, Bradley, WG: *"Benign" intracranial hypertension. A survey of the clinical and radiologic features, and long-term prognosis.* Brain 97:313, 1974.

14. Boden, G: *Radiation myelitis of the brain-stem.* J Fac Radiol 2:79, 1950.

15. Braunstein, GD, and Kohler, PO: *Pituitary function in Hand-Schuller-Christian Disease. Evidence for deficient growth-hormone release in patients with short stature.* N Engl J Med 286:1225, 1972.

16. Busch, W: *Die Morphologie der Sella turcica und ihre beziehungen zur Hypophyse.* Arch f Path Anat 320:437, 1951.

17. Calabrese, VP, Selhorst, JB, Harbison, JW: *Cerebrospinal fluid infusion test in pseudotumor cerebri.* Ann Neurol 4:173, 1978 (Abstract).

18. Carlow, TJ, and Glaser, JS: *Pseudotumor cerebri syndrome in systemic lupus erythematosus.* JAMA 228:197, 1974.

19. Ciric, I, and Zivin, I: *Neuroepithelia (colloid) cysts of the septum pellucidum.* J Neurosurg 43:69, 1975.

20. Colover, J: *Sarcoidosis with involvement of the nervous system.* Brain 71:451, 1948.

21. Cromptom, MR: *Hypothalamic lesions following the rupture of cerebral berry aneurysms.* Brain 86:301, 1963.

22. Crompton, MR, and Layton, DD: *Delayed radionecrosis of the brain following therapeutic x-radiation of the pituitary.* Brain 84:85, 1961.

23. Dargeon, HW: *Considerations in the treatment of reticuloendotheliosis. The Janeway Lecture, 1964.* Am J Roetgenol 93:521, 1965.

24. Dawson, BH, and Kothandaram, P: *Acute massive infarction of pituitary adenomas.* J Neurosurg 37:275, 1972.

25. Doniach, I, and Walker, AHC: *Combined anterior pituitary necrosis and bilateral cortical necrosis of kidneys following concealed accidental hemorrhage.* J Obstet Gynecol Br Emp 53:140, 1946.

26. Ezrin, C, Chaikoff, R, Hoffman, H: *Case report: Panhypopituitarism caused by Hand-Schuller-Christian disease.* Can Med Assoc J 89:1290, 1963.

27. Fadell, EJ: *Necrosis of brain and spinal cord following x-ray therapy.* J Neurosurg 11:353, 1954.

28. Fielder, R, and Krieger, DT: *Endocrine disturbances in patients with congenital aqueductal stenosis.* Acta Endocrinol 80:1, 1975.

29. Finn, JE, and Mount, LA: *Meningiomas of the tuberculum sellae and planum sphenoidale. A review of 83 cases.* Arch Ophthalmol 92:23, 1974.

30. Fischer, EG, Welch, K, Belli, JA, Wallman, J, Shillito, JJ, Jr, Winston, KR, Cassady, R: *Treatment of craniopharyngiomas in children: 1972–1981.* J Neurosurg 62:496, 1985.

31. Fishman, RA: *Brain edema.* N Engl J Med 293:706, 1975.

32. Fishman, RA: *The Cerebrospinal Fluid in Diseases of the Nervous System.* WB Saunders, Philadelphia, 1980, p 128.

33. Ghatak, NR, and White, BE: *Delayed radiation necrosis of the hypothalamus.* Arch Neurol 21:425, 1969.

34. Gjersoe, A, and Kjerule-Jensen, K: *Hypothalamic lesion caused by Boeck's sarcoid.* J Clin Endocrinol 10:1602, 1950.

35. Goldberg, MB, Sheline, GE, Malamud, N: *Malignant intracranial neoplasms following radiation therapy for acromegaly.* Radiology 80:465, 1963.

36. Greenhouse, AH: *Pituitary sarcoma: A possible consequence of radiation.* JAMA 190:269, 1964.

37. Hagar, H, Hirschberger, W, Briet, A: *Electron microscope observations on the x-radiated central nervous system of the Syrian hamster.* In Jaley, TJ, and Snidere, RS (eds): *Response of the Nervous System to Ionizing Radiation.* Academic Press, New York, 1962, p 783.

38. Hamilton, CR, Jr, Scully, RE, Kliman, B: *Hypogonadotropism in Prader-Willi Syndrome.* Am J Med 52:322, 1972.

39. Harlin, RS, and Givens, JR: *Sheehan's syndrome associated with eclampsia and a small sella turcica.* South Med J 61:900, 1968.

40. Harrop, JS, et al: *Pituitary function after treatment of intracranial tumors in children* (Letter to the editor) Lancet 2:231, 1975.

41. HODGSON, SF, RANDALL, RV, HOLMAN, CB ET AL: *Empty sella syndrome: Report of 10 cases* Med Clin North Am 56:897, 1972.
42. HOFF, J, AND BARBER, R: *Transcerebral mantle pressure in normal pressure hydrocephalus.* Arch Neurol 31:101, 1974.
43. HUCKMAN, MS, FOX, JS, RAMSEY, RG, PENN, RD: *Computed tomography in the diagnosis of pseudotumor cerebri.* Radiology, 119:593, 1976.
44. JORDON, RM, KENDALL, JW, KERBER, CW: *The primary empty sella syndrome: Analysis of the clinical characteristics, radiographic features, pituitary function and cerebrospinal fluid adeno-hypophysial hormone concentrations.* Am J Med 65:569, 1977.
45. JENKINS, JS, ET AL: *Hypothalamic pituitary-adrenal function after subarachnoid hemorrhage.* Br Med J 2:707, 1969.
46. JOHNSTON, I, AND PATERSON, A: *Benign intracranial hypertension. I. Diagnosis and prognosis.* Brain 97:289, 1974.
47. JOHNSTON, I, AND PATERSON, A: *Benign intracranial hypertension. II. CSF pressure and circulation.* Brain 97:301, 1974.
48. JOYNT, RJ, AFIFI, A, HARBISON, J: *Hyponatremia in subarachnoid hemorrhage.* Arch Neurol 13:633, 1965.
49. KAUFMAN, B: *The "empty" sella turcica — a manifestation of the intrasellar subarachnoid space,* Radiology 90:931, 1968.
50. KAUFMAN, B, PEARSON, OH, CHAMBERLIN, WB: *Radiographic features of intrasellar masses and progressive, asymmetrical nontumorous enlargements of the sella turcica, the "empty" sella.* In KOHLER, PO, AND ROSS, GT (EDS): *Diagnosis and Treatment of Pituitary Tumors.* Excerpta Medica, p 100.
51. KELLY, R: *Colloid cysts of the third ventricle. Analysis of twenty-nine cases.* Brain 74:23, 1951.
52. KEPES, JJ, AND KEPES, M: *Predominantly cerebral forms of histiocytosis-X. A reappraisal of "Gagel's hypothalamic granuloma," "granuloma infiltrans of the hypothalamus" and "Ayala's disease" with a report of four cases.* Acta Neuropathol 14:77, 1969.
53. KOVACS, K: *Necrosis of anterior pituitary in humans. I.* Neuroendocrinology 4:170, 1969.
54. KOVACS, K: *Necrosis of anterior pituitary in humans. II.* Neuroendocrinology 4:201, 1969.
55. LARKINS, RG, AND MARTIN, FIR: *Hypopituitarism after extracranial irradiation. Evidence for hypothalamic origin.* Br Med J 1:52, 1973.
56. LINDGREN, M: *On tolerance of brain tissue and sensitivity of brain tumors to irradiation.* Acta Radiol (Suppl) 170, 1958.
57. LISSER, H, AND CURTIS, LE: *Treatment of posttraumatic Simmonds' disease with methyl testosterone linguets.* J Clin Endocrinol 5:363, 1945.
58. LITTLE, JR, AND MACCARTY, CS: *Colloid cysts of the third ventricle.* J Neurosurg 39:230, 1974.
59. LOCKE, S, AND TYLER, HR: *Pituitary apoplexy.* Am J Med 30:643, 1961.
60. LOVE, JG, AND MARSHALL, TM: *Craniopharyngiomas (pituitary adamantinomas).* Surg Gynecol Obstet 90:591, 1950.
61. MANN, JD, JOHNSON, RN, BUTLER, AB, ET AL: *Impairment of cerebrospinal fluid circulatory dynamics in pseudotumor cerebri and response to steroid treatment.* Neurology 29:550, 1979 (abstract).
62. MATHEW, NT, MEYER, JS, OTT, EO: *Increased cerebral blood volume in benign intracranial hypertension.* Neurology 25:646, 1975.
63. MATSON, DD, AND CRIGLER, JR, JF: *Management of craniopharyngioma in childhood.* J Neurosurg 30:377, 1969.
64. MOLITCH, ME, HIESHIMA, GB, MARCOVITZ, S, ET AL: *Coexisting primary empty sella syndrome and acromegaly.* Clin Endocrinol 7:261, 1977.
65. MURDOCH, R: *Sheehan's syndrome. Survey of 57 cases since 1950.* Lancet 1:1327, 1962.
66. NEELON, FA, GROEE, JA, LEBOVITZ, HE: *The primary empty sella: Clinical and radiographic characteristics and endocrine function.* Medicine 52:73, 1973.
67. OLIN, P: *Growth hormone response to insulin induced hypoglycemia in a boy with diabetes insipidus and short stature before and after treatment with vasopressin.* Acta Paediatr Scand 59:343, 1970.
68. PECK, FC, AND MCGOVERN, ER: *Radiation necrosis of the brain in acromegaly.* Neurosurgery 25:536, 1966.
69. PENNELL, WH: *Boeck's sarcoid with involvement of the central nervous system.* Arch Neurol Psych 66:728, 1951.
70. PITTMAN, JA, JR, ET AL: *Hypothalamic hypothyroidism.* N Engl J Med 285:844, 1971.
71. PLAIR, CM, AND PERRY, S: *Hypothalamic-pituitary sarcoidosis.* Arch Path 24:527, 1962.
72. POULSEN, JE: *Diabetes and anterior pituitary insufficiency. Final course and postmortem study of a diabetic patient with Sheehan syndrome.* Diabetes 15:73, 1966.
73. PURNELL, DC, ET AL: *Postpartum pituitary insufficiency (Sheehan's syndrome): Review of 18 cases.* Mayo Clin Proc 39:321, 1964.
74. RAICHLE, ME, GRUBB, RL, JR., PHELPS, ME, ET AL: *Cerebral hemodynamics and metabolism in pseudotumor cerebri.* Ann Neurol 4:104, 1978.

75. RINGEL, SP, AND BAILEY, OT: *Rathke's cleft cyst.* J Neurol Neurosurg Psych 35:693, 1972.
76. ROPPER, AH, AND MARMAROU, A: *Mechanism of pseudotumor in Guillain-Barre syndrome.* Arch Neurol 41:259, 1984.
77. ROTHNER, AD, AND BRUST, JCM: *Pseudotumor cerebri. Report of a familial occurrence.* Arch Neurol 30:110, 1974.
78. ROVIT, L, AND FEIN, JM: *Pituitary apoplexy: A review and reappraisal.* J Neurosurg 37:280, 1972.
79. RUSH, JL, ET AL: *Intraventricular craniopharyngioma.* Neurology 25:1094, 1975.
80. RUSSELL, DS, AND RUBINSTEIN, LJ: *Pathology of Tumors of the Nervous System.* Williams & Wilkins, Baltimore, 1963.
81. RUSSO, RH, AND KINDT, GW: *A neuroanatomical basis for the bobble-head doll syndrome.* J Neurosurg 41:720, 1974.
82. RUSSMAN, BS, TUCKER, SH, SCHUT, L: *Slow tremor and macrocephaly: Expanded version of the bobble-head doll syndrome.* J Pediatrics 87:63, 1975.
83. SAHS, AL, AND JOYNT, RJ: *Brain swelling of unknown cause.* Neurology 6:791, 1956.
84. SCHOLZ, W, SCHOLTE, W, HIRSCHBERGER, W: *Morphologic effects of repeated low dosage and single high dosage application of x-irradiation to the central nervous system.* In HALEY, TJ, AND SNIDER, RS (EDS): *Response of the Nervous System to Ionizing Radiation.* Academic Press, New York, 1962.
85. SELENKNOW, HA, ET AL: *Hypopituitarism due to hypothalamic sarcoidosis.* Am J Med Sci 238:456, 1959.
86. SHALET, SM, ET AL: *Pituitary function after treatment of intracranial tumours in children.* Lancet 2:104, 1975.
87. SHEALY, CN, ET AL: *Hypothalamic-pituitary sarcoidosis.* Am J Med 30:46, 1961.
88. SHEEHAN, HL, AND MURDOCH, R: *Postpartum necrosis of anterior pituitary: Production of subsequent pregnancy.* Lancet 1:818, 1939.
89. SHEEHAN, HL: *The frequency of postpartum hypopituitarism.* J Obstet Gynecol Br Commonw 72:103, 1965.
90. SHEEHAN, HL, AND SUMMERS, VK: *Syndrome of hypopituitarism.* Quart J Med 18:319, 1949.
91. SHEEHAN, HL, AND WHITEHEAD, R: *The neurophypophysis in postpartum hypopituitarism.* J Pathol Bacteriol 85:145, 1963.
92. SHEEHAN, HL: *The repair of postpartum necrosis of the anterior lobe of the pituitary gland.* Acta Endocrinol 48:40, 1965.
93. SHEEHAN, HL: *Neurophypophysis and hypothalamus.* In BLOODWORTH, JMB (ED): *Endocrine Pathology.* Williams & Wilkins, Baltimore, 1968, p 12.
94. SHEEHAN, HL, AND STANFIELD, JP: *The pathogenesis of postpartum necrosis of the anterior lobe of the pituitary gland.* Acta Endocrinol 37:479, 1961.
95. SHEEHAN, HL, AND MURDOCH, R: *Postpartum necrosis of anterior pituitary: effect of subsequent pregnancy.* Lancet 2:132, 1938.
96. SHREEFTER, MJ, AND FRIENDLANDER, RL: *Primary empty sella syndrome and amenorrhea.* J Obstet Gynecol 46:535, 1975.
97. SHUCART, WA, AND WOLPERT, SA: *An aneurysm in infancy presenting with diabetes insipidus.* J Neurosurg 37:368, 1972.
98. SIMMONDS, M: *Ueber Hypophysisschwund mit Todichem ausgang.* Deut Med Wschr, 40:322, 1914.
99. SMITH, CW, JR, AND HOWARD, RP: *Variations in endocrine gland function in postpartum pituitary necrosis.* J Clin Endocrinol 19:1420, 1959.
100. SMOLIK, EA, ET AL: *Histiocytosis X in optic chiasm of an adult with hypopituitarism.* J Neurosurg 29:290, 196.
101. SONI, SS, ET AL: *Effects of central-nervous-system irradiation on neuropsychologic functioning of children with acute lymphocytic leukemia.* N Engl J Med 293:113, 1975.
102. TAYLOR, AL, ET AL: *Pituitary apoplexy in acromegaly.* J Clin Endocr 28:1784, 1968.
103. TILLGREN, J: *Diabetes insipidus as a symptom of Schaumann's disease.* Br J Dermat 47:223, 1935.
104. VELDHUIS, JD, AND HAMMOND, JM: *Endocrine function after spontaneous infarction of the human pituitary: Report, review, and reappraisal.* Endo Rev 1:100, 1980.
105. VOGEL, FS: *Effects of high dose gamma radiation on the brain and on individual neurones.* In HALEY, TJ, AND SNIDER, RS (EDS): *Response of the Nervous System to Ionizing Radiation.* Academic Press, New York, 1962, p 240.
106. VOGEL, JM, AND VOGEL, P: *Idiopathic histiocytosis: A discussion of eosinophilic granuloma, the Hand-Schuller-Christian syndrome and the Letterer-Siwe syndrome.* Sem Hemat 9:349, 1972.
107. WALL, M, AND WEISBERG, L: *Pseudotumor cerebri.* In JOHNSON, RT (ED): *Current Therapy in Neurologic Disease.* B C Decker, Philadelphia, 1985–1986, pp 226–230.
108. WEISBERG, LA: *The syndrome of increased ·intracranial pressure without localizing signs: A reappraisal.* Neurology 25:85, 1975.
109. WEISBERG, LA, HOUSEPIAN, EM, SAUR, DP: *Empty sella syndrome as complication of benign intracranial hypertension.* J Neurosurg 43:177, 1975.

HYPOTHALAMIC-PITUITARY DISEASE

110. Weisberg, LA: *A symptomatic enlargement of the sella turcica.* Arch Neurol 32:483, 1975.
111. White, JC: *Aneurysms mistaken for hypophyseal tumors.* J Clin Neurosurg 10:224, 1964.
112. Whitehead, R: *The hypothalamus in postpartum hypopituitarism.* J Pathol Bacteriol 86:55, 1963.
113. Wolman, L: *Pituitary necrosis in raised intracranial pressure.* J Pathol Bacteriol 72:575, 1956.
114. Zellweger, H, and Schneider, HJ: *Syndrome of hypotonia- hypomentia- hypogonadism-obesity (HHHO) or Prader-Willi Syndrome.* Am J Dis Child 115:588, 1968.
115. Rubinstein, LJ: *Embryonal central neuroepithelial tumors and their differentiating potential: A cytogenetic view of a complex neuro-oncological problem.* J Neurosurg 62:795–805, 1985.
116. Fishman, RA: *The patholophysiology of pseudotumor cerebri: An unsolved puzzle.* Arch Neurol 41:257–258, 1984.
117. Ebersold, MJ, Laws, RR, Jr, Scheithauer, BW, et al: *Pituitary apoplexy treated by transsphenoidal surgery: A clinicopathological and immunocytochemical study.* J Neurosurg 58:315–320, 1983.
118. Bernstein, M, Hegele, RA, Gentili, F, et al: *Pituitary apoplexy associated with a triple bolus test. Case report.* J Neurosurg 61:586–590, 1984.
119. Baskin, DS, and Wilson CB: *Surgical management of craniopharyngiomas: A review of 74 cases.* J Neurosurg 65:22–27, 1986.
120. Mechanick, JI, Hochberg, FH, LaRocque, A: *Hypothalamic dysfunction following whole-brain irradiation.* J Neurosurg 65:490–494, 1986.
121. Tindall, GT, and Barrow, DL: *Disorders of the pituitary.* In *Craniopharyngioma.* CV Mosby, St Louis, 1986, pp 321–348.
122. Manaka, S, Teramoto, A, Takakura, K: *The efficacy of radiotherapy for craniopharyngioma.* J Neurosurg 62:648–656, 1985.
123. Harsh, GR, IV, Edwards, MSP, Wilson, CB: *Intracranial arachnoid cysts in children.* J Neurosurg 64:835–842, 1986.
124. Fletcher, WA, Imes, RK, Hoyt, WF: *Chiasmal gliomas: Appearance and long-term changes demonstrated by computerized tomography.* J Neurosurg 65:154–159, 1986.
125. Lam, KSL, Wang, C, Yeung, RTT, et al: *Hypothalamic hypopituitarism following cranial irradiation for nasopharyngeal carcinoma.* Clin Endocrinol 24:643–651, 1986.
126. Lam, KSL, Tse, VKS, Wang, C, et al: *Early effects of cranial irradiation on hypothalamic-pituitary function.* J Clin Endocrinol Metab (in press).
127. Clark, WC, Acker, JD, Dohan, FC, Jr, et al: *Presentation of central nervous system sarcoidosis as intracranial tumors.* J Neurosurg 63:851–856, 1985.
128. Ludmerer, KM, Kissane, JM (eds): *Visual impairment, pituitary dysfunction and hilar adenopathy in a young man: Clinicopathologic conference.* Am J Med 80:259–268, 1986.
129. Martuza, RL, Miller, DC, MacLaughlin, DT: *Estrogen and progestin binding by cytosolic and nuclear fractions of human meningiomas.* J Neurosurg 62:750–756, 1985.
130. Jay, JR, MacLaughlin, DT, Riley, KR, et al: *Modulation of meningioma cell growth by sex steroid hormones in vitro.* J Neurosurg 62:757–762, 1985.

PART 5

Neuroregulatory Peptides and Their Clinical Implications

Chapter 18

NEUROREGULATORY PEPTIDES

INTRODUCTION

The discovery that identical peptides are present as secretory products in defined populations of neurons in the central and peripheral nervous system and in certain glandular cells of the pancreas and gut has been one of the most important advances in regulatory biology in the last two decades. This finding, together with new insights into the molecular evolution of neuropeptides, has broken down previous rigid classifications of the ways in which cellular function is integrated and has made it possible for scientists to apply the powerful tools of molecular biology to the understanding of brain function.

Substance P was the first of the peptides to be found in both gut and brain. It was initially isolated in crude form from intestinal extracts by Von Euler and Gaddum in 1931[183] on the basis of its biologic effects on smooth muscle, but its structure was not elucidated. More than 35 years later, while searching for corticotropin-releasing factor in hypothalamic extracts, Dr. Susan Leeman and colleagues[13] noted that a particular fraction induced intense salivation in assay animals. Using the sialogogic effect as a bioassay, these workers were able to isolate the active principle, to determine its structure, and to synthesize a peptide that had identical chemical and biologic properties to the sialogenic peptide. Further study of the pharmacologic effects of this compound led to the recognition that it was similar to the previously described substance P of Von Euler which was then shown to be an active sialogog. By this time specific immunologic techniques were available to show that intestinal substance P was immunologically identical to Leeman's "sialogen." The chemical structure of gut substance P is now known to be identical to hypothalamic substance P.

Immunohistochemical techniques demonstrated the presence of substance P in many different kinds of neurons and in certain glandular cells of the gut, thus establishing what appeared to be a new class of *gut-brain peptides.*[25,28,42,46,55,60,64,68,92]

The next advance in broadening our concepts of the significance of neuropeptides was the discovery in 1973 that thyrotropin-releasing hormone (TRH), functioning in the hypothalamus as the thyrotropin-releasing hormone, had a wide distribution in the extrahypothalamic brain of all mammalian species and in the brains of representatives of all animal classes down to the snail.[78,79,80] Thyrotropin-releasing hormone has more recently been demonstrated to be present in pancreas and gut and thus can be included in the list of classical gut-brain peptides.

The concept of the gut-brain peptides was broadened by discovery of somatostatin, reported in 1973 by Brazeau and colleagues.[23] Initially isolated from the hypothalamus where it functions as a hypophysiotropic hormone to inhibit growth hormone (GH) and thyroid-stimulating hormone (TSH) release, somatostatin was found to inhibit pancreatic and gut secretions and to be localized in certain gut and pancreatic cells.[53,142,146]

Perhaps the most electrifying advance in regulatory peptide physiology was the discovery of the endogenous opioids including the enkephalins, by Hughes, Kosterlitz and their collaborators in 1975,[74] and the subsequent identification of β-endorphin and of the family of molecules contained in the opiomelanocortin precursor.[91,106] Recognition of the widespread occurrence of peptides in brain and gut has led workers throughout the world to an enthusiastic effort to isolate traditional gut peptides from brain and brain peptides from gut. In fact, it has now become a matter of routine as new peptides are discovered for workers in this field to test for their presence in all tissues.

Additional new peptides continue to be described, owing to advances in peptide purification, sequencing, and synthesis procedures, and to development of new antibodies for radioimmunoassay and immunocytochemistry.[120] The development of molecular biology has revealed a new universe of potential neuropeptides, present in the sequences of prohormones, some of which have already been shown to have biologic activity.[65] For example, more than seven different peptide fragments of the somatostatin preprohormone have been identified. In some prohormones that contain more than one active peptide, for example, proopiomelanocorticotropin (POMC) and procalcitonin, alternative pathways are tissue specific.

The naming of peptides has not been systematic until recently. Some are named for their first recognized action, for example, somatostatin and motilin. Others have been named for the species in which they were first found, for example, bombesin. Substance P was so named for an activity in an intestinal powder. Mutt and collaborators[120] now suggest that peptides be named using the first and last amino acids and the number of amino acids; for example, PHI-27:peptide-histidine-isoleucine-27.

The list of peptides that can be found in both gut and brain is long and continues to grow (Table 1). There are few, if any, examples of regulatory peptides distributed in only one type of cell. Because it is estimated that conventional nonpeptide neurotransmitters may account for only 40 percent of the synapses in the central nervous system (CNS), it is apparent that elucidation of the role of peptides both discovered and unknown will provide major new insights into CNS function.

CONCENTRATION OF PEPTIDES IN BRAIN

All the peptides are found in brain in significantly lower concentrations (10^{-12}–10^{-15} M/mg protein) than are the classical biogenic amine neurotransmitters, such as acetylcholine, norepinephrine, and dopamine, which are found in concentrations of 10^{-9}–10^{-10} M/mg protein.[93,94] The amino acid neurotransmitters, gamma-amino butyric acid (GABA), glycine, and

TABLE 1. Categories of Neuropeptides

Hypothalamic Releasing Hormones
    Thyrotropin-releasing hormone (TRH)*
    Gonadotropin-releasing hormone (GnRH)
    Somatostatin*
    Corticotropin-releasing hormone (CRH)*
    Growth hormone releasing hormone (GHRH)
Neurohypophysial Hormones
    Vasopressin
    Oxytocin
    Neurophysin(s)
Gastrointestinal Peptides*
    Vasoactive intestinal polypeptide (VIP)
    Cholecystokinin (CCK-8)
    Gastrin†
    Substance P
    Neurotensin
    Methionine enkephalin
    Leucine enkephalin
    Dynorphin
    Insulin
    Glucagon
    Neuropeptide Y
    Bombesin
    Secretin
    Motilin
    Somatostatin
    TRH
    Pancreatic polypeptide
Pituitary Peptides
    Adrenocorticotropic hormone (ACTH)
    β-endorphin
    Melanocyte-stimulating hormone (α-MSH, β-MSH)
    Prolactin
    Growth hormone
    Luteinizing hormone
    Thyrotropin
Others, including growth factors
    Angiotensin
    Bradykinin
    Carnosine
    Sleep Peptide(s)
    Calcitonin and CGRP
    Insulin growth factor II (IGF/II)
    Nerve growth factor (NGF)
    Galanin

*Also found in gut
†Not conclusively shown to be present in brain

glutamate are found in even higher concentrations of 10^{-6}–10^{-8} M/mg protein. Hypothalamic and pancreatic concentrations of somatostatin are approximately equivalent, and the concentrations of brain adrenocorticotropin hormone (ACTH) is about 1/1000 that found in the anterior pituitary gland and that of brain insulin is approximately 1/1000 that present in pancreas.[94] Cholecystokinin (CCK) seems thus far to be the only peptide whose CNS concentration is greater than that described in the gastrointestinal tract. The recently discovered neuropeptide Y (NPY) appears to be found exclusively in neural tissues and is present in unusually high con-

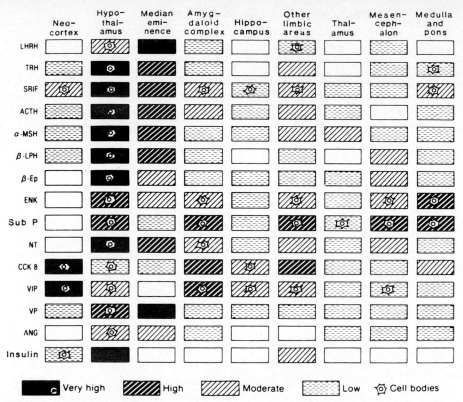

FIGURE 1. Regional distribution of neuropeptides in the mammalian central nervous system is represented here. This compilation is intended to show the selectivity of distribution of peptides, which presumably is related to specific functions. The hypothalamus contains the highest concentrations of most peptides, with the exception of CCK and VIP. Not shown is the distribution of neuropeptide Y, which is present in the cortex in the highest concentration of any peptide. (From Krieger, DT,[93] with permission.)

centrations in the CNS, exceeding by 10 times the concentration of CCK.[3,7] In general, however, CNS concentrations of peptides derived from homogenized tissue do not reliably indicate their functional importance. Concentration does not indicate turnover; additionally, regional, cellular, and subcellular distributions of peptides are likely of greater biologic importance than overall determinations of concentrations in whole regions of the brain or spinal cord. Aspects of the regional distribution of various neuropeptides in mammalian brain are summarized in Figure 1.

EVOLUTIONARY AND EMBRYOLOGIC ASPECTS OF NEUROPEPTIDES

Neuropeptides have undergone a fascinating evolutionary development. The families of neurohypophysial hormones illustrate this principle, in which evolution apparently gives rise to modifications of a common ancestral peptide.[2] Vasotocin, the ancient analog of vasopressin, has only a single amino acid substitution when compared with vasopressin. Lysine vasopressin, which also arose early in evolution, persists in the pig, where it exists as the major form. It is now known that marsupials, whether found in Australia, Africa, or North America or South America, are unique in containing both arginine and lysine vasopressin in the neural lobe of the pituitary gland, indicating their common ancestry.[2]

The family of tachykinins (which includes substance P, physalaemin, phyllomedusin, kassinin, and others) also occurs as a heterogeneous group of peptides, many of which are found in high concentrations in amphibian skin.[13] These patterns of peptide changes give valuable clues to the very nature and process of evolution.

Molecular biologic analysis also has traced divergent evolution of the neuropeptides. One example is that of somatostatin, represented by seven different genes in some species. It has been calculated that there is about 70 percent homology of somatostatin prohormones between fish and rat, species that may have diverged from a common ancestor 400 million years ago.[141,142]

The presence of similar peptides in different tissues and in different species indicates common evolutionary mechanisms, providing insight into gene structure and function and gene mutation and duplication. Neurotransmission and neurosecretion of peptides occur in coelenterates and annelids that have no recognizable endocrine tissue.[151,153] The presence of CCK and somatostatin in the gastrointestinal tract and brain has been noted as early in invertebrate evolution as the lamprey. Even more striking is the demonstration of substances similar to mammalian insulin, ACTH, and β-endorphin in unicellular eukaryotes (Tetrahymena paraformis, Neurospora crassa, Aspergilis fumigatis, E. coli).[151] These observations raise the possibility that most cells have a capacity for low-level expression of many peptides. In simpler organisms, peptides may have functions other than those that have evolved in higher organisms; with increasing evolutionary complexity, there may be selective enhanced expression of peptide biosynthesis in specific tissues.

Reports of similar peptides in different tissues also raise questions concerning the embryologic origins of peptides. Observations that peptide expression may be a common feature of many cells no longer make it necessary to attempt, as had been done previously, to establish a common embryologic origin for tissues that express the same peptides. For example, Pearse[133] postulated that all tissues containing similar peptides were of neural crest origin. It is now realized that many cells, regardless of embryologic origin, can express peptide-producing mechanisms.

BIOSYNTHESIS OF NEUROPEPTIDES

New methods in the rapidly emerging field of molecular biology and recombinant-DNA technology have now been applied to the study of several neuropeptides. These are reviewed in several publications[50,65,101,112] and are summarized in Figures 2 and 3.

In this chapter we summarize current understanding of the anatomy, biosynthesis, and function of the more important neuroregulatory peptidergic systems. How they may be implicated in the pathogenesis of disease, both neurologic and psychiatric, is discussed in chapter 19.

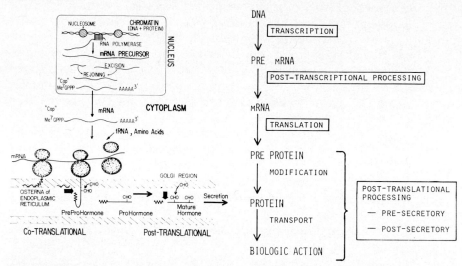

FIGURE 2. This is a schema of protein synthesis, showing steps in transfer of genetic information from DNA to RNA to protein. The schema specifically emphasizes the biosynthetic pathway for the synthesis of secretory proteins where posttranslational modifications of the polypeptide take place at the site of synthesis on the rough endoplasmic reticulum (RER). (From Habener, JF, and Potts, JT, Jr: *Biosynthesis of parathyroid hormone.* N Engl J Med 299:580–586, 635–642, 1978, with permission.)

COLOCALIZATION OF NEUROPEPTIDES AND CONVENTIONAL NEUROTRANSMITTERS

There is now extensive data documenting the colocalization of various neuropeptides and conventional neurotransmitters.[66,70,102-104,160] These data are summarized in Table 2. More extensive listings are found in recent publications of Hökfelt and coworkers.[192,193]

TABLE 2. Examples of Neurons and Endocrine Cells Containing Both a Classical Transmitter and a Peptide

Classical Transmitters	Peptide	Area (Species)
Serotonin	Substance P	Medulla oblongata (rat)
Serotonin	TRH	Medulla oblongata (rat)
Serotonin	Substance P + TRH	Medulla oblongata (rat)
Noradrenaline	Somatostatin	Sympathetic ganglia (guinea pig)
Noradrenaline	Enkephalin	Sup. cerv. ganglion (rat) Adrenal medulla (many species)
Noradrenaline	Neurotensin	Adrenal medulla (cat)
Noradrenaline	Somatostatin	Adrenal medulla (man)
Adrenaline	Enkephalin	Adrenal medulla (many species)
Dopamine	Enkephalin	Carotid body (cat, dog, monkey)
Dopamine	CCK	Ventral tegmental area (A9, A10) (rat, human)
Acetylcholine	VIP	Autonomic ganglia (exocrine glands) (cat)
Norepinephrine	NPY	Autonomic ganglia (sweat gland) (rat, cat)
Norepinephrine	NPY	Locus coeruleus (rat)
Acetylcholine	Calcitonin-gene-related peptide	Motor neurons, brainstem and spinal cord (rat)

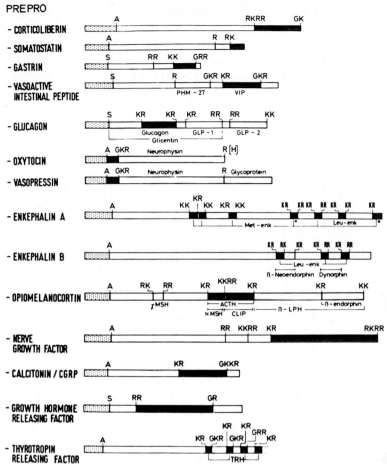

FIGURE 3. Structures of prohormones of previously characterized neuropeptides are shown here. Note that the capital letters indicate amino acids: K = lysine, R = arginine (basic amino acids usually conceived of as representing potential cleavage sites for processing by trypsin-like enzymes), H = histidine, G = glycine, representing a site as an amine donor for terminal amidation. The black bar indicates position within prohormone of originally described peptide. Note that VIP, PHM-27, depicted within the VIP prohormone, is (save for two amino acids) similar to a peptide recently isolated from porcine intestine and also has marked sequence homology to VIP. Other examples of repeat sequences of a given peptide within a prohormone are illustrated in the case of glicentin, which has marked similarity to glucagon; the enkephalin A and B precursor molecules, the MSH repeats in pro-opiomelanocortin, and the numerous repeats of the originally characterized peptide in the TRH precursor. (Reproduced from Richter, D: *Genes encoding hormones and regulatory peptides.* Humana Press, Clifton, NJ, 1985, with permission.)

THYROTROPIN-RELEASING HORMONE

The isolation of the tripeptide pyroglutamyl-histidyl-proline amide from hypothalamic extracts in 1969 ushered in the new era in neuroendocrinology (see chapter 2). The portal vessel chemotransmitter hypothesis was vindicated, and definitive studies of the neuropeptides' mechanism of action, hypothalamic localization, and specificity of effects could be initiated. Soon thereafter followed a number of observations that radically changed certain concepts of hypothalamic-pituitary regulation. Among these were the findings that the effects of TRH were not entirely specific,

Cerebral Cortex and Striatum

All parts of the cerebral cortex, including pyriform cortex and cingulate gyrus, contain somatostatinergic cell bodies which are located mainly, but not exclusively, in layers II, III, and VI.[84,96,182] These cells are principally bipolar or multipolar in shape and represent local interneurons (see chapter 19). Although concentrations in the cortex are low,[32,52] the total bulk of cortex (as compared with other parts of the brain) means that this part of the brain, in the aggregate, contains the largest percentage of total brain somatostatin.[32] None of the somatostatin in the cerebral cortex comes from the periventricular nucleus as shown by lesion experiments.[142] The existence of an intrinsic (presumably intraneuronal) system of cerebral cortical nerve cells separate from the hypothalamus is further established by studies in which the cerebral mantle of fetal rats is grown in dispersed cell culture. These cells synthesize and release somatostatin in response to modifications of the electrolyte and neurotransmitter milieu.[142]

Somatostatin is found in a subset of striatal neurons, called aspiny cells, owing to their lack of dendritic spines[61,172] (see chapter 19).

Circumventricular Organs

The system of ependyma-derived neurohemal organs arranged around the third ventricle (subfornical organ, pineal, subcommissural organ, median eminence, and organum vasculosum of the lamina terminalis) and in the floor of the fourth ventricle (area postrema) all contain nerve terminals of somatostatinergic neurons.[146] Their origin and function are unknown (see chapter 10).

GASTROINTESTINAL TRACT

Somatostatin is present in a population of cells in the pancreas (the "D" cell) as well as in nerve endings.[141,142] It is synthesized by islet cells in culture. The most important aspect of the D cell is its anatomic relationship to the other islet cells. Somatostatin cells are commonly found in direct contact with pancreatic β-cells. Fingerlike projections of somatostatin-secreting cells interdigitate with other cells in the islet.

Stomach and Intestine

Somatostatin-containing epithelial cells are present throughout the digestive tracts with a concentration gradient that decreases from the stomach to lower colon.

Somatostatin-secreting epithelial cells are found deep in the crypts of the stomach and intestine and contain microvilli, recognized as small processes directly opening into the gut lumen.[141,142] It is thought that such microvilli project into the lumen to provide a mechanism by which luminal content, particularly hydrogen ion and certain nutrients, can be sensed and can thereby regulate somatostatin secretion.

In addition to somatostatin-containing epithelial cells, the gut is innervated by separate systems of somatostatin neurons located in both the submucosal and the myenteric plexus. Cell bodies of the intrinsic system are located in the submucosal plexus, and the nerve endings come in contact with the interstitial space. The vagus nerve contributes an extrinsic somatostatinergic nerve fiber system. Because gut somatostatin content is unaltered by ligation of the nerve input to the intestine (or by transplantation), it has been concluded that the intrinsic system is the more important contributor to somatostatin nerve fiber activity in the gut.

It is not known at this time how the many somatostatin-containing elements of the gut — epithelia, nerve endings from vagus, and the intrinsic plexus — interact for physiologic control of the gut.

As a general rule, it can be stated that the brain somatostatin neural system has no direct effect on somatostatin systems outside the central nervous system. Lesions of the hypothalamus have no effect on pancreatic somatostatin.

OTHER VISCERAL DISTRIBUTION

Somatostatin immunoreactive D type cells have been identified in the salivary gland and in the parafollicular cells of the human thyroid.[115]Somatostatin is synthesized by medullary thyroid carcinoma cells.[169] In some studies, but not all, somatostatin appears to inhibit the secretion of calcitonin.[142] If this is part of a normal control system, it may be postulated that somatostatin is released from the cell and diffuses into the interstitial space where it comes in contact with somatostatin receptors on the cell membrane. This kind of control has been called *autocrine regulation.*

Immunoreactive somatostatin has been identified in collecting tubules of the kidney of the toad and in virtually all cells of toad bladder[21] and in the mammalian kidney. Human kidney contains immunoreactive somatostatin corresponding in molecular size to somatostatin 14. In both toad bladder and in the dog kidney, somatostatin interferes with vasopressin effects.[142]

BIOSYNTHESIS, PROCESSING AND TRANSPORT IN NEURONS

Somatostatin is biosynthesized from a prohormone. The amino acid sequence of preprosomatostatin has been elucidated in several tissues, and it is widely assumed that sequential processing of the peptide to smaller forms (corresponding to somatostatin 14, somatostatin 28, somatostatin 1-12 [of 1-28]), and larger molecular forms (prohormone, preprohormone) takes place within the endoplasmic reticulum and that the products are translocated to the Golgi apparatus for processing and assemblage into granule form (see chapter 8). In epithelial cells, the granules are then transported to the plasma membrane for exocytic secretion; in neurons the granules are transported from cell bodies via axons to nerve terminals for subsequent release. The transport of somatostatin in granules within the brain has been well documented in studies of effects of section of tuberoinfundibular axonal projections (which depletes the median eminence), by intraventricular injections of colchicine, and in ligation studies of the sciatic nerve of the rat.[142] Transport rate of the mobile fraction in sciatic nerve is approximately 400 mm per 24 hours, thus corresponding to the fast transport rate characteristic of secretory granules in neurosecretory fibers of the neurohypophysis, and in the sympathetic nerves. Only 20 percent of the somatostatin in sciatic nerve appears to be in the rapidly mobile fraction. Content of somatostatin in sensory ganglia of the sciatic nerve is estimated to turn over between 9 and 18 times in 24 hours.[140]

The relative amounts of the several forms of somatostatin secreted may have functional importance. All forms of somatostatin have growth hormone release inhibitory properties, and somatostatin 28 has been shown to be even more potent as a pancreatic and growth hormone release inhibitory peptide than somatostatin 14.[142]

The relative potency of the three different forms of somatostatin as neuromodulators has not been fully determined. It must be concluded that all three forms of somatostatin are secreted as such, and each can be regarded as a hormone, although the larger forms may be regarded as prohormones as well. In this respect, somatostatin resembles another gut-brain peptide, cholecystokinin (CCK), which is secreted as "big" CCK (33 amino acid residues) and "small" CCK (8 amino acid residues), both with biologic activity.

NEURAL FUNCTIONS OF SOMATOSTATIN

Regulation of Secretion

Depolarization of somatostatinergic nerve cells is followed by secretion of somatostatin in all preparations in which it has been studied. Depolarization-induced response is dependent upon the presence in the media of calcium and is blocked by agents that interfere with calcium entry. It is clear that membrane control of somatostatin release is mediated in the same way as all other neurotransmitter release processes.[142,145,146] Release of somatostatin is induced by veratridine, an agent that holds sodium channels in an open configuration[105,107] and that is blocked by the sodium channel blocker, tetrodotoxin.[17]

The extensive list of neurotransmitters and neuropeptides that will activate somatostatin release from various neural preparations are reviewed in Reichlin.[142] Contradictory effects have been reported, possibly due to differences in preparations and age of the donor animals.[142,145] For example, acetylcholine is stimulatory to dispersed fetal cells, but inhibitory in whole fragments of mature brains. Vasoactive intestinal peptide is also stimulatory to neurons in culture, but not to mature brains. The most convincing inhibitory effects were exerted by γ-aminobutyric acid (GABA), which suppressed somatostatin release.[51,145] Corticotropin-releasing factor stimulated somatostatin release from cultured brain cells.[134]

Little is known about factors that activate somatostatin secretion in extrahypothalamic neural tissues.

Electrophysiological Effects of Somatostatin

The earliest reports dealing with somatostatin effects on electrical activity of neurons indicated that in anesthetized cats or rats, "application of somatostatin by microiontophoresis decreases the spontaneous or glutamate evoked excitability of a proportion of neurons in the spinal cord, cerebral and cerebellar cortices and hypothalamus."[135] This action, which somewhat resembles that of GABA, was not blocked by the GABA antagonists, picrotoxin, or bicuculline.

> When iontophoresed onto cat spinal lamina V (the site of termination of dorsal root sensory nerves), spontaneous activity was depressed, and when perfused into isolated frog spinal cord, there followed "a small but immediate hyperpolarization in ventral root fibers, an action that shows desensitization and tachyphylaxis, enhancement of synaptic transmission between dorsal and ventral roots with considerable delay, and persistence after exposure to the peptide, and expression of glutamate evoked but not GABA evoked responses."[143,144] Hyperpolarization of hippocampal pyramidal cells *in vitro* by somatostatin was reported by Pittman and Siggins.[136]

Most of the more recent papers on somatostatin action report that this agent excites spontaneous neural activity.[40] Several unusual characteristics of the response to somatostatin may explain the discrepant reports in the literature. Delfs and Dichter[37] find that in response to somatostatin there is a "marked tachyphylaxis, an inverted U-shaped dose-response curve for membrane depolarization, and qualitatively different responses depending on the concentration of somatostatin." In their studies, somatostatin is predominantly an excitatory agent when applied to cortical neurons.

Effect of Somatostatin on Neurotransmitter Secretion

Somatostatin has been reported mainly to inhibit release of neurotransmitters. This has been shown to be true for acetylcholine release from intestine, norepinephrine release from hypothalamic neurons and from adrenal medullary cells, and TRH from rat hypothalamus. On the other hand, somatostatin is reported to stimulate release of acetylcholine from rat hippocampal synaptosomes,[121] norepinephrine release from cortex,[176] and serotonin release from several brain areas.[173] Somatostatin administered intracerebroventricularly is reported to increase acetylocholine turnover rate in diencephalon and hippocampus.[107]

Somatostatin Receptors

Membrane preparations from pituitary gland, pancreas, and brain have revealed specific binding sites. Different affinities for SS-14 and SS-28 are found in these tissues, suggesting that the two peptides may have different effects, depending upon their binding characteristics.[167,168] Tran and colleagues[175] recently characterized two different types of somatostatin receptors in brain. One, a high affinity receptor, called SS_A, was shown to have variable distributions in regions of brain. The other, SS_B, a low-affinity receptor, was present in brain but not in pituitary gland or pancreas. A complete mapping of CNS somatostatin receptors by autoradiography now has been published by Uhl and coworkers.[178]

Somatostatin Effects on Behavior

Many behavioral changes have been noted to follow the injection of somatostatin into brain or CSF. When given into the ventricles or hippocampus, somatostatin "has a general arousal effect, reducing both slow wave and paradoxical sleep, and in higher "pharmacological" doses (1-10 μg) it produces signs of pathological irritation such as hyperkinesia, stereotypic behavior, muscle tremor and rigidity, catatonia and finally, tonic-clonic seizures."[76] The term catatonia is really a misnomer and more properly should be referred to as catalepsy, a response similar to that observed after intracerebral injection of β-endorphin. Somatostatin-induced effects (unlike those of endorphins) are not reversed by naloxone and hence are presumed to act through nonopioid mechanisms.

> Other behaviors that have been observed after central administration are decreased sleep, excessive grooming and exploring, arrest of ongoing behaviors, motor incoordination, and analgesia. These findings are most compatible with reports of increased firing of neurons after local exposure to the peptide (see above) and indicate that somatostatin likely exerts important neural effects in many regions of the brain, including motor cortex, striatum, hippocampus, and limbic system. Somatostatin administration reverses post-ECT memory loss in the rat. In response to "kindling" brain somatostatin concentration rises.

Somatostatin in Cerebrospinal Fluid

As might be expected from the wide distribution of somatostatin-secreting cells throughout the brain and their proximity to the ventricles and subarachnoid space, this peptide is secreted into the CSF (see also chapter 19).[132] Levels in one large series of normal volunteers obtained between 8 and 9 AM gave means of 62.8 ± 6.38 SEM pg/ml. Similar values have been reported by others.[16] The peptide is relatively stable in CSF even at room temperature, showing only modest decline in immunoreactivity over days.

In an attempt to determine the site of entry of somatostatin into the CSF, comparisons have been made of the concentration of immunoreactive somatostatin in the first milliliter removed with that of later fractions. In the studies of Sorensen and associates[166] there was no difference in content in the 11th milliliter as compared with the first milliliter. In our own studies, comparisons were made of the 29th milliliter with a pool of the first to 12th milliliter.[142] Mean values were slightly but significantly higher in the later samples. The site of somatostatin release into the CSF is likely anatomically diffuse and not restricted to the hypothalamus. Berelowitz and colleagues[18] and Arnold and coworkers[10] have shown that CSF somatostatin concentration in the monkey varies with a distinct but small circadian rhythm, with lowest values observed during the day. The functional significance of this variation is not known. It is not correlated with GH regulation (as judged by known patterns of pulsatile GH secretion), nor is it correlated with the known alerting functions of somatostatin, because values are lowest during lighted hours. Acromegalic patients have normal CSF somatostatin levels.

> Published reports differ somewhat in their analysis of the molecular forms of somatostatin demonstrable in CSF. Our own studies, based on gel chromatography, indicate that forms with the characteristics of somatostatin 14, somatostatin 28, and a larger prohormone form are present in human CSF, in proportion to the forms secreted into the media of cerebral cells in tissue culture or in extracts of cortical cells. Similar findings have been made in CSF from the rhesus monkey.[10,18]

Pathologic Alterations in Brain Disease

Organic Brain Disease

In view of its wide distribution and important physiologic effects, studies of brain somatostatin secretion in various forms of brain disorder are of obvious importance. However, the limited approaches that are available to clinical investigators and problems of determining local secretion rates in functionally relevant brain regions make meaningful studies of the problem difficult. Hence, available studies have utilized the measurement of tissue concentrations in autopsy material or measurements in cerebrospinal fluid. Somatostatin concentration in brains of patients with Alzheimer's disease are reported to be markedly reduced in all regions tested: hippocampus, frontal cortex, parietal cortex, and superior temporal gyrus (see chapter 19). Of other neurotransmitters, only acetylcholinergic neurons are consistently involved. Neurons containing dopamine, norepinephrine, and serotonin are either maintained or mildly affected.

The validity of using postmortem brains for analysis was established by Cooper et al[32] who found little variations in concentration of somatostatin (or substance P and neurotensin) in brain tissue removed at different time periods up to 24 hours and then stored. This is in contrast to the rapid degradation of somatostatin in incubated extracts and suggests that in whole brain, somatostatin and virtually all other peptides are stored in a form compartmented from the peptidolytic enzymes. These studies do not exclude the occurrence of very early changes during the first two hours. Studies by Aronin et al[12] and Beal et al[15] have shown fourfold to fivefold increases in somatostatin in the basal ganglia of patients dying with Huntington's disease, data confirmed by others (see chapter 19). Somatostatin receptors are decreased in numbers in Alzheimer's disease proportional to the somatostatin deficit (see chapter 19). This finding has important implications when considering strategies for therapy in Alzheimer's disease.

In our laboratory, immunoreactive somatostatin was measured in 17 cultured cell lines derived from glioblastoma, medulloblastoma, neuroma, meningioma, craniopharyngioma, astrocytoma, hemangiomia, cordoma, and neuroblastoma. None showed any immunoreactivity.[142] The only human brain tumor to show immunoreactive somatostatin was that of a case of hamartoma of the hypothalamus. Somatostatin receptors are present in meningiomas; functional significance is unknown.

Somatostatin in Cerebrospinal Fluid in Neurologic Disorders

Pathologic increases in somatostatin concentration are observed in patients with a variety of structural CNS diseases including brain tumor, spinal cord compression, and metabolic encephalopathy, changes interpreted as indicating nerve cell damage, and possibly secretion by the tumor.[132] Several reports have appeared showing a decrease in CSF somatostatin levels in Alzheimer's disease[16] (see chapter 19). Patients with normal pressure hydrocephalus, with dementia, and with Huntington's disease have normal levels of somatostatin in CSF.

Decreased CSF somatostatin was reported in patients with multiple sclerosis in relapse.[166] The difference from normal was quite small, and as noted above, values in the normals were considerably higher than those reported by several other authors.

Somatostatin in Cerebrospinal Fluid in Psychiatric Disorders

CSF somatostatin was found to be significantly reduced in patients with unipolar depression.[54,154,195] Values returned to normal with recovery. Insufficient information is available to determine the significance of these findings. They may be indicative of a phase shift (values in primates, as noted above, are lowest during lighted hours), or a marker of state abnormality, or part of the mechanisms responsible for depression. Manic patients show CSF somatostatin levels indistinguishable from normal. Rubinow and colleagues[154] also have shown that administration of zimelidine (a serotonin agonist) raises CSF somatostatin; and carbamazepine, an anticonvulsant with antidepressant properties, lowers CSF somatostatin. The mechanisms of action of these agents are unknown.

Potential Therapeutic Use of Somatostatin in Brain Diseases

Intravenous somatostatin in the human was reported by Gerich to have a mild tranquilizing action.[53] Specific effects on extrapyramidal motor dysfunction and on paroxysmal electroencephalogram (EEG) were sought by Dupont et al,[41] who administered the peptide intravenously. No psychologic changes of any kind were noted. These authors point out the obvious fact that entry of the peptide into the brain is uncertain. An analog of somatostatin administered systemically had no effect in reversing memory loss in Alzheimer's disease, but measurements of CSF showed that the peptide had not entered brain substance.[202] The use of agents that enter the brain will be required before an adequate answer can be given to the question of therapeutic use in the human.[131] Alternatively, consideration may be given to methods of intracranial or CSF instillation. After intrathecal injection in the human being, somatostatin reduces pain.[203]

Cysteamine, a reducing agent, causes selective depletion of brain somatostatin after systemic administration in the rat.[155]

SUBSTANCE P

A dried powdered alcoholic extract of equine brain and intestine was shown by von Euler and Gaddum in 1931[183] to lower blood pressure and to stimulate muscular contractions in rabbit duodenum. That the effects were not due to acetylcholine was shown by lack of a blocking effect of atropine. The active principle was named substance *P*, for *powder*. Subsequent studies showed a similar material in the dorsal roots of the spinal cord, and several workers postulated that it might be a neurotransmitter involved in the axonal reflex.[13] However, it was not until 1970 that Chang and Leeman purified a sialogogic factor from bovine hypothalamus and characterized its structure as an 11-amino acid peptide.[13]

Substance P belongs to a family of related peptides called the *tachykinins*, which share vasodepressor and intestinal stimulatory effects (Fig. 4). These include eledoi-

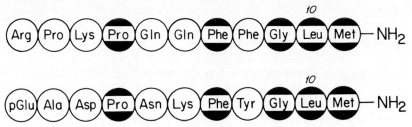

FIGURE 4. Structure of substance P *(top)* and physalaemin *(bottom)*.

sin, originally isolated from the salivary glands of an octopod, *Eledone moschata;* physalaemin, isolated from the skin of a South American amphibian, *Physalaemus bigilonigerus;* and uperolein, isolated from the skin of an Australian amphibian. The bioactive region of substance P resides in its carboxyl terminus; its sialogogic activity is abolished with oxidation of the terminal methionine. The carboxy-terminal three amino acids -Gly-Leu-Met-NH₂ are identical in each of the tachykinins. It is thought that substance P is the principal peptide of this group to be found in the mammalian central nervous system, although immunoreactive physalaemin-like peptides also recently have been found both in the gut and in the brain of several rodent species.

ANATOMIC DISTRIBUTION IN THE CENTRAL AND PERIPHERAL NERVOUS SYSTEMS

Radioimmunoassay and immunocytochemical studies provide complementary and confirmatory evidence of the regional and cellular localization of substance P in the nervous system. The highest concentrations in the central nervous system in the human are found in the pars reticulata of the substantia nigra, where it is located in the nerve terminals of the striatonigral system. There are also high concentrations in the inner segment of the globus pallidus, in the hypothalamus, in dorsal root sensory ganglia, and in the dorsal horn of the spinal cord. The peptide is also present in the ganglia and spinal nucleus of the trigeminal nerve, and in the ventral horn of the spinal cord.

> The habenulointerpeduncular system (of Meynert) contains substance P. Immunoreactive cell bodies that stain for substance P are found in the hypothalamus, striatum, globus pallidus, medial habenular nucleus, septal nucleus, and the nucleus of the tractus solitarius in the medulla oblongata. Electron microscopic studies of immunoreactive substance P have shown it to be associated with large secretory vesicles of approximately 115 to 120 nm diameter.

SUBSTANCE P AND PAIN PERCEPTION

In spinal dorsal root ganglia, substance-P-containing cells make up a subpopulation representing about 15 to 20 percent of the small bipolar cells. Central projections of these cells terminate in laminae I and II of the dorsal horn of the spinal cord. Similar terminations are abundant in the nucleus of the spinal tract of the trigeminal nerve in the medulla oblongata.

In addition to substance P, up to 20 percent of these small sensory cells contain somatostatin and a lesser number VIP.[81] A CCK-like peptide is found in others and may coexist in some cells with substance P. Other small dorsal root ganglion cells contain an angiotensin-like peptide, and yet others dopamine (see also chapter 19).

Of the potential functions of substance P, its relationship to pain perception has received the most attention. Substance P immunoreactivity can be visualized at the EM level in the central terminals of the dorsal horn in association with large dense core vesicles. Peripheral stimulation of A delta and C fibers (unmyelinated and small myelinated pain-transmitting fibers) results in release of substance P from these nerve terminals in the spinal cord. Substance P applied by microiontophoresis causes excitation and depolarization of neurons located in the dorsal horn, some of which are presumed to be second order pain transmission cells, which form the spino-thalamic tract. However, the activation induced by substance P is slow in onset and prolonged in duration, and it has been suggested that it acts to sensitize dorsal horn neurons to the actions of a more rapidly acting sensory transmitter which may coexist with substance P in sensory neurons. A similar slow excitatory action of substance P has been found to occur in neurons of the coeliac and inferior mesenteric ganglia.

> Attempts to elucidate the functions of substance P have taken advantage of the unusual effects of capsaicin, a molecule isolated from red peppers which gives rise to their characteristic pungent flavor. Administration of capsaicin causes degeneration of dorsal root neurons and depletion of substance P, an effect that is particularly apparent when the compound is given to neonatal animals. The intrathecal application of capsaicin to adult animals is reported to reduce behavioral responses to thermal noxious stimuli, presumed to be due to the neurotoxicity of the molecule on small sensory neurons.
>
> Problems in interpretation of these data arise from observations that neonatally treated animals when grown to adults show virtually no demonstrated loss of responsivity to noxious stimuli. These observations point to a role of substance P that is facilitatory rather than obligatory in pain transmission.

At the present time it remains uncertain what function(s) can be attributed to substance P in the transmission and perception of pain. Its electrophysiologic effects appear to be mediated via a slow excitatory potential.

BIOSYNTHESIS OF SUBSTANCE P

A prohormone precursor now has been identified for substance P.[81] The interesting outcome of this discovery was the identification of a second peptide of similar but not identical structure contained within the prohormone, which has been called substance K (kassenin). Both are active in CNS bioassays but appear to bind to separate receptor subtypes.

SUBSTANCE P IN THE GASTROINTESTINAL (GI) TRACT

Early studies of substance P, prior to its structural characterization, focused on its stimulatory effects on the motility of the small intestine of the rabbit and guinea pig. These bioassays confirmed abundant quantities of the material in the muscularis mucosae. By radioimmunoassay, substance P is found in highest concentrations in the duodenum and jejunum, and by immunohistochemistry it is localized in both neuronal cell bodies and in processes of Auerbach and Meissner plexuses. The fibers containing substance P in the gut are of both extrinsic and intrinsic origin and are distrib-

NEUROREGULATORY PEPTIDES

uted to all layers of the GI tract. Extrinsic fibers reach the gut primarily via the vagus and terminate principally adjacent to submucosal blood vessels and intrinsic ganglion cells. Intrinsic fibers that originate in the myenteric plexus distribute locally within the plexus and also are found in association with the circular muscle and the submucosal neuronal perikarya.

> No substance P-containing neuronal cell bodies were found in the submucosa. Terminals of the myenteric system that contain substance P also end on villi. These neuronal elements of the gut appear to interact closely with other neurons and fibers containing VIP, the enkephalins and somatostatin. Additionally, substance P immunoreactivity is found in "endocrine-like" cells throughout the small and large intestine.

The physiologic functions of substance P in the gut are poorly defined. Electrophoretic application of the peptide to neurons in ganglia of the myenteric plexus results in slow depolarization (excitation). The effect is not prevented by hexamethonium, atropine, naloxone, or enkephalin. There is also evidence that substance P acts directly on intestinal smooth muscle to cause contraction.

Substance P and the Autonomic Nervous System

Substance P is contained in a pathway arising in the small neurons of the dorsal root ganglia that innervate the sympathetic prevertebral ganglia (inferior mesenteric and coeliac).

> This pathway has been suggested to have a physiologic function in causing a slow depolarization of sympathetic postganglionic neurons, because a slow excitatory postsynaptic potential is evoked by application of substance P to ganglion cells. Electron microscopic studies indicate an axodendritic relationship of substance P-containing terminals on the postganglionic cells. In the adrenal medulla and in cells cultured from adrenal chromaffin cells (paraneurons), substance P causes inhibition of nicotinic-stimulated catecholamine release. Adrenal medullary tissue contains immunoreactive substance P, and it is possible that substance P exerts a regulatory function on sodium and potassium channels in chromaffin cells.

Substance P in Neuroendocrine Regulation

Immunoreactive fibers staining for substance P have been found in the median eminence in several species. Substance P is reported to stimulate prolactin (PRL) secretion in rats, both after intravenous and intraventricular administrations. A direct *in vitro* stimulatory effect of substance P on PRL has been reported. Both inhibitory and stimulatory effects on GH secretion have been recorded.[110] The data on effects of substance P on luteinizing hormone (LH) and TSH secretion are inconsistent. Taken as a whole, however—when routes of administration, magnitude of doses used, and inconsistency of results are all considered—it seems unlikely that substance P has an important direct neuroendocrine function.

Substance P in Endocrine and Neurologic Disorders

Carcinoid tumors of the gut and lung may, on rare occasion, contain and secrete substance P.[13,189] It remains to be demonstrated whether the circulating peptide has any physiologic effect. Decreased concentrations of substance P in the neostriatum, globus pallidus,and substantia nigra (pars reticulata) have been reported in Huntington's disease (see chapter 19) consistent with the death of substance P-containing cells. Small changes in concentration of substance P in the basal ganglia are found in Parkinson's disease (see chapter 19). Normal CSF contains low concentrations of substance P, ranging from 2.9 to 11.1 fmol/ml. Mean concentrations were found to be in the normal range in the CSF from patients with Huntington's disease, Parkinson's disease, and ALS. Patients with neuropathy (which presumably affects sensory fibers containing substance P) and with idiopathic postural hypotension with CNS signs (Shy-Drager syndrome) had significantly reduced SP concentrations in the CSF (see chapter 19).

NEUROTENSIN

In the course of isolation of substance P from bovine hypothalamic extracts, Carraway and Leeman[26] identified another peptide which caused vasodilation of exposed skin regions after intravenous injection. Subsequent biologic studies showed that the peptide also had a hypotensive effect, which led to their designating it as neurotensin (NT) (Fig. 5). They purified and sequenced the 13-amino acid linear peptide, which now has been synthesized and used widely for the development of radioimmunoassays and for immunocytochemistry.

ANATOMIC DISTRIBUTION OF NEUROTENSIN IN THE CENTRAL NERVOUS SYSTEM

The highest concentrations of NT in the human are found in the hypothalamus, substantia nigra, periaqueductal gray, locus coeruleus, nucleus accumbens, and amygdala.[11,86] Neurotensin also is found in the spinal cord and in the striatum and globus pallidus. Immunohistochemical studies have shown cell bodies that label for NT in the hypothalamus, amygdala, and the brainstem. A major system of NT is a projection from the amygdala which reaches the hypothalamus via the stria terminalis. Neurotensin is also found in perikarya of the periventricular zone of the hypothalamus, in the paraventricular nucleus, in the arcuate nucleus, and in the medial preoptic area. Positively stained fibers are also present in the external layer of the median eminence.

In the rat spinal cord, NT fibers appear in two discrete bands, a narrow one located at the border of laminae I and II and a second wider band in laminae II.[11] Cell bodies containing neurotensin are visible in the zone between laminae II and III. Immunoreactivity in the dorsal horn persists after dorsal rhizotomy in the rat suggesting that the NT neurons in the dorsal horn are intrinsic. Immunoreactive staining of NT in the dorsal horn of the monkey shows a somewhat different pattern of

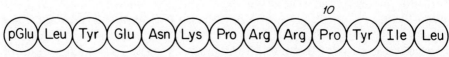

FIGURE 5. Structure of neurotensin.

localization. Reaction product was contained within laminae I-III, similar to the rat, but immunoreactive NT cell bodies were also found in the laminae II-VI, showing a more widespread distribution than found in the rat. This distribution of NT in the dorsal horn overlaps with the cell bodies and fibers that contain immunoreactive enkephalins. A possible function of NT in pain modulation has been suggested[11] (see below).

DISTRIBUTION OF NEUROTENSIN IN THE GASTROINTESTINAL TRACT

Neurotensin in extracts of gastrointestinal mucosa is identical chemically to that found in the brain.[11] It is concentrated in the intestinal epithelium of the jejunum and ileum in several species, including the human. Endocrine-like cells located in the muscosa of the small intestine contain neurotensin (N-cells). Immunoreactive fibers, but not neuronal cell bodies, are found in the esophagus, stomach, duodenum, and cecum. It thus appears potentially to have endocrine, paracrine, and neurotransmitter functions in the gut.

FUNCTIONS OF NEUROTENSIN IN THE CENTRAL NERVOUS SYSTEM

As is the case with many other neuropeptides, many different biologic effects have been observed after central or peripheral administration of neurotensin, but their physiologic significance is still uncertain. Three general kinds of activities have been reported: temperature homeostasis, anterior pituitary regulation, and pain perception. The role of peptides in temperature regulation is considered in chapter 11.

NEUROENDOCRINE CONTROL

Neurotensin-containing neurons are present in a well-defined subgroup of paraventricular cells that project to the median eminence. Their location makes it a virtual certainty, therefore, that NT is a hypophysiotropic factor, but a clear picture of its effects on the pituitary gland still has not emerged.[110] In the human, intravenous infusion of NT at concentrations of 104 ± 10 pmol/l had no effect on plasma levels of TSH, GH, PRL, LH, or FSH. In rats, on the other hand, systemic administration stimulates LH, PRL, GH, and TSH release. That the effect on TSH secretion is exerted directly on the pituitary gland is suggested by *in vitro* studies, but similar studies showed no effect on GH secretion.[11] Generally speaking, intraventricular injection of NT provokes the opposite kinds of effects on anterior pituitary secretion.

PAIN PERCEPTION

Both nerve cell bodies and terminals containing NT are localized in the dorsal horn of the spinal cord in regions known to receive sensory fiber input, but its function in pain perception has not been clarified.[126] In several species, intrathecal or intraventricular injection raises the pain threshold, an effect that is not apparently mediated by activation of central endorphinergic fibers because they are not blocked by naloxone. Electrophysiologic studies of the effects of neurotensin on neural activity in spinal cord have been inconclusive, both excitatory and inhibitory effects having been observed.

Neurotensin Receptors

Neurotensin receptors have been demonstrated in human brain by autoradiography.[11] The distribution corresponds closely to those of NT immunoreactivity found by radioimmunoassay and immunohistochemistry. One region of probable importance is the substantia nigra, where receptor levels are high and disappear by 90 percent after destruction of dopamine-containing cell bodies after administration of 6-OH dopamine. These findings suggest that most of the NT receptors in this region are present on dopamine neurons. These findings are suggested to have a functional importance in certain movement disorders; for example, in tardive dyskinesia, NT receptor density is markedly reduced.[178]

Function in the Gastrointestinal Tract

The intravenous administration of synthetic NT to dogs results in increased intestinal blood flow (mainly owing to dilatation of the mesenteric vascular bed), inhibition of gastric acid secretion, and suppression of gastric motility.[11] In some species, it appears to have a direct relaxing effect on the contractions of the small intestine, but the actions are biphasic and may interact with centrally mediated NT effects.

Neurotensin also may be involved in lipid homeostasis. Its secretion is stimulated by lipid feeding, and NT affects the secretion of pancreatic hormones, in some species, stimulating glucagon release and inhibiting insulin secretion, but appears to have little or no such effects in the human being.

ENKEPHALINS

The fact that binding sites for opiate narcotic substances occur naturally in the brain provided a strong rationale for the search for endogenous ligands.[74,170,174] Two pentapeptides with a capability to bind to endogenous opioid receptors were first identified in pig brain and named methionine-enkephalin (Tyr-Gly-Gly-Phe-Met) and leucine-enkephalin (Tyr-Gly-Gly-Phe-Leu) by Hughes and coworkers in 1975[74,89] (Fig. 6). The subsequent discovery of the endorphins, which are derived from the precursor pro-opiomelanocortin (POMC) (see chapter 6), and of dynorphin[56,57] and its precursor, gave additional evidence for the importance of this group of neuroactive substances.

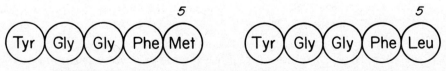

FIGURE 6. Structures of met-enkephalin (*left*) and leu-enkephalin (*right*).

Biosynthesis of the Enkephalins and Endorphins

Three separate precursors now are identified that give rise to opioid-receptor active peptides.[5,29,30,57,59,63,87,106,122,123] The first, proenkephalin A, gives rise to multiple copies of the enkephalins, including met- and leu-enkephalin[29,30,63,122] (see Figure 7). The second, proenkephalin B, gives rise to dynorphin and other opioid-binding peptides.[57,59,73,87,122,123] Pro-opiomelanocortin gives rise to MSH, β-endorphin, and to β-lipotropic hormone, ACTH, and a 16K glycoprotein (see chapter 6)[91,106] (Fig. 7). These precursor molecules occur in different neuronal perikarya and send nerve fibers to different regions of the CNS.

Anatomic Localization

Neurons that contain the enkephalins, dynorphins, and endorphins are dispersed widely in the CNS.[48,55,59,62,90,92,93,170,177,184,186] Met- and leu-enkephalin are found in interneurons in the dorsal horn of the spinal cord, in the nucleus of the fifth (trigeminal) nerve, in the raphe nuclei, in the periaqueductal gray matter of the brainstem, and in the amygdala, striatum, and cortex.[170] Opioid receptors are abundant in most of these areas, and their densities correspond closely, but not exactly, to the concentrations of the peptides as determined by radioimmunoassay.

The dorsal horn of the spinal cord has been studied carefully with respect to the localization of the enkephalins. Both enkephalin-containing cell bodies and axon terminals are found in superficial laminae I and II of the dorsal horn. Immunoreactive enkephalin present in the dorsal horn is not depleted after section of dorsal roots, indicating that the enkephalin contained there is not localized in afferent fibers. This is in contrast to substance P, the majority of which disappears in the dorsal horn after dorsal root transection. It has been proposed that enkephalin fibers make synaptic connections with substance-P-containing nerve terminals in the dorsal horn and that enkephalins inhibit the release of substance P to inhibit the relay of nociceptive signals. Experimental evidence strongly supports this contention.[81,117]

> In addition to the local interneurons of the superficial dorsal horn that contain the enkephalins, a long descending enkephalinergic pathway originating in a portion of the nucleus pars gigantocellularis of the medulla oblongata terminates in the dorsal horn close to local circuit neurons. Although not strictly proven, it is hypothesized that this pathway is one of several descending systems which function to modulate pain transmission at the level of the spinal cord.
>
> Several other enkephalin pathways have been described in the brain. The highest concentration of enkephalins is found in the basal ganglia, within the globus pallidus. The origin of the enkephalin found here is the caudate and putamen, which contain perikarya that stain for the peptide. Knife cuts that separate the striatum from the globus pallidus result in a decrease in pallidal enkephalin. Within the limbic system, a group of enkephalin cell bodies is located within the central nucleus of the amygdala with projections that reach the bed nucleus of the stria terminalis and the hypothalamus. In the hypothalamus, certain neurons of the supraoptic and paraventricular nuclei contain enkephalins; projections of these cells reach the neural lobe and probably the median eminence. Opioid receptors are found in the posterior pituitary gland, and enkephalins act to inhibit the release of vasopressin from the neural lobe. There is evidence that enkephalin coexists with vasopression and oxy-

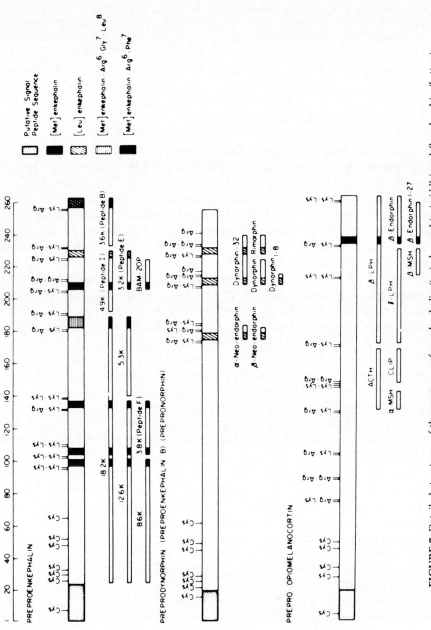

FIGURE 7. Detailed structures of the precursors for enkephalin (*top*), dynorphin (*middle*) and β-endorphin (*bottom*).

tocin in neurons of the hypothalamic-neurohypophysial system. Dynorphin also is found in neurons of this system and appears to coexist with the posterior pituitary peptides. Corticotropin-releasing factor (CRF) and dynorphin also are colocalized in a subset of periventricular hypothalamic neurons.[151]

Other regions containing enkephalin-staining cell bodies include the perifornical organ, the interpeduncular nucleus, the dorsal cochlear nuclei, the vestibular nuclei, the nucleus of the solitary tract, and certain cells of the cerebellum. Cells also have been described in the suprachiasmatic nucleus, the olfactory bulb, the pyramidal region of the hippocampus, the cerebral cortex, and the cingulate cortex.

The endorphins derived from POMC, in contrast to the enkephalins, are present in neuronal perikarya localized almost exclusively to the basal hypothalamus, primarily in the arcuate (infundibular) nuclei.[90,91] From this location, nerve fibers containing β-endorphin are distributed to the hypothalamus and to other regions of the CNS.[27] The distribution pattern is different from that containing the enkephalins. Lesions of the arcuate nucleus induced by monosodium glutamate (MSG) cause depletion of endorphins throughout the brain.

In the periphery, enkephalins are found in the sympathetic ganglia and in the peripheral nerves extending from them, in the adrenal medulla, and in the gut. Nerves containing the enkephalins are especially numerous in the outer layers of the gut, particularly of the myenteric plexus. Neuronal perikarya containing enkephalins also are found in the neurogenic plexuses of the gut. Enkephalins are not found in endocrine cells of the GI tract. Enkephalins are found in chromaffin cells of the adrenal medulla where they are colocalized with epinephrine.[150,181] Enkephalins are found in pheochromocytomas and are released along with catecholamines into the blood.[187,188]

RECEPTORS FOR THE ENDOGENOUS OPIOIDS

The original investigations that demonstrated the presence of opioid receptors in the CNS took advantage of the availability of tritiated ligands of opiate substances labeled to high specific activity.[89,170,174] These were shown to bind to cellular membranes prepared from brain tissues. The distribution of these "binding sites" was found to correspond to regions known to be associated with the pharmacologic actions of opiates. Kosterlitz and coworkers have described three types of opioid receptors, which they have called *mu, delta,* and *kappa*.[89] Morphine is the prototype ligand for the mu receptor, and its effects are blocked by low doses of the antagonist naloxone. The basis for a physiologic description of the mu receptor arose from experiments in the guinea pig ileum and the mouse vas deferens, whose contractile muscular elements show a response to the administration of morphine and other congeners. The kappa receptor has been defined pharmacologically by the selective effects of another group of narcotic agents of which *ketazocine* is the prototype. Substances that interact with this receptor and which are effective analgesics do not cross-react with the mu (morphine) receptor, made evident by the fact that ketazocine and other similar drugs will not substitute for morphine in the morphine-dependent monkey. Dynorphin favors the kappa receptor. The two enkephalins have no kappa receptor agonist effects, but neither are they pure mu receptor agonists; this additional binding effect is attributed to a separate class of receptor named the delta receptor.

Differences in the binding effects of the enkephalins and of β-endorphin have been demonstrated. For example, β-endorphin is equipotent in the guinea pig ileum and in the mouse vas deferens, whereas the enkephalins are 50-fold more potent in the mouse vas deferens. The interactions of the enkephalins with the delta receptors are not antagonized by naloxone to the same degree as is binding to the mu receptor. Consequently, larger doses of the antagonist are required, which gives rise to the additional problem of nonspecific effects when this drug is used. This discrepancy means that the use of naloxone is not an adequate means for excluding enkephalin-mediated responses. Other schemes of classification of opioid receptors have been suggested.

ACTIONS OF THE ENKEPHALINS

Direct application of enkephalins to the extracellular environment of neurons generally is found to inhibit the rate of firing. An apparent exception to this rule is found in the hippocampus, where firing rates are increased, but the possibility has been raised that this effect is secondary to the inhibition of inhibitory neurons so that the apparent excitatory effect is really indirect.

Application of enkephalins causes inhibition of the release of several other neurotransmitters including vasopressin, substance P, dopamine, acetylcholine (in the myenteric plexus), and somatostatin. It has been speculated by Snyder and colleagues[170] that this inhibition is due to an effect on calcium uptake, postulated to occur at a presynaptic site.

> Direct postsynaptic inhibitory effects also have been found in the locus coeruleus where opioids inhibit the firing rate of noradrenergic neurons. This effect is blocked by naloxone. Postsynaptic inhibitory effects also have been found on spinal cord neurons where intracellular recordings show enkephalin-mediated hyperpolarization.

Despite a large number of studies, there is no unifying hypothesis about the cellular mechanism of action of enkephalins on electrophysiologic responses of neurons.

Enkephalins and endorphins are speculated to act in the regulation of PRL (chapter 7), GH (chapter 8), and the gonadotropins (chapter 9).[88,116,149,150] Considerable evidence supports a function of opioid peptides in the regulation of temperature and of feeding behavior (see chapter 11).[33,88]

PROCESSING OF ENKEPHALINS

As described above, the enkephalins are synthesized first as large molecular weight precursors. Molecular cloning and sequencing techniques have now permitted precise structural identification of the precursors from the bovine adrenal gland and from human pheochromocytoma tissue (see above). The primary structure of proenkephalin A contains repeating sequences of the pentapeptides consisting of six copies of met-enkephalin and one of leu-enkephalin (see Figure 7). Dynorphin and alpha-neoendorphin are derived from proenkephalin B.

Studies are currently in progress to attempt to clarify the enzymatic cleavages that occur in the processing and degradation of the enkephalins. Central to this question is whether specific enzymes exist for the processing of the precursors or whether general trypsin-like and carboxypeptidase-like enzymes generate all the active peptides. Snyder and coworkers[170] have reported evidence for a carboxypeptidase B (an enzyme that removes a basic amino acid from the carboxyl terminus of a peptide) which may be selective for enkephalin biosynthesis, which they have termed "enkephalin convertase." It remains to be proven whether this enzyme acts only on enkephalins.

Investigators also have sought to define selective and specific enzymes for the degradation of enkephalins. Enzymes present in brain have been shown to remove the N-terminal tyrosine residue, but this activity is not considered to be specific for the enkephalins. Enkephalinase A is the name given to an enzyme activity that cleaves the carboxyl dipeptide of enkephalin. This enzyme is concentrated in brain membranes and has been partially purified. Enkephalinase B is the name given to an enzyme that degrades enkephalin by removal of the Tyr-Gly dipeptide. Neither of these enzymes has been convincingly demonstrated to be either selective or specific for the degradation of the enkephalins.

The role of enkephalins in neurologic and psychiatric diseases has been considered.[4] It is not surprising to note that the discovery of the enkephalins has encouraged numerous investigations of their possible role in disordered CNS function. Despite these efforts, conclusive (or consistent) data have been elusive, and to date it cannot be stated, without equivocation, that any abnormality has been identified. Human brain concentrations of the various endorphins have been examined. Only in Huntington's disease (HD), with the known death of spiny neurons in the striatum, some of which contain enkephalins, have definite reductions of the peptides been documented. In schizophrenia and manic-depressive disease, studies in brain and in CSF have not been rewarding (see review by Barchas[14]). A "hyperendorphenergic state" has been described in one case (see also chapter 19).

VASOACTIVE INTESTINAL PEPTIDE (VIP), MOTILIN, AND SECRETIN

For more than a century, physiologists studying the functions of the gastrointestinal tract were intrigued by the finding that acids entering the upper intestine produced an outpouring of copious secretion by the pancreas. Pavlov searched for a neural mechanism of pancreatic secretion but failed to find nerve fibers that he considered relevant. In 1902, Bayliss and Starling showed that extracts of intestinal mucosa obtained from the dog elicited, when administered intravenously, a stimulation of pancreatic secretion; they gave the name "secretin" to the active component without knowing its structure or mechanism of action. To this general principle of a substance eliciting effects after administration into the blood they gave the name "hormone" (on the recommendation of W.H. Hardy) from the Greek word meaning "I arouse to activity." Subsequently a number of other active peptides with similar properties have been isolated from gut extracts.

The chemical structures of secretin, VIP, and motilin were elucidated

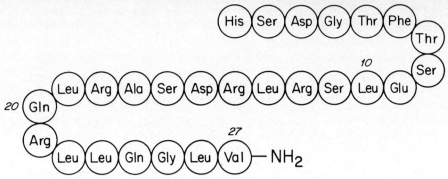

FIGURE 8. Structure of porcine secretin.

in the early 1970s. Porcine secretin, first characterized in 1970, was shown to contain 27 amino acid residues (Fig. 8). Bovine secretin is identical in structure, but that found in the chicken shows many differences. The structure of human secretin is unknown.

Porcine, bovine, and human VIP have the same amino acid composition and presumably the same sequences.[156] The structure of human VIP has been elucidated (Fig. 9). It contains 28 amino acids and is synthesized as part of a prohormone which also includes another related peptide, PHM-27, (Peptide-histidine-methionine-27).[66,77] Peptide-histidine-methionine has virtually the same biologic actions as VIP but is about one tenth as potent. Vasoactive intestinal peptide, growth hormone releasing hormone (GHRH), glucagon, secretin, and gastric inhibitory peptide (GIP) have similar structures (see chapter 8, Fig. 14). Motilin, which was purified from gut extracts on the basis of its stimulation of intestinal motility, has been characterized only in the pig and contains 22 amino acids.[120]

Vasoactive Intestinal Peptide

Anatomic Localization

Radioimmunoassay and immunocytochemistry studies have confirmed the presence of VIP-like material in several regions of the CNS.[104,156] It is

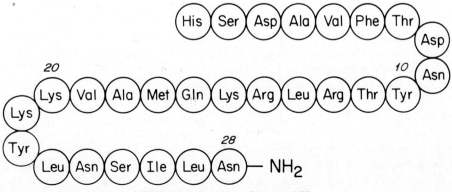

FIGURE 9. Structure of human VIP.

found in nerve cells of the cerebral cortex, hypothalamus, amygdala, hippocampus, and striatum.[104,156,157,159,161] In the human, unlike the rat, highest concentrations are found in the hypothalamus. The cerebellum contains very low concentrations. In the rat neocortex, VIP is present in a population of nonpyramidal neurons in layers II-IV, constituting 1 to 5 percent of the cells in these layers. Most cortical VIP-containing cells appear to project locally, and some fibers from these neurons appear to terminate on blood vessels. Brain VIP is identical in structure to intestinal VIP. Enkephalin and VIP are present in pheochromocytomas.[43]

Vasoactive intestinal peptide immunoreactivity also is found in cells and fibers of the suprachiasmatic and supraoptic nuclei of the rostral hypothalamus, in amacrine cells of the retina, in neurons of the periaqueductal gray matter, and in small bipolar neurons of the dorsal root ganglia of the spinal cord.[81,127,129] Vasoactive intestinal peptide prohormone is found in the same cells in the paraventricular nucleus that secrete CRH.[66] Although VIP neurons appear to be local interneurons, important exceptions occur. One is a VIP-containing projection from the mesencephalon, which ascends through the medial forebrain bundle to terminate in the amygdala. Another is the sacral nerve plexus which innervates the genital tract with VIPergic fibers that are known to be involved in penile erection.[9,34,35,38,137]

Subcellular fractionation studies show VIP to be concentrated in the synaptosomal fraction within synaptic vesicles. Electron microscopic immunocytochemistry reveals VIP within vesicles in presynaptic nerve terminals.

In the GI tract, VIP-containing nerve fibers are present in all layers of the gut. Most fibers are intrinsic, arising from local VIP-containing neurons found in the submucosal and myenteric plexuses. Vasoactive intestinal peptide is also present in nerve fibers of the urogenital tract, upper respiratory tract, and pancreas, and in the salivary and sweat glands.[103,127] VIPergic fibers also innervate the smooth muscle cells of blood vessels.

Release and Binding of VIP

Stimulation of preganglionic parasympathetic nerves causes release of VIP from tissues of the gut. In the CNS, depolarization causes VIP release, which is calcium dependent. Binding sites for VIP with similar characteristics of affinity and specificity have been found in brain and gut. Related peptides, like secretin, PHI, and PHM, show binding, but at lower affinity. The regional binding of VIP in the brain agrees closely to the anatomic distributions determined by radioimmunoassay. Of particular interest is the demonstration that VIP, unlike most other neuropeptides, acts to stimulate the accumulation of cyclic AMP. The functional significance of this observation is currently under study.

Functions of VIP

Of the many actions attributed to VIP, only a few are known to be of physiologic importance. A clue to its function as a vasodilator is derived from stimulation experiments of the vagal nerves. In the pig, such stimulation causes enhanced pancreatic secretion accompanied by vasodilation.

These effects are presumed to be the result of VIP released from autonomic nerve fibers that innervate the pancreas. Immunocytochemical coexistence of VIP with acetylcholine (ACh) in nerve fibers that innervate the salivary and sweat glands has been shown by Lundberg and colleagues.[102-104] In their elegant studies of the synergistic effects of VIP and ACh in these tissues, they showed that ACh stimulates sweat secretion from the acinar cells of the gland and VIP causes vasodilation; the resulting increased circulation to the gland facilitates further sweat production (see also chapter 1). The secretion of the sweat glands, but not the vasodilation, was blocked by atropine. Similarly, in the submandibular gland nerve stimulation enhances salivary secretion and causes vasodilation of blood vessels. Only the secretion was inhibited by atropine.

> VIP also inhibits muscular tone of the trachea in the guinea pig and counteracts the muscle contractions caused by histamine and carbachol. Bronchoconstriction induced by histamine and $PGF_{2\alpha}$ is reversed by VIP in the dog. Application by microiontophoresis onto cortical and hippocampal neurones has excitatory effects.

VIP is contained in sensory nerves of penis, clitoris, and vagina. Vasoactive intestinal peptide levels in blood taken from the dorsal vein of the penis increase during erection.[38] Peripheral blood VIP increases during clitoral stimulation in the human. Because VIP leads to vasodilation, it has been suggested that this peptide is an important mediator of tumescence. A patient with impotence caused by diabetic neuropathy was shown to have low VIP concentrations in the sacral sensory nerves.

Neuroendocrine Effects

Numerous endocrine effects of VIP have been described.[110] It is reported to cause release of glucagon, insulin, pancreatic polypeptide, and somatostatin. Recent attention directed to its effects on anterior pituitary secretion have focused on effects on PRL[1,156] (see chapter 7). Initially, reports of PRL stimulation by VIP after intraventricular or intravenous administration were attributed to indirect effects exerted on the hypothalamus, considered to be mediated by effects on dopamine synthesis and/or turnover. However, several recent reports document a direct stimulation of VIP on PRL secretion *in vitro.* Vasoactive intestinal peptide also stimulates PRL secretion from pituitary adenomas obtained at transsphenoidal surgery. Abe and coworkers[1] recently have shown that immunoneutralization of VIP delayed the onset of suckling-induced PRL secretion in the rat but did not prevent attainment of peak values. These results suggest that VIP is *a* physiologic PRF, but not the only one.

In clinical medicine, excess secretion of VIP has been implicated in the watery diarrhea syndrome, associated with pancreatic adenomas, carcinoids, or other intestinal tumors. Vasoactive intestinal peptide inhibits absorption of water, sodium and potassium and stimulates secretion of chloride in the GI tract. Vasoactive intestinal peptide levels in the cerebral cortex are normal in Alzheimer's disease; they are also unchanged in the striatum of HD (see chapter 19). A recent symposium reviewed current views of VIP's many effects.[194]

SECRETIN

Distribution

Whether brain secretin is identical in structure to that present in the gut has not been determined. Secretin-like immunoreactivity in pig and rat brain, with characteristics on high performance liquid chromatography (HPLC) identical to that of intestinal secretion, has been demonstrated.[120] The distribution of secretin in the rat brain differs from that of VIP. Particularly striking was the finding that secretin concentrations were low in the cortex, whereas VIP was high.

Actions of Secretin

Secretin has many effects, including stimulation of pancreatic duct cell secretion, stimulation of bile secretion, inhibition of lower esophageal sphincter tone, inhibition of gastric emptying and gastric acid secretion, inhibition of duodenal motility, stimulation of pepsin secretion, stimulation of insulin release, and stimulation of renal excretion of water, sodium, and potassium. Other described effects include stimulation of release of histamine from mast cells, stimulation of calcitonin secretion, and activation of hepatic bilirubin UDP-glucuronyl-transferase activity. It is recognized that many of these effects occur only after pharmacologic doses, and current investigations are directed toward measurement of and determination of factors that cause changes in plasma levels of the hormone. In this regard, Buchanan and coworkers[25] have reported that starvation produces high levels of the peptide in the circulation.

MOTILIN

Distribution and Actions

In experimental animals, motilin increases intestinal motility and stimulates secretion of pepsin, gastric acid, and pancreatic juice.[120] Motilin has no proven effects on pancreatic secretion in the human, however. The normal intestinal waves of contractility that occur in the gut between foods referred to as interdigestive myoelectric complexes (IMC) are initiated by motilin.[120] Its actions in this regard appear to be confined to the stomach and duodenum.

The evidence for the presence of motilin in the brain is limited. However, Yanaihara and coworkers[204] describe the presence of motilin-like immunoreactivity in the hypothalamus, neurohypophysis, anterior pituitary gland, and the pineal gland, with concentrations in several of these tissues exceeding those found in the intestine by 2 to 250-fold. Motilin antisera stain Purkinje cells in the cerebellum. Motilin was shown by Phillis and Kirkpatrick[135] to have potent depolarizing actions on dorsal and ventral root potentials in the spinal cord.

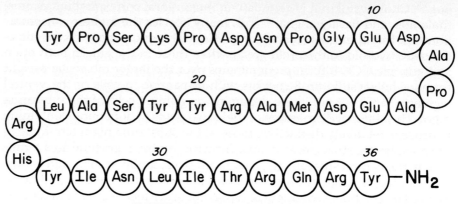

FIGURE 11. Structure of neuropeptide Y.

mammalian CNS.[3,6,7,36] To date it has been found exclusively in tissues of neuronal origin. In the brain it is found in high concentrations in cerebral cortex, striatum, and hypothalamus. Abundant numbers of neuronal cell bodies stain for NPY in the hypothalamic dorsomedial and arcuate nuclei.[124] In the striatum it appears to coexist with somatostatin; in cortex it coexists with somatostatin in some but not all cells (see chapter 19). It coexists with norepinephrine in one subgroup of cells in the locus coeruleus. In the peripheral nervous system NPY is found in autonomic nerves to the heart, and in the adrenal medulla where high concentrations are found in pheochromocytomas. Neuropeptide Y coexists with norepinephrine in postgangliomic cells and fibers of the autonomic nervous system.[124] Recent studies using pheochromocytoma have permitted isolation of mRNA and identification of the precursor to NPY.[113] Human NPY has a single amino acid sequence variation from porcine NPY.

Neuropeptide Y has effects in peripheral tissues, including reduction of coronary blood flow and stimulation of smooth muscle in the vas deferens. It is one of the most potent vasoconstrictors known. Its function in the brain remains obscure. It is present in abundant quantities in the arteries of the circle of Willis, presumably in nerve fibers. The possibility that it may elicit vasoconstriction of cerebral vessels is currently under investigation. A possible neuroendocrine function of NPY in regulating LH, GH, and FSH secretion has been suggested by McDonald and colleagues.[111]

BOMBESIN AND GASTRIN-RELEASING PEPTIDE (GRP)

Bombesin is a term now applied to several structurally related peptides isolated initially from amphibian skin. By bioassay, they are characterized functionally by possessing stimulatory effects on the smooth muscle of the gastrointestinal and urinary tracts. Bombesin itself, first isolated from skin of the frog *Bombina bombina* by Erspamer and colleagues in 1972, is a 14 amino acid peptide. A series of other peptides (now nine in number) show close homologies in structure, particularly of the C-terminus nonapeptide. These have been isolated from tissues obtained from amphibian, avian, and mammalian species. The carboxyl terminal nonapeptide contains the most important determinants for biologic activity. In 1978, McDonald and

NEUROREGULATORY PEPTIDES

coworkers[190] isolated a mammalian equivalent from porcine intestine and, by virtue of its potent effects on the stimulation of gastrin secretion, named the molecule gastrin-releasing peptide (GRP). This homologue, which contains 27 amino acid residues, has a 9 amino acid C-terminal peptide identical to bombesin, except for a single substitution. Gastrin-releasing peptide also has been sequenced from porcine brain.

LOCALIZATION OF BOMBESIN IN MAMMALIAN GUT AND BRAIN

Within the gut, bombesin-like peptides are found exclusively in nerve cells and nerve fibers. Fibers are found in the mucosa of the stomach and in the muscular layer of the intestine. Immunostaining nerve fibers also are found in the sympathetic prevertebral ganglia. Endocrine-type cells containing bombesin are found in the fetal lung, perhaps providing a clue to the fact that bombesin is commonly present in and secreted from oat cell carcinoma of the lung.

Bombesin in the brain is found in highest concentrations in the hypothalamus, nucleus of the solitary tract, trigeminal nucleus, interpeduncular nucleus, and dorsal horn of the spinal cord. Concentrations are low in the cerebellum. The peptide is concentrated in synaptosomal fragments, and it is released on depolarization. Bombesin receptors in CNS tissues have been partially characterized.

FUNCTIONS OF BOMBESIN IN BRAIN

Bombesin applied extracellularly to neurons in the hippocampus and the dorsal horn of the spinal cord causes excitation and depolarization. Administration of bombesin-14 or GRP-27 locally or into the lateral ventricles evokes a number of pharmacologic behavioral effects. One of the most potent effects is hypothermia, which occurs only when animals are exposed to a cold ambient temperature. The hypothermia is dose-dependent, rapid in onset, long-lasting, and reversible. It is antagonized by TRH, somatostatin, prostaglandin E_2, and naloxone. It is unaffected by agents that block biogenic amine receptors, and it is postulated that bombesin exerts its effects via mechanisms unrelated to the dopaminergic, adrenergic, or serotonergic systems. Local intracerebral injections indicate that the preoptic area is directly sensitive to bombesin in eliciting the hypothermic response. The physiologic significance, if any, of this effect for homeostatic maintenance of body temperature remains to be determined (see also chapter 11).

Bombesin also elicits hyperglycemia after injection into the brain. The response is similar to that caused by intravenous injection of epinephrine, because both are accompanied by a rise in glucagon and a decline in plasma insulin. The hyperglycemia effect of bombesin can be prevented by adrenalectomy, suggesting that the effect is mediated by release of catecholamines. Hyperglycemia is blocked by central administration of somatostatin, but not by treatment with angiotensin receptor blockers or by biogenic amine blocking drugs. Behavioral activation consisting of facial grooming, scratching, and inhibition of feeding and of water intake also occur after injection of bombesin into the brain. The inhibition of food

induce sleep (or sleep EEGs) following intracerebral injection, but it is not known whether these materials are contained in neurons or play a physiologic role in sleep. The two substances that have been isolated have been designated *delta-sleep-inducing-peptide (DSIP)*, which is a nonapeptide (Trp-Ala-Gly-Gly-Asp-Ala-Ser-Gly-Gly).[195,199] The sleep-inducing peptide isolated from urine is a muramyl dipeptide (acetylmuramyl-alanyl-isoglutaminyl-lysine).[196,198,200,201] Antisera developed against this material is cross-reactive with brain extracts. The muramyl dipeptides as a class are not synthesized in mammalian tissues but are a component of bacterial metabolism. It has been postulated that the material found in brain is of bacterial origin, incorporated into a bioactive material in a manner analogous to a vitamin.

OTHER PEPTIDES IN THE CNS

There is also evidence for glucagon[31] and insulin (see chapter 11) in the brain. Both likely are synthesized there rather than being transported from the periphery.

REFERENCES

1. ABE, H, ENGLER, D, MOLITCH, ME, ET AL: *Vasoactive intestinal peptide is a physiological mediator of prolactin release in the rat.* Endocrinology 111:1383–1390, 1985.
2. ARCHER, R: *Principles of Evolution: The neural hierarchy model.* In KRIEGER, DT, BROWNSTEIN, MJ, MARTIN, JB (EDS): *Brain Peptides.* John Wiley & Sons, New York, 1983, pp 135–164.
3. ADRIAN, TE, ALLEN, JM, BLOOM, SR, ET AL: *Neuropeptide Y distribution in human brain.* Nature 306:584–586, 1983.
4. AKIL, H, RICHARDSON, DE, BARCHAS, JD, ET AL: *Appearance of beta-endorphin-like immuno-reactivity in human ventricular cerebrospinal fluid upon analgesic electrical stimulation.* Proc Natl Acad Sci USA 75:5170–5172, 1978.
5. AKIL, H, WATSON, SJ, YOUNG, E, LEWIS, ME, KHACHATURIAN, H, WALTER, JM: *Endogenous opioids: Biology and function.* Ann Rev Neurosci 7:223–255, 1984.
6. ALLEN, JM, FERRIER, IN, ROBERTS, GW, CROSS, AJ, ADRIAN, TE, CROSS, TJ, BLOOM, SR: *Elevation of neuropeptide Y (NPY) in substantia innominata in Alzheimer type dementia.* J Neurol Sci 64:325–331, 1984.
7. ALLEN, YS, ADRIAN, TE, ALLEN, JM, TATEMOTO, K, CROW, TJ, BLOOM, SR, POLACK, JM: *Neuropeptide Y distribution in the rat brain.* Science 221:877–879, 1983.
8. AMIR, S, HAREL, M, SCHACHAR, S: *Thyrotropin-releasing hormone (TRH) improves survival in anaphylactic shock: A central effect mediated by the sympatho-adrenomedullary beta-adrenoceptive system.* Brain Res 298:219–224, 1984.
9. ANAND, P, GIBSON, SJ, McGREGOR, GP, ET AL: *A VIP-containing system concentrated in the lumbosacral region of human spinal cord.* Nature 305:143–145, 1983.
10. ARNOLD, MA, REPPERT, SM, RORSTAD, OP, SAGAR, SM, KEUTMANN, HT, PERLOW, MJ, MARTIN, JB: *Temporal patterns of somatostatin immunoreactivity in the cerebrospinal fluid of the rhesus monkey: Effect of environmental lighting.* J Neurosci 2:674–680, 1982.
11. ARONIN, N, CARRAWAY, RE, DIFIGLIA, M, LEEMAN, SE: *Neurotensin.* In KRIEGER, DT, BROWNSTEIN, M, MARTIN, JB (EDS): *Brain Peptides.* John Wiley & Sons, New York, 1983, pp 753–782.
12. ARONIN, N, COOPER, PE, LORENZ, LJ, BIRD, ED, SAGAR, SM, LEEMAN, SE, MARTIN, JB: *Somatostatin is increased in the basal ganglia in Huntington's disease.* Ann Neurol 13:519 526, 1982.
13. ARONIN, N, DIFIGLIA, M, LEEMAN, SE: *Substance P.* In KRIEGER, DT, BROWNSTEIN, MJ, MARTIN, JB (EDS): *Brain Peptides.* John Wiley & Sons, New York, 1983, pp 783–804.
14. BARCHAS, J, AND ELLIOTT, GR: *Neuropeptides: A new dimension in behavioral neurochemistry.* In MARTIN, JB, AND BARCHAS, J (EDS): *Neuropeptides in Neurologic and Psychiatric Disease (ARNMD #64).* Raven Press, New York, 1986, pp 215–258.
15. BEAL, MF, BIRD, ED, LANGLAIS, PJ, MARTIN, JB: *Somatostatin is increased in the nucleus accumbens in Huntington's disease.* Neurology 34:663–666, 1984.
16. BEAL, MF, MAZUREK, MF, BLACK, PMcL, MARTIN, JB: *Human cerebrospinal fluid somatostatin in neurological disease.* J Neurol Sci 71:91–104, 1986.
17. BENNETT, GW, EDWARDSON, JA, MARCANO DE COTTE, D, BERELOWITZ, M, PIMSTONE, BL, KRON-

HEIM, S: *Release of somatostatin from rat brain synaptosomas.* J Neurochem 32:1127–1130, 1979.

18. BERELOWITZ, M, PERLOW, MJ, HOFFMAN, HJ, FROHMAN, LA: *The diurnal variation of immunoreactive thyrotropin releasing hormone and somatostatin in the cerebrospinal fluid of the rhesus monkey.* Endocrinology 109:2102–2109, 1981.

19. BIENFELD, MC, MEYER, DK, BROWNSTEIN, MJ: *Cholecystokinin octapeptide in the rat hypothalamo-neurohypophysial system.* Nature 288:376–378, 1980.

20. BLACK, IB, AND KESSLER, JA: *Regulation of noradrenergic and peptidergic development: A search for common mechanisms.* In MARTIN, JB, REICHLIN, S, BICK, KL (EDS): *Neurosecretion and brain peptides: Implications for brain functions and neurological diseases.* Raven Press, New York, 1981, pp 287–297.

21. BOLAFFI, JL, REICHLIN, S, GOODMAN, DBP, FORREST, JN, JR: *Somatostatin: Occurrence in urinary bladder epithelium and renal tubules of the toad, Bufo marinus.* Science 210:644–646, 1980.

22. BOWKER, RM, WESTLUND, KN, SULLIVAN, MC, ET AL: *Descending serotonergic, peptidergic and cholinergic pathways from the raphe nuclei: A multiple transmitter complex.* Brain Res 288:33–48, 1983.

23. BRAZEAU, P, VALE, W, BURGUS, R, LING, N, BUTCHER, M, RIVIER, J, GUILLEMIN, R: Science 179:77–80, 1973.

24. BRECHA, NC, AND KARTEN, HJ: *Identification and localization of neuropeptides in the vertebrate retina.* In KRIEGER, DT, BROWNSTEIN, MJ, MARTIN, JB (EDS): *Brain Peptides.* John Wiley & Sons, New York, 1983, pp 437–463.

25. BUCHANAN, KD: *Gut hormones and the brain.* In BESSER, GM, AND MARTINI, L (EDS): *Clinical Neuroendocrinology,* vol 2. Academic Press, New York, 1982, pp 332–359.

26. CARRAWAY, R, AND LEEMAN, SE: *The isolation of a new hypotensive peptide, neurotensin, from bovine hypothalami.* J Biol Chem 248:6854–6861, 1973.

27. CLEMENT-JONES, V, AND REES, LH: *Neuroendocrine correlates of the endorphins and enkephalin.* In BESSER, GM, AND MARTINI, L (EDS): *Clinical Neuroendocrinology,* vol 2. Academic Press, New York, 1982, pp 140–204.

28. COLLU, R, BARBEAU, A, DUCHARME, J, ROCHEFORT, JG (EDS): *Nervous system effects of hypothalamic hormones and other peptides.* Raven Press, New York, 1979.

29. COMB, M, HERBERT, E, CREA, R: *Partial characterization of the mRNA that codes for enkephalins in bovine adrenal medulla and human pheochromocytoma.* Proc Natl Acad Sci USA 79:360–364, 1982.

30. COMB, M, SEEBURG, PH, ADELMAN, J, ET AL: *Primary structure of the human met- and leu-enkephalin precursor and its mRNA.* Nature 295:663–666, 1982.

31. CONLON, JM, SAMSON, WK, DOBBS, RE, ET AL: *Glucagon-like polypeptides in canine brain.* Diabetes 28:700–702, 1979.

32. COOPER, PE, FERNSTROM, JD, RORSTAD, OP, LEEMAN, SE, MARTIN, JB: *The regional distribution of somatostatin, substance P and neurotensin in human brain.* Brain Res 218:219–232, 1981.

33. COOPER, SJ, AND SANGER, DJ: *Endorphinergic mechanisms in food, salt and water intake: An overview.* Appetite 5:1–6, 1984.

34. CROWE, R, LINCOLN, J, BLACKLAY, PF, ET AL: *Vasoactive intestinal polypeptide-like immunoreactive nerves in diabetic penis. A comparison between streptozotocin-treated rats and man.* Diabetes 32:1075–1077, 1983.

35. DAIL, WG, MOLL, MA, WEBER, K: *Localization of vasoactive intestinal polypeptide in penile erectile tissue and in the major pelvic ganglion of the rat.* Neuroscience 101:1379–1386, 1983.

36. DAWBARN, D, HUNT, SP, EMSON, PC: *Neuropeptide Y: Regional distribution chromatographic characterization and immunohistochemical demonstration in postmortem brain.* Brain Res 296:168–173, 1984.

37. DELFS, JR, AND DICHTER, MA: *Effects of somatostatin on mammalian cortical neurons in culture: Physiological actions and unusual dose response characteristics.* J Neurosci 3:1176–1188, 1983.

38. DIXSON, AF, KENDRICK, KM, BLANK, MA, ET AL: *Effects of tactile and electrical stimuli upon release of vasoactive intestinal polypeptide in the mammalian penis.* J Endocrinol 100:249–252, 1984.

39. DOCKRAY, GJ: *Cholecystokinin.* In KRIEGER, DT, BROWNSTEIN, MJ, MARTIN, JF (EDS): *Brain Peptides.* John Wiley & Sons, New York, 1983, pp 851–870.

40. DODD, J, AND KELLY, JS: *Is somatostatin an excitatory transmitter in the hippocampus?* Nature 273:674–675, 1978.

41. DUPONT, EA, PRANGE HANSEN, F, JUUL-JENSEN, P, LUNDBACK, K, MAGNUSSEN, I, DEFINE, OLIVARIUS, B: *Somatotatin in the treatment of patients with extrapyramidal disorders and patients with EEG abnormalities.* Acta Neurol Scand 57:488–495, 1978.

42. EIDEN, LE, AND BROWNSTEIN, MJ: *Extrahypothalamic distributions and functions of hypothalamic peptide hormones.* Fed Proc 40:2553–2559, 1981.

43. EIDEN, LE, GIRAUD, P, HOTCHKIS, A, BROWNSTEIN, MJ: *Enkephalins and VIP in human pheochromocytomas and bovine adrenal chromaffin cells.* In COSTA, E, AND TRABUCCHI, M (EDS):

Regulatory peptides: From molecular biology to function. Raven Press, New York, 1982, pp 387–395.

44. ENGEL, WK, SIDDIQUE, T, NICOLOFF, JT: *Effect on weakness and spasticity in amyotrophic lateral sclerosis of thyrotropin-releasing hormone.* Lancet 2:73–75, 1983.

45. ETIENNE, T, GIRGIS, S, MACINTYRE, I, MORRIS, HR, PANICO, M, TIPPINS, FR: *An investigation of the activity of human and rat calcitonin gene-related peptide (CGRP) on isolated tissues from the rat and guinea pig.* J Physiol 351:489–499, 1984.

46. ERSPAMER, V, MELCHIORRI, P, EROCCARDO, M, ET AL: *The brain-gut-skin triangle: New peptides.* Peptides 2:7–16, 1981.

47. FADEN, AI, JACOBS, TP, HOLADAY, JW: *Thyrotropin-releasing hormone improves neurologic recovery after spinal trauma in cats.* N Engl J Med 305:1063–1067, 1981.

48. FINLEY, JCW, MADERDRUT, JL, PETRUSZ, P: *The immunocytochemical localization of enkephalin in the central nervous system of the rat.* J Comp Neurol 198:541–565, 1981.

49. FISHER, LA, KIKKAWA, DO, RIVIER, JE, ET AL: *Stimulation of noradrenergic sympathetic outflow by calcitonin gene-related peptide.* Nature 305:533–536, 1983.

50. GAINER, H: *Peptides in Neurobiology.* Plenum, New York, 1977.

51. GAMSE, R, VACCARO, DE, GAMSE, M, DEPACE, M, FOX, , TO, LEEMAN, SE: *Release of immunoreactive somatostatin from hypothalamic cells in culture: Inhibition by gamma amino butyric acid.* Proc Natl Acad Sci USA 77:5552–5556, 1980.

52. GEOLA, FL, YAMADA, T, WARWICK, RJ, TOURTELLOTTE, WW, HERSHMAN, JM: *Regional distribution of somatostatin-like immunoreactivity in the human brain.* Brain Res 229:35–42, 1981.

53. GERICH, JE: *Somatostatin.* In BROWNLEE, M, AND GARLAND, J (EDS): *Handbook of Diabetes Mellitus,* vol 1. STPM Press, New York, 1980, pp 297–354.

54. GERNER, RH, AND YAMADA, T: *Altered neuropeptide concentrations in cerebrospinal fluid of psychiatric patients.* Brain Res 238:298–302, 1982.

55. GOLDSTEIN, A: *Opioid peptides (endorphins) in pituitary brain.* Science 193:1081–1085, 1976.

56. GOLDSTEIN, A, FISCHLI, W, LOWNEY, LI, HUNKAPILLER, M, HOOD, L: *Porcine pituitary dynorphin: Complete amino acid sequence of the biologically active heptadecapeptide.* Proc Natal Acad Sci USA 78:7219–7223, 1980.

57. GOLDSTEIN, A, TACHIBANA, S, LOWNEY, LI, HUNKAPILLER, M, HOOD, L: *Dynorphin-(1-13), an extraordinarily potent opioid peptide.* Proc Natl Acad Sci USA 76:6666–6670, 1979.

58. GOLTZMAN, D, AND MITCHELL, J: *Interaction of calcitonin and calcitonin gene-related peptide at receptor sites in target tissues.* Science 227:1343–1345, 1985.

59. GOODMAN, RR, FICKER, LD, SNYDER, SH: *Enkephalins.* In KRIEGER, DT, BROWNSTEIN, MJ, MARTIN, JB (EDS): *Brain Peptides.* John Wiley & Sons, New York, 1983.

60. GOTTO, AM, JR, PECK, EJ, JR, BOYD, AE, JR (EDS): *Brain Peptides: A New Endocrinology.* Elsevier, New York, 1979.

61. GRAYBIEL, AM, AND RAGSDALE, CW, JR: *Biochemical anatomy of the striatum.* In EMSON, PC (ED): *Chemical Neuroanatomy.* Raven Press, New York, 1983, pp 427–504.

62. GROSSMAN, A: *Brain opiates and neuroendocrine function.* Clinics in Endocrinol Metab 12:725–746, 1983.

63. GUBLER, U, KILPATRICK, DL, SEEBURG, PH, GAGE, LP, UDENFRIEND, S: *Detection and partial characterization of proenkephalin mRNA.* Proc Natl Acad Sci USA 78:5484–5487, 1981.

64. GUILLEMIN, R: *Peptides in the brain: The new endocrinology of the neuron.* Science 202:390–402, 1978.

65. HABENER, J: *Genetic control of hormone formation.* In WILSON, JD, AND FOSTER, DW (EDS): *Williams' Textbook of Endocrinology,* ed 7. WB Saunders, Philadelphia, 1985, pp 9–32.

66. HÖKFELT, T, FAHRENKRUG, J, TATEMOTO, K, ET AL: *The PHI (PHI-27)/corticotropin-releasing factor/enkephalin immunoreactive hypothalamic neuron: Possible morphologic basis for integrated control of prolactin, corticotropin, and growth hormone secretion.* Proc Natl Acad Sci USA 80:895–898, 1983.

67. HÖKFELT, T, FUXE, K, JOHANSSON, O, JEFFCOATE, S, WHITE, N: *Thyrotropin releasing hormone (TRH)-containing nerve terminals in certain brain stem nuclei and in the spinal cord.* Neurosci Lett 1:133–139, 1975.

68. HÖKFELT, T, JOHANSSON, O, LJUNGDAHL, A, ET AL: *Peptidergic neurons.* Nature 284:515–521, 1980.

69. HÖKFELT, T, LUNDBERG, JM, SCHULTZBERG, M, ET AL: *Coexistence of peptides and putative transmitters in neurons.* Adv Biochem Psychopharmacol 22:1–23, 1980.

70. HÖKFELT, T, REHFELD, JF, SKIRBOLL, L, ET AL: *Evidence for coexistence of dopamine and CCK in meso-limbic neurons.* Nature 285:476–478, 1980.

71. HOLADAY, JW, AND D'AMATO, RJ: *Thyrotropin-releasing hormone improves cardiovascular function in experimental endotoxic and hemorrhagic shock.* Science 213:216–218, 1981.

72. HOLADAY, JW, TSENG, LF, LOH, HH, LI, CH: *Thyrotropin releasing hormone antagonizes beta-endorphin hypothermia and catalepsy.* Life Sci 22:1537–1543, 1978.

73. HORIKAWA, S, TAKAI, T, TOYOSATO, M, ET AL: *Isolation and structural organization of the human preproenkephalin B gene.* Nature 306:611–614, 1983.

NEUROREGULATORY PEPTIDES

74. HUGHES, JT, SMITH, W, KOSTERLITZ, HW, FOTHERGILL, LA, MORGAN, BA, MORRIS, HR: *Identification of two related pentapepties from the brain with potent opiate agonist activity*. Nature 258:577–579, 1975.

75. IMOTO, K, SAIDA, K, IWAMURA, K, ET AL: *Amyotrophic lateral sclerosis, a double-blind crossover trial of thyrotropin-releasing homone*. J Neurol Neurosurg Psych 47:1332–1334, 1984.

76. IOFFE, S, HAVLICEK, V, FRIESEN, H, CHERNICK, V: *Effect of somatostatin (SRIF) and L-glutamate on neurons of the sensorimotor cortex in awake habituated rabbits*. Brain Res 153:414–418, 1978.

77. ITOH, N, OBATA, K, YANAIHARA, N, ET AL: *Human preprovasoactive intestinalpolypeptide contains a novel PHI-27-like peptide, PHM-27*. Nature 304:547–549, 1983.

78. JACKSON, IMD: *Thyrotropin-releasing hormone (TRH): Distribution in mammalian species and its functional significance*. In GRIFFITH, EC, AND BENNETT, GW (EDS): *Thyrotropin-releasing hormone*. Raven Press, New York, 1983, pp 3–18.

79. JACKSON, IMD, AND LECHAN, RM: *Thyrotropin-releasing hormone (TRH)*. In KRIEGER, DT, BROWNSTEIN, M, MARTIN, JB, (EDS): *Brain Peptides*. John Wiley & Sons, New York, 1983, pp 661–686.

80. JACKSON, IMD, AND VALE, W: *Extrapituitary functions of hypothalamic hormones*. Fed Proc 49:2543–2544, 1981.

81. JESSELL, TM, AND DODD, J: *Neurotransmitters and differentiation antigens in subsets of sensory neurons projecting to the spinal dorsal horn*. In MARTIN, JB, AND BARCHAS, J (EDS): *Neuropeptides in Neurologic and Psychiatric Disease (ARNMD #64)*. Raven Press, New York, 1986, pp 111–134.

82. JOHANSSON, O, HOKFELT, T, PERNOW, B, ET AL: *Immunohistochemical support for three putative transmitters in one neuron: Coexistence of 5-hydroxy-tryptamine, substance P, and thyrotropin-releasing hormone-like immunoreactivity in medullary neurons projecting to the spinal cord*. Neuroscience 6:1857–1881, 1981.

83. JOHANSSON, O, AND HÖKFELT, T: *Thyrotropin-releasing hormone, somatostatin and enkephalin; distribution studies using immunohistochemical techniques*. J Histochem Cytochem 28:360–364, 1980.

84. JONES, EG, AND HENDRY, SHC: *The peptide containing neurons of the primate cerebral cortex*. In MARTIN, JB, AND BARCHAS, J (EDS): *Neuropeptides in Neurologic and Psychiatric Disease (ARNMD #64)*. Raven Press, New York, 1986, pp 163–178.

85. JOSEPH-BRAVO, P, CHARLI, JL, PALACIOS, JM, KORDON, C: *Effect of neurotransmitters on the in vitro release of immunoreactive thyrotropin-releasing hormone from rat mediobasal hypothalamus*. Endocrinology 104:801–806, 1979.

86. KAHN, D, ABRAMS, GM, ZIMMERMAN, EA, ET AL: *Neurotensin neurons in the rat hypothalamus: An immunohistochemistry study*. Endocrinology 107:47–54, 1980.

87. KAKIDANI, H, FURUTANI, Y, TAKAHASHI, H, NODA, M, MORIMOTO, Y, HIROSE, T, ASAI, M, INAYAMA, S, NAKANISHI, S, NUMA, S: *Cloning and sequence analysis of cDNA for porcine beta-neo-endorphin/dynorphin precursor*. Nature 298:245–249, 1982.

88. KASTIN, AJ, OLSON, GA, ZADINA, JE, OLSON, RD: *Disparate effects of peripherally administered endorphins and enkephalins in laboratory animals*. In MULLER, ER, AND GENAZZANT, AR (EDS): *Central and peripheral endorphins: Basic and clinical aspects*. Raven Press, New York, 1984, pp 99–108.

89. KOSTERLITZ, HW: *Endogenous opioid peptides: Historical aspects*. In HUGHES, J (ED): *Centrally acting peptides*. University Park Press, Baltimore, 1978. p 157.

90. KRIEGER, D: *Endorphins and enkephalins: Disease-a-month*. Year Book Medical Publishers, Chicago, 1982.

91. KRIEGER, DT: *The multiple faces of pro-opiomelanocortin, a prototype precursor molecule*. Clin Res 31:342–353, 1983.

92. KRIEGER, DT, BROWNSTEIN, M, MARTIN, JB: *Brain Peptides*. John Wiley & Sons, New York, 1983.

93. KRIEGER, DT: *Brain peptides: What, where, and why?* Science 222:975–985, 1983.

94. KRIEGER, DT, AND MARTIN, JB: *Brain peptides*. N Engl J Med 304:876–885, 944–951, 1981.

95. KRISCH, B: *Hypothalamic and extrahypothalamic distribution of somatostatin-immunoreactive elements in the rat brain*. Cell Tiss Res 195:499, 1978.

96. KRISCH, B: *Differing immunoreactivities of somatostatin in the cortex and the hypothalamus of the rat. A light and electron microscopic study*. Cell Tiss Res 212:457–464, 1980.

97. LAMBERTON, RR, LECHAN, RM, JACKSON, IMD: *Ontogeny of thyrotropin-releasing hormone and histidyl proline diketopiperazine in the rat central nervous system and pancreas*. Endocrinology 115:2400–2405, 1984.

98. LECHAN, RM, ADELMAN, LS, FORTE, S, JACKSON, IMD: *Organization of thyrotropin-releasing hormone (TRH) immunoreactivity in the human spinal cord*. Soc for Neurosci abstracts, 1984.

99. LECHAN, RM, SNAPPER, SC, JACKSON, IMD: *Evidence that spinal cord TRH is independent of the paraventricular nucleus*. Neurosci Lett, 43:61, 1983.

100. LECHAN, RM, SNAPPER, SB, JACOBSON, S, JACKSON, IMD: *The distribution of thyrotropin-releasing hormone (TRH) in the rhesus monkey spinal cord*. Peptides 5(Suppl 1):185–194, 1984.

101. LOH, YP, AND GAINER, H: *Biosynthesis and processing of neuropeptides.* In KRIEGER, DT, BROWNSTEIN, MJ, MARTIN, JB (EDS): *Brain Peptides.* John Wiley & Sons, New York, 1983, pp 79–116.

102. LUNDBERG, JM, ANGAARD, A, FAHRENKRUG, J: *Complementary role of vasoactive intestinal polypeptide (VIP) and acetylcholine for cat submandibular gland blood flow and secretion.* Acta Physiol Scand 3:329–337, 1982.

103. LUNDBERG, JM, ANGGARD, A, FAHRENKRUG, J, ET AL: *Vasoactive intestinal polypeptide in cholinergic neurons of exocrine glands: Functional significance of coexisting transmitters for vasodilation and secretion.* Proc Natl Acad Sci USA 77:1651–1655, 1980.

104. LUNDBERG, JM, HOKFELT, T, ANGGARD, T, ET AL: *Organizational principles in the peripheral sympathetic nervous system: Subdivision by coexisting peptides (somatostatin-, avian pancreatic polypeptide- and vasoactive intestinal polypeptide-like immunoreactive materials).* Proc Natl Acad Sci USA 79:1303–1307, 1982.

105. MAEDA, K, AND FROHMAN, LA: *Release of somatostatin and thyrotropin-releasing hormone from rat hypothalamic fragments in vitro.* Endocrinology 106:1837–1842, 1980.

106. MAINS, RE, EIPPER, BA, LING, N: *Common precursor to corticotropins and endorphins.* Proc Natl Acad Sci USA 74:3014–3018, 1977.

107. MALTHE-SORENSSEN, D,WOOD, PL,CHENEY, DL, COSTA, E: *Modulation of the turnover rate of acetylcholine in rat brain by intraventricular injections of thyrotropin-releasing hormone, somatostatin, neurotensin and angiotensin III.* J Neurochem 31:685–691, 1978.

108. MANAKER, S, WINOKUR, A, RHODES, CH, RAINBOW, TC: *Autoradiographic localization of thyrotropin-releasing hormone (TRH) receptors in human spinal cord.* Neurology 35:328–332, 1985.

109. MANAKER, S, WINOKUR, A, ROSTENE, WH, RAINBOW, TC: *Autoradiographic localization of thyrotropin-releasing hormone receptors in the rat central nervous system.* J Neurosci 5:167–174, 1985.

110. McCANN, SM: *The role of brain peptides in the control of anterior pituitary hormone secretion.* In MÜLLER, EE, AND MACLEOD, RM, (EDS): *Neuroendocrine Perspectives,* vol 1. Elsevier, Amsterdam, 1982, pp 1–22.

111. McDONALD, JK, LUMPKIN, MD,SAMSON, WK, McCANN, SM: *Neuropeptide Y effects secretion of luteinizing hormone and growth hormone in ovariectomized rats.* Proc Natl Acad Sci USA 82:561–564, 1985.

112. MILLER, WL, BAXTER, JD, EBERHARDT, NL: *Peptide hormone genes: Structure and evolution.* In KRIEGER, DT, BROWNSTEIN, MJ, MARTIN, JB (EDS): *Brain Peptides.* John Wiley & Sons, New York, 1983, pp 15–78.

113. MINTH, CD,BLOOM, SR, POLAK, JM, DIXON, JE: *Cloning, characterization and DNA sequence of a human cDNA encoding neuropeptide tyrosine.* Proc Natl Acad Sci USA 51:4577–4581, 1984.

114. MITSUMA, T, NOGUMOU, T, ADACHI, K, ET AL: *Concentrations of immunoreactive thyrotropin-releasing hormone in spinal cord of patients with amyotrophic lateral sclerosis.* Am J Med Soc 287:34–36, 1984.

115. MOLNAR, J, ARIMURA, A, KASTIN, A: Fed Proc 35:782, 1976.

116. MORLEY, JE: *Neuroendocrine effects of endogenous opioid peptides in human subjects: A review.* Psychoneuroendocrinology 8:361–379, 1983.

117. MUDGE, AW, LEEMAN, SE, FISCHBACH, G: *Enkephalin inhibits release of substance P from sensory neurons in culture and decreases action potential duration.* Proc Natl Acad Sci USA 76:526–530, 1979.

118. MUELLER, GP, ALPERT, L, REICHLIN, S, JACKSON, IMD: *Thyrotropin-releasing hormone and serotonin secretion from frog skin are stimulated by norepinephrine.* Endocrinology 106:1–4, 1980.

119. MUNSAT, TL, MORA, JS, ROBINTON, JE, JACKSON, IMD, LECHAN, R, HEDLUND, W, TAFT, J, REICHLIN, S, SCHEIFE, R: *Intrathecal TRH in amyotropic lateral sclerosis: Preliminary observations.* Neurology (Suppl 1) 34:239, 1984 (Abstract).

120. MUTT, V: *VIP, motilin, and secretin.* In KRIEGER, DT, BROWNSTEIN, MJ, MARTIN, JB (EDS): *Brain Peptides.* John Wiley & Sons, New York, 1983, pp 871–902.

121. NEMETH, EF, AND COOPER, JR: *Effect of somatostatin on acetylcholine release from rat hippocampal synaptosomes.* Brain Res 165:166–170, 1979.

122. NODA, M, FURUTANI, Y, TAKAHASHI, H, TOYOSATA, M, HIROSE, I, INAYAMA, S, NAKANISHI, S, NUMA, S: *Cloning and sequence analysis of cDNA for bovine adrenal proenkephalin.* Nature 295:202–208, 1982.

123. NODA, M, TERANISHI, Y, TAKAHASHI, H, TOYOSATO, M, NOTAKE, M, NAKANISHI, S, AND NUMA, S: *Isolation and structural organization of the human preproenkephalin gene.* Nature 297:431, 1982.

124. O'DONOHUE, TL, CHRONWALL, BM, PRUSS, RM, MEZEY, E, KISS, JZ, EIDEN, LE, MASSARI, VJ, TESSEL, RE, PICKEL, VM, DIMAGGIO, DA, HOTCHKISS, AJ, CROWLEY, WR, ZUKOWSKA-GROJEC, Z: *Neuropeptide Y and peptide YY neuronal and endocrine systems.* Peptides 6:755–768, 1985.

NEUROREGULATORY PEPTIDES

125. OGAWA, N, KABUTO, H, HIROSE, Y, NUKINA, I, MORI, A: *Up-regulation of thyrotropin-releasing hormone (TRH) receptors in rat spinal cord after codepletion of serotonin and TRH*. Regul Pept 10:85–90, 1985.

126. OSBAHR, AJ, NEMEROFF, CB, LUTTINGER, D, MASON, GA, PRANGE, AJ, JR: *Neurotensin-induced antinociception in mice: Antagonism by thyrotropin-releasing hormone*. J Pharmacol Exp Ther 217:645–651, 1981.

127. OTTESEN, B, ULRICHSEN, H, FAHRENKRUG, J, LARSEN, JJ, WAGNER, G, SCHIERUP, L, LONDERGAARD, F: *Vasoactive intestinal polypeptide and the female genital tract: Relationship to reproductive phase and delivery*. Am J Obstet Gynecol 143:414–420, 1982.

128. PALKOVITS, M: *Neuroanatomical techniques*. In KRIEGER, DT, BROWNSTEIN, MJ, MARTIN, JB (EDS): *Brain Peptides*. John Wiley & Sons, New York, 1983, pp 495–546.

129. PALKOVITS, M: *Topography of chemically identified neurons in the central nervous system: Progress in 1981-1983*. In MÜLLER, EE, AND MACLEOD, RM (EDS): *Neuroendocrine Perspectives*, vol 3. Elsevier, Amsterdam, 1984, pp 1–69.

130. PARKER, CR, JR. AND CAPDOVILA, A: *Thyrotropin-releasing hormone (TRH) binding sites in the adult human brain: Localization and characterization*. Peptides 8:701–706, 1984.

131. PARTRIDGE, WM, AND FRANK, HJL: *Mechanisms of peptide transport from blood to brain*. In MÜLLER, EE, AND MACLEOD, RM (EDS): *Neuroendocrine Perspectives*. Elsevier, Amsterdam, 1983, pp 107–122.

132. PATEL, YC, RAO, K, REICHLIN, S: N Engl J Med 296:529, 1977.

133. PEARSE, AGE: *The APUD concept and hormone production*. Clin Endocrinol Metab 9:211–222, 1980.

134. PETERFREUND, RA, AND VALE, WW: *Ovine corticotropin-releasing factor stimulates somatostatin secretion from cultured brain cells*. Endocrinology 112:1275–1278, 1983.

135. PHILLIS, J, AND KIRKPATRICK, JR: *The actions of motilin, luteinizing releasing hormone, cholecystokinin, somatostatin, vasoactive intestinal polypeptide and other peptides on rat cerebral cortical neurons*. Can J Physiol Pharmacol 58:612–623, 1980.

136. PITTMAN, QJ, AND SIGGINS, GR: *Somatostatin hyperpolarizes hippocampal pyramidal neurons in vitro*. Brain Res 121:402–408, 1981.

137. POLAK, JM, GU, J, MINA, S, ET AL: *Vipergic nerves in the penis*. Lancet 2:217–219, 1981.

138. PRANGE, AJ, JR, NEMEROFF, CB, LOOSEN, PT, ET AL: *Behavioral effects of thyrotropin-releasing hormone in animals and man: A review*. In COLLU, R, BARBEAU, A, DUCHARME, JR, ROCHEFORT, J-G (EDS): *Central nervous system effects of hypothalamic hormones and other peptides*. Raven Press, New York, 1979, pp 75–96.

139. PRANGE, AJ, JR, AND UTIGER, RD: *What does brain thyrotropin-releasing hormone do?* N Engl J Med 305:1089–1090, 1981.

140. RASOOL, CG, SCHWARTZ, AL, BOLLINGER, JA, REICHLIN, S, BRADLEY, WG: *Immunoreactive somatostatin distribution and axoplasmic transport in rat peripheral nerve*. Endocrinology 108:996–1001, 1981.

141. REICHLIN, S: *Somatostatin*. N Engl J Med 309:1495–1501, 1556–1563, 1983.

142. REICHLIN, S: *Somatostatin*. In KRIEGER, DT, BROWNSTEIN, MJ, MARTIN, JB (EDS): *Brain Peptides* John Wiley & Sons, New York, pp 711–752.

143. RENAUD, LP: In GOTTO, AM, JR, PECK, EJ, JR, BOYD, AE, III (EDS): *Brain Peptides: A New Endocrinology*. Elsevier, Amsterdam, 1979, pp 119–138.

144. RENAUD, LP, MARTIN, JB, BRAZEAU, P: *Depressant action of TRH LH-RH and somatostatin on activity of central neurons*. Nature 255:233–235, 1975.

145. ROBBINS, RJ, SUTTON, RE, REICHLIN, S: *Effects of neurotransmitters and cyclic AMP on somatostatin release from cultured cerebral cortical cells*. Brain Res 234:377–386, 1982.

146. RORSTAD, OP, MARTIN, JB, TERRY, LC: *Somatostatin and the nervous system*. In BARKER, JL, AND SMITH, TG, JR (EDS): *The role of peptides in neuronal function*. Marcel Dekker, New York, 1980, pp 573–614.

147. RORSTAD, OP, BROWNSTEIN, MJ, MARTIN, JB: *Immunoreactive and biologically active somatostatin-like material in rat retina*. Proc Natl Acad Sci USA 76:3019–3023, 1979.

148. ROSENFELD, MG, MERMOD, JJ, AMARA, SG, ET AL: *Production of a novel neuropeptide encoded by the calcitonin gene via tissue-specific RNA processing*. Nature 304:129–135, 1983.

149. ROSSIER, J: *Functions of beta-endorphin and enkephalins in the pituitary*. In MARTINI, L, AND GANONG, F (EDS): *Frontiers in Neuroendocrinology*, vol 7. Raven Press, New York, 1982, pp 191–209.

150. ROSSIER, J, DEAN, D, LIVETT, B, UNDENFRIEND, S: *Enkephalin congeners and precursors are synthesized and released by primary cultures of adrenal chromaffin cells*. Life Sci 28:781–789, 1981.

151. ROTH, KA, WEBER, E, BARCHAS, JD, CHANG, D, CHANG, J-K: *Immunoreactive dynorphin (1-8) and corticotropin-releasing factor in subpopulation of hypothalamic neurons*. Science 219:189–191, 1983.

152. ROTH, J, LEROITH, D, SHILOACH, J, ET AL: *The evolutionary origins of hormones, neurotransmitters and other extracellular chemical messengers*. N Engl J Med 306:523–527, 1982.

153. ROTH, J, LEROITH, D, SHILOACH, J, ET AL: *Intercellular communication: An attempt at a unifying hypothesis.* Clin Res 354–363, 1983.

154. RUBINOW, DR, GOLD, PW, POST, RM, BALLENGER, JC, COWDRY, R, BOLLINGER, J, REICHLIN, S: *CSF somatostatin in affective illness.* Arch Gen Psych 40:409–412, 1983.

155. SAGAR, SM, LANDRY, DL, MILLARD, WJ, BADGER, TM, ARNOLD, MA, MARTIN, JB: *Depletion of somatostatin-like immunoreactivity in the rat central nervous system by cysteamine.* J Neurosci 2:225–231, 1982.

156. SAID, SI: *Vasoactive intestinal polypeptide (VIP): Current status.* Peptides 5:143–150, 1984.

157. SAMSON, WK, SAID, SI, McCANN, SM: *Radioimmunologic localization of vasoactive intestinal peptide in hypothalamic and extrahypothalamic sites in the rat brain.* Neurosci Lett 12:265–269, 1979.

158. SCHMIDT-ACHERT, KM, ASKANAS, V, ENGEL, WKL: *Thyrotropin-releasing hormone enhanced choline acetyltransferase and creatine kinase in cultured spinal ventral horn neurons.* J Neurochem 43:586–589, 1984.

159. SHIMATSU, A, KATO, Y, MATSUSHA, N, KATAKAMI, H, YANIHARA, N, IMURA, A: *Immunoreactive VIP in hypophyseal portal blood.* Endocrinology 108:395–398, 1981.

160. SCHULTZBERG, M, HOKFELT, T, LUNDBERG, JM: *Coexistence of classical transmitters and peptides in the central and peripheral nervous system.* Br Med Bull 38:309–313, 1982.

161. SIMS, KB, HOFFMAN, DL, SAID, SI, ZIMMERMAN, EA: *Vasoactive intestinal polypeptide (VIP) in mouse and rat brain: An immunocytochemical study.* Brain Res 186:165–183, 1980.

162. SKOFITSCH, G, AND JACOBOWITZ, DM: *Calcitonin gene-related peptide coexists with substance P in capsaicin sensitive neurons and sensory ganglia of the rat.* Peptides 6:747–754, 1985.

163. SKOFITSCH, G, AND JACOBOWITZ, DM: *Calcitonin gene-related peptide: Detailed immunohistochemical distribution in the central nervous system.* Peptides 6:721–745, 1985.

164. SMITH, GP, GIBBS, J, JEROME, C, ET AL: *The satiety effect of cholecystokinin: A progress report.* Peptides 2:57–59, 1981.

165. SOBUE, I, TAKAYANAGI, T, NAKANISHI, T, ET AL: *Controlled trial of thyrotropin-releasing hormone tartrate in ataxia of spinocerebellar degenerations.* J Neurol Sci 61:235–248, 1983.

166. SORENSEN, KV, CHRISTENSEN, SE, HANSEN, AP, INGERSLEV, J, PEDERSEN, E, ORSKOV, H: *The origin of cerebrospinal fluid somatostatin: Hypothalamic or disperse central nervous system secretion?* Neuroendocrinology 32:335–338, 1981.

167. SRIKANT, CB, AND PATEL, YC: *Receptor binding of somatostatin-28 is tissue specific.* Nature 294:259–260, 1981.

168. SRIKANT, CB, AND PATEL, YC: *Somatostatin receptor identification and characterization in rat brain membranes.* Proc Natl Acad Sci USA 78:3930–3934, 1981.

169. SUNDLER, F, ALUMETS, J, HAKANSON, R, BJORKLUND, L, LJUNGBERG, O: *Somatostatin-immunoreactive cells in medullary carcinoma of the thyroid.* Am J Pathol 88:381–386, 1977.

170. SNYDER, SH: *Drug and neurotransmitter receptors in the brain.* Science 224:22–31, 1984.

171. TACHE, Y, LESEIGE, D, VALE, W, COLLU, R: *Gastric hypersecretion by intracisternal TRH: Dissociation from hypophysiotropic activity and role of central catecholamines.* Eur J Pharm 107:149–155, 1985.

172. TAKAGI, H, SOMOGYI, P, SOMOGYI, J, SMITH, AD: *Fine structural studies on a type of somatostatin-immunoreactive neuron and its synaptic connections in the rat striatum: A correlated light and electron microscopic study.* J Comp Neurol 214:1–16, 1983.

173. TANAKA, S, AND TSUJIMOTO, A: *Somatostatin facilitates the serotonin release from rat cerebral cortex, hippocampus and hypothalamus slice.* Brain Res 208:219–222, 1981.

174. TERENIUS, L, AND WAHLSTROM, A: *Physiological and clinical relevance of endorphins.* In HUGHES, J (ED): *Centrally acting peptides.* University Park Press, Baltimore, 161–178, 1978.

175. TRAN, VT, BEAL, MF, MARTIN, JB: *Two types of somatostatin receptors differentiated by cyclic somatostatin analogues.* Science 288:492–495, 1985.

176. TSUJIMOTO, A, AND TANAKA, S: *Stimulatory effect of somatostatin on norepinephrine release from rat brain cortex slices.* Life Sci 28:903–910, 1981.

177. UHL, GR, CHILDERS, SR, SNYDER, SH: *Opioid peptides and the opiate receptor.* Frontiers in Neuroendocrinology 5:289–328, 1978.

178. UHL, GR, TRAN, VT, SNYDER, SH, MARTIN, JB: *Somatostatin receptors: Distribution in rat central nervous system and human frontal cortex.* J Comp Neurol 240:288–304, 1985.

179. UHL, GR, KUHAR, MJ, SYNDER, SH: *Neurotensin: Immunohistochemical localization in rat central nervous system.* Proc Natl Acad Sci USA 74:4059–4063, 1977.

180. VANDERHAEGHEN, JJ, LOTSTRA, F, DEMEY, J, ET AL: *Immunohistochemical localization of cholecystokinin- and gastrin-like peptides in the brain and hypophysis of the rat.* Proc Natl Acad Sci USA 77:1190–1194, 1980.

181. VARNDELL, I, TAPIA, F, DEMEY, J, ET AL: *Electron immunocytochemical localization of enkephalin-like material in catecholamine-containing cells of the carotid body, the adrenal medulla, and in pheochromocytomas of man and other mammals.* J Histochem Cytochem 30:682–690, 1982.

182. Vincent, SR, Johansson, O, Hokfelt, T, et al: *Neuropeptide coexistence in human cortical neurons.* Nature 298:65–67, 1982.
183. Von Euler and Gaddum: *An unidentified depressor substance in certain tissue extracts.* J Physiol 72:74–83, 1931.
184. Watson, SJ, and Akil, H: *Alpha-MSH in rat brain: Occurrence within and outside of beta-endorphin neurons.* Brain Res 182:217–223, 1980.
185. Watson, SJ, Khachaturian, H, Taylor, L. Fischli, W, Goldstein, A, Akil, M: *Pro-dynorphin peptides are found in the same neurons throughout the rat brain: Immunocytochemical study.* Proc Natl Acad Sci USA 80:891–894, 1983.
186. Weber, E, and Barchas, JD: *Immunohistochemical distribution of dynorphin B in rat brain: Relation to dynorphin A and alpha-neo-endorphin systems.* Proc Natl Acad Sci USA 80:1125–1129, 1983.
187. Yoshimasa, T, Nakai, K, Li, S, et al: *Plasma methionine-enkephalins and leucine-enkephalins in normal subjects and patients with pheochomocytoma.* J Clin Endocrinol Metab 57:706–712, 1983.
188. Yoshimasa,T, Nakao, K, Ohtsuke, H, et al: *Methioine-enkephalins and leucine-enkephalin in human sympathoadrenal system and pheochromocytoma.* J Clin Invest 69:643–650, 1982.
189. Oates, JA: *The carcinoid syndrome.* N Engl J Med 315:702–704, 1986.
190. McDonald, TJ, Nilsson, G, Vagne, M, Ghatel, M, Bloom, SR, Mutt, V: *A gastrin-releasing peptide from the porcine nonantral gastric tissue.* Gut 19:767–774, 1978.
191. Walsh, JH: *Bombesin-like peptides.* In Krieger, DT, Brownstein, MJ, Martin, JB (eds): *Brain Peptides.* John Wiley & Sons, New York, 1983, pp 941–960.
192. Hökfelt, T, Melander, T, Staines, W, et al: *Neuropeptides and their possible role as auxilliary messengers.* In Frederiekson, RCA, Hendrie, HC, Hingtgen, JN, et al (eds): *Neuroregulation of Autonomic, Endocrine, and Immune Systems.* Wijholt Publishing, Boston, 1986, pp 61–87.
193. Hökfelt, T, Johansson, D, Goldstein, M: *Chemical anatomy of the brain.* Science 225:1326–1334, 1984.
194. Bataille, D, and Said, SI (eds): *VIP and related substances. Second international symposium.* Peptides 7 (Suppl 1): 1–293, 1986.
195. Yehuda, S, Mostofsky, DI: *Modification of the hypothermic circadian cycle induced by DSIP and melatonin in pinealectomized and hypophysectomized rats.* Peptides 5:495–497, 1984.
196. Karnovsky, ML: *Progress in sleep* [editorial]. N Eng J Med 315:1026–1028, 1986.
197. Chedid, L (ed): *Muramyl peptides as modulators of sleep, temperature, and immune responses.* Fed Proc 45:2531–2558, 1986.
198. Karnovsky, ML: *Muramyl peptides in mammalian tissue and their effects at the cellular level.* Fed Proc 45:2556–2558, 1986,
199. Schoenenberger, GA, Maier, PF, Tobler, HJ, et al: *The delta EEG (sleep)-inducing peptide (DSIP). XI Amino-acid analysis, sequence, synthesis and activity of the nonapeptide.* Pfleegers Arch 376:119–129, 1978.
200. Krueger, JM, Pappenheimner, JR, Karnovsky, ML: *The composition of sleep-promoting factor isolated from human urine.* J Biol Chem 257:1664–1669, 1982.
201. Krueger, JM, Pappenheimer, JR, Karnovsky, ML: *Sleep-promoting effects of muramyl peptides.* Proc Nat Acad Sci 79:6102–6106, 1982.
202. Cutler, Nr, Haxby, JV, Narang, PK, et al: *Evaluation of an analogue of somatostatin (L 363, 586) in Alzheimer's disease.* (letter) N Engl J Med 312:725, 1985.
203. Chrubasik, J, Meyadier, J, Blond, S, et al: *Somatostatin, a potent analgesic.* (letter) Lancet 2:1208–1209, 1984.
204. Yanaihara, C, Sato, H, Yanaihara, N, et al: *Motilin-substance P- and somatostatin-like immunoreactivities in extracts from dog, tupaia, and monkey brain and GI tract.* Adv Exp Med Biol 106:269–283, 1978.

Chapter 19

CLINICAL IMPLICATIONS OF NEUROPEPTIDES IN NEUROLOGIC DISORDERS

The discovery of many different peptides in the nervous system and the mounting evidence that they serve as neuroregulators raise the possibility that neuropeptides might be involved in neurologic diseases. Although the data accumulated to this time must be considered fragmentary and incomplete, it is already evident that methods used for the study of neuropeptides in experimental animals are also applicable to investigation of human tissue both normal and abnormal. The role of nigrostriatal dopamine deficiency in the pathophysiology[150] of Parkinson's disease (PD) has served as a model for pursuit of studies of neurochemical alterations in other neurodegenerative diseases.

Newly identified neuroanatomic systems, defined by immunohistochemical staining of peptide neuroregulators, have been described[74,90,92] (see chapter 18). As will be detailed in this chapter, there is ample evidence that abnormalities in neuropeptide concentrations occur in human diseases; however, there is as yet no direct evidence that these alterations play a significant role in the pathophysiology or etiology of any neurologic illness. There is, however, sufficient evidence implicating peptide abnormalities in neurologic disease to justify an effort to proceed further, to study dynamic aspects of peptide function, and to determine if peptide abnormalities are directly involved in the production of neurologic symptoms.

VALIDITY OF PEPTIDE MEASUREMENTS IN HUMAN DISEASE

The primary tools of peptide research, radioimmunoassay (RIA) and immunocytochemistry, have been applied to human brain tissue obtained at surgery and at autopsy. In general, the results have confirmed observations made in experimental animals, particularly primates and rodents, where tissue preparation is more satisfactory.

Measurements of neuropeptides in postmortem tissue show a degree of biologic variation in concentration; consequently, studies must include sufficient numbers of cases to be able to detect significant differences. Antemortem factors such as age, sex, time of death, drug treatment,[22] other coincident illness,[152] and cause of death must be considered as sources of peptide alterations.[152] For instance, virtually all patients dying with Huntington's disease or schizophrenia have been treated with long-term neuroleptic therapy. It is necessary, therefore, either to control for such therapy or to demonstrate that it is not the cause of any abnormalities recognized.

Peptides have been demonstrated to be quite stable in postmortem tissue. This stability probably is related to storage in vesicles with protection from lysosomal peptidases. Many studies show no correlation of peptide concentration with delay to autopsy. Substance P,[32,35,38,63] somatostatin,[32,35,40,41,53,65] cholecystokinin octapeptide (CCK-8),[63,64,122,135] met-enkephalin,[70] thyrotropin-releasing hormone (TRH),[26,114] gonadotropin-releasing hormone (GnRH),[28,114] neurotensin,[26,32,35,99] vasoactive intestinal polypeptide (VIP),[122] and bombesin,[68] all have been shown to be stable in human brain by this criterion.

Investigators have used chromatographic techniques to look for peptide degradation products in postmortem tissue and generally have failed to find them. Immunoreactive substance P,[8,50,103] CCK,[122,156] VIP,[51] neuropeptide Y (NPY),[1-3] met-enkephalin,[50] and neurotensin[99] in extracts of human brain all have been shown to migrate as single chromatographic peaks. In the case of somatostatin, where higher molecular weight forms of immunoreactive material generally can be found in extracts of animal tissue, it is encouraging that such presumed precursor forms are also present in extracts of human postmortem brain,[8,40,65] although conversion of high-molecular precursors to somatostatin 14 may continue slowly after death.[65]

The most convincing evidence of postmortem stability of neuropeptides has come from animal experiments. Substance P,[50] somatostatin,[40,42,65,97] CCK-8,[135] VIP,[51] and met-enkephalin[50] all have been shown to be stable in animal brains for at least 24 hours, and in some studies for as long as 72 hours postmortem.

It also has been possible to apply immunocytochemical techniques to human postmortem brain tissue.[74,100,101] Attachment of the antibody to antiperoxidase or to fluorescent-labeled probes has permitted double labeling experiments to examine for colocalization of two or more peptides or of peptides with other neurotransmitters or cellular markers.[96]

ANATOMIC OBSERVATIONS OF NEUROPEPTIDES IN THREE REGIONS OF BRAIN

Before proceeding to an account of certain abnormalities in neuropeptides that have been demonstrated in neurologic disorders, it is useful to review the relationship of neuropeptides to conventional neurotransmitters and to examine selected aspects of regional neuropeptidergic neuroanatomy. Three regions — cerebral cortex, basal ganglia, and spinal cord — have received sufficient attention to make the anatomic observations relevant for an understanding of certain disease states.

CEREBRAL CORTEX

Many of the currently known neuropeptides are found in neurons of the cerebral cortex in higher primates and man: VIP, somatostatin, CCK, NPY, corticotropin-releasing hormone (CRH), substance P, and dynorphin.[52,77-79,81,92] Each of these peptides has been demonstrated in cortex by immunocytochemistry both in intrinsic neurons and in fiber plexuses. The work of Jones, Hendry and collaborators[77-81,92,180] in the macaque monkey has provided detailed anatomic analysis of neuropeptide localization in cerebral cortex. Our own work in the human brain, although less extensive, shows nearly identical observations (Kowall, Beal and Martin, unpublished). Several generalizations now can be made from these observations.

All peptide-containing cortical neurons are fundamentally similar. Neuronal somata immunoreactive for each neuropeptide are found in all layers of the cortex but are particularly concentrated in two striata: layer II and the upper part of layer III, and in layer VI and the underlying white matter (Fig. 1). The neurons are small, 8 to 10 μ in diameter, and those containing VIP, CCK, somatostatin, and NPY each account for approximately 2 percent of the total population in most areas of cortex examined.[92] Immunoreactive cells staining for substance P, dynorphin, and CRH are found in far smaller numbers. The concentration of peptidergic neurons is greatest in the entorhinal and pyriform cortex, and more are found in the motor, premotor, and parietal cortices than in other neocortical areas.

The processes of all types of peptidergic cells for the most part project in a vertical orientation, interconnecting the various layers in a columnar fashion. The neuronal processes of peptidergic cells are beaded. Jones and Hendry[92] suggest that multiple axonal processes may arise from single individual cells. All form distinct plexuses, which arise from the vertical orientation of fibers, being concentrated in layers I and II and in layer VI and the subjacent white matter. The density of plexuses in the monkey is greatest for NPY and somatostatin. The cortical layer, IVC, containing thalamic afferents is devoid of peptidergic fibers.

Peptidergic fibers entering the cortex from other parts of the central nervous system (CNS) are strikingly absent. No peptidergic fibers are found in deeper white matter of the centrum semiovale or in the corpus callosum.[92] These observations taken together with the morphology of the cortical peptidergic somata suggest that all peptide containing cells of the cerebral cortex are local, intrinsic neurons without efferent projections.

Electron microscopic studies show that peptidergic cortical neurons form symmetric synapses. Most CCK and VIP synapses occur on somata of pyramidal cells.[92] Somatostatin and NPY synapses are found on small peripheral dendrites of pyramidal neurons. Terminals of CCK and VIP neurons ending on blood vessels have been described.

Studies in the monkey and our own observations in the human (Kowall and Martin, unpublished) indicate that over 80 percent of somatostatin positive cells colocalize with NPY. Similar findings are reported in rats.[34] In extensive double-staining studies in the monkey cortex, Jones and coworkers[92] found that at least 95 percent of cells containing somatostatin, NPY, and/or CCK are also immunoreactive for glutamic acid decarboxylase (GAD) or γ-aminobutyric acid (GABA). In rats, Eckenstein and Thoenen[49] showed that VIP and choline acetyltransferase are colocalized in a small number of peptidergic intrinsic neurons.

Because GABA is found in a high percentage of cortical neurons, it is important to consider whether all GABA-containing neurons also contain

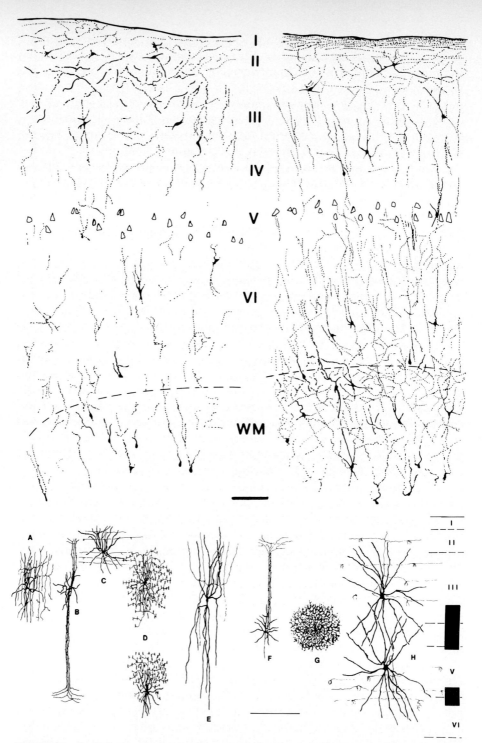

FIGURE 1. *(Top)* These camera lucida drawings from sections through the motor cortex of a monkey show the major concentrations of peptide immunoreactive cells in layers II-III and in layer VI and the subjacent white matter (WM). *(Left)* somatostatin immunoreactivity; *(right)* NPY immunoreactivity; bar 250 microns. (From Hendry et al,[15] with permission.) *(Bottom)* Morphologic types of intrinsic neurons in Golgi preparations of monkey sensory-motor cortex are shown here. A and B are basket cells, known to be GABAergic, as are the chandelier cells, D. Neurogliaform cell, C, cell with axonal arcades, E, and double bouquet cell, H, are likely to be GABAergic. Cell F is typical of all peptide-containing cells and shows colocalization of GAD and GABA with the peptides. Some such cells probably contain VIP and ChAT. Cell G is presumed to be an excitatory, spiny stellate cell. Bars, right, indicate layers of termination of thalamic afferents. (From Hendry and Jones,[12] with permission.)

neuropeptides.[84,145,146] The majority of the eight or nine morphologic types of cortical intrinsic neurons are GABAergic, but only one class described above contains neuropeptides.[139] The GABA-containing basket cells, which are much larger than the peptidergic neurons, have not, to date, shown any immunoreactivity to the known neuropeptides found in cortex. Certain of the same peptidergic cell types also contain acetylcholine. It can be concluded that data obtained to date suggest that all neuropeptides in primate cortex colocalize with either GABA or acetylcholine.

These anatomic considerations become important when considering the changes in neuropeptides (and acetylcholine) found in Alzheimer's disease.

Postmortem Studies of Cortex in Specific Neurologic Diseases

Alzheimer's Disease (AD). In Alzheimer's dementia and Alzheimer's-type senile dementia (AD), there is reduction of acetylcholine and its synthesizing enzyme, choline acetyltransferase (CAT), in the cerebral cortex to 60 to 90 percent of levels found in control brains.[6,40,41,130,131] This neurochemical abnormality reflects a loss of cholinergic terminals in the cortex and hippocampus. The cell bodies of origin of these terminals are found in the basal nucleus of Meynert, where loss of neuronal perikarya has been documented in AD.[136,170] Senile plaques, one of the cardinal neuropathologic signs of AD, contain degenerating cholinergic nerve terminals.[154] The degree of loss of CAT activity in the cerebral cortex correlates with the density of senile plaques, and both correlate with the degree of dementia.[37,121]

Measurements of neuropeptide concentrations in human brain regions dissected at autopsy have shown a selective loss of somatostatin-like immunoreactivity (SLI) in the neocortex and hippocampus of patients with AD when compared with controls[24,41,57,93,129,147] (Fig. 2). No consistent abnormalities of SLI concentration have been found in basal ganglia or hypothalamus in AD. In normal aging, there seems to be no loss of SLI from human cortex.[32,37,120] Cortical NPY and CRH concentrations are also reduced in AD.[175,181] Substance P, VIP, and CCK concentrations, as determined by radioimmunoassay, have not been found altered in AD.[6,37,38,120,122,133,135] The lack of alteration of VIP and CCK is of particular interest, because an alteration of somatostatin, NPY, and CRH and no change in other peptides found in similar cell types suggest a degree of selectivity of the cells that die in AD.

The degree of loss of SLI in cerebral cortex in AD correlates with the diminution in CAT activity.[41,134] The fall in SLI is presumed to represent a loss of somatostatin-containing neuronal elements in the cortex, presumably of intrinsic cortical neurons. The selectivity of somatostatin neuronal involvement in AD with sparing of other intrinsic peptidergic neurons containing CCK and VIP may provide clues to the pathogenesis of neuronal loss in AD.

Recent studies of NPY[157] in control and AD cortex are particularly interesting because of the colocalization of NPY and somatostatin.[1-3,96] Initial reports indicated that NPY levels are normal in cortex but elevated in substantia innominata in AD.[1] In our studies, concentrations of both soma-

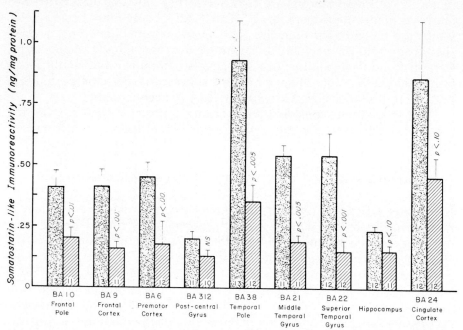

FIGURE 2. Decrease in somatostatin-like immunoreactivity in control *(left bar)* and Alzheimer's disease *(right)* cerebral cortex. (From Beal et al,[24] with permission.)

tostatin and NPY were measured in the same samples taken from AD and control brains.[181] Significant reductions in both peptides were found in 11 cortical regions and in the hippocampus and locus coeruleus. The most severely affected regions were the temporal and frontal lobes and the occipital cortex (Fig. 3). These observations have not, to date, been particularly instructive about the pathogenesis of Alzheimer's disease. They do suggest, as noted above, a certain degree of selectivity of cell involvement, namely, that certain classes of cells may be affected and that others are relatively or perhaps completely spared.

Somatostatin Receptor Binding to Membrane Preparations. Somatostatin receptor binding has been examined in rat, monkey, and human brain.[25,153,158,159] The regional distribution of somatostatin binding sites is similar in both human and monkey brain.[25] Binding is highest in cerebral cortex; intermediate in hippocampus, nucleus accumbens, striatum, and amygdala; and low in the thalamus, hypothalamus, and many brainstem areas. Comparison of somatostatin binding with concentration of somatostatin in human brain shows a rough correlation. Cingulate cortex, which contains the highest cortical concentrations of somatostatin, also has the highest somatostatin binding, and occipital cortex, which has the lowest somatostatin binding, has the lowest concentrations of somatostatin of any cortical region.

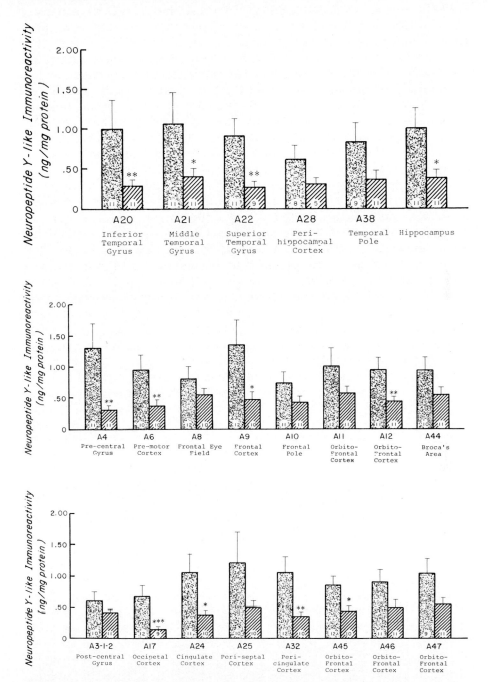

FIGURE 3. Neuropeptide Y-like immunoreactivity in temporal cortex (*top*), frontal cortex (*middle*), and remaining cortical regions (*bottom*). Control concentrations are on the left, and those in AD are on the right. The number of samples is indicated in parentheses. The error bars show standard error of the mean. Significant levels calculated using the Mann-Whitney U test are indicated (*p<0.05, **p<0.025, ***p<0.01). (From Beal et al, 1986, with permission).

Somatostatin receptors have been characterized in human brain using 125 I[Leu(8), DTrp(22) Tyr(25)]SS28.[24,25] These binding sites have many of the properties expected for a receptor.[24] To evaluate receptor concentrations in human tissue in disease states, it is necessary to establish postmortem stability of receptors. Receptors for several classical neurotransmitters are known to be stable postmortem, but much less is known about peptide receptors. No correlation was found between postmortem interval and somatostatin receptor concentrations in 8 cortical regions from 12 human control brains.[25] In addition, somatostatin receptor stability has been compared in an animal model simulating human autopsy conditions.[25] In these experiments, there was no significant loss of receptor binding in cerebral cortex, striatum, or hippocampus for up to 24 hours. Alzheimer brain tissue showed significant reductions in concentrations of somatostatin receptors to approximately 50 percent of control values in frontal cortex (Brodmann areas 6, 9, and 10) and temporal cortex (Brodmann area 21)[24] (Fig. 4). Cingulate cortex, postcentral gyrus, temporal pole, and superior temporal gyrus showed no significant changes. Concentrations of receptors were reduced approximately 40 percent in hippocampus, but this did not quite reach significance (p<0.10).

Several explanations could account for these results. Reduced somatostatin and reduced somatostatin receptors in the same regions could reflect loss of both presynaptic (somatostatin) and postsynaptic (somatostatinceptive) neurons in areas that have a predilection for the pathologic process. Neuronal loss in AD is greatest in frontal and temporal cortex, which are the regions in which the largest alterations in somatostatin and somatostatin receptors are found. Another possibility is that a proportion of somatostatin receptors are located on cortical afferents, such as the cholinergic system, which degenerate in AD. Another possibility is that somatostatin release is increased in AD, accounting for the reduced concentrations of

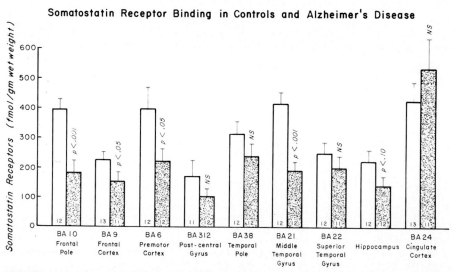

FIGURE 4. Decrease in somatostatin receptor binding in Alzheimer's disease compared with controls is illustrated here. SEM is shown for each group. Significant levels are shown above each bar.

somatostatin. If release was increased in AD, then one might expect a down regulation of somatostatin receptors in the same region. Arguing against this possibility, however, is the finding of reduced concentrations of CSF somatostatin in AD instead of the predicted increase if release had been increased (see below).

Recent autoradiographic studies of somatostatin receptors have provided more definitive cytologic localization. In studies in rat,[161] the highest binding was in cerebral cortex, particularly in layers III, IV, and layer VI. Binding was also demonstrated by autoradiography in human cerebral cortex.

Other neuropeptides also have been studied in Alzheimer's disease. Mazurek and coworkers measured the concentrations of vasopressin in control and AD brains.[182] Levels in most regions of the cerebral cortex were normal or slightly elevated (interpreted to signify preservation of vasopressin terminals in cortical atrophy). However, concentrations of vasopressin were significantly reduced in the hippocampus, a finding of considerable interest in view of the speculations concerning the role of vasopressin in memory.[104] Concentrations of vasopressin also were reduced in the globus pallidus and locus coeruleus in AD. Cerebrospinal fluid levels of vasopressin are also significantly reduced in AD.[179]

Histology of Alzheimer's Disease and Relationship of Neuropeptides to Senile Plaques. Many neuronal elements now characterized by immunocytochemistry or histochemistry appear to contribute to the neurites present in senile plaques. The enzyme acetylcholinesterase (AChE),[37,44] somatostatin,[44,108,127] NPY, NADPH diaphorase,[88] CCK, and VIP (Kowall and Martin, unpublished) all can be identified in plaques. What the relative contribution of each neuronal type is to plaque formation is unknown.

Huntington's Disease (HD) and Parkinson's Disease (PD). Neuropeptides in the cerebral cortex obtained from patients dying of HD and PD also have been studied. Two general sets of observations have emerged. First, no definitive abnormalities in conventional or neuropeptide neuroregulators have been found in HD.[27] Second, PD patients with dementia showed significant reduction in cortical somatostatin, whereas PD patients without dementia showed no change.[55] The question remaining to be resolved is whether those patients with PD and dementia also have Alzheimer's disease, or whether this neurochemical change accompanies the dementia of PD separate from AD. Changes in cortical neurotransmitters, neuropeptides, and receptor binding are summarized in Table 1.

BASAL GANGLIA

The anatomy of the basal ganglia has been investigated extensively in the past few years, and correlations of cell types with neurotransmitter content have been made.

A brief review of normal striatal histology and biochemistry is essential for an understanding of the implications of changes in neuropeptides. Nissl-stained sections of striatum reveal two neuronal populations: a medium-size (10 to 20 μ) cell group accounting for 90 percent of the total, and a

TABLE 1. Neurotransmitter, Neuropeptide, and Receptor Binding Changes in the Cerebral Cortex in Neurologic Diseases

Compound or Macromolecule	Levels	Neuroanatomic Location	Diseases
γ-Aminobutyric acid (GABA)	high	neurons	AD:decreased HD:unchanged
Glutamate	high	neurons	AD:unchanged
Aspartate	high	neurons	AD:unchanged
Acetylcholine	moderate	neurons and nerve fibers	AD:decreased PD:decreased or unchanged
Cholineacetyltransferase (CAT)	moderate	neurons and nerve fibers	AD:decreased
Muscarinic binding sites	moderate	—	AD:unchanged
Norepinephrine	moderate to low	nerve fibers	AD:unchanged or decreased PD:unchanged or decreased
Serotonin	low	nerve fibers	
Somatostatin	moderate	neurons	AD:decreased HD:unchanged PD:decreased in some patients
Somatostatin binding sites	high	—	—
Neuropeptide Y	high	neurons	AD:decreased or unchanged
Vasoactive intestinal polypeptide (VIP)	high	neurons	AD:unchanged
Cholecystokinin (CCK)	high	neurons	AD:unchanged
Substance P	low	neurons	AD:decreased or unchanged
Corticotropin releasing hormone (CRH)	low	neurons	AD:decreased
Dynorphin	low	neurons	—
Vasopressin	very low	nerve fibers	AD:decreased in some regions
Oxytocin	very low	nerve fibers	—

Abbreviations: AD, Alzheimer's disease; HD, Huntington's disease; PD, Parkinson's disease.

large-size group making up the remainder.[47,71,72] Golgi studies of various mammalian species, including the human, have defined five subsets of neurons with these categories.

> The majority are medium-size spiny neurons (type I) which in the human are larger,[47,71,72] have lower dendritic spine density, and greater dendritic fields than the corresponding type in the monkey (Table 2 and Fig. 5). They account for 70 to 80 percent of all cells. A second spiny type (type II) is medium to large, with sparse spiny dendrites (10 percent). Two types of aspiny cells are found: a medium (type I) and large size (type II); aspiny cells characteristically have an indented nucleus visible in Nissl-stained sections. This group accounts for 10 to 20 percent of striatal neurons in man.[56] A final category consists of small neurons with variable dendritic morphology (1 to 2 percent). Retrograde transport experiments in lower animals suggest that the medium-size spiny neurons account for most projecting neurons in striatum, whereas aspiny cells are involved *exclusively* in local intrinsic striatal circuits.[73,74,146]

Many compounds have been assayed in human striatum, including the classical neurotransmitters, amino acids, several peptides, and en-

TABLE 2. Principal Cell Types and Putative Cellular Messengers in the Striatum

Neuronal Classification	Transmitter/Neuroregulator
Spiny Type I	GABA/Enkephalin/Dynorphin*
Spiny Type II	Substance P
Aspiny Type I	Somatostatin/Neuropeptide Y
Aspiny Type II	Acetylcholine
Aspiny (?type)	CCK/VIP/CRH*

*These are largely within separate cell types. GABA and enkephalins coexist in some cells.

zymes[73,74] (Table 3). Histochemical methods permit the localization of these substances either to intrinsic cell groups or to extrinsic afferent fiber systems that project to the striatum.

Spiny type neurons contain GABA and the GABA synthetic enzyme, glutamic acid decarboxylase (GAD); half of these also contain enkephalin-like immunoreactivity.[73,74] Substance P and dynorphin also are localized in this group of neurons. *Aspiny neurons* contain a variety of neuroactive substances. Some contain GAD. The neuropeptides somatostatin, NPY, CCK, neurotensin, and CRH are found in this group as well.[45,46] The large aspiny neurons contain choline acetyl transferase (CAT) and the enzyme acetylcholinesterase (AChE).

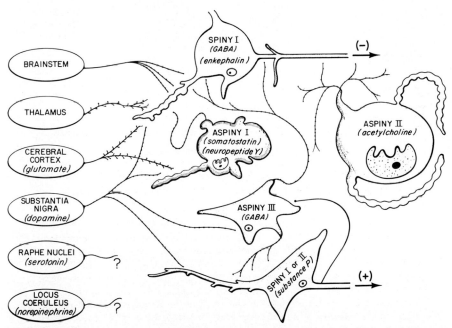

FIGURE 5. This is a schematic drawing of selected striatal cell types. Spiny I neurons (medium size) contain GABA and enkephalin (both transmitters coexist in some cells). Spiny I or II cells are believed to contain substance P. Both spiny I and II cells project from the striatum. Aspiny I cells contain somatostatin and neuropeptide Y and are positive for the enzyme reaction NADPH diaphorase. Large aspiny II cells probably contain acetylcholine. Aspiny III cells are postulated to contain GABA. Most aspiny cells appear to function as interneurons. Afferent inputs to the striatum are shown on the left. The details of the anatomic connections of afferent fibers to individual intrinsic cells of the striatum are largely unknown. (From Martin, JB,[102] with permission.)

TABLE 3. Neurotransmitter, Neuropeptide, and Receptor Binding Changes in Striatum in Neurologic Disorders

Compound or Macromolecule	Levels	Neuroanatomic Location	Diseases
Dopamine	highest in brain	nerve fibers of nigrostriatal pathway	HD:unchanged or increased PD:decreased
Tyrosine hydroxylase	very high	nerve fibers of nigrostriatal pathway	HD:unchanged
Dopamine binding sites	highest in brain	pre & post-synaptic sites	HD:decreased PD:decreased
Norepinephrine	very low	adrenergic nerve fibers	HD:unchanged or increased PD:decreased
Dopamine β-hydroxylase	low	adrenergic nerve fibers	HD:unchanged
Serotonin (5HT)	moderate	nerve fibers	HD:unchanged or increased PD:decreased
5HT binding sites	moderate	presynaptic and postsynaptic sites	HD:decreased PD:unchanged or decreased
γ-aminobutyric acid (GABA)	moderate to high	nerve cells and fibers	HD:decreased
Glutamic acid decarboxylase (GAD)	high	nerve cells and fibers	HD:decreased PD:decreased
GABA binding sites	moderate to high	presynaptic and postsynaptic sites	HD:decreased or unchanged PD:unchanged
Glutamate	high	nerve fibers	HD:decreased
Acetylcholine (ACh)	very high	neurons	HD:decreased
Cholineacetyltransferase (CAT)	very high	neurons	HD:decreased
Muscarinic ACh binding sites	highest in brain	—	HD:decreased PD:unchanged or increased
Met-enkephalin	high	neurons and nerve fibers	HD:unchanged in striatum: decreased in striatal efferents
Dynorphin	moderate	neurons	HD:decreased in striatal efferents
Angiotensin II	very high	neurons	—
Angiotensin converting enzyme (ACE)	highest in brain	neurons and nerve fibers	HD:decreased
Somatostatin	moderate	neurons and nerve fibers	HD:increased PD:unchanged
Somatostatin binding sites	moderate	—	—
Neuropeptide Y	moderate	neurons and nerve fibers	HD:increased
Cholecystokinin (CCK)	high	neurons and nerve fibers	HD:unchanged decreased in striatal efferents PD:unchanged
CCK binding sites	high	—	HD:decreased
Neurotensin	low to moderate	nerve fibers	HD:unchanged PD:unchanged
Substance P	moderate	neurons	HD:decreased PD:slightly decreased
Substance P binding sites	moderate	—	—
Thyrotropin releasing hormone	moderate	nerve terminals	HD:increased
Vasoactive intestinal polypeptide (VIP)	low to moderate	neurons and nerve fibers	HD:unchanged
VIP binding sites	highest in brain	—	—
Vasopressin	low	—	—

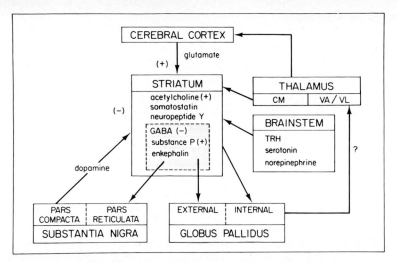

FIGURE 6. This diagram illustrates the principal anatomic connections of the basal ganglia. The neurotransmitters shown in each of the pathways are postulated on the basis of current evidence. Acetylcholine and somatostatin are present in interneurons of the striatum. The major efferent pathway from the striatum to the substantia nigra (pars reticulata) and to the external and internal segments of the globus pallidus contains GABA, substance P, and enkephalins. (From Martin, JB,[102] with permission.)

Recently the interrelationships between these peptides and enzymes have been studied in rat and human tissue.[96,163,165,166] The peptides somatostatin and NPY and the enzyme NADPH diaphorase colocalize in a single subset of aspiny neurons.[96,163,165] This population is distinct from the AChE-containing subset. They account for about 5 to 10 percent of the total striatal neuron population in the human brain. Vasoactive intestinal peptide and CCK also are found in aspiny cells, but these are rather infrequent.[96] It is not known at present if these latter two peptides are found in a separate aspiny population.

Many substances are located in fibers that project to the striatum. Midbrain tegmentum, locus coeruleus, and midbrain raphe neurons give rise to dopaminergic, noradrenergic, and serotonergic fibers, respectively.[73,74] Other peptides, including VIP, CRH, and vasopressin, originate from neurons in the hypothalamus and amygdaloid complex. Cortical fiber projections to the striatum contain the amino acids glutamate and aspartate (see Figures 5 and 6). Table 3 summarizes the distribution of several neuroactive substances in normal human striatum.

This rich neuronal and biochemical landscape is further organized into two major histochemical compartments. Graybiel and colleagues[73,74] first showed the compartmentalization with AChE staining, which in the cat and primate reveals a myriad of interconnected low AChE patches which they called *striosomes*. These patches contain high levels of opioid peptides and substance P and are surrounded by zones of AChE-rich neuropil.[66] Somatostatin neurons are found in the high-AChE zones, often near the striosomal boundaries.[96] Fiber connections to and from striatum also are segregated with respect to these zones.

Huntington's Disease

Huntington's disease (HD) is a hereditary disorder characterized by involuntary movements (termed chorea because of their dance-like quality) and changes in mental status ranging from altered mood and personality changes to profound dementia.[102] Inheritance follows an autosomal dominant pattern with complete penetrance. Using recombinant DNA techniques, the abnormal gene has been localized to the short arm of chromosome 4.[75] Most cases begin insidiously during the third to fifth decade. Interestingly, onset of the illness before age 21 is associated with paternal inheritance—an observation inconsistent with conventional Mendelian inheritance. Clinically, these early-onset patients often present with rigidity and seizures. Juvenile-onset cases have the same abnormal gene locus as later onset cases.[143] Late-onset HD cases (>50 years of age) have a more smoldering clinical course and less severe neuropathologic findings at autopsy.[109] Epidemiologic studies show a worldwide prevalence of 5 to 7 cases per 100,000 population. Seventy percent of cases occur in Caucasian populations. Detailed geneologic studies have traced the gene to a single mutation that probably originated in western Europe. No case of HD has been unequivocally proven to have arisen from a new spontaneous mutation (for reviews see Martin[102,178]).

Neuropathologic Findings in HD. Vonsattel and coworkers[167] have recently reported neuropathologic findings in more than 160 cases of HD. The most consistant neuropathologic observation, as first observed over 90 years ago, is striking atrophy of the caudate nucleus and putamen (together called the striatum). The nucleus accumbens and more anterior, lateral, and ventral parts of the striatum are generally less severely involved. In their series they found no consistent abnormalities in cerebral cortex or other brain regions. Others have reported abnormalities in frontal cortex, subthalamic nucleus, and brainstem. Microscopic neuronal loss and astroglial proliferation in the striatum parallel the degree of atrophy. They defined five grades of severity, which correspond with the clinical state of the patient. Grade 0 cases have typical clinical findings and a positive family history but normal gross and microscopic examinations at postmortem. Grade 1 cases have only microscopic abnormalities, with a 50 percent loss of caudate neurons. In grades 2 and 3, the head of the caudate is grossly atrophic. The grade 4 cases have pronounced atrophy of the caudate, which is reduced to a thin ribbon only a few millimeters wide, even at the level of its head. Ninety-five percent of neurons are lost by this stage.

Neurochemistry and Histology of HD. Many of the aforementioned peptides and enzymes have been measured in homogenates of frozen striatum obtained from patients with HD (reviewed in Bird[27] and Martin[102]). Several substances have been found to be diminished in quantity, as might be expected in a destructive process. These include GABA, substance P, and enkephalins. All of these compounds are found in the spiny population of neurons (GABA is in both). Graveland and coworkers[71] have reported that this spiny population of neurons appear to be disproportionately affected in HD. Golgi impregnations demonstrate recurved and distorted dendrites and alternations in the shape and density of dendritic spines.[71]

A second group of substances are either unchanged or somewhat increased in concentration in HD striatum. These substances are found in fibers that project to the striatum, their cell bodies safely removed from the destructive locus in the striatum. This group includes dopamine, serotonin, norepinephrine, and their related synthetic enzymes. Vasoactive intestinal peptide and TRH[151] also are found in afferent fibers, and they are preserved. Cholecystokinin is found mainly in fibers, and its concentration is preserved in the striatum despite depleted levels in the globus pallidus.[54]

Two peptides are strikingly enriched in HD striatum. Aronin and colleagues[8] reported a threefold to fivefold increase in striatal somatostatin content. This has been confirmed by Beal and associates[13] and Nemeroff and coworkers.[112] As would be expected based on colocalization studies, NPY and NADPH diaphorase activities also are increased.[43,56] It is possible that some striatal somatostatin is present in fibers that originate outside the striatum. Beal and associates performed a series of lesion experiments in order to answer this question.[14,15,18,19] Lesions that deafferent the striatum do not deplete somatostatin levels unless they involve the basal forebrain. It was concluded that the bulk of somatostatin arises from intrinsic striatal neurons. The degree of enrichment of somatostatin content is greater than that found for substances known to have extrinsic origins, such as dopamine. Immunocytochemical studies and enzyme histochemical studies have shown that the increase in somatostatin, NPY, and NADPH diaphorase content is due to selective preservation of this subset of neurons.[43,56] It is unknown if this subset is preserved alone or if other aspiny groups also are spared. Further immunocytochemical studies combined with enzyme histochemistry should answer this question. Table 3 summarizes the neurochemical changes in HD striatum. Somatostatin $28_{(1-12)}$ is also increased in the striatum in HD.[12]

It is important to consider whether these neurochemical findings have any clinical significance. Experimental studies provide a few intriguing clues. Somatostatin injected into rat striatum produces motor effects that mimic those seen with dopamine.[59] Push-pull cannula experiments have shown that somatostatin injections into rat and cat striatum cause increased dopamine release.[33]

It is known that in humans dopamine excess produces choreiform motor activity. This is most commonly seen in parkinsonian patients, who may develop chorea after excessive doses of levodopa. It is possible that surviving somatostatin neurons in the HD striatum contribute to the choreiform movements by virtue of their unopposed activity. One might, therefore, expect increased dopamine turnover in the striatum of HD patients.[21] Consideration has been given to measures that decrease somatostatin concentrations as an approach to ameliorate the movement disorder. Cysteamine, an agent that has been shown to deplete selectively brain somatostatin immunoreactivity when given systemically to rats, has received some initial evaluation.[20,138] Treatment for two weeks in five patients failed to show any benefit.[176]

Why do the somatostatin/NPY cells survive in HD? This question may be approached by examining what is unique about them. It is not known if peptides such as NPY or somatostatin can directly contribute protective effects. The enzyme NADPH diaphorase, on the other hand, is known to act as a detoxifying agent in other tissues.[169] We speculate that the unique biochemical makeup of this subset of neurons renders them resistant to a local toxin which is generated because of the abnormal HD gene product. It is of interest that the nucleus accumbens—which has higher levels of somatostatin, NPY, and NADPH diaphorase than the dorsal striatum—is less affected by the destructive process.[14,96] Several excitatory amino acid analogs have been found to produce neuronal cell death with axon-sparing lesions in rat striatum (reviewed in Schwarcz[140]). One such analog, quinolinic acid, is present endogenously and increases in concentration with age.[107,141] We have recently shown that the NPY-somatostatin-NADPH diaphorase neurons are resistant to this or to a similar endogenous toxin.

Further investigations into the distinct nature of these neurons may not only further clarify the pathogenesis of HD but suggest possible means of intervening biochemically to prevent the destructive process. Newly established gene detection methods could then be used to identify pre-symptomatic individuals and to allow the physician to offer these patients more than a gloomy prognostic verdict with an inevitable and irrevocable outcome.

Parkinson's Disease (PD)

Idiopathic Parkinson's disease (PD) is in many ways the archetypical neurodegenerative disease.[150] In PD there is a remarkably specific loss of the pigmented dopamine-containing neurons from the substantia nigra pars compacta and of their terminals in the caudate and putamen. Correlated with this loss is a depletion of dopamine, homovanillic acid, and tyrosine hydroxylase activity in substantia nigra and striatum.[150] Treatment of patients with PD with either the dopamine precursor L-dopa or dopamine agonists, such as bromocriptine, improves their symptoms but does not alter the progression of their disease.

The striato-nigral substance-P-containing pathway is thought to exert an excitatory influence on dopaminergic neurons in the substantia nigra. In brains of patients dying with PD, significant decreases in concentrations of substance-P-like immunoreactivity (SPLI) have been observed in the substantia nigra pars compacta and pars reticulata and in the globus pallidus external segment.[103] Substance-P-like immunoreactivity concentrations in caudate and putamen were reduced 24 and 27 percent, respectively—differences that were not statistically significant. The significant depletions of SPLI observed ranged from 32 percent in the pars compacta of the substantia nigra to 46 percent in the external division of the globus pallidus, considerably less than the 90 percent depletion of dopaminergic markers observed. Whether the loss of an excitatory substance P input to the substantia nigra contributes to the symptoms of PD is unknown.

Cholecystokinin-8 is of interest in PD in view of the evidence that a subset of dopamine-containing cells of the ventral midbrain tegmentum (the mesolimbic neurons) contain CCK-8. They project to the nucleus accumbens and frontal cortex. In PD, the pathologic observations of a virtual complete loss of pigmented neurons in the substantia nigra and ventral tegmentum and the near total depletion of dopamine in the midbrain suggest that all subdivisions of the midbrain dopaminergic system are involved in the disease. One would hypothesize, therefore, that PD would be associated with a loss of immunoreactive CCK-8 in the substantia nigra, ventral tegmentum, nucleus accumbens, and frontal cortex—the areas of projection of mesolimbic dopaminergic neurons thought to contain CCK-8. This hypothesis has been only partially verified. Concentrations of CCK-like immunoreactivity are reduced by about 40 percent in the substantia nigra in PD but are normal in nucleus accumbens, frontal cortex, and striatum.[156] Whether the loss in the substantia nigra reflects degeneration of some groups of neurons containing both dopamine and CCK-8 remains to be determined.

Met-enkephalin-like immunoreactivity also is reduced in the putamen, globus pallidus externa, substantia nigra pars compacta (but not the pars reticulata), and ventral tegmental area in PD.[122] Concentrations of met-enkephalin are normal in the caudate, nucleus accumbens, globus pallidus interna, and other forebrain areas examined. The clinical significance of these alterations in met-enkephalin concentration is unknown. No alteration of extrahypothalamic concentrations of immunoreactive arginine vasopressin (AVP) was found in PD.[132]

In dementia sometimes associated with PD, the pathologic findings are similar to those in AD, including the presence of senile plaques, neurofibrillary tangles, and neuronal loss from the basal nucleus or Meynert. Recent studies from Agid's group[55] show that somatostatin in the cerebral cortex is reduced in the dementia of PD, as it is in AD.

Schizophrenia

Several reports have searched for neuropeptide alterations in schizophrenia.[58,112] The findings have not been consistent.

SPINAL CORD

Studies of neuropeptides in the spinal cord have provided intriguing new hypotheses about sensory and motor mechanisms. It is now known that sensory neurons, particularly those of the C fiber and A delta categories, which conduct impulses for pain and temperature, contain a variety of neuropeptides.[91] Both the peripheral and central processes of these cells stain intensely for peptides.[110] The latter forms a dense band in layers I and II of the dorsal horn of the spinal cord. Certain intrinsic neurons of the spinal cord located in several regions also contain peptides. These regions include the gray matter of the dorsal horn, the intermediolateral cell column, and the vicinity of the central canal (Fig. 7).

Neuropeptides in Sensory Systems

Primary sensory neurons in the dorsal root ganglia (DRG) mediate transmission of sensory information from the periphery to the spinal cord. A combination of anatomic and electrophysiologic techniques has established that classes of afferent fibers that transmit specific sensory modali-

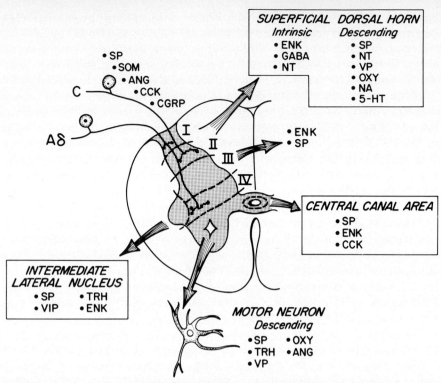

FIGURE 7. This diagram illustrates the diversity of neuropeptides found in the spinal cord. Abbreviations: A δ—A delta sensory fibers; ANG—angiotensin; C—C-sensory fibers; CCK—cholecystokinin; CGRP—calcitonin-gene related peptide; ENK—enkephalins; GABA—gamma aminobutyric acid; 5-HT—serotonin; NA—norepinephrine; NT—neurotensin; OXY—oxytocin; SOM—somatostatin; SP—substance P; VIP—vasoactive intestinal polypeptide; VP—vasopressin.

ties can be distinguished by their peripheral receptive properties, axonal conduction velocity, and central terminal organization.[31,76,89-91,125]

By morphologic criteria, DRG neurons can be classified into two major groups: large light cells and small dark cells. The small dark cells correspond to the slow conducting A delta or C fiber class, many of which are unmyelinated. These small cells and not the larger type are found to contain neuropeptides.[9,11] The central projections of the small dark cells terminate exclusively in laminae I and II of the dorsal horn, where their axon

TABLE 4. Neuropeptides in Subsets of Mammalian DRG* Neurons

	% DRG Neurons	Lamina Termination	Coexistence (Rat)
Substance P	20	I,,IIo	CCK,CGRP,VASO
Cholecystokinin	20	I,IIo	SP,CGRP,VASO
Calcitonin Gene Related Peptide	30	I,IIo	SP,CCK,VASO
Somatostatin	8	IIo	VASO
Angiotensin II	?	IIo	?

Modified from Jessel, T, and Dodd, J,[91] with permission.
*Dorsal root ganglia

terminals, as viewed in the electron microscope, contain both small clear and large granular (dense-core) vesicles. These observations suggest, but do not prove, that this class of fibers contains more than one neurotransmitter. Electrophysiologic studies suggest that fibers entering the dorsal horn can release transmitters with both fast and slow excitatory effects.[89-91]

More than a dozen neuropeptides have been identified within subsets of sensory neurons.[91] Included in this list are substance P,[116,160] somatostatin,[82] CCK, VIP, dynorphin, vasopressin, galanin, and oxytocin.[31,39,61,85,105] The percentage of DRG neurons containing each is summarized in Table 4. Coexistence of more than one peptide in a given DRG neuron appears to be the rule (Table 4). Individual DRG neurons may express five or six different peptides. Dopamine also is found in some cells.[124]

The identification of peptide receptors on dorsal horn neurons is an important next step in understanding the site of action of these substances. Although opioid receptors are abundant in the outer laminae of the dorsal horn, others have been less extensively studied.

The actions of neuropeptides in the mediation of transsynaptic events in the dorsal horn remain controversial and uncertain.[76] Neurotransmitters proposed to mediate fast excitatory potentials include adenosine triphosphate (ATP)[62] and glutamate. Substance P elicits an excitatory slow potential. The function of the other neuropeptides in the dorsal horn is unclear.[95]

The dorsal horn of the spinal cord is also the site of termination of several descending bulbospinal pathways that modify pain transmission. Transmitters in this system include serotonin, norepinephrine, substance P, neurophysin, and TRH[10] (see Figure 7). It is thought that these pathways modify transmission of sensory inputs at the level of the spinal cord.

Correlations with Sensory Abnormalities

Diseases that affect peripheral nerves and DRG neurons are reported to be associated with changes in neuropeptides in tissue or CSF (see below). Reductions in immunostaining for substance P have been reported in DRG cells in patients with congenital insensitivity to pain.

Neuropeptides Intrinsic to the Spinal Cord

Motor neurons of the spinal cord contain acetylcholine, and until recently no colocalized peptide had been identified. Recent studies indicate that calcitonin-gene-related peptide (CGRP)[128] is also present in anterior horn cells. Descending terminations on these cells from brainstem regions include fibers staining for substance P, TRH, and neurophysin (see Figure 7). TRH receptors are found in the anterior horns of the spinal cord.

Amyotrophic Lateral Sclerosis (ALS)

The anatomic observations of neuropeptide termination on anterior horn cells has led to a series of investigations of the therapeutic effects of TRH in ALS. After parenteral administration, this agent was reported to improve muscle function in several patients with ALS (see chapter 18).

NEUROPEPTIDES IN CEREBROSPINAL FLUID (CSF)

Measurements of peptides in CSF are generally valid because neuropeptide degradation is minimal and the immunoreactive material in CSF is chromatographically indistinguishable in most cases from the native peptide.[86] Certain factors must be borne in mind concerning the interpretation of CSF peptide concentrations. The evidence to date suggests that CSF peptides originate in the central nervous system and do not leak from the circulation.[4,7] Studies show that CSF peptide levels vary independently of circulating blood levels, and even large doses of peptides administered into the peripheral circulation fail to appear in the CSF, indicating a blood-CSF barrier, and presumably a blood-brain barrier (BBB), for peptides.[118] An exception to the general function of the BBB to exclude molecules occurs in the specialized circumventricular organs (see chapter 10).[106] At these locations, which comprise less than 0.02 percent of the entire capillaries of the brain, peptides can gain access slowly to the brain (and perhaps the CSF) from the blood. Specific receptors for transport of some hormones and peptides such as insulin and prolactin have been demonstrated. For others, like vasopressin, endogenous brain secretion is considered to occur.

The difficult issue is to identify which CNS regions contribute to the CSF peptide pool.[169] It is possible that regions deep in the brain supply a smaller proportion of CSF peptides than do regions close to the subarachnoid space. In one study,[149] in which lumbar punctures were performed and a total of 12 ml of CSF withdrawn, there was no difference in mean somatostatin concentration assayed in the first 2 ml and the final 2 ml, but albumin and gamma globulin concentrations were 20 percent less in the final milliliter than in the first milliliter.[149] The authors' conclusion from this data was that CSF somatostatin is supplied diffusely from the CNS, although it is also consistent with a predominant spinal cord source. A comparable study performed with substance P produced a similar result.[113] Consequently, peptides measured in lumbar CSF may be a more sensitive indicator of spinal cord disease than of brain disease.

The kinetics of peptide accumulation and clearance in the CSF have not been carefully studied. Some neuropeptides may be released specifically into the CSF and may use the CSF as a medium for transport to target sites,[70] but others may overflow passively into CSF. Several investigators have suggested that the tanycytes lining the third ventricle transport peptides from median eminence to CSF, although these cells seem, on anatomic grounds, to be more likely to be barriers than conduits and direct evidence for such transport is lacking.

Cerebrospinal fluid levels of neuropeptides also have been shown to be stable after withdrawal.[171] Immunoreactive substance P, somatostatin,[144] CCK,[126] TRH, and β-endorphin all have been shown to be stable under conditions of storage routinely used for clinical CSF samples and with no more precaution than refrigerating the samples. In addition, immunoreactive somatostatin and substance P in human CSF behave chromatographically as expected for the authentic peptides.

A number of neuropeptides have now been measured in human CSF (Table 5). Whether their presence in CSF indicates a functional role, that is, transport to distant sites to exert effects — or is merely a reflection of a

TABLE 5. Abnormalities of Peptides in the CSF*

	Normal Concentration	Disease State Altering Levels
Adenohypophysial Hormones		
GH	<1 ng/ml	
Prolactin	1–4 ng/ml	
TSH	<2 μU/ml	May be markedly elevated in pituitary
LH	<1 μU/ml	tumors with suprasellar extension
FSH	<1 μU/ml	
ACTH	20–80 pg/ml	
Posterior Pituitary Hormones		
AVP	<1.5–1.8 pg/ml	Slightly raised in anorexia nervosa, dehydration; slightly reduced in Alzheimer's disease
Oxytocin	7–15 pg/ml	Slightly raised after neuroleptic treatment (13 pg/ml); slightly reduced in bipolar depression (6 pg/ml)
Hypothalamic Releasing Factors		
TRH	2 ± 0.6 pg/ml	Unchanged in amyotrophic lateral sclerosis
GnRH	1 pg/ml	—
Somatostatin	40–65 pg/ml	Elevated in CNS Damage; lowered in Alzheimer's disease and multiple sclerosis (active phase)
GHRH	29 ± 2 pg/ml	Slightly reduced in idiopathic GH deficiency
CRH	60 pg/ml	Slightly raised in depression (75 pg/ml)
Opioid Peptides		
Endorphin	15 pg/ml	Elevated after local electrical brain stimulation; Nelson's syndrome
Met-enkephalin	5–29 pg/ml	Elevated after electroacupuncture; Leigh's syndrome
Leu-enkephalin	<5 pg/ml	—
Dynorphin	30 ± 2 pg/ml	—
Other Neuropeptides		
Histidyl Proline Diketopiperazine (His Pro DKP)	1 ng/ml	—
Substance P	25–45 pg/ml	Elevated in spina bifida and lumbar arachnoiditis (6–10 times); reduced in Shy-Drager syndrome and peripheral neuropathy
Neurotensin	34 ± 4 pg/ml	—
CCK	14 ± 3 pmol/ml 15 ± 2 pg/ml	Possibly increased in a subtype of schizophrenia
Gastrin	3 ± 1 pmol/l	—
Calcitonin	28 ± 14 pg/ml	Possibly reduced in mania and agitated schizophrenic subjects
Insulin	4 ± 1 μU/ml	—
VIP	68 pg/ml	Elevated following physostigmine administration; reduced in multiple sclerosis
Bombesin	33 ± 2 pg/ml	Slightly reduced in schizophrenia
HCG	Undetectable	Elevated in germinoma (ectopic pinealoma)
Other Peptides Reported in CSF	Basal levels not adequately characterized	
Angiotensin II		
Glucagon		

*The concentrations provided have been drawn from various sources, especially Jackson,[87] Wood,[171] Braunstein, et al,[30] and Post, et al.[123] Normal CSF peptide hormone levels should be established before inferences are made from a specific determination in an individual subject.

†Apart from the adenohypophysial hormones and HCG, the alterations cited in disease states should be viewed as tentative.

clearing away of substances deposited into brain extracellular spaces is a matter of continuing controversy.

Anterior Pituitary Hormones in the CSF

All anterior pituitary hormones have been demonstrated in the CSF in the human, usually in concentrations less than that present in blood.[30,98] The closest correlation between CSF and blood levels in pathologic states of anterior pituitary hypersecretion occurs with prolactin. Hyperprolactinemia is accompanied by elevated CSF prolactin levels. The other pituitary hormones, adrenocorticotropin hormone (ACTH) and β-lipotropin (in Cushing's disease), gonadotropin and thyroid-stimulating hormone (TSH) (in glycoprotein tumors), and GH (in acromegaly)[168] are not associated with increases of the hormone in CSF, unless the integrity of the subarachnoid space has been breached by a suprasellar extension of the tumor. Suprasellar or pineal region germinomas may secrete chorionic gonadotropin into the CSF.

Abnormalities of CSF Peptides in Neurologic and Psychiatric Diseases

There are now several interesting correlations between CSF peptide concentrations and certain neurologic diseases. Patients with advanced AD are found to have mean CSF somatostatin concentration lower than control groups[16,17,23,94,142,144,172] (Fig. 8), suggesting that the diminished level of cerebral cortical somatostatin is reflected in lumbar CSF. Cerebrospinal fluid somatostatin also has been reported to be reduced in multiple sclerosis during relapse. We find no alterations of somatostatin in the CSF of a number of other neurologic conditions, including HD and PD. This is in contrast to the reports of Cramer and coworkers,[36] who found decreased somatostatin in HD, and Dupont and coworkers,[48] who reported decreased levels in PD (see Figure 8). In multi-infarct dementia, levels are reduced to about 50 percent of normal.[16,60] Somatostatin elevation in CSF was reported in acute destructive lesions of brain, stroke,[119] meningitis, trauma, and in spinal cord disease. Cerebrospinal fluid somatostatin levels are reported to be decreased in some patients with depression.[67,123,137] Altered levels of plasma and CSF levels of vasopressin are found in anorexia nervosa[69] and in AD.[179] Another hypothalamic peptide, CRH, is reported to be elevated in depressed subjects, perhaps suggesting hyperactivity of the pituitary-adrenal axis as a consequence of CRH hypersection.[111] Corticotropin releasing hormone is actively cleared from the CSF to blood.[115]

Although TRH and gonadotropin hormone releasing hormone (GnRH) have been identified in CSF, no consistent alterations are present in disease states. Substance P levels in the CSF are reduced in patients with peripheral neuropathy and autonomic dysfunction (Shy-Drager syndrome). Because of the presence of substance P in dorsal root ganglia and dorsal horn, these findings suggest that lumbar CSF substance P arises from these structures and that damage to them causes reduced CSF substance P concentration. In contrast, patients with lumbar arachnoiditis have been reported to have elevated CSF substance P levels six to ten times

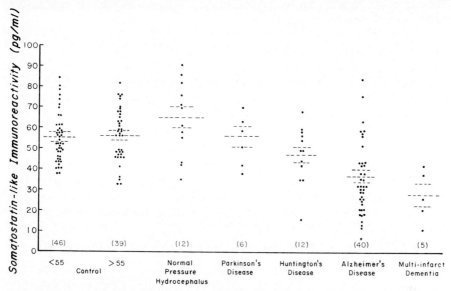

FIGURE 8. Cerebrospinal fluid concentrations of somatostatin in a number of neurologic diseases (From Beal, MF et al, with permission).

normal. Morphine administration which reverses the pain concomitantly reduces the substance P level in the CSF. It has been proposed that the chronic pain of lumbar arachnoiditis may be associated with or caused by release of substance P from nociceptive afferent fibers which can be inhibited by opioid substances.

Brandt and associates[29] reported a single case of a child with episodic coma, apnea, and pupillary miosis, along with a progressive neurologic degenerative illness culminating in death at 23 months of age. The pathologic findings were consistent with subacute necrotizing encephalomyelopathy (Leigh's syndrome), an autosomal recessive disease with prominent diencephalic involvement. The interest of the case is that some of the attacks of coma, apnea, and miosis could be transiently reversed with the narcotic antagonist naloxone. Moreover, the CSF levels of enkephalin-like material were elevated both during and between attacks and, at autopsy, met-enkephalin and leu-enkephalin concentrations in the cerebral cortex were greatly elevated over control values. The authors, therefore, make a case of this being a "hyperendorphin" syndrome. Although the transient and inconsistent nature of the response to naloxone calls this hypothesis into question, the abnormalities of peptide concentration reported are in magnitude far beyond those found in other pathologic states.

Peptide concentrations in CSF in demyelinating conditions have, in general, been uninformative. Levels of somatostatin are reduced during acute exacerbations.[148] Vasoactive intestinal peptide is normal.[5]

REFERENCES

1. ALLEN, JM, FERRIER, IN, ROBERTS, GW, CROSS, AJ, ADRIAN, TE, CROW, TJ, BLOOM, SR: *Elevation of neuropeptide Y (NPY) in substantia innominata in Alzheimer's type dementia.* J Neurol Sci 65:325–331, 1984.

2. ALLEN, JM, AND BLOOM, SR: *Neuropeptide Y: A putative neurotransmitter.* Neurochem Internat 8:1–8, 1986.

3. ALLEN, JM, FERRIER, IN, ROBERTS, GW, CROSS, AJ, ADRIAN, TE, CROSS, TJ, BLOOM, SR: *Elevation of neuropeptide Y (NPY) in substantia innominata in Alzheimer type dementia.* J Neurol Sci 64:325–331, 1984.

4. AMICO, JA, TENICELA, R, JOHNSTON, J, ROBINSON, AG: *A time-dependent peak of oxytocin exists in the cerebrospinal fluid but not in the plasma of humans.* J Clin Endocrinol Metab 57:947–951, 1982.

5. ANDERSON, O, FAHRENKRUG, J, WIKKELSO, C, JOHNSSON, BB: *VIP in cerebrospinal fluid of patients with multiple sclerosis.* Peptides 5:435–437, 1984.

6. ARAI, H, MOROII, T, KOSAKA, K: *Somatostatin and vasoactive intestinal polypeptide in postmortem brains from patients with Alzheimer-type dementia.* Neurosci Lett 52:73–78, 1984.

7. ARNOLD, MA, REPPERT, SM, RORSTAD, OP, SAGAR, SM, KEUTMANN, HT, PERLOW, MJ, MARTIN, JB: *Temporal patterns of somatostatin immunoreactivity in the cerebrospinal fluid of the rhesus monkey: Effect of environmental lighting.* J Neurosci 2:574–580, 1982.

8. ARONIN, N, COOPER, PE, LORENZ, LJ, BIRD, ED, SAGAR, SM, LEEMAN, SE, MARTIN, JB: *Somatostatin is increased in the basal ganglia in Huntington's disease.* Ann Neurol 13:519–526, 1983.

9. BARBER, RP, VAUGHN, JE, SLEMMON, JR, SABRATERRA, PM, ROBERTS, E, LEEMAN, SE: *The origin, distribution and synaptic relationships of substance P axons in rat spinal cord.* J Comp Neurol 184:331–352, 1979.

10. BASBAUM, AI, AND FIELDS, HL: *Endogenous pain control mechanisms: Review and hypothesis.* Ann Neurol 4:451–462, 1978.

11. BASBAUM, A, AND GLAZER, I: *Immunoreactive vasoactive intestinal polypeptide is concentrated in the sacral spinal cord: A possible marker for pelvic visceral afferent fibers.* Somatosensory Res 1:69–82, 1983.

12. BEAL, MF, BENOIT, R, BIRD, ED, MARTIN, JB: *Somatostatin 28 (1-12) immunoreactivity is increased in Huntington's disease.* Neurosci Lett 56:377–380, 1985.

13. BEAL, MF, BIRD, ED, LANGLAIS, PJ, MARTIN, JB: *Somatostatin is increased in the nucleus accumbens in Huntington's disease.* Neurology 34:663–666, 1984.

14. BEAL, MF, DOMESICK, VB, MARTIN, JB: *Regional distribution of somatostatin in the rat striatum.* Brain Res 278:103–108, 1983.

15. BEAL, MF, DOMESICK, VB, MARTIN, JB: *Effects of lesions in the amygdala and periventricular hypothalamus on striatal somatostatin-like immunoreactivity.* Brain Res 330:309–316, 1985.

16. BEAL, MF, GROWDON, JH, MAZUREK, MF, MARTIN, JB: *CSF somatostatin-like immunoreactivity in dementia.* Neurology 36(2):294–297, 1986.

17. BEAL, MF, GROWDON, JH, MAZUREK, MF, McENTEE, WJ, MARTIN, JB: *CSF somatostatin in dementia.* Neurology 34:120, 1984.

18. BEAL, MF, MARSHALL, P, BURD, GD, LANDIS, DMD, MARTIN, JB: *Excitotoxin lesions do not mimic the alteration of somatostatin in Huntington's disease.* Brain Res 361:135–145, 1985.

19. BEAL, MF, AND MARTIN, JB: *Effect of lesions on somatostatin-like immunoreactivity in the rat striatum.* Brain Res 266:67–73, 1983.

20. BEAL, MF, AND MARTIN, JB: *Depletion of striatal somatostatin by local cysteamine injection.* Brain Res 308:319–324, 1984.

21. BEAL, MF, AND MARTIN, JB: *The effect of somatostatin on striatal catecholamines.* Neurosci Lett 44:271–276, 1984.

22. BEAL, MF, AND MARTIN, JB: *Effects of neuroleptic drugs on brain somatostatin-like-immunoreactivity.* Neurosci Lett 47:125–130, 1984.

23. BEAL, MF, MAZUREK, MF, BLACK, PB, MARTIN, JB: *Human cerebrospinal fluid somatostatin in neurologic disease.* J Neurol Sci 71(1):91–104, 1985.

24. BEAL, MF, MAZUREK, MF, TRAN, VT, CHATTA, G, BIRD, ED, MARTIN, JB: *Somatostatin receptors are reduced in cerebral cortex in Alzheimer's disease.* Science 229:289–291, 1985.

25. BEAL, MF, TRAN, VT, MAZUREK, MF, CHATTA, G, MARTIN, JB: *Somatostatin binding sites in human and monkey brain: Localization and characterization.* J Neurochem 46(2):359–365, 1986.

26. BIGGINS, JA, PERRY, EK, McDERMOTT, JR, ET AL: *Post mortem levels of thyrotropin-releasing hormone and neurotensin in the amygdala in Alzheimer's disease, schizophrenia and depression.* J Neurol Sci 58:117–122, 1983.

27. BIRD, ED: *Chemical pathology of Huntington's disease.* Annu Rev Pharmacol Toxicol 20:533–551, 1980.

28. BIRD, ED, CHIAPPA, SA, FINK, G: *Brain immunoreactive gonadotropin-releasing hormone in Huntington's chorea and non-choreic subjects.* Nature 260:536–638, 1976.

29. BRANDT, NJ, TERENIUS, L, JACOBSEN, BB, KLINKEN, L, NORDIUS, A, BRANDT, S, BLEGVAD, K, YSSING, M: *Hyperendophin syndrome in a child with necrotizing encephalomyelopathy.* N Engl J Med 303:914–916, 1980.

30. BRAUNSTEIN, GD, HASSEN, G, KAMDAR, V, NELSON, JC: *Anterior pituitary hormone levels in the*

NEUROREGULATORY PEPTIDES

cerebrospinal fluid of patients with pituitary and parasellar tumors. Fertil Steril 36:164–171, 1981.

31. BROWN, AG: *The dorsal horn of the spinal cord.* Q J Exp Physiol 67:193–212, 1982.
32. BUCK, SH, DESHMUKH, P, BURKS, TF, YAMAMURA, HI: *A survey of substance P, somatostatin, and neurotensin levels in aging in the rat and human central nervous system.* Neurobiol Aging 2:257–264, 1981.
33. CHESSELET, MF, AND REISINE, TD: *Somatostatin regulates dopamine release in rat striatal slices and cat caudate nuclei.* J Neurosci 3:232–236, 1983.
34. CHRONWALL, BM, CHASE, TN, O'DONOHUE, TL: *Coexistence of neuropeptide Y and somatostatin in rat and human cortical and rat hypothalamic neurons.* Neurosci Lett 52:213–217, 1984.
35. COOPER, PE, FERNSTROM, MH, RORSTAD, OP, LEEMAN, SE, MARTIN, JB: *The regional distribution of somatostatin, substance P and neurotensin in human brain.* Brain Res 218:219–232, 1981.
36. CRAMER, H, KOHLER, J, OEPEN, G, SCHONBERG, G, SCHROTER, E: *Huntington's chorea-measurements of somatostatin, substance P, and cyclic nucleotides in the cerebrospinal fluid.* J Neurol 225:183–187, 1981.
37. COYLE, JT, PRICE, DL, DELONG, MR: *Alzheimer's disease: A disorder of cortical cholinergic innervation.* Science 219:1184–1190, 1983.
38. CRYSTAL, HA, AND DAVIES, P: *Cortical substance P-like immunoreactivity in cases of Alzheimer's disease and senile dementia of the Alzheimer type.* J Neurochem 38:1781–1784, 1982.
39. DALSGAARD, CJ, VINCENT, SR, HÖKFELT, T, LUNDBERG, JM, DAHLSTROM, A, SCHULTZBERG, M, DOCKRAY, GJ, CUELLO, AC: *Coexistence of cholecystokinin- and substance P-like peptides in neurons of the dorsal root ganglia of the rat.* Neurosci Lett 33:159–163, 1982.
40. DAVIES, P, KATZMAN, R, TERRY, RD: *Reduced somatostatin-like immunoreactivity in cerebral cortex from cases of Alzheimer disease and Alzheimer senile dementia.* Nature 288:279–280, 1980.
41. DAVIES, P, AND TERRY, RD: *Cortical somatostatin-like immunoreactivity in cases of Alzheimer's disease and senile dementia of the Alzheimer type.* Neurobiol Aging 2:9–14, 1981.
42. DAVIES, P, AND THOMPSON, A: *Postmortem stability of somatostatin-like immunoreactivity in mouse brain under conditions simulating handling of human autopsy material.* Neurochem Res 6:787–791, 1981.
43. DAWBARN, D, DEQUIDT, ME, EMSON, PC: *Survival of basal ganglia neuropeptide Y/somatostatin neurons in Huntington's disease.* Brain Res 340:251–260, 1985.
44. DELFS, JR, ZHU, CH, DICHTER, MA: *Coexistence of acetylcholinsterase and somatostatin-immunoreactivity in neurons cultured from rat cerebrum.* Science 223:61–63, 1984.
45. DIFIGLIA, M, AND ARONIN, N: *Quantitative electron microscopic study of immunoreactive somatostatin axons in the rat neostriatum.* Neurosci Lett 50:325–331, 1984.
46. DIFIGLIA, M, ARONIN, N, MARTIN, JB: *The light and electron microscopic localization of immunoreactive somatostatin in the rat caudate nucleus.* J Neurosci 9:1267–1274, 1982.
47. DIFIGLIA, M, PASIK, P, PASIK, T: *Ultrastructure of Golgi-impregnated and gold-toned spiny and aspiny neurons in the monkey neostriatum.* J Neurocytol 8:471–492, 1980.
48. DUPONT, E, CHRISTENSEN, SE, HANSEN, AP, OLIVARIAS, BF, ORSKOU, H: *Low cerebrospinal fluid somatostatin in Parkinson's disease: An irreversible abnormality.* Neurol 32:312–314, 1982.
49. ECKENSTEIN, F, AND THOENEN, H: *Cholinergic neurons in the rat cerebral cortex demonstrated by immunochemical localization of choline acetyltransferase.* Neurosci Lett 36:211–216, 1983.
50. EMSON, PC, ARREGUI, A, CLEMENT-JONES, V, ET AL: *Regional distribution of methionine-enkephalin and substance P-like immunoreactivity in normal human brain and in Huntington's disease.* Brain Res 199:147–160, 1980.
51. EMSON, PC, FAHRENKRUG, J, SPOKES, EGS: *Vasoactive intestinal polypeptide (VIP): Distribution in normal human and in Huntington's disease.* Brain Res 173:174–178, 1979.
52. EMSON, PC, AND HUNT, SP: *Anatomical chemistry of the cerebral cortex.* In SCHMITT, FO, WORDEN, FG, ADELMAN, G, DENNIS, SG (EDS): *The Organization of the Cerebral Cortex.* Cambridge, MA, MIT Press, 1981, pp 325–345.
53. EMSON, PC, ROSSOR, M, LEE, CM: *The regional distribution and chromatographic behavior of somatostatin in human brain.* Neurosci Lett 22:319–324, 1981.
54. EMSON, PC, REHFELD, JF, LANGEVIN, H, ROSSOR, M: *Reduction in cholecystokinin-like immunoreactivity in the basal ganglia in Huntington's disease.* Brain Res 198:497–500, 1980.
55. EPELBAUM, J, RUBERG, M, MOYSE, E, JAVOY-AGID, F, DUBOIS, B, AGID, Y: *Somatostatin and dementia in Parkinson's disease.* Brain Res 278:376–379, 1983.
56. FERRANTE, RJ, KOWALL, NW, BEAL, MF, RICHARDSON, EP, BIRD, ED, MARTIN, JB: *Selective sparing of a class of striatal neurons in Huntington's disease.* Science 230:561–563, 1985.
57. FERRIER, IN, CROSS, AJ, JOHNSON, JA, ROBERTS, GW, CROW, TJ, CORSELLIS, JAN, LEE, YC, O'SHAUGHNESSY, D, ADRIAN, TE, McGREGOR, GP, BARACESE-HAMILTON, AJ, BLOOM, SR: *Neuropeptides in Alzheimer type dementia.* J Neurol Sci 62:159–170, 1983.
58. FERRIER, IN, ROBERTS, GW, CROW, TJ, JOHNSTONE, EC, OWENS, DGC, LEE, YC, O'SHAUGHNESSY, DO, ADRIAN, TE, POLAK, JM, BLOOM, SR: *Reduced cholecystolinin-like and somato-*

statin-like immunoreactivity in limbic lobe is associated with negative symptoms in schizophrenia. Life Sci 33:475–483, 1983.

59. FINK, S, AND MARTIN, JB: *Behavioral effects of intrastriatal infusions of somatostatin and somatostatin analogues.* Neurosci Abst 10:174, 1984.

60. FRANCIS, PT, BOWEN, DM, NEARY, D, PALO, J, WIKSTROM, J, OLNEY, J: *Somatostatin-like immunoreactivity in lumbar cerebrospinal fluid from neurohistologically examined demented patients.* Neurobiol Aging 5:183–186, 1984.

61. FUXE, K, AGNATI, LF, McDONALD, T, LOCATELLI, V, HÖKFELT, T, DALSGAARD, CJ, BATTISTINI, N, YANAIHARA, N, MUTT, V, CUELLO, AC: *Immunohistochemical indications of gastrin releasing peptide-bombesin-like immunoreactivity in the nervous system of the rat. Codistribution with substance P-like immunoreactive nerve terminal systems and coexistence with substance P-like immunoreactivity in dorsal ganglion cell bodies.* Neurosci Lett 37:17–22, 1983.

62. FYFFE, REW, AND PERL, ER: *Is ATP a central synaptic mediator for certain primary afferent fibers from mammalian brain?* Proc Natl Acad Sci USA 81:6890–6893, 1984.

63. GALE, JS, BIRD, ED, SPOKES, EG, ET AL: *Human substance P: Distribution in controls and Huntington's chorea.* J Neurochem 30:633–634, 1978.

64. GEOLA, FL, HERSHMAN, JM, WARWICK, R, ET AL: *Regional distribution of cholecystokinin-like immunoreactivity in the human brain.* J Clin Endocrinol Metab 53:270–275, 1981.

65. GEOLA, FL, YAMADA, T, WARWICK, RJ, TOURTELLOTTE, WW, HERSHMAN, JM: *Regional distribution of somatostatin-like immunoreactivity in the human brain.* Brain Res 229:35–42, 1981.

66. GERFEN, CR: *The neostriatal mosaic: Compartmentalization of corticostriatal input and striatonigral output systems.* Nature 311:461–463, 1984.

67. GERNER, RH, AND YAMADA, T: *Altered neuropeptide concentrations in cerebrospinal fluid of psychiatric patients.* Brain Res 238:298–302, 1982.

68. GHATEI, M, BLOOM, SR, LANGEVIN, H, McGREGOR, GP, LEE, YC, ADRIAN, TE, O'SHAUGHNESSY, DJ, BLANK, MA, UTTENTHAL, LO: *Regional distribution of bombesin and seven other regulatory peptides in human brain.* Brain Res 292:101–109, 1984.

69. GOLD, PW, KAYE, W, ROBERTSON, GL, ET AL: *Abnormalities in plasma and cerebrospinal-fluid arginine vasopressin in patients with anorexia nervosa.* N Engl J Med 308:1117–1123, 1983.

70. GRAMSCH, C, HOLLT, V, MEHRAEIN, P, ET AL: *Regional distribution of methionine-enkephalin- and beta-endorphin-like immunoreactivity in human brain and pituitary.* Brain Res 171:261–270, 1979.

71. GRAVELAND, GA, WILLIAMS, RS, DIFIGLIA, M: *Evidence for degenerative and regenerative changes in neostriatal spiny neurons in Huntington's disease.* Science 227:770–773, 1985.

72. GRAVELAND, GA, WILLIAMS, RS, DIFIGLIA, M: *A Golgi study of the human striatum: Neurons and afferent fibers.* J Comp Neurol 234:317–333, 1985.

73. GRAYBIEL, AM, AND RAGSDALE, CW: Proc Natl Acad Sci USA 75:5723–5726, 1978.

74. GRAYBIEL, AM, AND RAGSDALE, CW: *Biochemical anatomy of the striatum.* In EMSON, PC (ED): *Chemical Neuroanatomy.* Raven Press, New York, 1983, pp 427–504.

75. GUSELLA, JF, WEXLER, NS, CONNEALLY, PM, ET AL: *A polymorphic DNA marker genetically linked to Huntington's disease.* Nature 306:234–238, 1983.

76. HARPER, AA, AND LAWSON, SN: *Electrical properties of rat dorsal root ganglion neurons with different peripheral nerve conduction velocities.* J Physiol 359:47–63, 1985.

77. HENDRY, SHC, HOUSER, CR, JONES, EG, VAUGHN, JE: *Synaptic organization of immunocytochemically identified GABA neurons in the monkey sensory-motor cortex.* J Neurocytol 12:639–660, 1983.

78. HENDRY, SHC, AND JONES, EG: *Sizes and distributions of intrinsic neurons incorporating tritiated GABA in monkey sensory-motor cortex.* J Neurosci 1:390–408, 1981.

79. HENDRY, SHC, JONES, EG, BEINFELD, MC: *CCK immunoreactive neurons in rat and monkey cerebral cortex make symmetric synapses and have intimate associations with blood vessels.* Proc Natl Acad Sci USA 80:2400–2404, 1983.

80. HENDRY, SHC, JONES, EG, DEFLIPE, J, SCHMECHET, D, BRANDON, C, EMSON, PC: *Neuropeptide-containing neurons of the cerebral cortex are also GABAergic.* Proc Natl Acad Sci USA 81:6526–6530, 1984.

81. HENDRY, SHC, JONES, EG, EMSON, PC: *Morphology, distribution, and synaptic relations of somatostatin-and neuropeptide Y-immunoreactive neurons in rat and monkey neocortex.* J Neurosci 4:2497–2517, 1984.

82. HÖKFELT, T, ELDE, R, JOHANSSON, O, LUFT, R, NILSSON, G, ARIMURA, A: *Immunohistochemical evidence for separate populations of somatostatin-containing and substance P-containing primary afferent neurons in the rat.* Neuroscience 1:131–136, 1976.

83. HONDA, CN, RETHELYI, M, PETRUSZ, P: *Preferential immunohistochemical localization of vasoactive intestinal polypeptide (VIP) in the sacral spinal cord of the cat: light and electron microscopic observations.* J Neurosci 3:2183–2196, 1983.

84. HOUSER, CR, HENDRY, SHC, JONES, EG, VAUGHN, JE: *Morphological diversity of immunocytochemically identified GABA neurons in monkey sensory-motor cortex.* J Neurocytol 12:617–638, 1983.

85. Hunt, SP, and Rossi, J: *Peptide and non-peptide containing unmyelinated primary afferents: The parallel processing of nociceptive information.* Phil Trans R Soc Lond B 308:283–289, 1985.

86. Jackson, IMD: *Significance and function of neuropeptides in cerebrospinal fluid.* In Wood, JH, (ED): *Neurobiology of Cerebrospinal Fluid.* Plenum, New York, 1980, pp 625–650.

87. Jackson, IMD: *Neuropeptides in the cerebrospinal fluid.* In Müller, EE, and MacLeod, RM (EDS): *Neuroendocrine Perspectives,* vol 3. Elsevier, Amsterdam, 1984, pp 121–159.

88. Jacobs, RW, Farivar, N, Butcher, LL: *Alzheimer dementia and reduced nicotinamide adenine dinucleotide (NADH)-diaphorase activity in senile plaques and the basal forebrain.* Neurosci Lett 53:39–44, 1985.

89. Jahr, CE, and Jessell, TM: *Synaptic transmission between dorsal root ganglion and dorsal neurons in culture: Antagonism of EPSPs and glutamate excitation by kynurenate.* J Neurosci 5: in press, 1985.

90. Jessell, TM: *Nociception.* In Krieger, D, Brownstein, M, Martin, JB (EDS): *Brain Peptides.* John Wiley & Sons, NY, 1983, pp 315–352.

91. Jessell, TM, and Dodd, J: *Neurotransmitters and differentation antigens in subsets of sensory neurons projecting to the spinal dorsal horn.* In Martin, JB, and Barchas, J, (EDS): *Implications of Neuropeptides in Neurological and Psychiatric Diseases.* Assoc Res Nerv Ment Dis, vol 64. Raven Press, New York, 1986, pp 111–134.

92. Jones, EG, and Hendry, SHC: *The peptide containing neurons of the primate cerebral cortex.* In Martin, JB, and Barchas, J (EDS): *Implications of Neuropeptides in Neurological and Psychiatric Diseases.* Assoc Res Nerv Ment Dis, vol 67. Raven Press, New York, 1986, pp 163–178.

93. Joynt, RJ, and McNeill, TH: *Neuropeptides in aging and dementia.* Peptides (Suppl 1) 5:269–274, 1984.

94. Kohler, J, Schroter, E, Cramer, H: *Somatostatin-like immunoreactivity in the cerebrospinal fluid of neurological patients.* Arch Phychiat Nervenkr 231:503–508, 1982.

95. Konishi, S, Akagi, H, Yanagisawa, M, Otsuka, M: *Enkephalinergic inhibition of slow transmission in the rat spinal cord.* Neurosci Lett (Suppl) 13:S107, 1983.

96. Kowall, N, and Martin, JB: *Patterns of cell loss in Huntington's disease.* Trends in Neurosci, November, 1986.

97. Lee, CM, Emson, PC, Iversen, LL: *Chromatographic behaviour and post-mortem stability of somatostatin in the rat and mouse brain.* Brain Res 220:159–166, 1981.

98. Lenhard, L, and Deftos, LJ: *Adenohypophyseal hormones in the CSF.* Neuroendocrinology 34:303–308, 1982.

99. Manberg, PJ, Youngblood, WW, Nemeroff, CB, et al: *Regional distribution of neurotensin in human brain.* J Neurochem 38:1777–1780, 1982.

100. Marshall, PE, and Landis, DMD: *Huntington's disease is accompanied by changes in the distribution of somatostatin-containing neuronal processes.* Brain Res 329:71–84, 1985.

101. Marshall, PE, Landis, DMD, Zalneraitis, E: *Immunocytochemical studies of substance P and leucine-enkephalin in Huntington's disease.* Brain Res 298:11–26, 1983.

102. Martin, JB: *Huntington's disease: New approaches to an old problem.* Neurology 34:1059–1072, 1984.

103. Mauborgne, A, Javoy-Agid, F, Legrand, JC, et al: *Decrease of substance P-like immunoreactivity in the substantia nigra and pallidum of parkinsonian brains.* Brain Res 268:167–170, 1983.

104. Mazurek, MF, Beal, MF, Martin, JB: *Vasopressin in postmortem Alzheimer brain.* Annals of Neurol 18:143–144, 1985.

105. Melander, T, Staines, WA, Hökfelt, T, Rokaeus, A, et al: *Galanin-like immunoreactivity in cholinergic neurons of the septum-basal forebrain complex projecting to the hippocampus of the rat.* Brain Res 360:130–138, 1985.

106. Mezey, E, and Palkovits, M: *Two-way transport in hypothalamo-hypophyseal system.* Frontiers in Neuroendocrinology, vol 7, 1982.

107. Moroni, F, Lombardi, G, Moneti, G, Aldino, C: *The excitotoxin quinolinic acid is present in the brain of several mammals and its cortical content increases during the aging process.* Neurosci Lett 47:51–55, 1984.

108. Morrison, JH, Rogers, J, Scherr, S, Benoit, R, Bloom, FE: *Somatostatin immunoreactivity in neuritic plaques of Alzheimer's patients.* Nature 31:490–492, 1985.

109. Myers, RH, Sax, DS, Schoenfeld, M, et al: *Late onset of Huntington's Disease.* J Neurol Neurosurg Psych 48:530–534, 1985.

110. Nagy, JI, and Hunt, SP: *The termination of primary afferents within the rat dorsal horn: Evidence for rearrangement following capsaicin treatment.* J Comp Neurol 218:145–158, 1983.

111. Nemeroff, CB, Widerlov, E, Bissette, G, Walleus, H, Karlsson, I, Eklund, K, Kitts, CD, Loosen, PT, Vale, W: *Elevated concentrations of CSF corticotropin-releasing factor-like immunoreactivity in depressed patients.* Science 226:1342–1344, 1984.

112. Nemeroff, CB, Youngblood, WW, Manberg, PJ, Prange, AJ, Kizer, JS: *Regional brain con-*

centration of neuropeptides in Huntington's chorea and schizophrenia. Science 221:972–975, 1983.

113. Nutt, JG, Mroz, EA, Leeman, SE, et al: *Substance P in human cerebrospinal fluid: Reductions in peripheral neuropathy and anatomic dysfunction.* Neurology 30:1280–1285, 1980.

114. Okon, E, and Koch, Y: *Localisation of gonadotropin-releasing and thyrotropin-releasing hormone in human brain by radioimmunoassay.* Nature 263:345–347, 1976.

115. Oldfield, EH, Schulte, HM, Chrousos, GP, Rock, JP, Kornblith, PL, O'Neil, DL, Poplack, DG, Gold, PW, Cutler, GB, Jr, Loriaux, L: *Active clearance of corticotropin-releasing factor from the cerebrospinal fluid.* Neuroendocrinology 40:84–87, 1985.

116. Otsuka, M, Konishi, S, Yanagisawa, M, Tsunoo, A, Akagi, H: *Role of substance P as a sensory transmitter in spinal cord and symapthetic ganglia.* Ciba Found Symp 91:13–34, 1982.

117. Otten, U, and Lorez, HP: *Nerve growth factor increases substance P, cholecystokinin and vasoactive intestinal polypeptide immunoreactivity in primary sensory neurons of newborn rats.* Neurosci lett 34:153–158, 1983.

118. Pardridge, WM: *Neuropeptides and the blood brain barrier.* Ann Rev Physiol 45:73–82, 1983.

119. Patel, YC, Rao, K, Reichlin, S: *Somatostatin in human cerebrospinal fluid.* N Engl J Med 296:529–533, 1977.

120. Perry, EK, Blessed, G, Tomlinson, BE, Perry, RH, Crow, TJ, Cross, AJ, Dockray, GJ, Dimaline, R, Arregui, A: *Neurochemical activities in human temporal lobe related to aging with Alzheimer-type changes.* Neurobiol Aging 2:251–256, 1981.

121. Perry, EK, Tomlinson, BE, Blessed, G, Bergman, K, Gibson, PH, Perry, RH: *Correlation of cholinergic abnormalities with senile plaques and mental test scores in senile dementia.* Br Med J 2:1457–1459, 1978.

122. Perry, RH, Dockray, R, Dimaline, R, et al: *Neuropeptides in Alzheimer's disease, depression and schrizophrenia: A post mortem analysis of vasoactive intestinal peptide and cholecystokinin in cerebral cortex.* J Neurol Sci 51:465–472, 1981.

123. Post, RM, Gold, R, Rubinow, DR, Ballenger, JC, Bunney, WE, Jr, Goodwin, FK: *Peptides in the cerebrospinal fluid of neuropsychiatric patients: An approach to central nervous system peptide function.* Life Sciences 31:1–15, 1982.

124. Price, J, and Mudge, AW: *A subpopulation of rat dorsal root ganglion neurons is catecholaminergic.* Nature 301:241–243, 1983.

125. Ralston, JH, III: *Distribution of dorsal root axons in laminae I, II, and III of the macaque spinal cord.* J Comp Neurol 184:643–684, 1979.

126. Rehfeld, JF, and Kruse-Larsen, C: *Gastrin and cholecystokinin in human cerebrospinal fluid. Immunochemical determination of concentrations and molecular heterogeneity.* Brain Res 155:19–26, 1978.

127. Roberts, GW, Crow, TJ, Polak, JM: *Location of neuronal tangles in somatostatin neurons in Alzheimer's disease.* Nature 314:92–94, 1985.

128. Rosenfeld, MG, Mermod, J-J, Amara, SG, Swanson, LW, Sawchenko, PE, Rivier, J, Vale, WW, Evans, RM: *Production of a novel neuropeptide encoded by the calcitonin gene via tissue-specific RNA processing.* Nature 304:129–135, 1983.

129. Rossor, MN, Emson, PC, Mountjoy, CQ, Roth, M, Iversen, LL: *Reduced amounts of immunoreactive somatostatin in the temporal cortex in senile dementia of Alzheimer type.* Neurosci Lett 20:373–377, 1980.

130. Rossor, MN, Fahrenkrug, J, Emson, PC, et al: *Reduced cortical choline acetyltransferase activity in senile dementia of Alzheimer type is not accompanied by changes in vasoactive intestinal polypeptide.* Brain Res 201:249–253, 1980.

131. Rossor, MN, Garrett, NJ, Johnson, AI, Roth, M, Mountjoy, CQ, Iversen, LL: *A postmortem study of the cholinergic and GABA systems in senile dementia.* Brain 105:313–330, 1982.

132. Rossor, MN, Hunt, SP, Iversen, LL, et al: *Extrahypothalamic vasopressin is unchanged in Parkinson's disease and Huntington's disease.* Brain Res 253:341–343, 1982.

133. Rossor, MN, Iversen, LL, Hawthorn, J, et al: *Extrahypothalamic vasopressin in human brain.* Brain Res 214:349–355, 1981.

134. Rossor, MN, Iversen, LL, Reynolds, GP, Mountjoy, CQ, Roth, M: *Neurochemical characteristics of early and late onset types of Alzheimer's disease.* Br Med J 288:961–964, 1984.

135. Rossor, MN, Rehfeld, JF, Emson, PC, et al: *Normal cortical concentration of cholecystokinin-like immunoreactivity with reduced choline acetyltransferase activity in senile dementia of Alzheimer type.* Life Sci 29:405–410, 1981.

136. Rossor, MN, Svendsen, S, Hunt, SP, et al: *The substantia innominata in Alzheimer's disease: A histochemical and biochemical study of cholinergic marker enzymes.* Neurosci Lett 28:217–222, 1982.

137. Rubinow, DR, Gold, PW, Post, RM, Ballenger, JC, Cowdry, R, Bollinger, J, Reichlin, S: *CSF somatostatin in affective illness.* Arch Gen Psych 40:409–412, 1983.

138. Sagar, SM, Landry, D, Millard, WJ, et al: *Depletion of somatostatin-like immunoreactivity in the rat central nervous system by cysteamine.* J Neurosci 2:225–231, 1982.

139. Schmechel, DE, Vickrey, BG, Fitzpatrick, D, Elde, RP: *GABAergic neurons of mammalian cerebral cortex: Widespread subclass defined by somatostatin content.* Neurosci Lett 47:227–232, 1984.

140. Schwarcz, R, Foster, AC, French, ED, Whetsell, WO, Kohler, C: *Excitotoxic models for neurodegenerative disorders.* Life Sci 35:19–32, 1984.

141. Schwarcz, R, Whetsell, WD, Mangano, RM: *Quinolinic acid: An endogenous metabolite that produces axon-sparing lesions in rat brain.* Science 219:316–318, 1983.

142. Serby, M, Richardson, SB, Twente, S, Siekerski, J, Corwin, J, Rotrosen, J: *CSF somatostatin in Alzheimer's disease.* Neurobiol Aging 5:187–189, 1984.

143. Sharma, S, Svec, P, Mitchell, GH, Godson, GN: *Diversity of circumsporozoite antigen genes from two strains of the malarial parasite Plasmodium knowlesi.* Science 229:779–782, 1985.

144. Soinin, HS, Jolkkonen, JT, Reinikainen, KJ, Halonen, TO, Riekkinen, PJ: *Reduced cholinesterase activity and somatostatin-like immunoreactivity in the cerebrospinal fluid of patients with dementia of the Alzheimer type.* J Neurol Sci 63:167–172, 1984.

145. Somogyi, P, Hodgson, AJ, Smith, AD, Nunzi, MG, Gorio, A, Wu, J-Y: *Differential populations of GABAergic neurons in the visual cortex and hippocampus of the cat contain somatostatin or cholecystokinin immunoreactive material.* J Neurosci 4:2590–2603, 1984.

146. Somogyi, P, and Smith, AD: *Projection of neostriatal spiny neurons to the substantia nigra. Application of a combined Golgi-staining and horseradish peroxidase transport procedure at both light and electron microscopic levels.* Brain Res 178:3–15, 1979.

147. Sorensen, KV: *Somatostatin: Localization and distribution in the cortex and the subcortical white matter of the human brain.* Neuroscience 7:1227–1232, 1982.

148. Sorensen, KV, Christensen, SE, DuPont, E, Hansen, AP, Pedersen, E, Oskov, A: *Low somatostatin content in cerebrospinal fluid in multiple sclerosis.* Acta Neurol Scand 61:186–191, 1980.

149. Sorensen, KV, Christensen, SE, Hansen, AP, Ingerslev, J, Pedersen, E, Orskov, H: *The origin of cerebrospinal fluid somatostatin: Hypothalamic or dispersed central nervous system secretion?* Neuroendocrinology 32:335–338, 1981.

150. Sourkes, TL: *Parkinson's disease and other disorders of the basal ganglia.* In Siegel, GJ, Albes, RW, Agranoff, BW, Katzman, R (eds): *Basic Neurochemistry, ed 3.* Boston, Little, Brown & Co, 1981, pp 719–733.

151. Spindel, ER, Wurtman, RJ, Bird, ED: *Increased TRH content of the basal ganglia in Huntington's disease.* N Engl J Med 303:1235–1236, 1980.

152. Spokes, EGS: *Neurochemical alterations in Huntington's chorea: A study of post-mortem brain tissue.* Brain 103:179–210, 1980.

153. Srikant, CB, and Patel, YC: *Cysteamine-induced depletion of brain somatostatin is associated with up-regulation of cerebrocortical somatostatin receptors.* Endocrinology 115:990–995, 1984.

154. Struble, RG, Cork, LC, Whitehouse, PJ, Price, DL: *Cholinergic innervation in neuritic plaques.* Science 216:413–415, 1982.

155. Struble, RG, Kitt, CA, Walker, LC, Cork, LC, Price, DC: *Somatostatinergic neurites in senile plaques of aged non-human primates.* Brain Res 324:394–396, 1984.

156. Studler, JM, Javoy-Agid, F, Cesselin, F, et al: *CCK-8-immunoreactivity distribution in human brain: Selective decrease in the substantia nigra from Parkinsonian patients.* Brain Res 243:176–279, 1982.

157. Tatemoto, K, Carlquist, M, Mutt, V: *Neuropeptide Y—A novel brain peptide with structural similarities to peptide YY and pancreatic polypeptide.* Nature 296:659–660, 1982.

158. Tran, VT, Beal, MF, Martin, JB: *Two types of somatostatin receptors differentiated by cyclic somatostatin analogues.* Science 228:492–495, 1985.

159. Tran, VT, Uhl, G, Perry, DC, Manning, DC, Vale, WW, Perrin, MH, Rivier, JE, Martin, JB, Snyder, SH: *Autoradiographic localization of somatostatin receptors in rat brain.* Eur J Pharm 101:307–309, 1984.

160. Tuchscherer, MM, and Seybold, VS: *Immunohistochemical studies of substance P, cholecystokinin-octapeptide and somatostatin in dorsal root ganglia of the rat.* Neuroscience 14:593–605, 1985.

161. Uhl, GR, Tran, VT, Snyder, SH, Martin, JB: *Somatostatin receptors: Distribution in rat central nervous system and human frontal cortex.* J Comp Neurol 240:288–304, 1985.

162. Veber, DF, Freidinger, RM, Perlow, DS, Paleveda, WJ, Holly, FW, Strachan, RG, Nutt, RF, Arison, BH, Homnick, C, Randall, WC, Glitzer, MS, Saperstein, R, Hirschmann, R: *A potent cyclic hexapeptide analogue of somatostatin.* Nature 292:55–58, 1981.

163. Vincent, SR, and Johansson, O: *Striatal neurons containing both somatostatin- and avian pancreatic polypeptide (APP)-like immunoreactivities and NADPH-diaphorase activity. A light and electron microscopic study.* J Comp Neurol 217:264–270, 1983.

164. Vincent, SR, Johansson, O, Hökfelt, T, Meyerson, B, Sachs, C, Elde, RP, Terenius, L, Kimmel, J: *Neuropeptide coexistence in human cortical neurons.* Nature 298:65–67, 1982.

165. Vincent, SR, Johansson, O, Hökfelt, T, Skirboll, L, Elde, RD, Terenius, L, Kimmel, J,

Goldstein, M: *NADPH-diaphoras: A selective histochemical marker for striatal neurons containing both somatostatin-and avian pancreatic polypeptide (APP)-like immunoreactivities.* J Comp Neurol 217:252–263, 1983.

166. Vincent, SR, Staines, WA, Fibiger, HC: *Histochemical demonstration of separate populations of somatostatin and cholinergic neurons in the rat striatum.* Neurosci Lett 35:111–114, 1983.

167. Vonsattel, JP, Myers, RH, Stevens, TJ, et al: *Neuropathological classification of Huntington's disease.* J Neuropath Exp Neurol 44:559–577, 1985.

168. Wass, JAH, Penman, E, Medbak, S, Rees, LH, Besser, GM: *CSF and plasma somatostatin levels in acromegaly.* Clin Endocrinol 13:235–241, 1980.

169. Wermuth, B: *Purification and properties of an NADPH-dependent carbonyl reductase from human brain. Relationship to proglandin 9-ketoreductase and xenobiotic ketone reductase.* J Biol Chem 256:1206–1213, 1981.

170. Whitehouse, PJ, Price, DL, Struble, RG, Clark, AW, Coyle, JT, DeLong, MR: *Alzheimer's disease and senile dementia: Loss of neurons in the basal forebrain.* Science 215:1237–1239, 1982.

171. Wood, JH: *Neuroendocrinology of cerebrospinal fluid: Peptides, steroids and other hormones.* Neurosurgery 11:293–305, 1982.

172. Wood, PL, Etienne, P, Lal, S, Gauthier, S, Cajal, S, Nair, NPV: *Reduced lumbar CSF somatostatin levels in Alzheimer's disease.* Life Sci 31:2073–2079, 1982.

173. Beal, M, and Growden, JH: *CSF neurotransmitters markers in Alzheimer's disease.* Prog Neuropsychopharmacol Biol Psychiatry 10:259–270, 1986.

174. Beal, MF, Uhl, G, Mazurek, MF, Kowall, N, Martin, JB: *Somatostatin: Alterations in CNS in neurological diseases.* In Martin, JB, and Barchus, J (eds): *Neuropeptides in Neurological Disease* (ARNMD 64). Raven Press, New York, pp 215–258, 1986.

175. Beal, MF, and Martin, JB: *Neuropeptides and neurological disease.* Ann Neurol 20:547–565, 1986.

176. Shults, C, Steardo, L, Barone, P, et al: *Huntington's disease: Effect of cysteamine, a somatostatin-depleting agent.* Neurology 36:1099–1102, 1986.

177. Beal, MF, Kowall, NW, Ellison, DW, et al: *Replication of the neurochemical characteristics of Huntington's disease with quinolinic acid.* Nature 321:168–171, 1986.

178. Martin, JB, and Gusella, J: *Huntington's disease: Pathogenesis and management.* N Engl J Med 315:1267–1276, 1986.

179. Mazurek, MF, Growden, JH, Beal, MF, Martin, JB: *CSF vasopressin concentration is reduced in Alzheimer's disease.* Neurology 36:1133–1136, 1986.

180. Jones, EG: *Neurotransmitters in the cerebral cortex.* J Neurosurg 65:135–153, 1986.

181. Beal, MF, Mazurek, MF, Chattha, GK, et al: *Neuropeptide Y immunoreactivity is reduced in cerebral cortex in Alzheimer's disease.* Ann Neurol 20:282–288, 1986.

182. Mazurek, MF, Beal, MF, Bird, ED, Martin, JB: *Vasopressin in Alzheimer's disease: A study of postmortem concentrations.* Ann Neurol (in press).

183. Sagar, SM, Beal, MF, Marshall, PE, Landis, DMD, Martin, JB: *Implications of neuropeptides in neurological diseases.* Peptides (Suppl 1) 5:255–262, 1984.

PART 6

Psychoneuroendocrinology

Chapter 20

EFFECTS OF HORMONES ON THE BRAIN AND BEHAVIOR

The interactions between hormones and behavior are the major focus of the field of *psychoneuroendocrinology*. Virtually every hormone exerts effects on brain function and behavior, and emotional states can influence many endocrine functions. The endocrine disturbances that occur in the major psychiatric disorders, depression, and schizophrenia have been considered as markers of central neurotransmitter abnormalities potentially useful in providing a clue to the underlying nature of the disease. This chapter considers the effects of hormones on the brain and behavior and psychologic aspects of endocrine disease. Chapter 21 deals with the effects of psychologic stress on endocrine function and the endocrine abnormalities that are associated with the major psychiatric disorders—manic depressive illness, schizophrenia, anorexia nervosa, and other eating disorders.

EFFECTS OF HORMONES ON THE BRAIN

Hormones can influence brain function in many different ways. Some act by disturbing the constancy of the internal milieu, which is necessary for normal functioning of nerve cells. Others act directly on nerve cell membrane receptors to modulate electrolyte flux or to change the concentration of a second messenger, such as $3',5'$ cyclic AMP. Yet others react with nuclear hormone receptors to change the rate of transcription of genetic information directing synthesis of neurotransmitters. Some hormones can act in more than one way. For example, adrenal cortical steroids can produce hypokalemia, can modulate cell membrane potentials directly, and can activate nuclear cortisol receptors (Fig. 1). To be emphasized is that neurons share most of the properties of parenchymal cell targets of hormones, including specific receptors, coupling mechanisms in cell membranes, identical second messengers, and identical systems for activation or inhibition of the genome.

During development, hormones can exert an effect on the process of differentiation and organization of structure and function. For example, gonadal hormones are essential for the normal *development* of the capacity for normal mating behavior. These effects are permanent and involve structural changes in the central nervous system. These can be looked upon as *organizing* or *differentiating* functions of hormones. Hormones also can

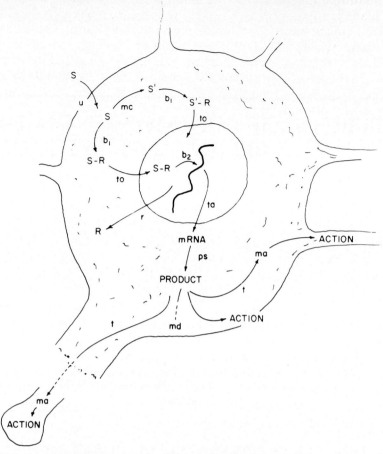

FIGURE 1. This schematic representation illustrates the steps in steroid hormone action on development of a steroid responsive neuron. The steroid "s" binds to a cytoplasmic receptor to form a complex S'-R which in turn binds to nuclear DNA. The complex then regulates the synthesis of mRNA, which leads to changes in many products, which in turn influence a wide variety of hormone actions. In the case of estrogen binding it is now clear that receptors are in the nucleus and not in cytoplasm. (From Gorski, RA,[45] with permission.)

exert effects on brain function to modify already established patterns of activity. Such actions are called *activating* functions and are exemplified by the effects of testosterone on sex drive.

THYROID HORMONES

Neurons contain nuclear receptors for both thyroxine (T_4) and triiodothyronine (T_3). When the receptors are occupied by thyroid hormones, specific mRNA synthesis is activated, which is responsible for growth, differentiation of function, and formation of neurotransmitter synthesizing and other enzymes (Fig. 2). The developing brain is rich in thyroid hormone receptors (about the same as in adult liver[84]), and the number of receptors falls as development proceeds, but even in the adult brain there is a relatively high concentration of receptors second only to the pituitary gland and the liver. During development, thyroid hormones exert a significant and crucial effect on differentiation.[30,93] In the adult, the mechanism of thyroid hormone action is still uncertain. Despite the presence of receptors, oxidative metabolism in the brain is not stimulated by thyroid hormones, in contrast to the situation in most other tissues. In the adult brain, thyroid hormone can influence the concentration of several enzymes, including enzymes involved in the metabolism of thyroid hormone itself.[61] As in other parts of the body, T_3 is more potent than T_4, and this is at least in part due to the higher affinity of the receptors for T_3 than for T_4.

T_4 is actively deiodinated to T_3 within the brain. This is functionally important because T_3 is more potent than T_4; and the rate of conversion is adaptively regulated by thyroid state so as to stabilize the concentration of T_3 in the brain. This adaptive response involves two deiodinating enzymes; one of which deiodinates T_4 and is more active in the hypothyroid state, and the other, which deiodinates T_3 and is less active, thereby increasing the concentration of T_3 in the brain. The reverse reaction is induced by hyperthyroidism. Under normal conditions, about 80 percent of the T_3 found attached to the brain T_3 nuclear receptor is derived from T_4 *in situ*. The various types of deiodinases and their adaptive function are reviewed

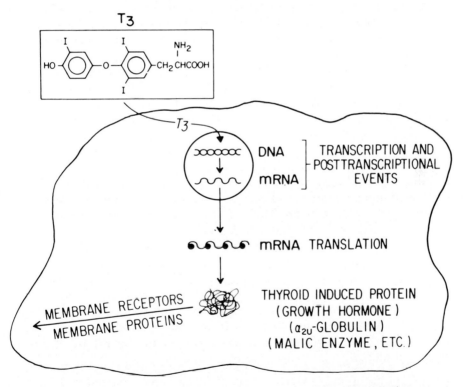

Summary of the current concepts of thyroid hormone action.

FIGURE 2. T_3 (triiodothyronine) is shown as binding to chromosomal DNA which in turn regulates the rate of mRNA transcription. Variations in mRNA concentration in turn regulate the synthesis of proteins, which mediate cell activity. In neurons they regulate the formation of several enzymes, including those that degrade T_4, and synthesize neurotransmitters and probably modify membrane receptors. (From Samuels, HH: *Identification and characterization of thyroid hormone receptors and action using cell culture techniques.* In Oppenheimer, JH, and Samuels HH: *Molecular Basis of Thyroid Hormone Action.* Academic Press, New York, 1983, pp 35–65, with permission).

by Kaplan.[61] In afferent nerves, thyroid state appears to regulate the rate of fast axoplasmic transport and of the synthesis of somatostatin.[117]

Thyroid Hormones in Development

Thyroid deficiency beginning *in utero* is termed *cretinism*.[26] The manifestations depend on the time of onset of hypothyroidism and the severity of hormone deficiency in the infant and become more recognizable as the infant grows. The diagnosis may be difficult to make at birth. Screening methods measuring cord-blood thyroid hormone thyroid-stimulating hormone (TSH) indicate an incidence of 1 in 4000 newborns.

The most important characteristic of cretinism is mental and growth retardation, which may not become obvious until later infancy. The first recognizable symptoms include peristent physiologic jaundice of the newborn, poor appetite, failure to thrive, torpid behavior, hypothermia, dry and thickened skin, muscle laxness, umbilical hernia, and a hoarse cry. There is a high correlation between early and adequate thyroid replacement therapy and ultimate intelligence quotient (IQ) attained, but some cretins fail to respond. It is crucial, therefore, that diagnosis and hormone treatment be early, and persistence of treatment also is important. Although thyroid therapy early in life will prevent most manifestations of cretinism, there is some evidence that even early therapy does not restore brain development fully to normal.

Thyroid hormone is essential for normal development of the central nervous system.[26] In the brains of cretins, perikarya of neurons in the sensorimotor cortex are decreased in size and closely packed; axons, dendrites, and synapses are hypoplastic. The early postnatal period is critical for brain development in the rat, and in this species, induced thyroid deficiency leads to an analogous abnormal maturation of the cerebral and cerebellar cortexes, the principal features of which are decreased size of cell bodies, increased packing density, decreased dendritic development, and decreased myelinization.[30] All of these features are reversed by thyroxine administration. The concentrations of dopamine, norepinephrine, and serotonin are reduced, and the development of the rate-limiting enzymes tyrosine hydroxylase and tryptophan hydroxylase is also retarded by hypothroidism and reversed by thyroid hormone administration.

In the cretin, the electroencephalogram (EEG) shows a decreased basic frequency and a flat, uneventful record, features that are normalized by replacement of thyroid hormone. Hyperthyroidism appears to have little effect on growth and development in the human, although cell formation and glial development can be increased in the rat by thyroxine administration.[30]

STEROID HORMONES

Steroid hormones exert their effects on neurons, as in other target tissues, in part, by diffusing through the lipid phase of the cell membrane and reacting with specific protein receptors (see Figure 1).[11,17,50,59,71] The receptor-steroid complex binds to a specific regulatory gene sequence in the nucleus to activate or to repress the formation of mRNAs coding for various proteins, including structural proteins, enzymes, and steroid receptors themselves. Certain steroid-activated behaviors can be blocked by the administration of drugs that interfere with gene transcription. It has long been believed that the specific receptors were located in the cytoplasm, and after activation were translocated to the nucleus. However, immunohistochemical studies using antiestrogen receptor antisera indicate that the estrogen receptor is localized to the nucleus *in situ*, thus suggesting that the earlier differentiation of cellular from nuclear receptor may have been an artifact of the extraction and separation process used.[17,63] Glucocorticoid receptors also are located on specific sequences of DNA.

Although most steroid effects appear to be mediated through activation of nuclear transcription of mRNA, and hence have an appreciable delay time (hours or days), some steroid effects appear to be mediated at the level of the cell membrane and are almost instantaneous. These include electrophysiologic effects of glucocorticoids and estrogens on single cell neuron action potentials and, for example, the short latency inhibition of ACTH release (see chapter 6). The mechanism of these membrane-mediated effects is not well understood.[69]

The chemical structure of steroid receptors is unique for each steroid and apparently is similar or identical in all tissues in the same animal. Each class of steroid receptor is chemically distinct, but the structure of steroid receptors is highly conserved throughout the animal kingdom. This important observation means that steroid hormone action appeared very early in evolution. A striking example of this is the finding of estrogen-like steroid molecules in organisms as primitive as yeast. During embryologic development, brain receptors appear in a well-defined sequence, following a genetically and steroid-modulated program.

Steroid receptors in brain have a wide but relatively specific distribution corresponding to their sites of physiologic action.[25,96]

> Estrogen receptors are localized predominantly to the hypothalamus, preoptic area, amygdala, and anterior pituitary gland; progesterone receptors to hypothalamus, preoptic area, anterior pituitary and cerebral cortex; androgen receptors to hypothalamus, preoptic area, septum, amygdala, and anterior pituitary gland; glucocorticoids to hippocampus, amygdala, septum, and anterior pituitary gland. Mineralocorticoids are distributed to the same regions as are glucocorticoids. Some binding can be demonstrated in other regions.[71] The distribution of glucocorticoid receptors in the limbic system has been demonstrated by immunohistochemical methods.[38]

As in the case of thyroid hormones, the brain has the capacity to alter the chemical structure of steroid hormones by enzymatic action. For example, aromatases can convert testosterone to estradiol, androstenedione to estrone, and reductases can convert testosterone to 5-alpha dihydroxytestosterone.[71] These interactions are important because certain of the actions of the hormones may require conversion to the derived form.

Another important aspect of steroid action is that steroids can regulate the formation of steroid receptors. For example, in certain peripheral tissues, estrogens induce progestin receptors, and progestin administration can inhibit the production of progestin receptors in the pituitary gland.[6,17]

Physiologic Effects of Sex Steroid Action on the Brain

Progesterone affects the brain directly.[10,71] This steroid acts on the hypothalamic temperature-regulating area to raise the "setpoint" for body temperature control. This reaction is the basis for the postovulatory rise in the basal body temperature of normal women. Together with other hormones, it has a synergistic effect on aspects of reproductive function, facilitating sexual behavior and gonadotropin secretion. Some progesterone is essential for the normal induction of the luteinizing hormone (LH) surge in rats and guinea pigs and in the human being. Progesterone depresses the excitability threshold of hypothalamic neurons to reflex stimuli from the genital area and to direct electrical stimulation. In fact, sexual behavior can be considered to be a sex-hormone-dependent secondary sexual characteristic. Widespread binding of radioactive progesterone in brain tissue has been demonstrated with a gradient of increasing concentrations from anterior hypothalamus through posterior hypothalamus to the region of the cerebral peduncle in the mesencephalon. Corticosterone competes for these binding sites, which appear therefore, to be glucocorticoid receptor sites. Specific progesterone receptor sites have been found only in the hypothalamus, where they undoubtedly underlie progesterone-induced responses.

Estradiol is localized to specific neurons in the preoptic area, hypothalamus, and amygdaloid region (areas previously shown to be involved in gonadotropin and behavioral regulation).[71,96] The upper tegmental-posterior mammillary region of the female rhesus monkey is sensitive to estrogen; implants produce an increase in sexual receptivity and, in the male partner, an increase in mounting attempts and ejaculations.[74]

Estrogen binds primarily to nuclear receptor sites in neurons, where it may produce effects by an alteration in RNA synthesis (see above). Estrogen-induced gonadotropin inhibition is blocked by treatment with actinomycin D, which inhibits RNA transcription. Estrogen administration also increases monoamine oxidase and alters the turnover of ^{3}H-norepinephrine. An alternative (or complementary) mechanism of estrogen action on brain is the conversion of estradiol to catechol-estradiol by brain enzyme systems.[36] It is postulated that the catechol-estrogen and the catecholamines (both of which have a dihydroxy-substituted benzene ring) may compete for common substrates and binding sites.

Sex Steroid Effects on Brain Development. In all subprimate animal species that have been studied, androgens exert an early organizing effect on brain mechanisms influencing both gonadotropin regulation and sexual behavior. The primate, including the human being, may be quite different in this regard (see below). The rat, which is the best understood species from this point of view, shows (in the absence of hormones) female patterns of sexual behavior and of gonadotropin regulation. In the male rat the small amounts of testosterone secreted by the developing testicle during the first 10 days of life masculinize the "female" brain. The term *female brain* refers to the capacity of the rat (when sexual maturity is achieved under the appropriate treatment with estrogenic hormones) to display female receptive mating patterns in response to a sexually active male, and

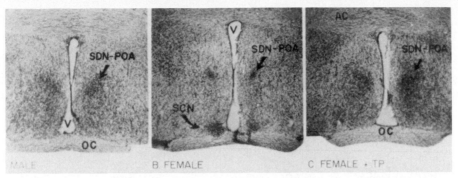

FIGURE 3. The sexually dimorphic nucleus of the preoptic area (SDN-POA) of the rat is illustrated in this coronal section. *(Left)* The area in the male, *(center)* the area in the female, and *(right)* the area of a female exposed to testosterone during development. (From Gorski, RA,[45] with permission.)

to show recurring cycling of gonadotropic secretion in the presence of a normal ovary. The *"male"* brain is associated with active male mating behavior (after treatment with testosterone) and a tonic, noncyclic pattern of gonadotropin secretion.[29,45]

Testosterone induces the male brain pattern, at least in part, by stimulating the growth and function of specific nuclei in the central nervous system which are termed sexually dimorphic; that is, they are anatomically different in male and female rats. The two most important regions are the sexual dimorphic nucleus of the preoptic area (SDN-POA) (Fig. 3) and the region in the sacral cord that supplies the bulbocavernosus muscle. One of the best bits of evidence to indicate that the SDN-POA is crucial to the response to androgens is the finding that transplantation of this region to the brains of either female rats, or male castrates, restores mating and gonadotropin-regulating activity.[4,5]

The differentiating action of testosterone on the brain is not a direct effect. Testosterone probably acts after being converted within the hypothalamus to estradiol-17 β. The reason for believing that this is true is that neonatal "androgenization" can be brought about by treatment of male infant rats with large doses of estradiol (whereas the testosterone metabolite dihydroxytestosterone is ineffective). Aromatase, the enzyme that converts testosterone to estradiol, is present early in the postnatal period. It is therefore reasonable to ask why the newborn female rat, which has relatively high blood levels of estradiol, is not masculinized. It appears that estradiol is excluded from the developing brain because of the presence in the blood of young rats of the estrogen binding protein alpha-fetoprotein, which therefore acts in a protective fashion.

Animals display a wide variety of sexually dimorphic behaviors, some of which are not specifically sexual; an example is the leg-raising reflex in male dogs during urination (see Gorski[45] for review). Sexual dimorphism of the brain also has been demonstrated in primates[15] (Fig. 4).

Sexual dimorphisms are not limited to the brain and behavior. Several enzyme systems in the rat are "feminized" by early hormone exposure into a pattern of steroid hydroxylation that remains fixed into adult life. The feminizing factor is of pituitary origin and is probably growth hormone

---

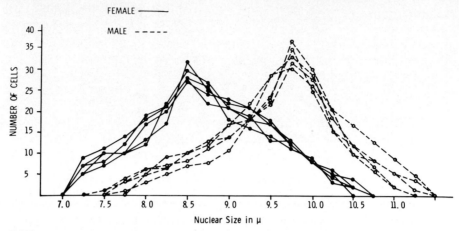

FIGURE 4. Sexual dimorphism in the nuclear size of amygdalar neurons in the squirrel monkey. (From Bubenik, GA, and Brown, GM,[15] with permission.)

(GH). Jansson and colleagues have shown that androgens determine the pulsatile pattern of GH secretion at a critical stage.[113]

Because sexual dimorphisms are widespread in mammals, much interest has been shown in the role of early hormonal organizing effects in primates, including man. In the monkey, prenatal androgenization of female monkeys causes the development of ambiguous genitalia, but the female monkey is capable of normal cyclical ovarian function and normal receptive behavior in a mating situation. However, such monkeys are reported to be more aggressive and "tomboyish" than normal female monkeys.[47] Analogous *in utero* androgenization occurs in the human in disorders such as the adrenogenital syndrome or as a toxic side effect of maternal treatment with progestins that have androgenic effects. As adults, neonatally androgenized human female patients show normal menstrual function, ovulation, and the capacity to become pregnant. If raised as girls, they assume female gender identification, and, generally speaking, take normal female roles in mating. However, it has been shown that there is an increase in aggressive, tomboyish behavior, a tendency as children to be more active in male stereotypic activity, such as contact sports, and as a group a higher IQ[33] and greater mathematical ability.[12]

Further clinical evidence that the human (in contrast to other animal forms) is much less dependent upon *in utero* endocrine factors for gender orientation has come from the study of a rare congenital disorder of testosterone metabolism in which individuals lack the enzyme that converts testosterone to the tissue active form, dihydroxytestosterone. In this condition, those structures which are virilized by testosterone itself develop normally (epididymis, vas deferens, seminal vesicle, and ejaculatory duct), but the external genitalia that are dihydroxytestosterone dependent do not develop normally, leaving the patient with a small penis and a vagina. At puberty, these individuals (who have normal testes) develop the normal pubertal levels of testosterone and show partial development of the penis.[49,57] What makes these cases especially instructive from the point of view of hormonal determination of gender role is that they are generally considered to be girls at the time of birth and are raised as girls. At the time

PSYCHONEUROENDOCRINOLOGY

of puberty, when the penis and other male secondary sexual features appear, most of the individuals with this disorder (who have been studied in a small Dominican Republic community) assume the female role. One interpretation of these events is that gender role is virtually independent of hormonal status except insofar as gonad status determines the external appearance of genitalia, which in turn defines sex role, and the gender of rearing.[109]

The role of sex hormones in determining intelligence and nonsexual behavior in man has received much study. High mathematical ability is more likely to be expressed in male persons. For example, in the work of Benbow and Stanley,[12] among students below the age of 13 who scored higher than 700 on the mathematics Scholastic Aptitude Test, the ratio of boys to girls was 13:1. As pointed out by Geschwind and Behan,[40] boys have a higher incidence of left-handedness and a greater tendency to dyslexia. A large somewhat controversial literature has grown up on the role of selective right- and left-sided brain development in men as compared with women. It has been suggested that men have a relatively greater development of the right side of the brain than do women.

The role of prenatal sex hormone status in determining sexual orientation has extended to inquiries into factors leading to homosexuality and transsexualism. As noted above, prenatal androgenization in female persons may lead to an increased incidence of some male hormone dependent behaviors (aggressive play, for example) but does not lead to an increased incidence of homosexuality.[31,32,77] Some male homosexuals may have lower than average male hormones,[42] and their pituitary gonadotropin response to estrogen administration may be intermediate between male and female, but they may be subpopulations, because most studies indicate that male homosexuals are not hormonally different from male heterosexuals.[90] Similarly, although some subpopulations of female homosexuals may have gonadotropin-regulatory differences, as a group no abnormalities can be consistently shown.[73] In one report, female to male transsexuals were described as showing "male" patterns of estrogen priming in response to LHRH, that is, males normally are inhibited by estrogen and females are sensitized,[95] but subsequent studies failed to confirm this report.[109] The differences in estrogen feedback effects on the pituitary gland which are sex specific were shown to be a consequence of blood testosterone levels.[115,116] It must be concluded, therefore, that prenatal hormone milieu does not determine sexual orientation.

Gonadal Steroids and Human Sexual Function

Male Sexual Function. Increased levels of androgenic hormone at puberty are required for normal development of libidinal drive and potency. Once established, acquired androgenic deficiency must be severe before normal male sexual function is seriously impaired, and the onset of impotence and loss of libido lag behind the loss of androgenic function.[23,56,89] Both boys and girls have significant increases in circulating androgens at the onset of puberty. In girls, these steroids come mainly from the adrenal gland; in boys the increase in adrenal androgen secretion is paralled by a much larger increase (about 10 times as great) in the secretion of testosterone by the

relatively constant in almost all men until the sixth decade. The normal decline in male sexual vigor with age probably represents maturation and aging of neural or gonadal structures involved in sexual behavior.[52] The role of modest decline in androgens (within the normal range) over long periods in the course of "normal" decline in potency and vigor of men is unknown. It is folk knowledge that the aging man not uncommonly seeks to maintain and to demonstrate his youthful sexual vigor by seeking out new (and younger) sex partners.

A male climacteric does occur, but it is much less dramatic than the female counterpart, the menopause.[52] Beginning in the fifth decade, a gradual rise in plasma levels of LH and follicle-stimulating hormone (FSH) occurs in most men. This rise indicates reduced feedback signal from the testes. A gradual diminution in sexual competence occurs in later years. The efficacy of androgen treatment of this decreased libido remains to be established. In addition, approximately 15 percent of older men show evidence of testicular aging by biopsy and by chemical studies of testosterone. A proportion of these men lose libido and manifest autonomic and nervous changes similar to those of menopause, with restoration of these function after testosterone administration. This syndrome is not a normal part of the aging process and is uncommon. Although some workers dispute the existence of the male climacteric and dismiss the syndrome as being a manifestation of psychoneurosis, it appears reasonable to look for pituitary and testicular deficiency as causes of loss of libido or potency in men suspected of having the syndrome of the male climacteric and to judge each case on its merits.

Female Sexual Function. Hormonal regulation of psychosexual function in women is far more complex than in men, involving adrenal androgens as well as cyclic changes in estrogen and progesterone secretion. Most endocrine literature related to hormones and female sexuality concerns the importance of adrenal androgens. Adrenalectomy or hypophysectomy leads to almost complete loss of libido and sex drive, and the reversal of this loss by treatment with testosterone supports the conclusion that androgen, not estrogen, is the major determinant of sexual behavior in female humans.[89,90,91] However, these findings are not necessarily applicable to all women, inasmuch as the patients studied were for the most part suffering from cancer. Analogous findings are observed in spontaneously occurring pituitary-adrenal disease. High-dosage androgen therapy leads in some cases to enhanced, even pathologic, sex drive. These pathologic changes may be due only to clitoral enlargement and hypersensitivity, or to an additional central component which has not been clearly established.

With respect to estrogens, the situation in the human may differ from that in experimental animals, including both rats and monkeys. In the rat, estrogen alone administered to the adrenalectomized female rat produces typical lordosis behavior (sexually accepting). Estrogens administered to female monkeys result in their accepting male sexual advances. This appears to be due to two factors which operate together: (1) an increased frequency of the female monkey presenting to the male monkey, and (2) the release of pheromone by the female monkey.[74] The pheromone in the female rhesus monkey which stimulates male sexual activity appears to be a mixture of fatty acids synthesized by bacteria in the vagina as a result of estrogen-induced changes in vaginal pH and secretion. The appearance of this pheromone actually stimulates male courting behavior prior to the appearance of the heightened sexual receptivity of the female monkey, suggesting that the neural response to estrogens in the female monkey has a higher threshold of hormone effect than does the biochemical change in vaginal secretion. Michael and coworkers[76] have demonstrated similar fatty acids in the preovulatory phase in 30 percent of normal women in their sample, which are absent in women on oral contraceptives. It remains to be determined whether attractant pheromones play a role in human sex behavior, but the use of perfumes has long tradition as a stimulator of sexual arousal. The bases of many perfumes are musk or civet, substances which are pheromones in certain animals.

In the female human, sexual function is less dependent on hormonal influences than in lower forms. The greater role of the psychic component in female sexuality as compared with male sexuality makes it difficult to evaulate the effects of estrogen and progesterone. Spontaneous or induced menopause produces a marked diminution in the levels of both progesterone and estrogen.[35] Not only are there physical signs of estrogen deficiency—such as vaginal atrophy, osteoporosis, and hot flashes—but frequently there are depressive symptoms ranging from "blues" to an inability to work and a sense of hopelessness.[35,58] Coupled with these, there may be a loss of interest in sexual activity. The hot flashes and associated mental symptoms are due to estrogen deficiency, because they are also observed with administration of the antiestrogen clomiphene as well as occasionally in hypopituitarism. The regressive changes in the female genitalia induced by estrogen deficiency—thinning and friability of the vulva and vagina and decrease in secretions—may cause dyspareunia. Loss of a sense of well-being also contributes to the loss of sexual feeling. Continued sexual activity is said to be an important factor in maintenance of sexual function in older women, but adequate replacement therapy is needed to prevent vulvovaginal involution.[67,70] Most physicians are conservative in their use of endocrine replacement in menopausal women and fail to take into account the affective state, the sexual functioning of the patient, and the presence of unpleasant vasomotor menopausal symptoms. Reports linking estrogen therapy to an increased incidence of uterine[68] and possibly breast cancer have made it even more mandatory that the diagnosis of behavioral or affective disorder caused by estrogen deficiency be established with certainty and that the possible disadvantages as well as the benefits of estrogen therapy be carefully considered.

Another estrogen deficiency state is Turner's syndrome, or gonadal dysgenesis. In this syndrome, patients lack one X chromosome and frequently have short stature, webbing of the neck, and deformity of the forearms (cubitus valgus). Individuals with this syndrome are described as being warm-hearted, friendly, pleasant, and lacking in aggression. They are also reported to have low sex drive. These patients do not have adrenal insufficiency and apparently have normal levels of circulating androgens. The low sex drive, therefore, appears to be due to the low level of estrogen and is probably related, at least in part, to lack of development of female secondary sex characteristics. Therapy with estrogens restores sex drive.

EFFECTS OF HORMONES ON THE BRAIN AND BEHAVIOR   651

Changes in female sexuality that accompany the normal menstrual cycle are even more complex.[1-3,7,8] These are deeply intertwined with conscious and unconscious conflicts over the significance of the menses themselves. Studies with animals in which sex drive is closely associated with high estrogen levels would lead one to suppose that women should show heightened sexual receptivity at midcycle, at a time when gonadal readiness might be expected to coincide with behavioral acceptance. This supposition, based on work in lower animals, appears to hold in part in the human. In a now classic study using a unique longitudinal approach and double-blind methodology, Benedek and Rubenstein[13] examined mood changes during 152 menstrual cycles in 15 women undergoing psychoanalytic treatment. Vaginal exfoliative cytology was examined and used to divide the cycle into five stages: follicle ripening phase, early ovulation phase, ovulatin phase, progesterone (luteal) phase, and premenstrual phase. Although sexual feeling varied throughout the menstrual cycle, and on the average was maximum on the 14th day of the cycle, not all women had a peak of sexual interest around the time of ovulation, and some demonstrated increased sexual desire just before and just after the menses. Most women had a decline in sexual feeling during the luteal (postovulatory) phase of the cycle. Hormone changes during these stages of the menstrual cycle have subsequently been well characterized. Estrogen levels rise during the first two stages, peak in the ovulatory phase, remain high in the progesterone phase, and drop rapidly in the premenstrual phase. Progesterone level rises only after ovulation and drops together with estrogen in the premenstrual phase.

In a series of married women studied by Udry and Morris,[105] peak frequency of coitus and orgasm was between the 14th and 16th days of the cycle, with minimum frequency on the fourth day. It is now known that testosterone levels during the menstrual cycle also fluctuate, being significantly higher during the midcycle period than during the follicular or luteal phase.

Premenstrual Syndrome. There are few topics that are as difficult to evaluate as the premenstrual syndrome (PMS).[51,88,90] Although many women show variations in mood and irritability in relationship to their periods, the occurrence of major disability occurs in only a few, although some workers in this field claim that the incidence is much higher than generally recognized, and in those women affected there is often serious disability and even profound disruption of normal interpersonal relations, the committing of illegal acts, and the exercise of poor judgment. The problem has become entangled with feminist issues as well; on one hand, many women feel that it is wrong to single out women as being especially vulnerable and periodically under par because they are women, whereas on the other hand, if there is a physical disability, treatment should be given to correct hormonal or other difficulties. Another problem that has developed recently is that the lay press has publicized this problem, especially following legal cases in which PMS was claimed as an extenuating circumstance in capital crime.[22] Normally, menstruating women show maximum "negative" affect immediately after and immediately before their menses.[98] This is true for both anxiety and hostility. There is a report that 84 percent of crimes of violence committed by women in Paris occurred during the premenstrual and menstrual phases. About half of the occurrences of industrial sickness, acute psychiatric admission, and acute medical and surgical admissions coincide with the four premenstrual and four menstrual days. Specialty PMS clinics which provide comprehensive psychologic and endocrinologic evaluation have grown up in the United States.[83]

As defined, PMS is characterized as a disorder manifesting depression or anxiety, fatigue, irritability, swelling of legs and abdomen, tenderness of breasts, significant weight gain, increased acneiform eruptions, and interference with usual work and social activities.[90] To be considered as part of the syndrome, the changes must be cyclic and relatively predictable. The actual timing suggests that the term PMS may be a misnomer, because some of the symptoms complained of may not begin or reach their peak until the second or third day of the period.

Much attention has been focused on premenstrual retention of salt and water as an important factor in premenstrual tension. However, many sufferers show no evidence of weight gain, and dehydration measures do not lead to relief except in those cases in which fluid retention is obvious.

The hormonal basis of the syndrome is poorly understood.[8,88,106] Patients with PMS have no abnormalities in secretion or in blood levels of estrogen, progesterone, or PRL; hence if there is a hormonal abnormality it is an abnormal response to normal levels of hormone. Nevertheless, the role of hormones in this syndrome is well demonstrated. When ovarian function is completely abolished by treatment with GnRH superagonists, the symptoms of PMS are almost completely abolished.[81] This finding demonstrates its dependence upon sexual steroid secretion and provides a new tool for therapy and clinical investigation. Most studies show that PRL is not elevated in PMS and that bromocriptine, which lowers PRL levels, is no better than placebo.[88]

Proponents of progesterone therapy for treatment of PMS advocate the use of extremely high doses of progesterone — given usually as vaginal suppositories in doses from 100 to 500 mg per day — and claim that in those cases with "true" PMS there is a high rate of remission.[83] One double-blind study of the progesterone treatment of PMS reported some benefit,[27] but others have been equivocal.[88] Other medications have been tried — birth control pills of various types, duphaston, a progesterone-related drug, bromocriptine (to treat the alleged prolactin excess); good effects have been reported for a proportion of cases in all studies. Diuretics have been used with only minimal success, and various tranquilizers form the basis of common clinical practice. The clinician does not have any firm therapeutic guidelines to follow. The validity of programs of high progesterone administered in specialized clinics remains to be established; but even if they are successful, the combination of group psychotherapy, special diets (low cholesterol, low salt), and the special mystique of such programs makes them hard to evaluate objectively. Bromocriptine is useful for treatment of mastodynia even when prolactin levels are in the normal range. Diuretics are useful for excessive fluid but do not relieve the psychologic symptoms. If the PMS-like syndrome is brought on by delayed menses or anovulatory cycles, the use of a progestin—for example, medroxyprogesterone (Provera) 5 to 10 mg for 5 days, or progesterone, 100 mg intramuscularly—will usually relieve the situation.

The normal fluctuating pattern of anxiety and hostility is observed in women taking sequential contraceptives but not in those taking combined therapy with estrogens and gestagens (progesterone-like drugs).[21,43,55,60] It appears that gestagens prevent the occurrence of the usual midcycle peak of well-being. There is also a slight decrease in menstrual symptomatology. Oral contraceptives of the combined type are said to frequently, but not uniformly, inhibit libido. Up to 10 percent of women taking oral contraceptives are liable to develop symptoms of depression or increased irritability that require discontinuation of treatment, but a higher percentage (62 percent in one study) develop lesser symptoms. Risk of depression is higher in those with a history of depressive disorders and in those with premenstrual or menstrual disorders. The relationship of these symptoms to estrogen and progesterone levels is not clear because a unitary relationship has not been established. Controlled double-blind studies emphasize that placebo effects may play a major role in changing mood and affect.

Influences of Hormones on Headache

Migraine shows a distinct sex difference in adults (but not children), occurring two to three times as often in women as compared with men. Headaches and migraine tend to occur at times of hormonal change: around the time of menstruation, as part of the premenstrual syndrome, at ovulation, at the menarche, at menopause, and during pregnancy, although in some cases pregnancy has no effect.[34]

In a few female patients with migraine (probably less than 20 percent), repeated exacerbation of migraine coincides with the fall in circulating estrogen in the immediate premenstrual phase of the cycle. Headaches in such patients can be delayed by administration of long-acting estrogens, the symptoms developing as estrogen levels fall.[99,100] The management of such patients remains difficult, because continued administration of estrogens is usually not feasible.

One major side effect of the contraceptive pill is an increased incidence of migraine in susceptible women, particularly with progestogenic pills containing estrogen in low dosage.[28] This combination is the commonest type of oral contraceptive now in use because it results in a lower incidence of thrombosis. Various mechanisms have been invoked for this migraine susceptibility. Alterations in metabolism of serotonin and norepinephrine (which are implicated in migraine attacks) or effects in monoamine oxidase activity, and catechol-O-methyltransferase activity are possible contributory factors.[48]

Effects of GnRH on the Brain

Studies in the rat suggest that GnRH is involved in regulation of sexual activity. Administration of GnRH to the female rat produces an increase in lordosis behavior, even in hypophysectomized recipients; evidently this action is not mediated through pituitary gonadotropins but is a direct one.[79]

The administration of GnRH directly into the preoptic area has the same effect, suggesting that there is a GnRH-sensitive "center" for sex drive in the anterior hypothalamus. Several studies of LHRH as a libido-producing substance have been carried out. The initially promising reports of Moss[79] have not been supported by subsequent studies.[24]

Adrenal Steroid Effects on Brain Development

The mechanism of glucocorticoid effects on the brain were considered previously. Cortisol administration delays development of behavioral responses in rats and causes a delay in central nervous system maturation when given in the first seven postnatal days; thereafter, glucocorticoids accelerate maturation. In tissue culture glucocorticoids caused increased branching of neurons, an increased migration of glia cells, and the induction of several enzymes. Effects of brain development in the human are not known.

PSYCHOLOGIC DISTURBANCE IN ENDOCRINE DISEASE

BEHAVIORAL CHANGES IN THYROID DISEASE

Abnormalities in mentation and behavior are invariable in patients with abnormally elevated or reduced thyroid function, and in some cases they dominate the clinical picture.[26,75,87,90]

In thyrotoxic states a minority of patients, particularly the elderly, become depressed, withdrawn, apathetic, and anorectic. In extremely "toxic" patients, delirium and coma may supervene; indeed, the occurrence of organic delerium in *thyrotoxicosis* is one of the hallmarks of thyroid storm. Detailed psychologic testing reveals "organic brain damage" in many. These features improve following treatment. The organic deficit persists after treatment in a minority of patients, suggesting that severe hyperthyroidism may cause irreversible brain damage.

The role of premorbid personality disturbance in the pathogenesis of Graves' disease is still subject to debate. A few authors report a high incidence of psychologic abnormality, with a specific type of personality associated with premature assumption of responsibility and a martyr-like suppression of dependency wishes. Others report precipitation by emotional stress, especially with object loss. Still others claim that such abnormalities are due to the disease itself.

The neurophysiologic basis of *thyrotoxic encephalopathy* has not been established and is in fact enigmatic. Surprisingly, cerebral oxygen consumption is not increased in Graves' disease; brain tissue oxygen consumption (measured in laboratory animals), unlike that of liver and skeletal muscle, is unaltered by thyroid administration, and isolated brain mitochondria (unlike those from muscle, kidney, or liver) fail to swell or "uncouple" when exposed to excess thyroxine. These results indicate that hyperthyroid encephalopathy is probably not due to a simple increase in cellular metabolism. Thyroxine appears to produce direct effects on neuronal electric activity. Iontophoretic application produces activation of most

panied by personality disorder. In one review of 78 cases of hypopituitarism, only six patients were free of psychologic disturbances. Many hypopituitary patients are extremely dependent and psychologic invalids. Early symptoms include fatigability, impotence, and loss of libido, together with loss of body hair and intolerance to cold. Later, apathy, depression, drowsiness, loss of initiative and drive, and mental torpor are the most common manifestations. As pointed out by Michael and Gibbons,[75] "apathy, indifference and inactivity may become so profound that patients rarely leave their living quarters, they lie in bed for much of the day and they neglect even their personal hygiene." Flexor spasm, upper motor neuron signs, and severe contractures may occur. Chronic diffuse brain disturbance with disorientation and loss of memory is common, with delirium and stupor ending in hypopituitary coma in the extreme form.

Adrenal cortical deficiency is the major factor contributing to the mental disturbance of patients with hypopituitarism, as exemplified by the confused or stuporous patients who may rapidly become alert and mentally clear following intravenous therapy with hydrocortisone. Thyroxine, although important, is usually less crucial. For individuals of both sexes, return of libido requires replacement doses of androgenic hormones. In women, an increased sense of well-being often follows estrogen administration.

It is noteworthy that even after all of these replacements have been supplied, certain patients with panhypopituitarism still show residual symptoms such as apathy, lack of drive, and chronic fatigue. The basis for this residual deficiency is unknown; it may be related to deficiency of growth hormone or prolactin, or another unknown pituitary factor, but data to prove this point are lacking. It is also possible that long-standing pituitary insufficiency leads to irreversible brain damage. Little is known about GH psychologic effects. Possible behavioral effects of prolactin are also unknown. Inasmuch as prolactin affects a wide range of behaviors in lower forms, including the induction of maternal behavior and migratory drive, it is not unreasonable to suppose that there are behavioral effects in the human and that eventually these will be established.

BRAIN DYSFUNCTION SECONDARY TO HORMONALLY MEDIATED CHANGES IN THE INTERNAL MILIEU

Virtually all the important plasma constituents whose constancy is normally guarded by homeostatic mechanisms (including those dependent upon hormone action) influence brain function. The major controlled variables are the concentrations in blood of glucose, carbon dioxide, hydrogen, calcium, sodium, potassium, and osmotically active particles. Gross disturbance of any of these variables can produce metabolic disorder in the brain, with diffuse impairment of higher functions ranging from mild disturbance in consciousness, memory, and judgment to confusion, disorientation, stupor, coma, and death. A variety of symptoms resembling neurasthenia, neurosis, and functional psychosis also can be seen in these syndromes. A detailed account of organic brain disorders is given by Plum.[87] In this section only disturbances in calcium and glucose will be considered.

Abnormalities in Plasma Calcium

Hypercalcemia

High blood calcium levels can result from hyperparathyroidism, from vitamin D intoxication, and from carcinomas causing either massive destruction of bone or a parathyroid-hormone-like syndrome. One of the most dramatic endocrine causes of acute hypercalcemia is infarction of a parathyroid adenoma, which leads to an outpouring of parathyroid hormone. In addition to the relatively unspecific signs of encephalopathy, hypercalcemic patients manifest a variety of poorly defined neurotic symptoms, fatigue, headache, and organic psychosis. Seizures are exceedingly rare. In an extensive study of the psychiatric aspects of hyperparathyroidism, Peterson[85] evaluated 54 patients. As summarized by Smith and collaborators:[98]

> Personality changes noted in the majority of these patients began with an affective disturbance characterized by lack of initiative and spontaneity and by depression. This depression was sometimes combined with moroseness, irascibility lity, or explosiveness. Suicidal tendencies were occasionally noted, although none of the patients had to be hospitalized because of this. Generalized fatigue was a common complaint. Memory impairment, with reduced ability to concentrate, was less common. All these changes developed slowly, sometimes over several years. Acute organic psychosis generally appeared as disorientation, delirium, confusion, paranoid ideas, and hallucinations. Severe acute organic psychosis often began abruptly and necessitated rapid surgical correction of hyperparathyroidism. Peterson carefully correlated the degree of psychiatric disturbance with the level of serum calcium. As the level of serum calcium rose, the severity of mental changes increased. This was true whether hypercalcemia was caused by hyperparathyroidism or other causes. When eucalcemia was attained, as by hemodialysis, mental abnormalities disappeared, despite persisting hyperparathyroidism. The serum calcium per se was the determining factor.

Cope,[19] a surgeon with vast experience in the surgical treatment of hyperparathyroidism, emphasized the importance of neurologic and psychiatric symptoms as clues in the evaluation and diagnosis of hyperparathyroidism. The clinical picture of paranoid schizophrenia has been seen in hyperparathyroidism, and its relationship to the illness proven by complete cure after surgery. In Peterson's series,[85] serum calcium levels of 12 to 16 mg/dl were associated with neurasthenic changes, and acute psychosis at values above 16 mg/dl. Calcium levels of 16 to 19 mg/dl were associated with alterations in consciousness; somnolence or coma occurred with values over 19 mg/100ml.

Although many kinds of psychologic disturbance can be seen in patients with hypercalcemia, and blood calcium levels should be measured in all patients with psychiatric problems, it must be emphasized that a modest elevation in blood calcium level is not necessarily the cause of psychiatric illness in a given patient. The true incidence of significant mental impairment is not known. The recent finding of numerous patients with mild hypercalcemia following the application of the multiphasic screening methods has shown that most are asymptomatic. As a practical matter, the likelihood that one is dealing with asymptomatic mild hypercalcemia in a

Initial effects of hypoglycemia are due to cortical depression with headaches, faintness, confusion, restlessness, clouded consciousness, hunger, irritability, and visual disturbances. Other symptoms, related to epinephrine release, are anxiety, tremor, perspiration, tachycardia, pallor, and tingling of the fingers or around the mouth. With more severe hypoglycemia, or a more rapid onset, progressive changes include loss of environmental contact, myoclonic twitching, clonic spasms, and increased sensitivity to stimulation. Still further central nervous system depression leads to tonic spasms, torsion spasms, independent movement of the eyes, and the appearance of long-tract signs. Death may occur. Treatment with glucose alleviates the symptoms, in reverse order, but prolonged or repeated severe hypoglycemia may not be compatible with complete recovery. Unfortunately, the lay public has discovered hypoglycemia as a convenient diagnosis to explain chronic fatigue and depression and other psychoneurotic symptoms, and in recent years an extraordinarily large number of patients are seen whose chief complaint is hypoglycemia.

Crucial to the diagnosis of true hypoglycemia is the demonstration that (1) symptoms are correlated with either a rapid fall in blood sugar level or with a low absolute value (less than 50 mg/dl), and (2) they respond to treatment with glucose. Many people when tired or bored get a "pick-up" from a carbohydrate-rich snack, and this is particularly true of those on weight-reducing diets. This is not evidence of hypoglycemia and is more likely a normal response. Complete analysis of the diagnostic approach to hypoglycemia is dealt with in the endocrine and metabolic literature. It is important to emphasize here that a minimum workup includes a 5-hour glucose tolerance test after appropriate preparation (300 g carbohydrate intake daily for 3 days or more). The only test that completely excludes the diagnosis of insulinoma is a 3-day fast under observation in a hospital setting. Few, if any, patients with pancreatic insulin-producing tumors will fail to show diagnostically low levels of glucose (less than 40 mg/dl) and symptoms by this time. This test is mandatory in cases in which so-called hypoglycemic symptoms are causing significant disturbance in brain function.

Hyperglycemia

High blood sugar levels appear in untreated or poorly treated diabetics, and occasionally in extremely stressed individuals. Values above 1000 mg/dl are seen almost exclusively in patients with associated renal insufficiency. High blood glucose levels in this range cause cerebral disease through a hyperosmolar mechanism, because gross encephalopathy can be observed even in the absence of ketosis or ketonemia. When severe, hyperosmolar coma is fatal in a high proportion of cases. Even when treated successfully, patients who have experienced a period of hyperosmolar coma may continue to show impairment of higher functions indefinitely, indicating that irreversible neuronal damage has taken place. Autopsy in such cases shows loss of nerve cells. A similar hyperosmolar state is seen in severe water deficiency, as in untreated diabetes insipidus. Persistent hyperosmolarity or hypoosmolarity can lead to permanent brain damage. Rapid restoration of hypoosmolarity can cause brain damage.

REFERENCES

1. ABPLANALP, JM, DONNELLY, AF, ROSE, RM: *Psychoendocrinology of the menstrual cycle. I. Enjoyment of daily activities.* Psychosom Med 41:587–604, 1979.
2. ABPLANALP, JM, ROSE, RM, DONNELLY, AF, LIVINGSTON-VAUGHN, L: *Psychoendocrinology of the menstrual cycle. II. Relationship between enjoyment of activities, moods and reproductive hormones.* Psychosom Med 41:605–615, 1979.
3. ADAMS, DB, AND GOLD, AR: *Rise in female-initiated sexual activity at ovulation and its suppression by oral contraceptives.* N Engl J Med 229:1145–1150, 1978.
4. ARANDASH, G, AND GORSKI, R: *Enhancement of sexual behavior in female rats by neonatal transplantation of brain tissue from males.* Science 217:1276–1278, 1982.
5. ARANDASH, GW: *Brain tissue transplantation, a new tool for exploring the sexual differentation of the brain.* IBRO News 11:7–12, 1983.
6. ATTARDI, B: *Progesterone modulation of the luteinizing hormone surge: Regulation of hypothalamic and pituitary progestin receptors.* Endocrinology 115:2113–2122, 1984.
7. BACKSTROM, T, SANDERS, D, LEASK, R, ET AL: *Mood, sexuality, hormones and the menstrual cycle: II. Hormone levels and their relationship to the premenstrual syndrome.* Psychosom Med 45:503–507, 1983.
8. BANCROFT, J, AND BACKSTROM, T. *Premenstrual syndrome.* Clin Endocrinol (Oxf) 22:313–335, 1985.
9. BANCROFT, J, SANDERS, D, DAVIDSON, D, ET AL: *Mood, sexuality, hormones and the menstrual cycle: III. Sexuality and the role of androgens.* Psychosom Med 45:509–516, 1983.
10. BARFIELD, RJ, GLASER, JH, RUBIN, BS, ETGEN, AM: *Behavioral effects of progestin in the brain.* Psychoneuroendocrinology 9:217–231, 1984.
11. BAXTER, JD, AND FUNDER, JW: *Hormone Receptors.* N Engl J Med 301:1149–1161, 1979.
12. BENBOW, CP, STANLEY, JC: *Sex differences in mathematical reasoning ability: More facts.* Science 222:1029–1031, 1983.
13. BENEDEK, T, AND RUBENSTEIN, BB: *The sexual cycle in women. Psychosomatic medicine monographs, vol. 3, nos. 1 and 2.* National Research Council, Washington, DC, 1942.
14. BERLIN, FS, AND MEINECKE, CF: *Treatment of sex offenders with antiandrogenic medication: Conceptualization, review of treatment modalities and preliminary findings.* Am J Psychiatry 138:601–607, 1981.
15. BUBENIK, GA, AND BROWN, GM: *Morphologic sex differences in primate brain areas involved in regulation of reproductive activity.* Experientia 29:619–621, 1973.
16. CARPENTER, WT, JR, STRAUSS, JS, BUNNEY, WE, JR: *The psychobiology of cortisol metabolism: Clinical and theoretical implications.* In SHADER, RI, (ED): *Psychiatric complications of new drugs.* Raven Press, New York, 1972, p 49–72.
17. CLARK, JH, SCHRADER, WT, O'MALLEY, BW: *Mechanisms of steroid hormone action.* In *Williams Textbook of Endocrinology,* ed 7. WB Saunders, Philadelphia, 1985, p 33–75.
18. COOPER, AJ, ISMAIL, AA, PHANJOO, AL, LOVE, DL: *Antiandrogen (cyproterone acetate) therapy in deviant hypersexuality.* Br J Psychiatr 120:59–63, 1972.
19. COPE, OE: *Hyperparathyroidism: Diagnosis and management.* Am J Surg 99:394–403, 1960.
20. CRYER, P: *Glucose homeostasis and hypoglycemia.* In WILSON, JD, AND FOSTER, DW (EDS): In *Williams Textbook of Endocrinology,* ed 7. WB Saunders, Philadelphia, 989–1017, 1985.
21. CULLBERG, J: *Mood changes and menstrual symptoms with different gestagen/estrogen combinations.* Acta Psychiatr Scand (Suppl) 236:1, 1972.
22. DALTON, K: *The Premenstrual Syndrome and Progesterone Therapy.* William Heinemann, London.
23. DAVIDSON, JM: *Hormones and sexual behavior in the male.* In KRIEGER, DT, AND HUGHES, JC (EDS): *Neuroendocrinology.* Sinaver Associates, Sunderland, MA, 1980, pp 232–239.
24. DAVIES, TF, MOUNTJOY, CQ, GOMEZ-PAN, A, ET AL: *A double, blind cross over trial of gonadotropin releasing hormone (LHRH) in sexually impotent men.* Clin Endocrinol 5:601–607, 1976.
25. DE KLOET, ER: *Function of steroid receptor systems in the central nervous system.* Clin Neuropharm 7:272–280, 1984.
26. DEGROOT, LJ, LARSEN, PR, REFETOFF, S, STANBURY, JB: *The thyroid and its diseases.* John Wiley & Sons, New York, 1984.
27. DENNERSTEIN, L, SPENCER-GARDNER, C, GOTTS, G, BROWN, JB, SMITH, MA, BURROWS, GD: *Progesterone and the premenstrual syndrome: A double blind crossover trial.* Br Med J 290:1617–1621, 1985.
28. DESROSIERS, JJ: *Headaches related to contraceptive therapy and their control.* Headache 13:117–124, 1973.
29. DONOVAN, BT: *Role of hormones in perinatal brain differentiation.* In MOTTA, M (ED): *The Endocrine Functions of the Brain.* Raven Press, New York, 1980, pp 117–141.
30. EAYRS, JT: *Developmental relationships between brain and thyroid.* In MICHAEL, RP (ED): *Endocrinology and Human Behaviour.* Oxford University Press, London, 1968, p 239–255.

Chapter 21

ENDOCRINE RESPONSE TO STRESS AND PSYCHIATRIC DISEASE

The term stress as commonly used in the biomedical literature has an ambiguous meaning. It can be defined as a factor such as pain, trauma, cold exposure, fear, and personal loss that markedly disturbs functioning in an individual, or it can be defined as the physiologic and psychologic state produced in an individual subjected to a stressful factor. The definition of stress is somewhat circular in that a stressful factor will be a stress only if it produces a stressed state in an individual. There is not much difficulty in defining most physical stresses such as burns, laparotomy, bone fracture, or pyrogen administration, but much more difficulty in defining psychologic stressors.[37,48,49,59]

The secretion of each of the known pituitary hormones is affected by both physical and psychologic stress.[49] These responses are mediated through specific neural pathways that ultimately impinge upon the hypophysiotropic hormonal pathways in the hypothalamus.[23] Stress responses are of importance because they may have teleologic value, and they serve as markers of hormonal regulatory function and have been widely utilized for evaluation of hypothalamic-pituitary disease. Because the pituitary-adrenal stress response was the earliest to be recognized and in many ways served as the conceptual model for other hormonal reactions, it will be considered first.

ADRENOCORTICOTROPIC HORMONE (ACTH)- ADRENAL STRESS RESPONSE

The long history of research on adrenal stress response has distinguished conceptual roots in the work of Claude Bernard[3] and Walter Cannon.[9] Bernard emphasized the constancy of the internal milieu as the requirement for survival; Cannon pointed out the importance of the adrenal medulla and sympathetic nervous system in coping with stressful stimuli both physical and psychologic. Selye[54] extended Cannon's theme to include the function of the pituitary-adrenal axis. Both Cannon and Selye believed, with Bernard, that these autonomic and endocrine responses had a positive survival value; Selye added the concept that in the general alarm reaction, the adaptive responses might become excessive and in themselves become part of the damaging process.

To these workers, the adrenal response had teleologic value in preventing deficiency of one or more life-supporting substances. This view has undergone considerable refinement in recent years, Munck and colleagues[45] in particular pointing out that pituitary-adrenal activation in stress is not a teleologic response to rectify an induced chemical deficiency but, rather, a response of the body to *suppress* certain deleterious effects of stress. In brief, Munck has proposed that glucocorticoids "generally suppress rather than enhance our normal defense mechanisms." He and colleagues have proposed that, "(1) the physiological function of stress-induced increases in glucocorticoid levels is to protect not against the source of stress itself but against the normal defense reactions that are activated by stress; and (2) the glucocorticoids accomplish this function by turning off those defense reactions, thus preventing them from overshooting and themselves threatening homeostasis." These normal defense reactions include the release of lymphokines from lymphocytes, release and biologic effects of the endogenous pyrogen (which stimulates fever and acute phase reactants), and the release of inflammatory mediators such as prostaglandins, leukotrienes, and many other active compounds with potentially tissue-damaging effects. From this point of view the stress response may have been developed in evolutionary time to deal with invading viruses and bacteria. Mechanisms so developed have, in higher forms including the human, been co-opted to respond to symbolic threats. Psychic stress-induced cortisol secretion in the human probably serves no useful teleologic purpose; its significance to the psychoneuroendocrinologist lies in these responses as markers of archetypical function of the limbic system-hypothalamic mechanism, and potentially as providing a window to the abnormalities of central neurotransmitter control in psychiatric disorder (see below.)

Although the biologic significance of the pituitary-adrenal stress response may still be subject to speculation, the phenomenon itself has been studied exhaustively; indeed, many workers have regarded this response as defining stress. Virtually all severe physical damage such as surgery, leg fracture, toxic chemical administration, histamine injection, pyrogens, exercise, and hypoglycemia induce a marked and abrupt increase in blood adrenocorticotropin hormone (ACTH) followed shortly by an increase in plasma cortisol and aldosterone.

The response to psychologic stress is more complex. Acute situational change, symbolic or physical, may trigger an adrenal response. The work of Mason and colleagues[41] has emphasized the importance of the *novelty* of psychologic stressors. In a classical study, they showed that the parents of children with leukemia (who were clearly upset and stressed) did not have increased adrenocortical secretion unless an unexpected incident occurred. They suggested that as long as individuals are coping psychologically, they do not show increased pituitary-adrenal function. Extensive studies in stressed individuals and those anticipating stress[19,27,49,52] reinforce this view.

GROWTH HORMONE

In the human, both physical and emotional stresses lead to an increase in growth hormone (GH) secretion (see chapter 8).[5,27,52] This is in contrast to several rodent species in whom stress causes an inhibition of GH release. In rats, early fondling can lead to increased rates of growth and to increased GH levels, the reverse of the stress response. In a study in which patients were undergoing cardiac catherization, the occurrence of a GH rise appeared to correlate with poor coping behavior.[27] There is no clearly defined physiologic advantage of the GH stress response. Although Selye published a series of papers showing that inflammatory responses are reduced by GH, others have speculated that GH, through its anabolic effects on muscle and bone, is protective against steroid-induced and interleukin-I-induced negative nitrogen balance. Under certain circumstances the GH stress response is deleterious. It counters the effects of insulin, and in diabetic patients it increases insulin resistance.

PROLACTIN

Prolactin (PRL) secretion is activated by many of the same stressful stimuli that trigger cortisol secretion — physical trauma, pain, exercise (see chapter 7).[4] As pointed out by Hökfelt and colleagues,[31] PRL-releasing factors vasoactive intestinal peptide (VIP), peptide histidine isoleucine-27 (PHI) are cocontained in the CRF containing neurons: It would be expected, therefore, that any stress that increased ACTH release should be accompanied by PRL secretion. However, the psychologic factors that lead to PRL secretion have not been well defined. In an instructive experiment by Nesse and colleagues,[62] serial measurements were made of blood PRL levels during the course of "flooding" therapy, a form of treatment of phobic individuals by forcing them to come into physical contact with the objects of phobia such as small furry animals and snakes. Despite the self-recorded occurrence of severe, overwhelming anxiety, blood PRL did not rise. This observation has not been explained but does indicate that PRL stress pathways are not nonspecific and require a particular constellation of psychic inducers.

The elevation of PRL known to accompany temporal lobe seizures suggests that electrical discharges in specific regions of the limbic system can activate PRL release.[57]

GONADOTROPINS

Severe acute or chronic stress leads to an inhibition of gonadotropin-gonadal function. In women, anovulation, amenorrhea, and gonadal atrophy can be seen in "stress amenorrhea," and a comparable suppression of testosterone can be observed in severely stressed men. The changes in men are less evident than the changes that occur in women.

PITUITARY-THYROID

In experimental animals and in the human, chronic physical stress leads to a depression in thyroid function. In the human, this is made evident by the syndrome of the sick euthyroid state (see chapter 5), a complex disorder which includes alterations in the circulating thyroid hormone carrier proteins, changes in tissue utilization of thyroid hormone, and inappropriately reduced TSH secretion. Increased thyroid function (as inferred from elevated levels of T_4) is observed in about a third of psychiatric patients shortly after admission.[16,56] Loosen and colleagues have postulated that this is due to inappropriate increase in TRH secretion (see below).[39,40]

ENDOCRINE CHANGES IN PSYCHIATRIC DISEASE

Psychoneuroendocrinologists have been interested in endocrine responses to psychiatric illness for two main reasons, one physiologic and the other symbolic. The physiologic rationale is based on the knowledge that the secretion of the tuberohypophysial neuron system is regulated by an array of neurotransmitters—adrenergic, cholinergic, serotonergic, peptidergic—and that the same neurotransmitters may be involved in the pathophysiology of depression and schizophrenia.[23] The suggestion has been made, therefore, that the pituitary gland is a "window to the brain" and that one can infer from pituitary changes the nature of the disturbance in brain function. Furthermore, the finding that pituitary function is disturbed in any psychologic disorder gives credence to the idea that there is an organic basis to its origin.

There are significant problems with these assumptions.[22,43,58] The most important is that the neural pathways that subserve the emotional state may not be the same as those that regulate the anterior pituitary gland. The best example, and perhaps the most important, is the tuberoinfundibular dopamine (TIDA) system. The reason that this system is important stems from the fact that the major neuroleptic agents are dopamine receptor antagonists, and their clinical potency in reversing psychotic symptoms in schizophrenia parallels closely their ability to raise resting PRL levels (Fig. 1).[36a] In fact, one of the screening tests used by pharmaceutical companies to select neuroleptic agents is their effect in modulating PRL levels. However, there are well-documented differences between the tuberoinfundibular system and the mesolimbic system, which is thought to be involved in psychosis. Turnover of dopamine in TIDA neurons is inhibited by PRL (but mesolimbic neurons are not so inhibited), and there are no postreceptor dopamine receptors on TIDA neurons, whereas these are well demonstrated in the mesolimbic system.[43] Therefore, changes in dopamine-related pituitary functions cannot be used as indicators of dopamine-related mesolimbic activity.

Another example is illustrated by ACTH secretion. At least four neurotransmitters are involved in ACTH regulation—serotonin, epinephrine, GABA, and acetycholine—and there is no clear indication that those fibers that innervate the hypothalamus have the same activity as those terminating in the limbic system.

Psychoendocrine responses also are studied for their symbolic significance. By this is meant the correlation between a given endocrine response and a given psychologic state, without necessary consideration of the intermediate steps in between. Loosely put, this ignores the contents of the "black box" that intervenes between input and output. An example of the symbolic use of pituitary tests is the inference about coping behavior as discussed above. The nature of the coping reaction emerged from studies of individuals under stress or those anticipating stress; for example, soldiers

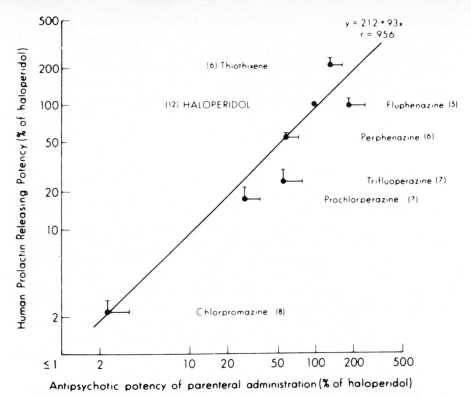

FIGURE 1. Correlation between the antipsychotic potencies and prolactin-stimulating potencies of a series of neuroleptic agents known to act by blocking dopamine receptors. The potencies are given relative to haloperidol. (From Langer, G, et al,[36a] with permission.)

entering combat, paratroopers anticipating a jump, and from the parents of children with leukemia in whom death was feared or expected.[48,49] In all of these studies it has emerged that urinary corticoid excretion, a measure of hypothalamic-pituitary-adrenal corticoid activity, is not increased when the individuals are prepared for the event. On the other hand, steroid excretion is enhanced when unexpected traumatic events occur. Normal steroid secretion thus is an indicator of normal coping behavior, and increased steroid excretion means that coping mechanisms have been overcome.

Psychoendocrine tests have also been used as an empirical indicator of specific psychiatric disease. The best example of this use is the dexamethasone suppression test, an empirical indicator of active depression (see below).

A number of hormonal secretory abnormalities occur in the major psychiatric disorders, depression and schizophrenia, and in an important nonpsychotic illness, anorexia nervosa, in which pituitary abnormalities are a striking feature of the disease. It is important to point out that few if any abnormalities of endocrine function are observed in anxiety or other forms of psychoneurosis, thus indicating that emotional state alone does not have sustained effects of endocrine function. These topics have been reviewed in detail in several publications.[8,48]

Psychoneuroendocrinology of Depression

As summarized by Rubin and Poland,[50] endogenous depression has clearly defined attributes. These include "anhedonia (inability to experience pleasure), lack of energy, fatiguability, reduced sexual drive, anorexia, weight loss, sleep disturbance (especially early morning awakening), depression worse in the morning, self-reproach, excessive guilt, psychomotor agitation or retardation, lack of reactivity to the environment, etc. Delusions or hallucinations (often of a depressive, somatic nature) also may be present, giving an additional, psychotic dimension to the illness."

This illness has a high incidence in families, usually begins in a setting of ordinary psychologic life but can be precipitated by psychologic factors, usually does not respond to psychotherapy, and requires active intervention with drugs or electroshock therapy. Endogenous depression can occur at any age, often leads to suicide, and can alternate with manic periods. The natural history of the disease is usually to have recurring episodes, but in a few, the disease remains relatively constant, resistant to therapy.

The main endocrine abnormalities that have been observed in patients with endogenous depression are (1) increased pituitary-adrenal secretion, (2) resistance to the inhibitory effects of exogenous steroids (abnormal DST, (3) blunted TSH response to injection of thyrotropin-releasing hormone (TRH) and (4) reduced responsiveness of GH to several provocative stimuli.

Hypersecretion of Cortisol

As first recognized by the late Edward Sachar, many patients with endogenous depression have increased blood levels of cortisol throughout the 24

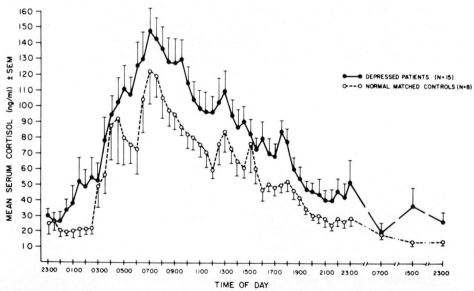

FIGURE 2. Mean half-hourly serum cortisol concentrations ± SEM for 15 primary endogenous depressives and 8 normal control subjects matched to the patients on age, sex, race, and menstrual status. (Figure and legend reproduced from Rubin, RT, and Poland, RE,[50] with permission).

hours.[52,53] They show the normal circadian pattern, but sustained at an increased level[50] (Fig. 2). The levels of cortisol achieved in a few cases approach those seen in Cushing's disease, but, paradoxically, depressed patients do not usually show physical evidence of this disorder, a finding that has not been well explained. Such patients also display marked disturbance in the structure of their sleep patterns.

Abnormal Dexamethasone Supression Test (DST)

Reasoning that the sustained hypersecretion of cortisol in depressive patients must be due to an altered setpoint of feedback control (see also chapter 6), Carroll and colleagues[10-12] determined the efficacy of dexamethasone in inhibiting cortisol secretion in depression. This test was a modification of the approach originally used by Liddle and colleagues, which showed that patients with Cushing's disease had an elevated setpoint of feedback inhibition of ACTH. Normally, cortisol is suppressed for 24 hours after oral administration of 1 mg. As presently carried out, the DST is executed by administering a single dose of 1 mg of dexamethasone by mouth at 11 PM or midnight, and measuring blood cortisol at 4 PM and at 11 PM the following day. If one defines a cortisol level of 5 μg/dl as being the upper limit of normal, Carroll concludes that the test has a 96 percent specificity and 67 percent sensitivity in the diagnosis of severe depressive illness.[35] That is, abnormal tests will be found in only 4 percent of nondepressive patients, and normal tests in only 33 percent of depressive patients.

Following the description of the DST, a number of clinicians adopted this test as part of their workup for depression.[1,2,7,8] However, because the frequency of abnormal tests has not proven to be as high in some clinics as in Carroll's original study, it does not appear to have the specificity and sensitivity required for a diagnostic test. In the compilation of Arana and colleagues[1] the sensitivity of the DST in major depression was 44 percent in 5000 cases from the literature and higher in psychotic affected disorder (67 to 78 percent). However, there are many medical factors that confound the results. The diagnosis of depressive disorder is best made by following diagnostic critera, helped by a family history. A committee of the National Institutes of Health (NIH) has recommended that this test be used only as a research tool and should not be used for routine diagnosis.[29,30] The DST is under continuing review and refinement. Greater specificity is endowed by expressing blood cortisol as a function of dexamethasone level achieved.

Reversal of the abnormality indicates that it marks *state disturbance*, not *trait disturbance*. The abnormal DST test usually reverts to normal with the recovery of the patient, and appearance of an abnormal DST may herald a relapse of the disorder (Fig. 3). The test must be interpreted with caution and cannot be used in patients suffering from medical illness, alcoholism, or who have been taking barbiturates. Carroll and associates[11-13] have shown that the abnormal responsiveness is not due to impaired absorption of dexamethasone, and they have mobilized arguments to indicate that this is not simply a stress response. Precautions must also be taken to ensure that the cortisol levels are measured with precision.

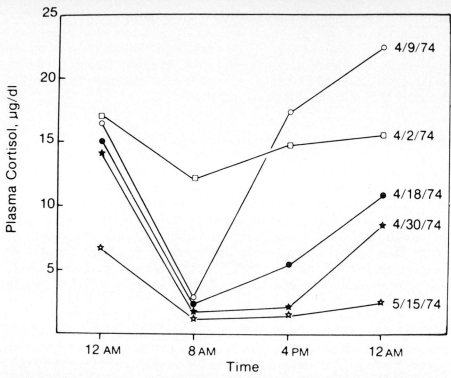

FIGURE 3. Time course of recovery of the abnormal dexamethasone suppression test (DST) in a 49-year-old depressed woman before antidepressant treatment (curves labeled 4/2/74, 4/9/74), and after. The patient was given dexamethasone, 1.0 mg at midnight. Note that the first curve obtained showed virtually no suppression, that the second curve showed normal suppression but with an early escape, and the last curve showed a normal suppressive course. (From Carroll, BJ, Curtis, GC, Mendels, J: *Neuroendocrine regulation in depression. I Limbic system-adrenocortical dysfunction.* Arch Gen Psychiatr 33:1039–1044, 1976, with permission.)

Thyroid Function in Depression

The majority of patients with depression have thyroid hormone blood levels within the normal range, although several reports indicate that values tend to be at the upper limit of normal (see above). On the other hand, transient hyperthyroxinemia has been reported to occur in some acutely disturbed patients over the first few days of hospitalization (see above). The most convincing evidence that there may be abnormalities of pituitary-thyroid regulation in depression is the observation that approximately 25 percent of patients with depression show a blunted TSH response to TRH, that is, an increment of less than 5 μU/ml[39,40] (Fig. 4). The true frequency of this abnormality has been debated; a few reports have failed to confirm this finding, whereas other observers confirm it. Whether it is a marker of the state of depression or of a trait is not certain. In a few studies, remission in the mental disturbance was accompanied by return of normal TRH response, but in other studies the abnormality persisted. That the abnormal test may be a trait marker also is suggested by studies showing an increased incidence of blunted responses in first-order relatives of patients with unipolar depression. The mechanism underlying the blunted response is obscure. The abnormality is not due to excess cortisol secretion

676   PSYCHONEUROENDOCRINOLOGY

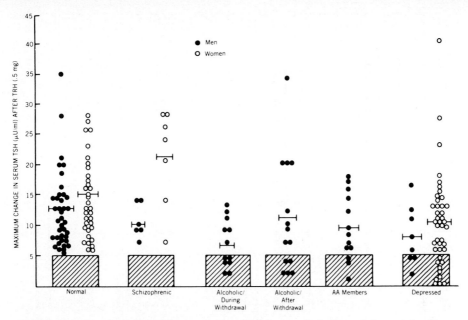

FIGURE 4. TSH responses to TRH in normal, schizophrenic, alcoholic, and depressed subjects. Plotted is maximum TSH increment. The shaded area shows values that were blunted, that is, less and 5 μU/ml, which is the absolute cutoff for the normal group. Note that the mean response was reduced in alcoholic patient at all stages of treatment and recovery and in depressive patients, and that blunting was noted in these groups as well. (From Loosen, PT, and Prange, AJ, Jr,[40] with permission.)

(as was reported at one time), because a number of studies have since shown that abnormal DST or elevated cortisol levels are not correlated with the blunting response. It has been proposed by Loosen and Prange[40] that blunting may be due to chronic hyperstimulation with TRH, that is, a state of chronic hypersecretion of TRH.

In favor of this view is the fact that long continued TRH administration does bring about blunted TRH responses[33] (Fig. 5). In such patients blood levels of T_4 and T_3 are elevated *above the baseline for the patient* but are not elevated into the abnormal range. Hence, one could see blunted TRH responses owing to chronic TRH stimulation without abnormally elevated blood levels of either TSH, T_3, or T_4. Alternative hypotheses are that somatostatin secretion is enhanced in depression (thus inhibiting TSH responsiveness) or that dopamine secretion is increased in the tuberinfundibular dopamine pathways. Although neither hypothesis can be confirmed or excluded, it is of possible relevance that CSF somatostatin is actually decreased in depression.[25,51,58,59] However, the significance of this finding in relation to pituitary regulation is obscure. The incidence of blunted TRH responses is so low (25 percent in most studies) that it is not a useful diagnostic test and is of interest mainly as a research tool. At least one group has proposed that TRH responses can be used as a prognostic tool.

The finding of blunting of TRH-induced TSH response arose as an incidental finding in studies of the effect of TRH on affective state. Prange and colleagues[46] had been studying the effects of thyroid hormones and of TSH in the treatment of depression for several years when TRH was dis-

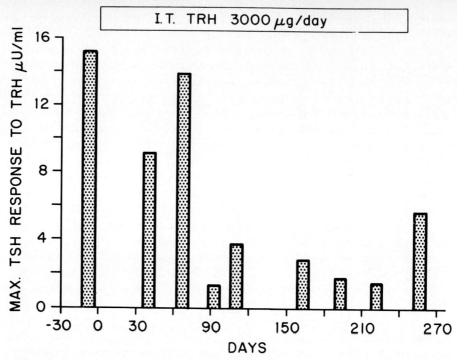

FIGURE 5. Blunting of TSH responses to TRH in a patient receiving sustained infusion of TRH, intrathecally (3000 μg/day) as treatment for amyotrophic lateral sclerosis (ALS). (From Kaplan, et al,[33] with permission.)

covered and became available for clinical testing. It was a logical next step for this group to determine the effect of TRH on affective state, and in their first report they noted that the majority of patients given TRH showed transient psychologic improvement. Similar results were reported almost simultaneously by Kastin and colleagues.[34] Since then a large and controversial literature has evolved,[39,40,45a] variously reporting that some depressed patients (usually a minority of subjects studied) do show some benefit. Treatment has been by subcutaneous injection, intravenous injection, and by mouth, and results are too variable to make a coherent pattern. Whether there are some subgroups that are responsive remains to be proved. Blunting of TRH-induced TSH (see above) does not correlate with reported benefits. At this time, it seems reasonable to conclude that the relationship between TRH abnormalities or responses and depression is too uncertain to have clinical value, and its importance as a tool for understanding the pathophysiology of depression is still unknown. Thyrotropin-releasing hormone does produce significant activation of the sympathetic nervous system in animals and humans; possibly this activating effect could have antidepressant action.

Secretion of GH and PRL in Depression

Extensive studies have been carried out of the neuroendocrine responses of GH and PRL in depression. These have been extensively reviewed.[14,15,50]

In most studies, GH secretion provoked by hypoglycemia shows blunting in depression, but the significance of this finding is qualified by the fact that depressed patients are more resistant to insulin-induced hypoglycemia. One report that controlled for the degree of hypoglycemia still showed that depressive patients had lower responses. Other stimuli to which depressed individuals have lower GH responses are amphetamine, clonidine (an α-adrenergic stimulator), desipramine, serotonin, sleep, and thermal stimulation. On the other hand, responses were normal to L-DOPA and apomorphine. Checkley and Arendt[15] infer from these findings that dopamine receptors are normal in depression but that there may be an abnormality in α-adrenergic responsiveness, but they emphasize the reservations that must be made in interpretation of data of this type.

A few depressed patients show a paradoxical increase in GH following TRH administration (in contrast to the normal patient, in whom GH levels do not rise after TRH). Other conditions in which GH responds paradoxically to TRH are malnutrition, anorexia nervosa, and somatotrope hyperplasia owing to sustained hyperstimulation with growth hormone releasing factor (GHRH) (as in the ectopic GHRH syndrome) (see chapter 8).

Prolactin regulation in depression has not been adequately studied in a controlled manner, but the bulk of experiments that have been done fail to show any consistent abnormalities in 24-hour secretory patterns, or responses to pharmacologic agents, or to TRH. Prolactin levels were normal in a series of patients with mild depression tested in an outpatient setting.[1]

Abnormalities in Melatonin Secretion in Depression

Melatonin, the principal secretion of the pineal gland, is normally secreted mainly at night in response to lights out. Because of a growing interest in the role of external lighting on affective state (see chapter 10), there has been a corresponding interest in possible abnormalities in melatonin secretion in depression. The controversial literature on this topic is discussed by Rubin and Pollard,[50] and the possible neuropharmacologic basis of these effects have been reviewed by Brown and colleagues.[6,7]

PSYCHONEUROENDOCRINOLOGY OF SCHIZOPHRENIA

In contrast to the depressive disorders in which a number of endocrine abnormalities can be demonstrated, there are few convincing reports of abnormal endocrine function in this disease. These studies are summarized by Meltzer[42] and by Davis and colleagues.[20] Among the secretions found to be normal are 24-hour secretory patterns of GH, GH response to dopamine receptor stimulation with apomorphine, response to d-amphetamine, and insulin-induced hypoglycemia; most also show normal nocturnal secretion. Schizophrenics have been reported to show paradoxical GH responses to TRH and to GnRH. It is almost impossible for a normal person to drink oneself into a state of water intoxication, but 47 such cases in schizophrenic persons were reported by Smith and Clark.[55] Twelve of the 47 were not taking any drugs that could have caused the syndrome of inappropriate antidiuretic hormone (ADH) secretion. There has been much interest in PRL secretion in schizophrenics because of the fact that the principal antipsychotic drugs are dopamine antagonists, and because the TIDA system secretes dopamine, which inhibits PRL secretion. Reasons for questioning the possible relevance of PRL secretion to mesolimbic dopamine function are discussed above, and, indeed, little useful information has come from study of basal PRL secretion or responses to dopamine agonists — the bulk of results suggesting that there is little or no abnormality in any of these functions.

Pituitary-gonadal secretion may be reduced in schizophrenia, but the roles of chronic hospitalization, chronic illness, and lack of psychosexual stimulation have not been adequately controlled.

ANOREXIA NERVOSA

Anorexia is a severe psychiatric disorder characterized by an intense fear of becoming obese and a preoccupation with body image and food intake. It can be associated with severe symptoms of depression and anxiety and with compulsive eating behavior (bulimia). It is usually accompanied by endocrine disturbances and has an appreciable mortality — the highest of any psychiatric disease. The disease appears to arise in a context of social pressure for slimness and intense intrafamilial conflicts. It is notoriously difficult to treat. Anorexia nervosa, though primarily a psychologic disease, is always considered in textbooks of medicine and endocrinology because of the profound medical disturbances in this condition which often dominate the picture, and because of the historical fact that this disease (recognized clinically by Sir William Gull) was for many years confused with hypopituitarism with which it shares many features in common. In fact, the first description of hypopituitarism and cachexia in postpartum pituitary infarction by Simmonds now appears in retropect to have been that of a case of anorexia nervosa. This disorder has been extensively reviewed.[7,8,18,21,24,28,48,60]

Diagnostic criteria of anorexia nervosa have been published in the *Diagnostic and Statistical Manual of Mental Disorders*, volume III, published by the American Psychiatric Association, Washington, DC, 1980. They are:

1. Intense fear of becoming obese, which does not diminish as weight loss progresses.
2. Disturbance of body image, e.g., claiming to "feel fat" even when emaciated.
3. Weight loss of at least 25 percent of original body weight or if under 18 years of age, weight loss from original body weight plus weight gain expected from growth charts may be combined to make the 25 percent.
4. Refusal to maintain body weight over a minimal normal weight for age and height.
5. No known physical illness that would account for the weight loss.

Anorexia nervosa is largely a disease of women in their "teens" and twenties, but about 5 percent of cases occur in boys and men, and the disorder can begin before puberty and persist into maturity. Because depression and anxiety may occur in anorexia nervosa, there may be diagnostic confusion with the eating disturbance that occurs in patients with depression or in psychoneurosis. However, the distinction is usually easy to make because the eating disturbance in anorexia nervosa is so severe and so pervasive that it dominates the clinical picture.

Societal factors predispose to this disorder. It is much more common in caucasians and individuals of the higher socioeconomic class, and the norm of beauty in Western society puts a premium on thinness in its models. This view is epitomized in the statement that, "one can never be too rich or too thin." There is evidence that the frequency of anorexia nervosa is increasing in Western society; an incidence of between 1 and 3 percent has been cited, but it is much higher in some populations. If one encounters anorexia nervosa in a male patient, it is more likely that the person will have a typical disease with prominent psychologic disturbance, including schizoid or other psychotic features.

A common sequence of events in the onset of the disease has been outlined by Crisp[18] (Fig. 6). In early adolescence, the teenager finds herself gaining weight (a common occurrence that is due to early secretion of estrogens which promote fat deposition in areas of secondary sex characteristics, that is, buttocks, abdomen, breasts). The adolescent goes on a diet and does not stop when ideal body weight is reached. The disturbed feeding mechanism, combined with a distorted body image, may persist, waxing and waning throughout the patient's life, or it may be resolved after a single episode.

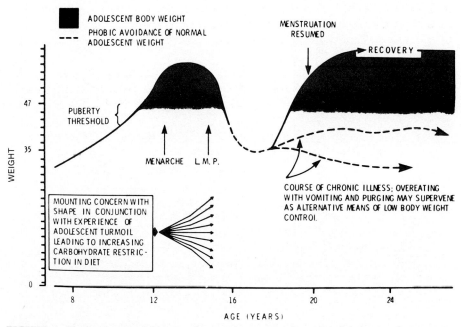

FIGURE 6. Idealized natural history of anorexia nervosa. In early adolescence, the teenager finding herself gaining weight (a common occurrence that is due to developing estrogen secretion) goes on a diet and does not stop when ideal body weight is reached. The disturbed feeding mechanism combined with a distorted body image may persist, waxing and waning throughout the patient's life, may be resolved after a single episode, or may terminate fatally. (From Crisp,[18] with permission).

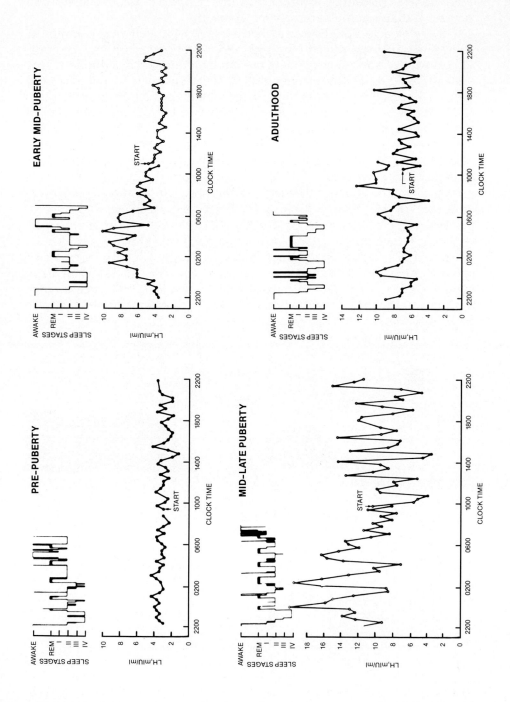

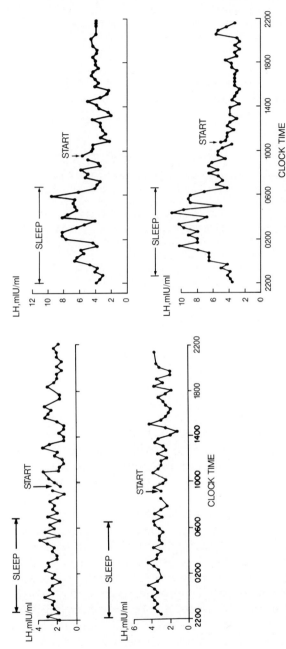

FIGURE 7. (*Top*) Age-related changes in the secretory patterns of luteinizing hormone (LH) to show stages associated with changes in maturation. The upper left panel shows the low and modest pulsations in a prepubertal girl. The upper right panel shows the increased amplitude of nocturnal pulses in a girl in early puberty, progressing through striking pulsatile secretions both during the day and the night at mid-late puberty (*lower left panel*). Finally, the adult pattern (*lower right panel*) shows relatively high amplitude pulses during the night and low amplitude pulses during the day. These normal stages are to be compared with patterns in patients with anorexia nervosa (see below). (*Bottom*) Patterns of gonadotropin secretion in two women with anorexia nervosa compared with normal secretory patterns in younger women. The curves on the *left* show the pattern in a 21-year-old patient with anorexia nervosa (*upper curve*) and the normal pattern in a 9-year-old (*lower curve*). The curves on the *right* compare the pattern in a 17-year-old woman with anorexia nervosa (*upper curve*) and the normal pattern in a 12-year-old pubertal girl (*lower curve*). (From Katz, JL, Boyar, RM, Weiner, H, et al: *Toward an elucidation of the psychoneuroendocrinology of anorexia nervosa.* In Sachar, EJ (ed): *Hormones, Behaviour and Psychopathology.* Raven Press, New York, 1978, pp 263–283, with permission.)

The psychologic setting of the disease is very important, and different workers have formulated this in different terms.

> "Factors within the patient include a strong need for perfection and control, masking a sense of overall helplessness, and perceptual and conceptual disturbances. A confused sense of autonomy and identity appears to be at the root of the psychopathology. The patients feels a lack of self-control and a sense of personal mistrust of her body, and experiences conflict regarding her identity."[21]

This may be caused by a combination of constitutional factors and those learned from early parent-daughter interactions. It has been suggested that disturbances in body image and disturbances in the recognition of internal visceral and affective states are closely related to these general feelings of ineffectiveness.[24]

> "The psychodynamics are not clear and in fact may not be fixed. Whatever other factors operate in the genesis of the disease, the families tend to be 'enmeshed'; there are blurred generational boundaries so that parents and children are constantly involved in each other's problems. Some workers suggest that both major eating disorders — anorexia nervosa and obesity — have as fundamental characteristic a paralysing sense of ineffectiveness induced by early events in family life. Subjects experience themselves as acting only in response to demands coming from others, and as not doing anything because they want to. The family structure of bulemic subjects has a higher prevalance of affective disorders, alcoholism and drug use than is the case with classic anorexia nervosa."[21]

Hormonal Disturbances in Anorexia Nervosa

The most common endocrine disturbance in this disorder is amenorrhea secondary to GnRH deficiency, although minor degrees of gonadotropin failure can give rise to anovulation or irregular periods. The amenorrhea initially begins in most cases as part of the hypothalamic disturbance that is part of the syndrome. In approximately 10 percent, amenorrhea precedes, and in about 50 percent amenorrhea accompanies, the first signs of the disorder. In the remainder, amenorrhea ensues when malnutrition has become severe. Twenty-four hour gonadotropin patterns of anorexic patients show a reversion to a more immature cyclic pattern or, if severe, to complete loss of gonadal stimulation (Fig. 7).

The final common pathway for neuroendocrine abnormality in anorexia nervosa (and other forms of hypothalamic amenorrhea) appears to lie in the arcuate nucleus of the hypothalamus.[36] Lesions of this nucleus in the rhesus monkey lead to marked suppression of gonadotropin secretion, which can be restored to normal by administration of repetitive pulses of GnRH corresponding in time to the normal spontaneous rhythm of GnRH release. Because malnutrition per se can cause amenorrhea, there has been some confusion as to the role of psychogenic factors in the amenorrhea as compared with amenorrhea secondary to anorexia-induced malnutrition. Both factors do play a role after the disorder has been established, and menses will not return until malnutrition has been rectified. The interaction between nutrition and amenorrhea has been well demonstrated by Frisch and colleagues, who have shown that the onset of menses (in development) coincides with the attainment of a critical weight, which is a function of fat storage (see also chapter 9). In some way, body fat depots can determine hypothalamic function; in this instance, the secretion of GnRH.

Although gonadotropin failure in anorexia nervosa is due to GnRH deficiency, pituitary responses to GnRH range from none to normal, depending upon the severity of the disease.

It is reasonably certain that the impaired GnRH responsiveness and restoration to normal when weight is regained is due to the effects of GnRH deficiency on pituitary responsiveness, presumably through changes in GnRH receptors, because repeated doses of GnRH can restore responsivity to normal even when weight remains low. The suppression of GnRH may be due to excessive endogenous opioid activity, because it can be reversed in some cases by administration of naloxone, an opioid antagonist.[47]

The role of gonadal deficiency in the course of anorexia nervosa has not been determined. In one study, pregnancies induced by gonadotropins led to reversal of the disease in two out of three cases.

The other endocrine disturbances in anorexia nervosa are secondary to malnutrition (Table 1). These include low T_3, elevated reverse T_3, marginally low T_4, elevated GH levels, exaggerated ACTH response to metyrapone, elevated basal levels of cortisol, normal prolactin, and paradoxical GH release to TRH. Patients with severe anorexia have an apparent difficulty in excreting a water load, now shown by Gold and colleagues[26] to be due to inappropriate secretion of ADH (see chapter 4) (Fig. 8). This appears to be a marker of state, inasmuch as it clears following restitution of weight to normal. It likely is a consequence of malnutrition.

Other evidence of hypothalamic disorder has been reported in this disorder, including difficulties in thermoregulation in response to either excessive heat or cold. Patients show marked peripheral vasoconstriction (cold hands and feet) with reddish purple discoloration of extremities

TABLE 1. Endocrine Findings in Normal Women and in Patients with Anorexia Nervosa and with Simple Weight Loss

Item Tested	Patients with Simple Weight Loss	Patients with Anorexia Nervosa
GH	↑	↑
PRL	NI*	NI
TSH	NI	NI
LH	NI	↓
FSH	↓	↓
Cortisol	NI	NI
Free thyroxine	NI	NI
3,5,3'-Tri-iodothyronine	↓	↓
LH response to GnRH	Late peak	Later peak
FSH response to GnRH	NI	Late peak
TSH response to TRH	Late peak	Later peak
PRL response to TRH	NI	Late peak
Rate of change in core temperature	↓	↓

(From Warren, MP: *Effects of undernutrition on reproductive function in the human.* Endocr Rev 4:363–377, 1983.)
*Normal.

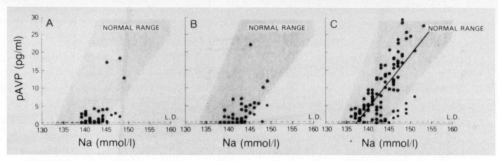

FIGURE 8. Impaired clearance of water and regulation of vasopressin secretion in anorexia nervosa. This figure illustrates changes in serum arginine vasopressin levels as a function of blood sodium in a group of patients with anorexia nervosa who have been infused with intravenous saline. The normal range of responses is shown in the shaded areas. *(A)* Response in patients with active disease, *(B)* partially recovered, and *(C)* recovered patients. It is clear that patients with active disease have a form of physiologic diabetes insipidus. (From Gold, PW, et al,[26] with permission.)

owing to venous pooling of blood. The possible central neurotransmitter abnormalities are reviewed by Liebowitz.[38]

Differentiation from Hypopituitarism

In most cases the clinical history permits a distinction between amenorrhea of pituitary disease and anorexia nervosa. In addition, maintenance of adrenal function in the anorexic patient leads to retention of normal axillary and pubic hair. The anorexic person shows an increased amount of lanugo type body hair (in contrast to hypopituitarism, in which it is lost).

Treatment

The treatment of anorexia nervosa is extremely unsatisfactory, and measures directed at the eating disorder itself are usually futile. This includes

TABLE 2. General Principles of Treatment of Anorexia Nervosa

1. It is preferable to hospitalize patients for initial treatment; the usual period is six to eight weeks.
2. The immediate aim is to induce weight gain; psychotherapy is of little benefit until nutritional status has improved.
3. The patient should never eat alone; food must be taken in the company of a nurse or with groups of patients and staff.
4. It is preferable to have a single staff person ("special") carry out primary interactions with the patient.
5. The support staff should be friendly and reassuring about the "safety" of eating, but lengthy intellectualizing about food and weight should be avoided.
6. Parenteral or enteral nutrition should be prescribed only as a life-saving measure; hyperalimentation is never indicated as a primary treatment.
7. Caloric intake should be increased gradually over seven to ten days from 1000 calories to a level twice that of a normal adult (3000 to 5000 calories, depending on size).
8. Psychoactive drugs should be used if needed for depression or anxiety.
9. As nutritional status improves, social therapy should be initiated (arts, crafts, games).
10. Parental involvement should be started early either as family units (patient and family) or in groups of involved parents.
11. Following discharge the patient should be seen at least biweekly for support and guidance.

(From Foster, DW,[21] with permission.)

PSYCHONEUROENDOCRINOLOGY

hormonal treatments such as insulin, thyroid hormone, and appetite stimulants. Similarly ineffective are tranquilizers and antipsychotic measures, antidepressants, and electroconvulsive therapy. The essential features of therapy now advocated are urgent attention to physical state in order to avoid fatal malnutrition (which can terminate in cardiac arrhythmia), psychotherapy and behavioral modification, and family counseling. Foster[21] has formulated a useful table setting forth the basic tenets of management (Table 2). However, it is a regrettable fact that long-term followup shows that therapy is not highly successful. In one series of 100 patients, only 64 attained and maintained normal weight (over 4 to 7 years), 18 were improved, 14 were below pubertal weight, and 2 had died. In another series, 6 percent were dead. Between 50 and 75 percent of patients resume normal menses, but more than half continue to have psychologic difficulties even when their weight has been returned to normal.

BULIMIA

Bulimia is defined as compulsive gorging, sometimes associated with anorexia nervosa (preceding it, following it, alternating with it), usually accompanied by efforts to lose weight by forced vomiting and cathartic abuse.[21,28] Cathartic abuse and vomiting can lead to profound, even fatal, electrolyte abnormalities with hypokalemia, hyponatremia, and volume contraction. In a series of 40 patients cited by Foster,[21] "the mean duration of gorging was 1.2 hours but could last as long as eight hours. On average gorging occurred 12 times a week, but the range was from as few as one to as many as 46 times. The mean number of calories ingested per episode was 3415 but could reach 11,500 at one sitting." Gorging is carried out in private. Individuals may steal food, and this kind of behavior bears many resemblances to the behavior of alcoholics. Bulimic patients have been called foodaholics. Once they have begun to eat (usually a carbohydrate-rich meal), they will eat compulsively until the episode is terminated by enormous satiety and a sense of guilt. Unless accompanied by anorexia, bulimics usually do not have abnormalities in endocrine function. Treatment is mainly behavioral and psychiatric.

Other psychogenic disorders of gonadotropin secretion are considered in chapter 9.

PSYCHONEUROIMMUNOLOGY, NEUROIMMUNOLOGY, AND IMMUNONEUROENDOCRINOLOGY

Along with the nervous and endocrine systems, the immune system is one of the three major integrating and adaptive systems in higher organisms. Immunocompetent cells, such as particular classes of lymphocytes, bear cell surface receptors that endow them with the ability to recognize foreign molecules such as toxins, constituents of infectious organisms, and nonself tissues (including neoplasms).[78] In response to these molecules, these cells secrete an extraordinary range of peptide and protein substances whose function it is to neutralize, to inactivate, and to sequester these external materials. These secretions include the immunoglobulins and *lymphokines.*

brain hormones that reach the blood directly may also modify immune responses.[81] An extensive literature has grown up detailing the effects of most of these compounds on various elements of the immune reaction.[81,83] Unfortunately, these findings have not been integrated into a comprehensive model of neuroimmunomodulation and applied to specific clinical situations to date. Even if it can be shown that endocrine secretions can influence the immune response, it still remains to be shown that in specific psychologic states, characteristic patterns of hormone secretion are manifest and that they are of a magnitude sufficient to influence immune functions.

IMMUNONEUROENDOCRINOLOGY

Starting with the initial premise that neuroendocrine regulation of the pituitary gland, generally speaking, usually involves some form of feedback mechanism, several investigators have proposed that lymphokines secreted during the immune response may in turn exert effects on the hypothalamus and pituitary gland. For example, Besedowsky and colleagues[74,75] have shown that during the process of immunization, a characteristic pattern of hypothalamic-pituitary-adrenal response is elicited, which conceivably could be part of a feedback immunoregulatory circuit to moderate the exuberance of inflammation. Among the candidate regulators is Interleukin-1, (IL-1, endogenous pyrogen) released from pyrogen-activated lymphocytes, which has been shown to stimulate the release of ACTH and secondarily of adrenal corticoids.[75] IL-1 has been shown to act directly on the pituitary to release ACTH, but its possible effects on hypothalamic regulation of releasing factors have not been determined. It is known that IL-1 activates prostaglandin generation in hypothalamic and cerebral cortical slices (a mechanism presumed to be crucial to fever induction).[79] On the other hand, as noted below, Newcastle virus activated leukocytes in the mouse have been shown to contain biologic activities that resemble both ACTH and corticotropin-releasing factor (CRF).[76,86,87] These findings indicate that there are several mechanisms by which activated lymphocytes could modulate hypothalamic-pituitary function. They also have been interpreted to mean that the peripheral lymphocyte system has the ability to sense foreign molecules and to communicate this information to the neuroendocrine system.

Blalock and colleagues[76] and others have carried out extensive studies of the secretion of neuropeptides and pituitary hormones by activated lymphocytes. They have, for example, reported that Newcastle virus invasion of leukocytes in the mouse leads to the formation of ACTH-like peptides, detectable by immunocytochemistry, demonstrable by bioassay, and capable of maintaining adrenal function in hypophysectomized animals.[82,85,87] In addition, they report that activated leukocytes secrete a compound indistinguishable from CRF, and that other secretory products of monocytes, for example, hepatocyte-stimulating factor, are at least as potent as CRF itself.[89] Moreover, these effects on ACTH release are inhibited by glucocorticoids such as dexamethasone. On the basis of this finding, these workers propose that in parallel with the hypothalamic-pituitary-adrenal axis there is a lymphocyte-pituitary-adrenal axis. Receptors for both

CRF and dexamethasone have been identified in lymphocytes. Production of ACTH-like peptides by lymphocytes reportedly are increased by exposure to CRF.

A possible clinical example of this phenomenon was reported in a patient with the ectopic ACTH syndrome thought to be due to inflammatory tissue.[76] It should be recalled that in sarcoidosis, a disease characterized by formation of foci of granulomas, hypersecretion of 1,25-dihydroxy-Vit D is the consequence of excessive, uncontrolled conversion of its precursor by the mass of lymphocytes.

Delineation of a lymphocyte-pituitary-adrenal axis has led Blalock and colleagues and others to search for other classical hormones and hormone receptors in lymphocytes. They have reported that lymphocyte extracts contain, in addition to ACTH-like substances, other factors that cross-react with antisera to TSH, endorphins, chorionic gonadotropin, GH, FSH, and LH. They propose that "the immune and neuroendocrine systems represent a totally integrated circuit by virtue of sharing a common set of hormones."[76]

It is still too early to draw firm conclusions from these studies. The physiologic relevance of the observation of generation of hormones by lymphocytes, and neuroendocrine effects of classical lymphokines, remains to be demonstrated, especially in the human being. It has been shown that Interleukin-2, for example, brings about the release of cortisol, PRL, and GH in the human being,[70] but these may be nonspecific stress effects. Nevertheless, the concept that the lymphocyte system constitutes a potent sensory organ, capable of responding to the antigen milieu and signaling appropriate homestatic responses is an exciting one.

Perhaps the most surprising of the suggestions of overlap has been that immune responses may act directly to mediate or to induce sleep. Isolation from human urine of a slow-wave sleep-inducing peptide, called muramyl peptide (known to be a monomer of bacterial cell-wall material), has been followed by the observation that the peptide can also stimulate macrophages to release IL-1 and prostaglandin E_2 and that these substances also are capable of inducing slow-wave sleep when introduced intraventricularly. Karnovsky describes evidence that such immune modulators may be important in the regulation of sleep.[90] There is preliminary evidence that muramyl peptides may compete with serotonin at receptors on macrophages and by extrapolation at sites in the CNS.

REFERENCES

1. ARANA, GW, BALDESSARINI, RJ, ORNSTEEN, M: *The dexamethasone suppression test for diagnosis and prognosis in psychiatry.* Arch Gen Psychiatry 42:1193–1204, 1985.
2. ARANA, GW, WILENS, TE, BALDESSARINI, RJ: *Plasma corticosterone and cortisol following dexamethasone in psychiatric patients.* Psychoneuroendocrinology 10:49–60, 1985.
3. BERNARD, C: *Leçons de physiologie experimentale appliqués a la mèdicine* (2 vols). J. B. Balliére, Paris, 1855–1856.
4. BOYD, AE, AND REICHLIN, S: *Neural control of prolactin secretion in man.* Psychoneuroendocrinology 3:113–130, 1978.
5. BROWN, GM, SEGGIE, JA, CHAMBERS, JW, ETTIGI, PG: *Psychoendocrinology and growth hormone: A review.* Psychoneuroendocrinology 3:131–153, 1978.
6. BROWN, GM, AND NILES, LP: *Studies on melatonin and other pineal factors.* In BESSER, GM, AND MARTINI, L (EDS): *Clinical Neuroendocrinology,* vol 2. Academic Press, New York, 1982, pp 205–265.

7. BROWN, GM, GARFINKEL, PE, GROF, E, GROF, OM, CLEGHORN, JM, BROWN, P: *A critical appraisal of neuroendocrine approaches to psychiatric disorders.* In MÜLLER, EE, AND MACLEOD, RM (EDS): *Neuroendocrine Perspectives.* Elsevier, Amsterdam, 1983, p 329–364.

8. BROWN, GM, KOSLOW, SH, REICHLIN, S: *Neuroendocrinology and psychiatric disorder.* Raven Press, New York, 1984.

9. CANNON, WB: *Bodily changes in pain, hunger, fear and rage. An account of researches into the function of emotional excitement,* Harper, New York, 1929. (Reprinted 1963).

10. CARROLL, BJ, FEINBERG, M, GREDEN, JF, TARIKA, J, ALBALA, AA, HOSLETT, RF, JAMES, NM, KRONFOL, Z, LOHR, N, STEINER, M, deVIGNE, TP, YOUNG, E: *A specific laboratory test for the diagnosis of melancholia.* Arch Gen Psychiatry 38:15–22, 1981.

11. CARROLL, BJ: *Dexamethasone suppression test: A review of contemporary confusion.* J Clin Psychiatry 46:13–24, 1985.

12. CARROLL, BJ: *The dexamethasone suppression test for melancholia.* Br J Psych 140:292–304, 1982.

13. CARROLL, BJ: *In discussion: Affective disorders-endocrine features.* In BROWN, GM, KOSLOW, SH, REICHLIN, S (EDS): *Neuroendocrinology and Affective Disorder.* Raven Press, New York, 1984, p 228.

14. CHECKLEY, SC: *Endocrine changes in psychiatric illness.* In BESSER, GM, AND MARTINI, L (EDS): *Clinical Neuroendocrinology,* vol 2. Academic Press, New York, 1982, p 226–282.

15. CHECKLEY, S, AND ARENDT, J: *Pharmacoendocrine studies of GH, PRL, and melatonin in patients with affective illness.* In BROWN, GW, KOSLOW, SH, REICHLIN, S (EDS): *Neuroendocrinology and Psychiatric disorder.* Raven Press, New York, 1984, pp 115–190.

16. COWDRY, RW, WEHR, TA, ZIS, AP, GOODWIN, FK: *Thyroid abnormalities associated with rapid-cycling bipolar illness.* Arch Gen Psychiatry 40:411–420, 1983.

17. CREESE, I, BURT, DR, SNYDER, SH: *Dopamine receptor binding predicts clinical and pharmacological potencies of antischizophrenic drugs.* Science 192:481–483, 1976.

18. CRISP, AH: *Some aspects of the evolution, presentation, and follow-up of anorexia nervosa.* Proc Roy Soc Med 58:814, 1965.

19. CZEISLER, CA, EDE, MC, REGESTEIN, QR, ET AL: *Episodic 24-hour cortisol secretory patterns in patients awaiting elective cardiac surgery.* J Clin Endocrinol Metab 42:273–283, 1976.

20. DAVIS, JM, VOGEL, C, GIBBONS, R, PAVKOCIC, I, ZHANG, M: *Pharmacoendocrinology of schizophrenia.* In BROWN, GM, KOSLOW, SH, REICHLIN, S (EDS): *Neuroendocrinology and Psychiatric Disorder.* Raven Press, New York, 1984, pp 29–54.

21. FOSTER DW: *Eating disorders: Obesity and anorexia nervosa.* In *Williams Textbook of Endocrinology,* ed 7. WB Saunders, Philadelphia, 1985, pp 1081–1107.

22. FROHMAN, LA: *Evaluation of neuropharmacologic strategies in schizophrenia.* In BROWN, GM, KOSLOW, SH, REICHLIN, S (EDS): *Psychoneuroendocrinology and Psychiatric Disorder.* Raven Press, New York, 1984, pp 67–74.

23. GANONG, WF: *Neurotransmitter mechanisms underlying stress responses.* In BROWN, GM, KOSLOW, SH, REICHLIN, S (EDS): *Neuroendocrinology and Psychiatric Disorder.* Raven Press, New York, 1984, pp 133–144.

24. GARFINKEL, PE: *Anorexia nervosa: An overview of hypothalamic-pituitary function.* In BROWN, GM, KOSLOW, SH, REICHLIN, S (EDS): *Neuroendocrinology and Psychiatric Disorder.* Raven Press, New York, 1984, pp 301–314.

25. GERNER, RH, YAMADA, T: *Altered neuropeptide concentrations in cerebrospinal fluid of psychiatric patients.* Brain Res 238(1):298–302, 1982.

26. GOLD, PW, KAYE, W, ROBERTSON, GL, EBERT, M: *Abnormalities in plasma and cerebrospinal fluid arginine vasopressin in patients with anorexia nervosa.* N Engl J Med 308:117–1123, 1983.

27. GREENE, WA, CONRON, G, SCHALCH, DS, ET AL: *Psychological correlates of growth hormone and adrenal secretory responses of patients undergoing cardiac catheterization.* Psychosom Med 32:599–614, 1970.

28. HERZOG, DB, AND COPELAND, PM: *Eating Disorders.* N Engl J Med 313:295–303, 1985.

29. HIRSCHFELD, RMA, KOSLOW, SH, KUPFER, DJ: *Clinical utility of the dexamethasone test.* US Department of Health and Human Services, Public Health Service, Alcohol, Drug Abuse, and Mental Health Administration, National Institute of Mental Health, Rockville, Maryland.

30. HIRSCHFELD, RMA, KOSLOW, SH, KUPFER, DJ: *The clinical utility of the dexamethasone suppression test in psychiatry.* JAMA 250:2172–2174, 1983.

31. HÖKFELT, T, FAHRENKRUG, J, TATEMOTO, K, MUTT, I, WERNER, S, HULTING, AL, TERENIUS, L, CHANG, KJ: *The PHI (PHI-27)/corticotropin-releasing factor/enkephalin immunoreactive hypothalamic neuron: Possible morphological basis for integrated control of prolactin, corticotropin, and growth hormone secretion.* Proc Natl Acad Sci USA 80:895–899, 1983.

32. HOU, S: *Syndrome of inappropriate antidiuretic hormone secretion.* In REICHLIN, S (ED): *The Neurohypophysis.* Plenum, 1984, pp 165–189.

33. KAPLAN, MM, TAFT, JA, REICHLIN, S, MUNSAT, TL: *Sustained rises in serum thyrotropin, thyrox-*

ine and triiodothyronine during long term, continuous thyrotropin-releasing hormone treatment in patients with amyotrophic lateral sclerosis. J Clin Endocrinol Metab 63:808–814, 1986.

34. KASTIN, AJ, EHRENSING, RH, SCHALCH, DS, ANDERSON, MS: *Improvement in mental depression with decreased thyrotropin response after administration of thyrotropin-releasing hormone.* Lancet II: 740–742, 1972.

35. KENDALL, JW: *Pituitary-adrenocortical dysfunction in severe depressive illness.* In BROWN, GM, KOSLOW, SH, REICHLIN, S (ED): *Neuroendocrinology and Psychiatric Disorder.* Raven Press, New York, 1984, pp 201–208.

36. KREY, LC: *Neuronal and endocrine mechanisms involved in the control of gonadotropin secretion.* In BROWN, GM, KOSLOW, SH, REICHLIN, S (EDS): *Neuroendocrinology and Psychiatric Disorder.* Raven Press, New York, 1984, pp 325–338.

37. LEVENE, S: *Stress (discussion):* In BROWN, GM, KOSLOW, SH, REICHLIN, S (EDS): *Neuroendocrinology and Psychiatric Disorder.* Raven Press, New York, 1984, pp 145–150.

38. LIEBOWITZ, SF: *Brain monoamine projections and receptor systems in relation to food intake, diet preference, meal patterns, and body weight.* In BROWN, GM, KOSLOW, SH, REICHLIN, S (EDS): *Neuroendocrinology and Psychiatric Disorder.* Raven Press, New York, 1984, pp 383–400.

39. LOOSEN, PT: *The TRH-induced TSH response in psychiatric patients: A possible neuroendocrine marker.* Psychoneuroendocrinology 10:237–260, 1985.

40. LOOSEN, PT, AND PRANGE, AJ: *Serum thyrotropin response to thyrotropin-releasing hormone in psychiatric patients.* Am J Psych 139:405–416, 1982.

41. MASON, JW: *A review of psychoendocrine research on the pituitary adrenal cortical system.* Psychosom Med 30:576–607, 1968.

42. MELTZER, HY: *Neuroendocrine abnormalities in schizophrenia: Prolactin, growth hormone and gonadotropins.* In BROWN, GM, KOSLOW, SH, REICHLIN, S (EDS): *Neuroendocrinology and Psychiatric Disorder.* Raven Press, New York, 1984, pp 1–28.

43. MOORE, KE, AND DEMAREST, KT: *Prolactin secretion and dopaminergic neurons: An evaluation of neuropharmacologic strategies.* In BROWN, GM, KOSLOW, SH, REICHLIN, S (EDS): *Psychoneuroendocrinology and Psychiatric Disorders.* Raven Press, New York, 1984, pp 75–84.

44. MORLEY, JE, AND SHAFER, RF: *Thyroid function screening in new psychiatric admissions.* Arch Intern Med 142:591–593, 1982.

45. MUNCK, A, GUYRE, PM, HOLBROOK, NJ: *Physiological functions of glucocorticoids in stress and their relation to pharmacological actions.* Endo Rev 5:25–44, 1984.

46. PRANGE, AJ, WILSON, IC, LARA, PP, ALLTOP, LB, BREESE, GR: *Effects of thyrotropin releasing hormone in depression.* Lancet II: 999–1002, 1972.

47. QUIGLEY, ME: *Hypothalamic inhibitory influences on gonadotropin secretion in normal cycling and hypogonadotropic amenorrheic women.* In BROWN, GM, KOSLOW, SH, REICHLIN, S (EDS): *Neuroendocrinology and Psychiatric Disorder.* Raven Press, New York, 1984, pp 357–370.

48. ROSE, RM: *Psychoneuroendocrinology.* In WILSON, JD, AND FOSTER, DW (EDS): *Williams Textbook of Endocrinology,* ed 7. WB Saunders, Philadelphia, 1985, pp 653–681.

49. ROSE, RM: *Overview of endocrinology of stress.* In BROWN, GM, KOSLOW, SH, REICHLIN, S (EDS): *Neuroendocrinology and Psychiatric Disorder.* Raven Press, New York, 1984, pp 95–122.

50. RUBIN, RT, AND POLAND, RE: *The chronoendocrinology of endogenous depression.* In MÜLLER, EE, AND MACLEOD, RM (EDS): *Neuroendocrine Perspectives.* Elsevier Amsterdam, 1982, pp 305–338.

51. RUBINOW, DR, GOLD, PW, POST, RM, ET AL: *CSF somatostatin in affective illness.* Arch Gen Psych 40:409–412, 1983.

52. SACHAR, EJ, *Hormonal changes in stress and mental illness.* In KRIEGER, DT, AND HUGHES, JC (EDS): *Neuroendocrinology.* Sinauer Associates, Sutherland, MA, 1980, pp 177–183.

53. SACHAR, EJ: *Neuroendocrine abnormalities in depressive illness.* In SACHAR, EJ (ED): *Topics in Psychoendocrinology.* Grune & Stratton, New York, 1975, pp 135–156.

54. SELYE, H: *General adaption syndrome and disease of adaption.* J Clin Endocrin Met 6:117–230, 1946.

55. SMITH, CK, ET AL: *Psychiatric disturbance in endocrinologic disease.* Psychosom Med 34:69–86, 1972.

56. SPRATT, DI, PONT, A, MILLER, MB, ET AL: *Hyperthyroxinemia in patients with acute psychiatric disorders.* Am J Med 73:41–48, 1982.

57. STOCKIGT, JR: *Euthyroid hyperthyroxinemia.* Thyroid Today 7:1–7, 1984.

58. THORNER, MO, AND EVANS, WS: *Is prolactin a marker for brain dopamine function?* In BROWN, GH, KOSLOW, SH, REICHLIN, S (EDS): *Neuroendocrinology and Psychiatric Disorder.* Raven Press, New York, 1984, pp 55–66.

59. URSIN, H, AND MURISON, RCC: *Classification and description of stress.* In BROWN, GM, KOSLOW, SH, REICHLIN, S (EDS): *Neuroendocrinology and Psychiatric Disorder.* Raven Press, New York, 1984, p 123.

60. VIGERSKY, RA, LORIAUX, DL, ANDERSON, AE, ET AL: *Anorexia nervosa: Behavioral and hypothalamic aspects.* Clin Endocrin Metab 5:517–535, 1976.

61. LANGER, G, SACHAR, EJ, GRUEN, PH, HALPERN, FS: *Human prolactin responses to neuroleptic*

drugs correlate with antischizophrenic potency. Nature 266:639–648, 1977.

62. NESSE, RM, CURTIS, GC, BROWN, GW, RUBIN, RT: *Anxiety induced by flooding therapy for phobias does not elicit prolactin secretory response.* Psychosom Med 42:25–31, 1980.

63. PRANGE, A, JR, NEMEROFF, CB, LOOSEN, PT, BISSETTE, G, OSBAHR, A, III, WILSON, IC, LIPTON, MS: *Behavioral effects of thyrotropin-releasing hormone in animals and man: A review.* In COLLU, R, BARBEAU, A, DUCHARME, JR, ROCHEFORT, JG (EDS): *Central nervous system effects of hypothalamic hormones and other peptides.* Raven Press, New York, 1979, pp 75–96.

64. WYLLIE, E, LUDERS, H, MACMILLAN, JP, ET AL: *Serum prolactin levels after epileptic seizures.* Neurology 34:1601–1604, 1984.

65. NEMEROFF, CB, WALSH, TJ, BISSETTE, G: *Somatostatin and behavior: Preclinical and clinical studies.* In REICHLIN, S (ED): *Somatostatin: Fourth International Symposium.* Plenum, New York (in press).

66. BISSETTE, G, WIDERLOV, E, WALLEUS, J, KARLSSON, I, EKLUND, K, FORSMAN, A, NEMEROFF, CB: *Alterations in cerebrospinal fluid concentrations of somatostatin-like immunoreactivity in neuropsychiatric disorders.* Arch Gen Psychiatr (in press).

67. RUBINAW, DR. In REICHLIN, S (ED): *Fourth International Symposium on Somatostatin.* Plenum, New York (in press).

68. ADER, R: *Behaviorally conditioned modulation of immunity.* In GUILLEMIN, R, COHN, M, MELNUCHUK, T (EDS): *Neural Modulation of Immunity.* Raven Press, New York, 1985, pp 55–72.

69. ANDER, R (ED): *Psychoneuroimmunology.* Academic Press, New York, 1981.

70. ATKINS, MB, GOULD, JA, ALLEGRETTA, M, ET AL: *Phase I evaluation of recombinant Interleukin-2 in patients with advanced malignant disease.* J Clin Oncology 4:1380–1391, 1986.

71. ANGELL, M: *Disease as a reflection of the psyche* (editorial) N Engl J Med 312:1570–1572, 1985.

72. BEHAN, PO, AND GESCHWIND, N: *Hemispheric laterality and immunity.* In GUILLEMIN, R, COHN, M, MELNUCHUK, T (EDS): *Neural Modulation of Immunity.* Raven Press, New York, 1985.

73. BEHAN, PO, AND SPREAFICO, F (EDS): *Neuroimmunology.* Serono Symposia Publications, vol 12. Raven Press, New York, 1984.

74. BESEDOVSKY, HO, DEL RAY, AE, SORKIN, E: *Immune-neuroendocrine interactions.* J Immunol. 135:750s–754s, 1985.

75. BESEDOVSKY, H, DEL RAY, A, SORKIN, E, DINARELLO, CA: *Immunoregulatory feedback between Interleukin-1 and glucocorticoid hormones.* Science 233:652–654, 1986.

76. BLALOCK, JE, HARBOUR-MCMENAMIN, D, SMITH, EM: *Peptide hormones shared by the neuroendocrine and immunologic systems.* J Immunol 858s–861s, 1985.

77. BULLOCH, K: *Neuroanatomy of lymphoid tissue: A review.* In GUILLEMIN, R, COHN, M, MELNUCKHUK, T (EDS): *Neural Modulation of Immunity.* Raven Press, New York, 1985, pp 111–142.

78. COHN, M: *What are the "must" elements of immune responsiveness?* In GUILLEMIN, R, COHN, M, MELNUCHUK, T (EDS): *Neural Modulation of Immunity.* Raven Press, New York, 1985, pp 3–28.

79. DINARELLO, CA: *An update on hyman interleukin-1: From molecular biology to clinical relevance.* J Clin Immunol 5:1–11, 1985.

80. GUILLEMIN, R, COHN, M, MELNUCHUK, T (EDS): *Neural Modulation of Immunity.* Raven Press, New York, 1985.

81. MACLEAN, D, AND REICHLIN, S: *Neuroendocrinology and the immune process.* In ADER, R (ED): *Psychoneuroimmunology.* Academic Press, New York, 1981, pp 475–520.

82. MARTIN, JB: *Neuroendocrine regulation of the immune response.* In BEHAN, PO, AND SPREAFICO, F (EDS): *Neuroimmunology.* Serona Symposia Publications, vol 12. Raven Press, New York, 1984, pp 433–444.

83. PIERPAOLI, W: *Immunoregulatory and morphostatic function of bone marrow-derived factors.* In GUILLEMIN, R, COHN, M, MELNUCHUK, T (EDS): *Neural Modulation of Immunity.* Raven Press, New York, 1985.

84. ROSZMAN, TL, CROSS, RJ, BROOKS, WH, ET AL: *Neuroimmunomodulation: Effects of neural lesions on cellular immunity.* In GUILLEMIN, R, COHN, M, MELNUCHUK, T, (EDS): Raven Press, New York, 1985, pp 95–110.

85. SMITH, EM, HARBOUR-MCMENAMIN, D, BLALOCK, JE: *Lymphocyte production of endorphins and endorphin-mediated immunoregulatory activity.* J Immunol 135:779s–782s, 1985.

86. SMITH, EM, MEYER, WJ, BLALOCK, JE: *Virus-induced corticosterone in hypohpysectomized mice: Possible lymphoid adrenal axis.* Science 218:1311–1312, 1982.

87. SMITH, EM, MORRILL, AC, MEYER, WJ, BLALOCK, JE: *Corticotropin releasing factor induction of leukocyte-derived immunoreactive ACTH and endorphins.* Nature 321:881–882, 1986.

88. STEIN, M: *Bereavement, depression, stress, and immunity.* In GUILLEMIN, R, COHN, M, MELNUCHUK, T (EDS): *Neural Modulation of Immunity.* Raven Press, New York, 1985, pp 29–44.

89. WOLOSKI, MRNJ, SMITH, EM, MEYER WJ, ET AL: *Corticotropin-releasing activity of monokines.* Science 230:1035–1037, 1985.

90. KARNOVSKY, ML: *Progress in sleep* (editorial) N Engl J Med, 315:1026–1028, 1986.

INDEX

Page numbers followed by F indicate figures; page numbers followed by T indicate tables.

Amino acid structures, hypophysiotropic
hypothalamic hormones and, 26,
26F, 27F
α-Aminobutyric acid (GABA), 56T, 61, 204
anterior pituitary function and, 45
neurons containing, peptidergic neurons
and, 609, 611
somatostatin secretion and, 572
TSH secretion and, 140
L-Aminodecarboxylase, 58
Aminoglutethimide, Cushing's syndrome
treatment with, 191
Amiodarone, thyroid hormones and, 127
Amitriptyline (Elavil), 57T
reuptake process and, 55
serotonin reuptake and, 59
Amnestic syndrome, hypothalamus and, 413
AMP. *See* Adenosine monophosphate
Amphetamine(s), 57T
ACTH and, 176
food intake regulation and, 403
release of preformed granules and, 53–54
reuptake process and, 55
thyroxine and, 125, 139
Amygdala, 38, 38F
ACTH regulation and, 175, 176F
afferents of, 39
bilateral lesions of, food intake regulation
and, 406
efferents of, 39
electrical stimulation of, cardiovascular
system and, 394
growth hormone secretion and, 247, 247F
neurotensin in, 580
vasopressin in, 69
Amygdaloid complex, subdivisions of, 39
Amyotrophic lateral sclerosis (ALS),
thyrotropin-releasing hormone
and, 143, 568, 625
Anatomy
hypothalamic, 17–19, 18F
limbic system, 37–40, 38F
nerve fiber, visual pathway, 448F
neurophypophysial, 68–72, 69F, 70F,
71F
optic, 446–447
pineal gland, 351–352, 352T
pituitary, 12–17, 13F, 14F, 16F, 17F
posterior, 68–72, 69F, 70F, 71F
Androgen(s), 297. *See also* Sex hormones;
specific androgen
adrenal, 163
female sexual function and, 650
aggressive behavior and, 648
brain development and, 644–645
gonadotropin secretion and, 28
male sexual function and, 647–650
personality effects of, 648–649
psychologic side effects of, 648
sexually dimorphic nucleus and, 645
spermatogenesis and, 313
Androgenization, estradiol and, 645
Androstenedione, secretion of, 163–164
Androsterone, secretion of, 163–164
Anemia, syndrome of inappropriate ADH
secretion and, 101

Anesthesia
malignant hyperthermia and, 392
prolactin release and, 209–210
Aneurysm(s)
adenoma vs., radiologic assessment of,
472F–473F, 475–476
berry
pituitary apoplexy vs., 538
rupture of, hypothalamic damage
following, 537
circle of Willis, diabetes insipidus and, 93
parasellar, magnetic resonance imaging
of, 467
radiologic assessment of, 472F–473F,
475–476
cerebral angiography in, 471F, 480
sellar enlargement and, 460
Angiography
adrenal disease diagnosis and, 191
carotid, left, 471F
cerebral, 471F, 480
Angiotensin II, vasopressin regulation and,
89
Angiotensinogen, CRF and, 165
Angiotensinogen mRNA, thirst and, 81–82
Anorexia
lateral hypothalamic lesions and, 407
tumors causing, 406
Anorexia nervosa
amenorrhea and, 316, 324, 684
antidiuretic hormone excretion and, 79
chronic hypothermia and, 391
diagnostic criteria of, 680
epidemiologic factors in, 680–681
glucose growth hormone suppression test
and, 501
GnRH response in, 489, 505
growth hormone secretion and, 239,
268–269
hormonal disturbances in, 682F–683F,
684–686, 685T, 686F
hypopituitarism vs., 686
lateral hypothalamic lesions and, 407
natural history of, 681, 681F
psychologic setting of, 684
symptoms of, 680
treatment of, 686–687, 686T
Anorexigenic peptide, food intake
regulation and, 405–406
Anosmia, 453
craniopharyngioma and, 531
Anovulation, nursing and, 319–320
Anovulatory menses, clomiphene and, 523
Antabuse (disulfiram), 57T
5-hydroxytryptophan conversion and, 58
Antagonist(s)
α-adrenergic, 54
growth hormone regulation and,
249–250
thyrotropin secretion and, 139
β-adrenergic, growth hormone secretion
and, 250
angiotensin II, thirst and, 82
cortisol, 165
definition of, 54
dopamine, 54

Arginine vasopressin. *See also* Antidiuretic
    hormone
  plasma, plasma osmolality and, 78F
  preprohormone for, 73F
  structure of, 72F
Argonz del Castillo syndrome, 215
Argyll Robertson pupils, 454
Aromatase, 645
Arrhythmias
  central nervous system lesions and,
    395–396
  pathophysiology of, 396
Arterial blood pressure
  neural control of, 393
  noradrenergic control of, 395
  vasopressinergic control of, 395
Arterial hypertension, pseudotumor cerebri
    and, 550
Artery(ies), carotid
  ectasia and, acromegaly and, 536
  internal
    aneurysms of, sellar enlargement and,
      460
    calcification of, 460, 460F
Arthritis, rheumatoid,
    psychoneuroimmunology and,
    689
Aspiny neurons, 617
Aspirin
  fever and, 389
  pituitary-thyroid function and, 127
Assessment. *See also* Diagnosis; *specific*
    assessment; specific disorder
  neurologic, hypothalamic-pituitary
    disorders and, 445
  olfactory, 453–454
  radiologic
    acromegaly in, 472–473
    ACTH producing tumors in, 472
    advances in, 457
    aneurysms in, 472F–473F, 475–476
    brain scan in, 479
    calcification in, 473–474
    CAT scans in, 462–463
      axial images in, 467
      coronal, 463, 465–467
      metrizamide with, 467, 468F
    cerebral angiography in, 471F, 480
    importance of, 457
    magnetic resonance imaging in, 467,
      469F
    nonsecretory adenomas in, 470F–471F,
      473
    pituitary adenomas in, differential
      diagnosis of, 474
      aneurysm in, 472F–473F, 475–476
      craniopharyngioma in, 476, 477F,
        478F
      hypothalamic glioma in, 476,
        478–479
      metastasis in, 479
      tuberculum sellae meningioma in,
        474F–475F, 476
    pituitary apoplexy in, 473
    prolactinoma in, 471
    secretory adenomas in, 471–473

sella turcica in, 457, 458F, 459F
  calcification in, 460, 460F
  increased intracranial pressure and,
    461–462
  size in, 458–459
    causes of enlargement and,
      460–461
  visual acuity, 446–447
  visual field, 447–453, 453T
Asthma, psychoneuroimmunology and, 689
Astrocytoma(s), 92
  diencephalic syndrome and, 407–408,
    408F
  malignant, 534
  pineal gland, 362
Ataxia, TRH and, 143
Athetoid movements, hypocalcemia and, 660
ATP. *See* Adenosine triphosphate
Atriopeptins, 79, 84–86
  actions of, 83
  cardiac failure and, 83, 87F
  sodium excretion and, 86F
  structure of, 83, 84F
  system of, 85F
Atrophy
  adrenal, idiopathic, 182
  Huntington's disease and, 620
Atropine, 57T
  acetylcholine and, 61
  muscarinic receptors and, 61
  ovulation and, 304
  temperature regulation and, 385
  thirst and, 81
Autocrine regulation, 571
Autoimmune diseases, 689
Autoimmune disorder, Addison's disease
    and, 182
Autonomic epilepsy, diencephalic,
    391–392, 414
  hypertension in, 395
Autonomic nervous system
  neuropeptide Y in, 594
  substance P in, 579
Avian pancreatic polypeptide, 593
Axon(s)
  monoaminergic pathway, 45, 46F
  tuberoinfundibular neurons and, 25
Axon terminals, median eminence, 22
Axonal transport, catecholamine, 55

Baldness, testosterone therapy and, 521
Barbiturates
  Addison's disease and, 657
  chronic hypothermia and, 391
  thirst and, 81
  vasopressin regulation and, 89
Basal ganglia, 615–619, 617F, 617T
  anatomic connections of, 619F
  neuropeptides in, Parkinson's disease
    and, 622–623
  thyrotropin-releasing hormone in, 131
Basis pendunculi, 19
Basolateral amygdala, 39
Basophilism, pituitary, 178–179
  corticotropin-releasing hormone
    responses in, 492, 506

metastasis from
  pituitary, 440, 535
  radiologic assessment of, 479
oat-cell, lung, Cushing's syndrome and,
    179–180
pineal gland and, 361
pituitary, primary, 440
proopiomelanocortin and, 162
psychoneuroimmunology and, 689
Cardiovascular system
electrical stimulation of hypothalamus
    and, 394
neural regulation of, 393–394
thyroid hormone complications in, 525
Cardiac arrhythmias, central nervous
    system lesions and, 395–396
Cardiac disturbance(s)
pathophysiology of, 396
thyroid hormone replacement and, 525
Cardiac failure, atriopeptins and, 83, 87F
Cardiac overload, furosemide and, 103
Carotid angiogram, left, 471F
Carotid artery
aneurysms of
  radiologic assessment of, 472F–473F
  sellar enlargement and, 460
calcification of, 460, 460F
ectasia of, acromegaly and, 536
Carter-Robbins test, 95
Castration, sexual function and, 648
CAT. See Choline acetyltransferase
CAT scanning. See Computerized axial
    tomography
Catalepsy, somatostatin and, 574
Catapres (clonidine), 56T. See also Clonidine
Catecholamine(s). See also Dopamine;
    Epinephrine; Norepinephrine
adrenocorticotropin regulation and, 176
amenorrhea and, 322
anterior pituitary function and, 45
axonal transport of, 55
biosynthesis and degradation of, 51–55
cardiac abnormalities and, 396
gonadotropin-releasing hormone
    regulation and, 304
growth hormone secretion and, 248–251
hypertension and, 395
hypothalamic-pituitary function and, 55,
    56T–57T
immune process and, 689
inactivation of, 55
median eminence and, 22
nonshivering thermogenesis and, 389
receptors on postsynaptic neuron and,
    interaction of, 54
temperature regulation and, 384–385,
    389
thyroid hormones and, chronic cold
    exposure and, 122
thyrotropin secretion and, 139–140
Catecholamine storage, 52–53
Catechol-estradiol, 644
Catechol-O-methyltransferase (COMT), 55
Cathartic abuse, bulimia and, 687
Catheterization, venous, adrenal disease
    diagnosis and, 191

Caudate nucleus, Huntington's disease and,
    620
Cavernous sinus
coronal CAT scans of, 466
pituitary fossa and, anatomic relations of,
    447F
Cavernous sinus invasion, CAT scan of,
    463, 464F
CBG (cortisol-binding globulin), 165
CCK. See Cholecystokinin
Cell(s). See also Neuron(s)
containing conventional
    neurotransmitters and
    neuropeptides, 564T
corticotrope, 423
CRF-immunoreactive, 32F
dopamine-containing, Parkinson's disease
    and, 622–623
dorsal root ganglion, substance P in,
    577–578
endocrine, 4
  gene expression of, mechanism for, 34F
ependymal, 21, 368
exocrine, 4
glial, pineal, 353
gonadotrope, 423
hormone-secreting adrenal medulla, 5F
hypothalamic, 19, 20T
immunocompetent, 687
juxtaglomerular, renal, renin and, 4
lactotrope, 201, 423
Leydig, 313
median forebrain bundle, 19
myoepithelial, periacinar, 72
  oxytocin and, 86
nerve, bombesin in, 595
neural crest, tumors arising from, ACTH
    secretion and, 180–181
neuroendocrine transducer, 8
neurohormonal, 4
neurohypophysial, 68
neuromodulator, 4
  neurosecretion and, 6–7
neuronal, 4
neuropeptide, site of, 4
neurosecretory
  hypothalamus and, 4, 5F
  pituitary and, 4
neurotransmitter
  neurosecretion and, 6–7
  site of, 4
  structures of, 47F
nononcocytic, 439
oncocytic, 439
pars distalis, 13–14
parvocellular, 69
pineal, 351
pituitary, dopamine and, 33
secretory
  anterior pituitary hormone, 13–14
  capillary and, ultrastructural
    relationship of, 33F
  classification of, 4
  function of, 4
  regulation of, 4
Sertoli, 313

Endorphin(s)—*Continued*
  biosynthesis of, 583, 584F
  discovery of, 582
  growth hormone secretion and, 253
  receptors for, 586
  vasopressin regulation and, 89
β-Endorphin
  corticotropin-releasing hormone and,
    166, 168
  discovery of, 560
  food intake regulation and, 405
  temperature regulation and, 387
Endorphinergic neurons, 162
Endotoxin, antidiuretic hormone secretion
    and, 79
Endoxin, 82
  metabolism of salt and water and, 83
Enkephalin(s). *See also* Opioid peptides;
    specific enkephalin
  actions of, 586
  anatomic localization of, 583, 585
  biosynthesis of, 583, 584F
  discovery of, 560, 582
  growth hormone secretion and, 253
  Huntington's disease and, 587
  processing of, 586–587
  receptors for, 585–586
Environmental stimuli, prolactin release
    and, 208
Environmental temperature
  hypothalamic sensing of, 382
  thermal discomfort and, 383, 383F
Enzymatic synthesis, 52. *See also specific*
    substance
Enzyme(s)
  cellular, activation of, 33
  Huntington's disease and, 620–622
  melatonin-forming, 355
  membrane-bound, phosphoinositol
    mechanism and, 34
  peptides and, 619
Eosinophilic granuloma, 542
  CAT scan in, 479
  course of, 543–544
  diabetes insipidus and, 93
  diagnosis of, 543
  treatment of, 544
Ependymal structures, periventricular, 351,
    369F
  organum vasculosum of the lamina
    terminalis, 369–370
  subcommissural, 368–369
  subfornical, 370–371
Ependymal zone, inner, 22, 23–24
Ependymoma(s), 534
  pineal gland, 364
Epidemic encephalitis, 409–410
Epidermoid tumors, 532
Epilepsy. *See also* seizure(s)
  diencephalic, 391–392, 407–408, 408F,
    414
    clinical features of, 409T
    hypertension in, 395
    tumors producing, 409T
Epinephrine
  adrenergic innervation of hypothalamus
    and, 49–50

biosynthesis and degradation of, 51–55,
    51F
CRF and, 168
growth hormone regulation and, 248–249
hypoglycemia and, 661, 662
ovulation and, 45, 304
release of, regulation of, 4
vasopressin regulation and, 88
Epiphysin, 361
Episodic hypercortisolemia, 414
Erosion, sellar floor, 461
Essential hypernatremia, 97–98
Estradiol
  androgenization with, 645
  GnRH response and, 306F
  normal levels of, 339
  physiologic brain effects of, 644
  structure of, 297F
Estinyl estradiol, growth hormone
    responsiveness and, 503
Estrogen(s), 269–297
  acromegaly treatment with, 281
  amenorrhea evaluation and, 340
  clomiphene and, 341
  conjugated, gonadal deficiency and, 272
  deficiency of
    diagnosis of, 338
    signs and symptoms of, 651
    Turner's syndrome and, 651
  dexamethasone suppression test and, 190
  feedback effect of, 305, 306F
  female sexual behavior and, 650–652
  gonadotropin secretion and, 28, 521–522
  growth hormone secretion and, 28
  male sexual function and, 648
  menstrual cycle and, 309–313, 652
  migraine and, 654
  physiologic brain effects of, 644
  pituitary adenomas and, 425–426
  prolactin release and, 208, 209
  TRH response and, 141
  TSH secretion and, 120, 126
Estrogen inunctions, skin patches in, 522
Estrogen therapy, cancer and, 651
Estrus, 296
Ethinyl estradiol, replacement therapy with,
    521
"Euthyroid" Graves' disease. *See also* Sick
    euthyroid syndrome
  TRH response in, 142
Evoked response, visual, 454–455
Evolution
  neuropeptide, 562–563
  regulatory systems, 4
Exercise
  growth hormone secretion and, 239,
    271–272
  impotence and, 649
  puberty and, 316, 318
Exhibitionism, treatment of, 648
Exocrine cells, 4
Exocrine gland(s), 5F
  regulation of, 4
Exocytosis, 35
  growth hormone secretion and, 234–235
Extrahypothalamic pedptidergic neuron
    systems, 7

Extrahypothalamic regulation
ACTH and, 175–176, 176F
antidiuretic hormone and, 90
food intake and, 406
growth hormone and, 246–248, 247F, 248F
hypothalamic-adenohypophysial system and, 36
limbic system and, 37–40
Extrahypothalamic thyrotropin-releasing hormone, distribution of, 130–131
Eye(s). *See also* Optic *entries*; Vision; Visual *entries*
adduction of, 453
examination of, 446–453
pineal tumors and, 454
Eyelid edema, pituitary apoplexy and, 538

Factitious hypercortisolism, 181
Factril (gonadotropin-releasing hormone), 489. *See also* Gonadotropin-releasing hormone
False pregnancy, 313, 322, 324
Familial diabetes insipidus, 91
Familial pineoblastoma, 364
Familial testotoxicosis, 333
Fasting, growth hormone secretion and, 239
Fasting hypoglycemia, causes of, 661
Fat mass, appetite sensory mechanism and, 401–402. *See also* Anorexia nervosa
Fat tissue, menarche and, 316, 318. *See also* Anorexia nervosa
Fatigue
hypercalcemia and, 659
hypopituitarism and, 658
premenstrual syndrome and, 653
Fatty acids, preovulatory, 651
Feedback
glucocorticoid, 174–175, 174F
corticotropin-releasing hormone and, 168–169
negative, gonadotropin secretion and, 305, 307F, 308F
pituitary-thyroid, 114–115
positive, estrogen and, gonadotropin secretion and, 310, 311F
prolactin secretion, 208–209
short-loop, growth hormone and, 253–254
Female brain, definition of, 644–645
Female hypogonadotropic hypogonadism, 322, 324–325
management of, 521–522
Female infertility, management of, 522–524, 523T
Female puberty, 315F
Female sex hormones, 296–297
feedback controls and, 308F
headache and, 654
menstrual cycle and, 308–313
physiologic brain effects of, 644
Female sexual function
gonadal steroids and, 650–652
premenstrual syndrome and, 652–654

Fenfluramine, ACTH regulation and, 176
Fertility. *See also* Infertility
promotion of, bromocriptine in, 222
Fetus
sex hormones in, 316
thyroid deficiency in, 642
thyrotropin-releasing hormone in, 136
Fever, mechanism of, 388–389, 389F
Fibrillation, ventricular, CNS lesions and, 395
Fludrocortisone (Florinef), Addison's disease management with, 182
Fluid(s). *See also* Water *entries*
retention of, premenstrual, 653
Fluoxymesterone, gonadotropin deficiency treatment with, 521
Fluorohydrocortisone, Cushing's disease treatment and, 192
Flutter, ventricular, CNS lesions and, 395
Focal myocytolysis, 396
Focal subendocardial necrosis, 396
Follicle-stimulating hormone (FSH), 12, 295–296. *See also* Gonadotropin(s)
cells secreting, 423
GnRH effects on, 298–299, 299F, 488–491, 488T–490T, 505
menstrual cycle and, 309–310
normal levels of, 323T
secretion of, 300
GnRH neurons and, 301
spermatogenesis and, 313
tumors secreting, 338
Folliculostatin (inhibin), 298, 314
Food intake regulation. *See also* Obesity
anorexia nervosa and, 680, 681. *See also* Anorexia nervosa
appetite control and
anorexigenic peptide in, 405–406
neuropharmacologic, 403
peptide hormones in, 403–405
TRH in, 405
bombesin and, 595–596
cholecystokinin in, 593
diencephalic syndrome and, 407–408, 408F, 409T
external vs. internal factors in, obesity and, 406–407
extrahypothalamic, 406
hypothalamic factors in obesity and, 406–407
lateral hypothalamic lesions and, 407
neural control of, 396–399, 397F, 398F
physiologic sensors of caloric state and
long-term, 401–402
short-term, 399–401, 400F
Prader-Willi syndrome and, 415
temperature and, 383
tumor anorexia and, 406
Foodaholics, bulimic patients as, 687
Fornix, 37–38
Foster-Kennedy syndrome, 450
Free-running pineal rhythms, 357
FSH. *See* Follicle-stimulating hormone
Functional amenorrhea, 322, 324–325
clomiphene and, 341
treatment of, 522–523

Furosemide
  pseudotumor cerebri and, 551
  SIADH treatment with, 103–104
Furth thyrotropic tumor, 146
Fusaric acid, 57T

GABA. *See* γ-Aminobutyric acid
GAD (glutamic acid decarboxylase), 61
Gait disturbances, pineal neoplasms and, 366
Galactorrhea
  adenomas and, 216
  amenorrhea and, 215
    bromocriptine therapy for, 221–224,
      221F
    GnRH and, 299F
    hypothyroidism and, 217
    postpill, 217
    radiation therapy and, 516
  diagnosis in, 218
  hypothyroidism and, 217
  nonpuerperal, 213–215, 214F
  pituitary isolation and, 216
Ganglia
  basal, 616–619, 617F, 617T
    anatomic connections of, 619F
    neuropeptides in, Parkinson's disease
      and, 622–623
    thyrotropin-releasing hormone in, 131
  dorsal root, neuropeptides in, 623–625,
    624T
    substance P, 577–578
    somatostatin in, 569
Gangliocytoma(s)
  hypothalamic, 533
    CRF-secreting, 179
  sellar
    CRF-secreting, 431, 431F
    GH-secreting adenoma and, 428F
Gangliomas, ACTH secretion and, 180
GAP (gonadotropin-releasing factor
    associated peptide), 28, 205, 205F
Gastric emptying, cholecystokinin and, 399
Gastric juice, regulation of, 4
Gastrin, 592
  structure of, 592F
Gastrin-releasing peptide (GRP), 595
Gastrointestinal (GI) tract
  bromocriptine and, 222
  neurotensin in
    distribution of, 581
    function of, 582
  somatostatin in, 570–571
  substance P in, 578–579
  vasoactive intestinal peptide in, 589
Gastroscopy, prolactin release and, 210
Gaze
  downward, defects in, 454
  upward, conjugate, paralysis of, 454
Gender identification, sex steroids and,
    646–647
Genes, POMC, 161, 162
Gene expression
  endocrine cell, cellular mechanism for, 34F
  vasopressin, glucocorticoids and, 78
General anesthesia, prolactin release and,
    209–210

General paresis, diurnal variations in ACTH
    and, 171
Genetics
  Huntington's disease and, 620
  pituitary adenomas and, 425
Genitourinary system, TRH effects on, 138
Geriatric patients
  chronic hypothermia in, 391
  drug-induced SIADH in, 101
  growth hormone levels in, 238
  null cell adenomas in, 439
  osmolar regulation in, 81
  sella turcica calcification in, 460
  stress tests for ACTH abnormalities in, 186
  thyroid hormone replacement therapy in,
    520–521
  thyrotoxic states in, behavioral changes
    in, 655
  water excretion in, ADH secretion and, 89
Germ-cell tumors, intracranial, prognosis
    of, 367, 368F
Germinoma(s)
  intracranial, 364
  metastasis of, 362–363
  pineal gland, 362
  pineal region, treatment of, 366, 367, 367T
Gestagens, premenstrual syndrome and, 654
GH. *See* Growth hormone
GHRH. *See* Growth hormone releasing
    hormone
GI tract. *See* Gastrointestinal tract
Gigantism
  cerebral, 269
  pathophysiology of, 266–268
Gland(s). *See also specific gland*
  exocrine, 5F
    regulation of, 4
  influences on, 4
Glandular secretion(s), neural control of
  neurosecretion and, 6–9
  secretomotor, 4, 6
Glial cells, pineal gland, 353
Glioblastoma(s), 534
  pineal gland, 362
Glioma, 92
  hypothalamic, pituitary adenoma vs.,
    476, 478–479
  optic nerve, 476, 478–479
Gliosis, spontaneous periodic hypothermia
    and, 392
Globus pallidus, GABA in, 61
Glucagon
  central nervous system, 598
  growth hormone secretion and, 253
Glucocorticoid(s), 162, 164
  Addison's disease and, 182, 657
  antidiuretic hormone secretion and, 77–78
  blood, diurnal variations of, 170–171
  brain development and, 655
  Cushing's syndrome and, 177
  excess of, diagnosis of, 188–190, 189F
  feedback regulation by, 174–175
    corticotropin-releasing hormone and,
      168–169
  growth hormone secretion and, 270
  hypersecretion of, 429

Growth hormone releasing hormone
(GHRH), 26, 245, 245F. *See also*
GnRH-associated peptide
acetylcholine and, 61
acromegaly and, GH-secreting adenomas
and, 427–428
actions of, 257
anatomy of, 31F
clinical studies with, 257, 258F
ectopic, 268
glutamate and, 62
hypothalamic, 255
normal response to, 494, 495F, 506
pituitary growth hormone release and, 260
structure of, 26F
structure-function relations of, 256–257,
256F
synthetic, 257
Growth hormone releasing hormone test,
275
growth hormone deficiency and,
273–274, 273F
Growth hormone-inhibiting factor, 568
acromegaly and, 282, 428
actions of, 259–260, 259F
Alzheimer's disease and, 611, 612F
analogs of, 262–263, 263F
behavioral effects of, 573–574
biosynthesis of, 571
brain disease and, 575–576
cerebral cortical, 570
cerebrospinal fluid, 574
psychiatric disorders and, 576
circumventricular, 570
degradation of, 262
discovery of, 257–258, 560
electrophysiological effects of, 572–573
enkephalins and, 586
gastrointestinal, 570–571
mechanism of action of, 261–262
molecular forms of, 258–259
neural functions of, 572–574
neurotransmitter secretion and, 573
pituitary growth hormone release and,
260
processing of, 571
regulation of, 572
sensory system, 569
striatal, 570
Huntington's disease and, 621
temperature regulation and, 388
therapeutic potential of, 576
tuberoinfundibular system, 569
visceral distribution of, 571
Growth hormone-inhibiting factor receptor
binding, 612
Alzheimer's disease and, 614–615, 614F
Growth hormone-inhibiting factor
receptors, 261, 573
Growth retardation, cretinism and, 642
Growth spurt
normal age of
female, 329, 329T
male, 329, 329T
GRP (gastrin-releasing peptide), 595
Guillemin peptide, 255

Guinuclidinyl benzilate, muscarinic
receptors and, 61
Gut
bombesin in, 595
cholecystokinin in, 593
substance P in, 578–579
thyrotropin-releasing hormone in,
566–567
Gut-brain peptides, 559–560
Gynecomastia
neurogenic hypogonadism and, 327
prolactin excess and, 216

H_1 receptors, 60
H_2 receptors, 60
Hair, anorexia nervosa and, hypopituitarism
vs., 686
Hair loss, radiation therapy and, 517
Haldol (haloperidol), 56T. *See also*
Haloperidol
Hallucinations
Cushing's syndrome and, 656
pituitary tumor and, 446
Haloperidol (Haldol), 54, 673F
temperature regulation and, 384–385
Hamartoma(s), 92, 532
hypothalamic
obesity and, 397–398, 398F
precocious puberty and, 331–332
somatostatin in, 575
symptoms of, 533
Hand-Schuller-Christian disease, 543
chemotherapy for, 544
Hard wiring, point-to-point, 4
Hashimoto's disease
Addison's disease and, 182
plasma TSH and, 146
HCG. *See* Human chorionic gonadotropin
Head injury, diabetes insipidus and, 91–92
Head tremor, arachnoid cysts and, 533
Headache
benign intracranial hypertension and, 548
colloid cyst and, 535
craniopharyngioma and, 531
empty-sella syndrome and, 547
hormonal influences on, 654
hypercalcemia and, 659
pituitary apoplexy and, 538
pituitary tumor and, 445–446
sleep and, 446
Heart disease, vasopressin and, 94
Heart failure, congestive, furosemide and,
103
Heart rate, neural regulation of, 393
Heat exposure, poikilothermia and, 381
Heat production. *See also* Temperature
regulation
brown fat and, 389–390
Heat stroke, body temperature in, 388
Heavy particle therapy, 518–519
Hematoma, subdural, SIADH and, 100
Hemianopsia
bitemporal, 449
hypothyroidism and, 146
craniopharyngioma and, 531
Hemiplegia, 454

drug effects on, 127
  plasma, plasma TSH and, 114, 114F
  secretion of, 115–116
  thyrotropin secretion and, 120
Hormone-secreting cells, adrenal medulla, 5F
Hormonogenesis, 111
Horseradish peroxidase (HRP), median
      eminence and, 21
Hostility, premenstrual syndrome and, 654
Hot flashes, menopause and, 651
Houssay phenomenon, 541
hpGRF. *See* Human pancreatic growth
      hormone releasing factor
HPL (human placental lactogen), 211
HRP (horseradish peroxidase), median
      eminence and, 21
5-HT (5-hydroxytryptamine), adrenergic
      innervation of hypothalamus
      and, 50–51, 51F
Human chorionic gonadotropin (HCG),
      295–296
  ovulation induction and, 523
  pineal gland tumors and, 363
Human growth hormone (hGH). *See also*
      Growth hormone
  biosynthetic, 524–525
  injections of, 275
  secretion of, spontaneous fluctuations in,
      236–238, 237F
  structure of, 233, 235F
Human menopausal gonadotropin (HMG),
      296
  ovulation induction and, 523
Human pancreatic growth hormone
      releasing factor (hpGRF), 255
  growth hormone secretion and, 258F
  structure of, 256
Human placental lactogen (HPL), 211
Huntington's disease
  enzymes and, 620–622
  grades of atrophy in, 620
  inheritance of, 620
  manifestations of, 620
  neuropathologic findings in, 620
  neuropeptides and, 620–622
    cortical, 615, 616T
    enkephalins, 587
    somatostatin, 575
    substance P, 580
  TRH distribution in, 131
HVA (homovanillic acid), 55
Hydrocephalus
  arachnoid cysts and, 533
  craniopharyngioma and, 531
  internal, pineal neoplasms and, 365–366
  lipomas and, 534
Hydrochlorothiazide, polyuria and, 96
Hydrocortisone
  ACTH deficiency treatment with, 520
  mental disturbance in hypopituitarism
      and, 658
  severe hypopituitarism treatment with,
      525
γ-Hydroxybutyrate, dopamine release and,
      54
17-Hydroxycorticosteroids
  ACTH hypersecretion and, 188

ACTH test and, 184–185
  electroconvulsive therapy and, 172F
  metyrapone test and, 186
5-Hydroxyindoleacetic acid (5-HIAA), 59
Hydroxyindole-O-methyltransferase
      (HIOMT), 354–355
  pineal parenchymal tumor and, 365
11-β-Hydroxylase, metyrapone test and,
      185
5-Hydroxytryptamine (5-HT), adrenergic
      innervation of hypothalamus
      and, 50–51, 51F
5-Hydroxytryptophan, 56T
  growth hormone and, 59–60
  prolactin and, 59, 207
5-Hydroxytryptophol, 353
Hypercalcemia
  acute management of, 660
  brain dysfunction and, 659–660
Hypercortisolism, 177–178
  causes of, CRH response and, 494
  CRH responses in, 492, 492F, 493T, 494
  depression and, 674–675, 674F
  differential diagnosis of, 180–181,
      188–190, 189F
  diurnal variations and, 184
  ectopic ACTH secretion and, 179–181
  episodic, 414
  psychologic disturbance in, 656
  treatment of, 191
Hyperepinephrinemia, reactive
      hypoglycemia and, 661
Hyperhidrosis, disabling, intermittent
      hypothermia with, 391–392
Hyperglycemia
  bombesin and, 595
  brain dysfunction and, 662
Hypergonadotropic hypogonadism,
      definition of, 320
Hyperinsulinemia, obesity and, 404
  growth disturbances and, 269
Hyperkinesia, somatostatin and, 574
Hypernatremia. *See also* Sodium regulation
  essential, 97–98
Hyperosmolar coma, hyperglycemic, 662
Hyperosmolarity
  age and, 81
  hypernatremia and, 97–98
  thirst and, 81
Hyperosmotic hypodipsia, 81
Hyperparathyroidism, hypercalcemia and,
      659
Hyperphagia. *See also* Food intake regulation
  cyproheptadine and, 191
  obesity and, hypothalamic lesions and,
      397–398, 398F
  pathophysiology of, 407
Hyperprolactinemia
  acidophil stem cell adenoma and, 436
  causes of, 214–215, 215T
  CSF prolactin in, 628
  differential diagnosis of, 219
  galactorrhea and, 218
    thoracic spinal cord lesions and, 217
  hypothyroidism and, 217
  idiopathic, 218
  management of, 219

anovulatory, clomiphene and, 523
Menstrual cycle
  female sexual function and, 652
  GnRH response and, 488
  headache and, 654
  premenstrual syndrome and, 652–654
  regulation of, 308–313, 310F, 311F,
      312F
  temperature regulation and, 384
Menstruation
  induction of
    clomiphene and, 522
    progestin and, 521–522
  precocious, definition of, 329
Mental disturbance
  adrenocortical disease and, 656–657
  anorexia nervosa and, 680–681, 684
  bulimia and, 687
  depression and, 674
  endocrine changes in, 672–673
  hypercalcemia and, 659–660
  hypocalcemia and, 660–661
  hypoglycemia and, 661–662
  hypopituitarism and, 657–658
  schizophrenia and, 679–680
  thyroid disease and, 655
Mental retardation
  cretinism and, 642
  Prader-Willi syndrome and, 415
Mesolimbic system, tuberoinfundibular
      system vs.,
      psychoneuroendocrinology and,
      672
Messenger signals, 34, 35F
Metabolic degradation, thyrotropin-
      releasing hormone, 129–130,
      130F
Metabolic encephalopathy, CSF
      somatostatin in, 575
Metabolic factors, 4
Metabolic pathways
  catecholamine synthesis, 51–52, 52F
  phosphoinositol mechanism and, 34
Metabolic regulation, growth hormone,
      238–239
Metabolism
  carbohydrate, disorders of, brain
      dysfunction and, 661–662
  thyrotropin-releasing hormone, 132
Metastatic tumor(s), 535
  diabetes insipidus and, 92–93
  pituitary gland and, 440
  SMS 201–995 in, 263
Metastasis
  germinomas and, 362–363
  pituitary adenomas vs., 479
Met-enkephalin, 162
  anatomic localization of, 583
  structure of, 582F
Met-enkephalin-like immunoreactivity,
      Parkinson's disease and, 623
Methionine, biosynthetic hGH containing,
      524
Methionine-enkephalin, 162
  anatomic localization of, 583
  structure of, 582F

Methionine-enkephalin-like
      immunoreactivity, Parkinson's
      disease and, 623
3-Methoxy-4-hydroxyphenylglycol
      (MHPG), 55
3-Methoxy-4-hydroxyphenylglycol sulfate
      (MHPG-sulfate), 55
3-Methoxytyramine, 55
α-Methyldopa (Aldomet), 57T
  prolactin release and, 207, 217
α-Methyl-p-tyrosine, 57T
Methylscopolamine, 57T
Methysergide (Sansert), 56T
  growth hormone secretion and, 250
  serotonin and, 59
Metoclopramide
  gonadotropin secretion and, 304
  prolactin and, 204
  thyrotropin secretion and, 120
Metrizamide, CAT scanning with, 462
Metrizamide cisternography, 467, 468F
Metyrapone
  anorexia nervosa and, 685
  Cushing's syndrome treatment and, 191
Metyrapone test, 185–186, 185F
Meynert, nucleus basalis of, 39
  acetylcholine and, 60
MFB. See Medial forebrain bundle
MHPG (3-methoxy-4-hydroxy-
      phenylglycol), 55
MHPG-sulfate (3-methoxy-4-
      hydroxyphenylglycol sulfate), 55
Microadenoma(s). See also Adenoma(s)
  CAT scans of, 190, 462–463
    coronal, 465
  definition of, 433
  differential diagnosis of
      hyperprolactinemia and, 219
  pituitary
    CAT scans of, 190
    Cushing's disease and, 429
    pathogenesis of, 423–424
  pregnancy and, 223
  prolactin-secreting, 216
    nonintervention in, 220
    selective transsphenoidal
        adenomectomy for, 220–221
  radiation therapy for, 516–517
  sellar enlargement and, 461
  silent, 424
    incidence of, 465
  surgery for, 220–221, 510, 511F, 512
    corticotropin-releasing hormone after,
        432
    Cushing's disease and, 179
    mortality and morbidity with, 513
Microsurgery. See also Surgery
  acromegaly management with, 279–281
  pineal tumors and, 366–367
  pituitary, Cushing's disease and, 192
  transsphenoidal, 510, 511F
Midbrain, limbic connections in, 40
Migraine
  female sex hormones and, 654
  symptoms of, pituitary tumor symptoms
      vs., 446

Neuropathology, chronic hypothermia and, 391T
Neuropathy, substance P and, 580
Neuropeptide(s). *See also* Peptide(s); *specific neuropeptide*
  ACTH regulation and, 176–177
  anterior pituitary function and, 45
  basal ganglia, Parkinson's disease and, 622–623
  biosynthesis of, 563, 564F, 565F
  brain concentration of, 560–562, 562F
  categories of, 561T
  cerebrospinal fluid, 626
    abnormalities of, 627T
    diseases and, 628–629, 629F
  conventional neurotransmitters and, colocalization of, 564, 564T
  cortical, 608–610, 610F
    Alzheimer's disease and, 611, 612F, 613F, 616T
      senile plaques and, 615
      somatostatin receptor binding to membrane preparations and, 612, 614–615, 614F
    Huntington's disease and, 615, 616T
    Parkinson's disease and, 615, 616T
  discovery of, 559–560
  embryologic aspects of, 563
  enzymes and, 619
  evolutionary aspects of, 562–563
  food intake regulation and, 403
  Huntington's disease and, 615, 616T, 620–622
  immune responses and, 689–690
  lymphocyte secretion of, 690
  neurologic disorders and, 607–608
  pineal gland, 353
  site of, function and, 4
  sleep, 597–598
  spinal cord, 624F
    intrinsic, 625
    sensory abnormalities and, 625
    sensory neuron, 623–625, 624T
  striatal, 617
    neurologic disorders and, 618T
Neuropeptide Y, 593–594
  Alzheimer's disease and, 611–612, 613F
  striatal, Huntington's disease and, 621–622
  structure of, 594F
Neurophysin(s), 73, 74F
Neurophysin I, 74
Neurophysin II, 74
  structure of, 73F
Neurosecretion, 7F, 8F, 9F
  definition of, 6
  neurohypophysis and, 6
Neurosecretomotor neurons, 5F
Neurosecretory cell(s)
  hypothalamus and, 4, 5F
  pituitary and, 4
  supraoptic system, 5F
Neurosecretory dysfunction
  diagnosis of, GHRH in, 497
  growth hormone, 271
Neurosis

endocrine function and, 673
hypercalcemia and, 659–660
hypocalcemia and, 660
Neurotensin
  central nervous system
    distribution of, 580–581
    functions of, 581
  discovery of, 580
  gastrointestinal tract
    distribution of, 581
    function of, 582
  neuroendocrine regulation by, 581
  pain perception and, 581–582
  structure of, 580F
  temperature regulation and, 387.
Neurotensin receptors, 582
Neurotransmitter(s). *See also specific neurotransmitter*
  ACTH regulation and, 176–177
  amino acid, 61–62
  conventional, neuropeptides and, colocalization of, 564, 564T
  cortical, neurologic disease and, 616T
  degradation of, 55
  endocrine changes in psychiatric disease and, 672
  food intake regulation and, 403
  free, reuptake of, 54–55
  gonadotropin regulation and, 304–305
  immune responses and, 689
  neuromodulators vs., 6–7
  regulation and, 4
  site of, function and, 4
  somatostatin and, 573
  striatal, neurologic disorders and, 618T
  structures of, 47F
  temperature regulation and, 384–385
  TRH as, 136–137
  TSH secretion and, 139–140
Neurotransmitter specificity, 4
Newborn. *See also* Infant(s)
  thyrotropin-releasing hormone in, 136
Nicotine test, diabetes insipidus and, 95
Nicotinic acid receptors, stimulation of, 88
Nicotinic receptors, acetylcholine and, 61
Nipple stimulation, 318–319
NM (normetanephrine), 55
Nocturia, diabetes insipidus and, 93
Nodular goiter, toxic, tumors causing, 148
Nonapeptides, neurohypophysial, 73
Nononcocytic cells, 439
Nonpuerperal galactorrhea, 213–215, 214F
Nonsecretory adenomas, radiologic assessment of, 470F–471F, 473
Nonshivering thermogenesis, 389
  chronic cold exposure and, 122
Noradrenergic activity, drugs increasing, 55
Noradrenergic agents, vasopressin regulation and, 88
Noradrenergic impulses, 47
Noradrenergic synapse, 53F
Noradrenergic system, blood pressure control and, 395
Norepinephrine
  adrenergic innervation of hypothalamus and, 49

and, 89–90
Osmoreceptor neuron system,
    hypothalamic, 76–77
Osmoreceptor setpoint
    essential hypernatremia and, 98
    volume regulation and, 77
Osmoreceptor-ADH-renal reflex, 75
Osteoporosis, menopause and, 651
Ouabain, endogenous digitalis-like
    compounds and, 82
Outer palisade zone, 22
Ovaries, hyperstimulation of, clomiphene
    and, 523
Overhydration, schizophrenia and, 79
OVLT (organum vasculosum of the lamina
    terminalis), 369–370
Ovulation
    atropine and, 61
    drugs influencing, 304
    epinephrine and, 45
    headache and, 654
    hormonal events in, 308–313
    induction of
        clomiphene in, 341, 523
        menopausal gonadotropin and human
            chorionic gonadotropin in, 523
        pulsatile GnRH in, 523, 523T
    neurotransmitters and, 304
    sex drive and, 652
    suckling and, 212
Ovulatory surge, gonadotropin secretion
    and, 300
Oxotremorine, muscarinic receptors and, 61
Oxytocic effects, neurohypophysial, 72
Oxytocin
    cerebrospinal fluid, 69
    fibers containing, 69
    lactation and, 319, 319F
    neurohypophysis and, 68
    prolactin release and, 206
    secretion of, 6
        labor and, 87–88
        milk let-down reflex and, 86–87
        neuropharmacologic regulation of, 89
    structure of, 72, 72F
Oxytocinergic pathways, 69

Pain perception
    neurotensin and, 581–582
    substance P and, 577–578, 625
Pain transmission, dorsal horn and, 625
Palisade zone(s)
    inner, 23
    outer, 22
Palsy
    ocular, pituitary tumors and, 453
    sixth-nerve, craniopharyngioma and, 531
Pancreas, thyrotropin-releasing hormone in,
    135, 566–567
Pancreatectomy, TSH and, 135
Pancreatic growth hormone releasing
        factor, human, 255
    growth hormone secretion and, 258F
    structure of, 256
Pancreatic hormones, secretion of, 6
Pancreatic islets, 6
Pancreatic polypeptide, 593

Pancreatic tumors, vasoactive intestinal
        peptide and, 590
Panhypopituitarism
    Addison's disease and, 182
    aqueduct stenosis and, 536
    empty-sella syndrome and, 547
    growth hormone deficiency and,
        264–265
    idiopathic, TRH response in, 142, 143F
    prolactin deficiency and, 218
    psychologic disturbance in, 658
    secondary to pituitary infarction, TRH
        response in, 142, 142F
Papilledema. See also Benign intracranial
        hypertension
    chiasm lesion and, 450
    craniopharyngioma and, 531
    increased intracranial pressure and, 446
Papillitis, chiasm lesions vs., 449
Parachlorophenylalanine
    diurnal variations in plasma cortisol and,
        171
    prolactin and, 59
Paralysis, conjugate upward gaze, pineal
        tumors and, 454
Paranoid delusions, Cushing's syndrome
        and, 656
Paranoid schizophrenia
    hyperparathyroidism and, 659
    thyroxine and, 125
Parasellar aneurysm, magnetic resonance
        imaging of, 467
Parasellar lesion(s)
    adenoma vs., 474–475
    visual disturbance in, 449
Parasellar tumor(s), 439–440, 440T, 461T
    meningioma, radiologic assessment of,
        474F–475F
    pinealoma, diagnosis of, 366
Parasympathetic nervous system,
        secretomotor nerve fibers and, 6
Parasympathetic neurons, parotid and
        sweat glands and, 6
Parathyroid adenoma, infarction of,
        hypercalcemia and, 659
Paraventricular nuclei, 68, 70F
    input to, 36
    TSH secretion and, 116, 117
Paraventricular-hypophysial nerve tract, 68,
        69F
Paresis, general, diurnal variations in ACTH
        and, 171
Pargyline
    noradrenergic activity and, 55
    serotonin and, 59
Parinaud's syndrome, pineal tumors and,
        366, 454
Parkinsonism, bromocriptine therapy and,
        222
Parkinson's disease
    cortical neuropeptides and, 615, 616T
    dopamine receptors and, 54
    L-dopa and, 52
    melatonin and, 359
    neuropeptides and, basal ganglia,
        622–623
    substance P in, 580

INDEX   737

Periventricular organ(s), 351, 369F
  organum vasculosum of the lamina
        terminalis, 369–370
  somatostatin in, 570
  subcommissural, 368–369
  subfornical, 370–371
Perphenazine, 54
Persistent adenoma, surgical management
        of, 513–514
Personality
  androgens and, 648–649
  immune function and, 689
Personality disorder(s)
  adrenocortical disease and, 656–657
  anorexia nervosa and, 680–681, 684
  bulimia and, 687
  depression and, 674
  growth hormone and, 657
  hypercalcemia and, 659–660
  hypocalcemia and, 660–661
  hypoglycemia and, 661–662
  hypopituitarism and, 657–658
  premorbid, Graves' disease and, 655
  septal lesions and, 39
  thyroid disease and, 655–656
pGLU-His-Gly-OH, food intake regulation
        and, 405–406
Pharmacology. See also Drug(s); specific drug
  tuberoinfundibular dopamine system
        and, 48
Phenobarbital, pituitary-thyroid function
        and, 127
Phenothiazines
  acute hyperthermia and, 392
  amenorrhea and, 322
  prolactin and, 204, 207, 217
Phenoxybenzamine (Dibenzylene), 54, 56T
  ovulation and, 304
Phentolamine (Regitine), 54, 56T
  growth hormone secretion and, 249, 250,
        250F
  pituitary-adrenal function and, 176
Phenylalanine, growth hormone secretion
        and, 251
Phenylethanolamine-N-methyltransferase
        (PNMT), 49
  epinephrine formation and, 52
Phenytoin
  antidiuretic hormone and, 89, 104
  dexamethasone suppression test and, 190
  pituitary-thyroid function and, 127
  TSH secretion and, 127
  vitamin D deficiency and, 660
Pheochromocytoma, ACTH secretion and,
        180
Pheromone, 650–651
PHI (peptide histidine isoleucine-27), 28, 206
Phlebotomy, blood volume and, vasopressin
        and, 77
PHM-27, 588
Phosphatidylinositol, 34
  thyrotropin-releasing hormone and, 134
Phosphorylation, protein kinase, 33
Photosensitivity, desmocycline and, 104
Phylogenetic distribution, thyrotropin-
        releasing hormone, 131–132,
        131T, 567

Physalaemin, structure of, 577F
Physostigmine, acetylcholinesterase and, 61
PI (phosphatidylinositol), 34, 134
PIF (prolactin-inhibiting factor), 204–205.
        See also Dopamine
Pigeon milk, prolactin and, 212–213
Pigmentation, ectopic ACTH secretion and,
        180
Pimozide, 54, 56T
Pineal gland
  anatomy of, 351–353, 352F
  aplasia of, 362
  apoplexy of, 364
  calcification of, 361–362
  circadian rhythms and, 353, 354F,
        357–359, 358F
  development of, 351–353, 352T
  diurnal variations in prolactin secretion
        and, 211
  endocrine effects of, 360–361
  growth hormone regulation and, 248
  hypoplasia of, 362
  innervation of, 358F
  lesions of, male sexual precocity and, 334
  malignancy and, 361
  melatonin and, 4
  thyroid regulation and, 121
  thyrotropin-releasing hormone in, 131
Pineal secretion, 352
  neural regulation of, 353–357, 354F,
        355F, 356F
Pineal tumor(s), 362
  classification of, 363T
  hCG-secreting, 335
  management of, 366–367, 367T
  manifestations of, 365–366
  neurologic function and, 454
  precocious puberty and, 364–366
  prognosis of, 367, 368F
Pinealectomy, melatonin and, 359
Pinealocyte(s), 351
  synapses on, 352F, 353
Pinealoma
  ectopic, 362
  seminomatous, 362
  third ventricular, diagnosis of, 366
Pineoblastoma, 362
  familial, 364
Pineocytoma, 362
Pinocytosis, reverse, 35
Piperoxane, 54
Pitressin (vasopressin), diabetes insipidus
        and, 94, 96
Pituicytomas, 533
Pituita, 12
Pituitary adenoma(s)
  CAT scans of, 462–463, 463F, 464F, 469
  cell types and, 423
  classification of, 424, 424T
  Cushing's disease and, 178–179
  differential diagnosis of
        aneurysm in, 472F–473F, 475–476
        craniopharyngioma in, 476, 477F, 478F
        hypothalamic glioma in, 476, 478–479
        metastasis in, 479
        tuberculum sellae meningioma in,
        474F–475F, 476

Polyostotic fibrous dysplasia
  acromegaly with, radiation therapy and,
        278
  sexual precocity with, 332–333
Polypeptide, pancreatic, 593
Polyuria
  control of, 96
  diagnosis and, 95
POMC. *See* Proopiomelanocortin
Porcine secretin, structure of, 588, 588F
Portal vessels, pituitary, 16, 17F
Positive feedback system, 48
  estrogen and, gonadotropin secretion
        and, 310, 311F
Postabsorptive hypoglycemia, symptoms of,
        661
Postcommissural fibers, 21
Posterior pituitary gland, 6, 12, 351. *See also*
        Pituitary *entries*
  anatomy of, 68–72, 69F, 70F, 71F
  blood pressure and, 72
  insufficiency of, water deprivation test of,
        507–508
  neurons of
    cholinergic pathways and, 61
    electrophysiology of, 89–90
  research on, 67–68
  thyrotropin-releasing hormone in, 566
  tumors of, 533
    diabetes insipidus and, 92
Posterior pituitary hormones, 22–23,
        72–74. *See also specific hormone*
  evolution of, 562–563
Posterior pituitary nerve terminal, 9F
Postfixed chiasm, 450
Postganglionic sympathetic fibers, 5F
Postmortem tissue, neuropeptides in,
        607–608
  Alzheimer's disease and, 611, 612F, 613F,
        616T
    senile plaques and, 615
    somatostatin receptor binding to
        membrane preparations and,
        612, 614–615, 614F
  Huntington's disease and, 615, 616T
  Parkinson's disease and, 615, 616T
Postpartum pituitary necrosis, 539–540
  clinical manifestations of, 540–541
  diabetes insipidus and, 93
Postpill amenorrhea, 214
  galactorrhea and, hyperprolactinemia
        and, 217
Postradiation necrosis, 541–542
Postradiation thyroiditis, plasma TSH in, 146
Postreceptor effects, activation pathways of,
        33–34
Postsynaptic membrane, receptors on,
        serotonin and, 59
Postsynaptic neuron, receptors on,
        catecholamine interaction with,
        54
Posttraumatic diabetes insipidus, 91–92
Postural hypotension
  bromocriptine and, 222
  idiopathic, substance P in, 580
Potassium level, furosemide and, 104

Prader-Willi syndrome, 415
  food intake in, naloxone and, 405
Precocious adrenarche, 329
Precocious menstruation, definition of, 329
Precocious pubarche, 329
Precocious puberty, 314, 328
  diagnosis of, 333–335
    GnRH superagonists in, 491
  differential diagnosis of, 330T
  female, clinical diagnosis of, 334–335
  hypothyroidism and, 217, 332
  idiopathic, 331
  incidence of, 329–330
  male, clinical diagnosis of, 334
  management of, 335–337, 336F
  neurogenic, 331–332
  pineal gland and, 364–366
  polyostotic fibrous dysplasia and,
        332–333
Precocious thelarche, 329
Precoma, pituitary, treatment of, 525–526
Prednisone
  ACTH deficiency treatment with, 520
  Addison's disease management with, 182
Prefixed chiasm, 450
Prefrontal cortex, electrical stimulation of,
        cardiovascular system and, 394
Preganglionic sympathetic fibers, 5F
Pregnancy
  false, 313, 322, 324
    hyperprolactinemia vs., 218
  headache and, 654
  hormonal events in, 211
  induction of, bromocriptine in, 222
    complications with, 223
  multiple, clomiphene and, 523
  pituitary necrosis following, 539
    clinical manifestations of, 540–541
  prolactin levels in, 202–203, 203F, 209
Premarin (conjugated estrogens), gonadal
        deficiency and, 272
Premenstrual syndrome (PMS), 652–654
Premorbid personality disturbance, Graves'
        disease and, 655
Preoptic area
  electrical stimulation of, luteinizing
        hormone and, 303F
  sexually dimorphic nucleus of, 645, 645F
Preprosomatostatin, 571
Pressor effects, neurohypophysial, 72
Primary hypothalamic polydipsia, 95
Primary hypothyroidism, 146
  differential diagnosis of, 145
  TRH response and, 141
PRL. *See* Prolactin
Proctoscopy, prolactin release and, 210
Proenkephalin, 162
Proenkephalin A, 583, 586–587
Proenkephalin B, 583, 587
Progesterone
  acromegaly treatment with, 281
  amenorrhea evaluation and, 340
  body temperature and, 384
  gonadotropin secretion and, 28
  male sexual function and, 648
  menstrual cycle and, 308–313, 311F, 652

physiologic brain effects of, 644
premenstrual syndrome treatment with,
653–654
structure of, 297F
Progestin(s), 297. *See also specific progestin*
menstrual period induction with, 521–522
premenstrual syndrome treatment with,
653, 654
Prohormones
hypothalamic hypophysiotropic
hormone, 28
neurohypophysial, 74
neuropeptide, 565F
Prolactin (PRL), 12
abnormal secretion of,
adenomas and, 216
diagnosis of, 218–219
hypothyroidism and, 217
idiopathic, 218
neuroleptic drugs and, 217
nonpuerperal galactorrhea and,
213–215, 214F
peripheral receptor control and,
216–217
pituitary isolation and, 216
psychogenic, 218
acromegaly and, 267–268
breastfeeding and, 202F, 203
cells secreting, 423
cerebrospinal fluid, 628
deficiency of, 218
drug effects on, 56T–57T
effects on nonmammals of, 212–213
episodic secretion of, 211
excess secretion of, management of, 219
macroadenomas and, 224–225
microadenomas and, 220–224
radiation therapy in, 225
feedback regulation of, 208–209
hypothalamic control of, 203–207, 204F
insulin hypoglycemia test and, 502, 503
lactation and, 211–212, 319F
male sexual function and, 649
milk production and, 318
neural pathways and, 208
normal levels of, 218
pituitary secretion of, 201–203, 202F, 203F
pseudopregnancy and, 313
schizophrenia and, 679–680
secretion of
factors influencing, 210T
seizure-associated, 210–211
sleep-associated, 211
stimuli of, 201, 202F
stress-associated, 209–210, 671
serotonergic neurons and, 59
substance P and, 579
TRH and, 134, 487
tuberoinfundibular dopamine system
and, 48
vasoactive intestinal peptide and, 590
Prolactin-inhibiting factor(s) (PIF),
204–205. *See also* Dopamine
Prolactinoma(s), 432–433
pathology of, 436, 437F
pituitary, CAT scan of, 464F

radiologic assessment of, 471
treatment of, 512
radiation therapy in, 225
conventional, 515–516, 516T
Prolactin-releasing factor(s), 205–207, 206F
TRH as, 134
Proopiomelanocortin (POMC), 161–162,
161F, 583
cells secreting, 423
Prooxyphysin, 73
Propranolol (Inderal), 56T
food intake regulation and, 403
growth hormone secretion and, 250
pituitary-adrenal function and, 176
thyroid hormones and, 124F, 127
Propressophysin, 73
Propylthiouracil
sexual precocity and, 332
thyroid hormones and, 127
Prostaglandin E$_2$
fever and, 389
sleep and, 691
Prostaglandins, stress response and, 670
Protein(s)
neurophysins, 73–74
regulatory, cellular, 164–165
Protein kinases, phosphorylations of, 33
Protein metabolism, growth hormone
secretion and, 239
Protein synthesis, 33, 564F
TSH secretion and, 114–115
Protein-steroid complex, 165
Proton beam irradiation, 518
acromegaly management with, 278–279
advantages and disadvantages of, 519
Cushing's disease treatment and, 192
visual field and, 453
Provera (medroxyprogesterone acetate). *See
also* Medroxyprogesterone
acetate
premenstrual syndrome treatment with,
654
Pseudocyesis, 313, 322, 324
hyperprolactinemia vs., 218
Pseudo-Cushingoid disorder,
hypercortisolism vs., 177
Pseudohypoparathyroidism, hypocalcemia
in, psychologic disturbance in,
660
Pseudoprecocious puberty, 329
Pseudotumor cerebri, 461
differential diagnosis of, 549T
etiology of, 548–549
pathophysiology of, 550–551
treatment of, 551
Psychiatric disease
anorexia nervosa
diagnostic criteria of, 680
epidemiologic factors in, 680–681
hormonal disturbances in, 682F–683F,
684–686, 685T, 686F
hypopituitarism vs., 686
natural history of, 681, 681F
psychologic setting of, 684
symptoms of, 680
treatment of, 686–687, 686T

Radiation therapy
  acromegaly and, 277–279, 517
  alpha particle, 518, 519
  complications of, 517
  craniopharyngioma and, 532
  Cushing's disease and, 192, 517
  heavy particle, 518–519
  microadenoma and, 516–517
  pineal tumor and, 366
  pituitary adenoma and, 514–516, 515T, 516T
  prolactinoma and, 515, 516, 516T
  proton beam, 518–519
  visual effects of, 453
Radioimmunoassay (RIA)
  antidiuretic hormone, 95
  β-lipotropic hormone, 184
Radioiodine treatment, hypothyroidism following, 145
Radioisotope brain scan, 479
Radiologic assessment
  acromegaly and, 472–473
  ACTH-producing tumors on, 472
  advances in, 457
  aneurysms in, 472F–473F, 475–476
  brain scan in, 479
  calcification in, 473–474
  CAT scans in, 462
    axial images in, 467
    coronal, 463, 465–467
    metrizamide with, 467, 468F
  cerebral angiography in, 471F, 480
  importance of, 457
  magnetic resonance imaging in, 467, 469F
  nonsecretory adenomas in, 470F–471F, 473
  pituitary adenomas in, differential diagnosis of
    aneurysm in, 472F–473F, 475–476
    craniopharyngioma in, 476, 477F, 478F
    hypothalamic glioma in, 476, 478–479
    metastasis in, 479
    tuberculum sellae meningioma in, 474F–475F, 476
  pituitary apoplexy in, 473
  prolactinoma in, 471
  secretory adenomas in, 471–473
  sella turcica, 457, 458F, 459F
    calcification in, 460, 460F
    increased intracranial pressure and, 461–462
    size in, 458–459
      causes of enlargement and, 460–461
Radiosensitivity, relative, regions of brain and, 542
Raphe nucleus(i)
  electric stimulation of, 59
  growth hormone secretion and, 247
Rathke's cleft cysts, 529–530
Rathke's pouch, 12
Reactive hypoglycemia, symptoms of, 661
Receptor(s)
  α-adrenergic, 54
    food intake regulation and, 403
    growth hormone regulation and, 240, 249–250

β-adrenergic, 54
    food intake regulation and, 403
    growth hormone secretion and, 250
  breast, suckling and, 36
  cold peripheral, 121
  cortisol, 165
  dopamine, 54
    psychoneuroendocrinology and, 672, 673F
  glucocorticoid, 175
  glutamate, 62
  histamine, 60
  hypophysiotropic hormone binding to, 33
  hypothalamic, thirst sensation, 80
  muscarinic, acetylcholine and, 61
  neurotensin, 582
  nicotinic, acetylcholine and, 61
  nicotinic acid, stimulation of, 88
  opioid, 585–586
  pituitary membrane, CRF and, 169
  postsynaptic membrane, serotonin and, 59
  postsynaptic neuron, catecholamine interaction with, 54
  somatostatin, 261, 573
    binding of, 612
      Alzheimer's disease and, 575, 614–615, 614F
  specialized, on target cells, 4
  steroid, 643
  thyrotropin-releasing hormone, 136–137
  volume control, vasopressin and, 78–79
Receptor specificity, 4
Receptor-blockers
  angiotensin II, thirst and, 82
  definition of, 54
  dopamine, 54
  muscarinic, 61
  nicotinic, 61
Recurrent adenoma, surgical management of, 513–514
Reflex(es)
  cold-receptor, 121
  mediation of, 36
  milk let-down, 86–87, 212, 318–319
  osmoreceptor-ADH-renal, 75
Regional enteritis, psychoneuroimmunology and, 689
Regitine (phentolamine), 56T
Regulation. See also specific substance
  autocrine, 571
  blood volume, 77
  cholinergic pathways in, 61
  endocrine system, 4
  extrahypothalamic pathways in, 40
  feedback, glucocorticoid, CRF and, 168–169
  hypothalamic pathways in, 40
  hypothalamic-adenohypophysial system, extrahypothalamic, 36
    limbic system and, 37–40
  hypothalamic-pituitary-thyroid axis, 112F
  neural, 4
  neuronal, 4
  neurotensin in, 581
  osmolar, age and, 81
  pituitary, 4

visual effects of, 453

Saline, hypertonic
  diabetes insipidus and, 95
  SIADH and, 103
  thirst and, 80, 81
Saliva, regulation of, 4
Salt metabolism, endoxin and, 83
Salt regulation
  disorders of
    central "essential" hypernatremia,
      97–98
    diabetes insipidus, 90
      diagnosis of, 93
      etiology of, 91–93, 91T
      management of, 96–97
    syndrome of inappropriate ADH
      secretion, 98
      clinical manifestations of, 101–103
      diagnosis of, 103
      etiology of, 99–101, 99T
      management of, 103–104
      pathophysiology of, 101, 102T
  subfornical organ and, 370
Salt retention, premenstrual, 653
Sansert (methysergide), 56T
Saralasin, drinking behavior and, 82
Sarcoid granuloma, CAT scan of, 479
Sarcoidosis, 93
  hypothalamic-pituitary, 544–546, 545F
  immunoneuroendocrinology and, 691
  polydipsia and, 95
Sarcoma, radiation-induced, 278, 279
Satiety. See also Food intake regulation
  behavioral changes accompanying,
    403–404
  cholecystokinin and, 404, 593
  short-term signals of, 399–401
  VMN mechanism for, 402–403
Sauvagine, corticotropin-releasing hormone
    and, 165
Schilder's disease, adrenoleukodystrophy
    vs., 183
Schizophrenia
  antidiuretic hormone excretion and, 79
  endocrine function in, 679–680
  hypoglycemia and, 661
  paranoid
    hyperparathyroidism and, 659
    thyroxine and, 125
  stress-induced prolactin release and, 210
  thyrotropin-releasing hormone response
    in, 677F
Schizophreniform illness, bromocriptine
    and, 222
Schmidt's syndrome, 182
Schwartz-Bartter syndrome, 98
  clinical manifestations of, 101–103
  diagnosis of, 103
  etiology of, 99–101, 99T
  management of, 103–104
  pathophysiology of, 101, 102T
SCN (suprachiasmatic nuclei), 21, 68, 71F
Scopolamine, 61
Scotoma(ta)
  assessment of, 447–448
  hemianopic, bitemporal, 449

tangent screen evaluation of, 448
  unilateral, central, 449–450, 451F
Sebum, regulation of, 4
Secondary hypothyroidism, 146
  differential diagnosis of, 145
Secondary sex characteristics, normal age of
    development of, 329, 329T
Secretin
  actions of, 591
  distribution of, 591
  structure of, 587–588, 588F
Secretion(s). See also specific substance
  anterior pituitary, 5F
    drugs affecting, 55, 56T–57T
  cell, calcium and, 34
  mechanisms of, 9F
  neural control of
    neurosecretion and, 6–9
    secretomotor, 4, 6
  neural lobe, 6
  neuronal, study of, 4
  osmoreceptor function and, 89–90
  pancreatic hormone, 6
  peptide hormone, 5F
  pineal, 353–357, 354F, 355F, 356F
  thyroid hormone, 115–116
Secretomotor control, 4, 6
Secretomotor fibers, exocrine glands and, 4
Secretory cells, 4
  capillary and, ultrastructural relationship
    of, 33F
  pars distalis, 13–14
Seizure(s), 454
  hypocalcemia and, 660
  prolactin release and, 210–211
  somatostatin and, 574
  syndrome of inappropriate ADH
    secretion and, 102
Selective transsphenoidal adenomectomy,
    microprolactinoma and, 220–221
Sella turcica
  abnormal, Cushing's disease and, 178
  chiasm location relative to, visual
    symptoms and, 450
  craniopharyngioma and, 531
  enlargement of, 459
    causes of, 460–461
    empty-sella syndrome and
      endocrine manifestations of, 547
      etiology of, 546
      management of, 547–548
      neurologic manifestations of, 547
  floor of
    coronal CAT scans of, 467
    erosion of, 461
  primary hypothyroidism and, 146
  radiologic assessment of, 457, 458F, 459F
    calcification in, 460, 460F
    CAT scanning in, 462F, 463, 463F,
      464F, 467
    increased intracranial pressure and,
      461–462
    size in, 458–459
      causes of enlargement and, 460–461
  tumors of, 431, 431F, 439–440, 440T,
    461T
  volume of, 459